Psychiatric Consultation in Long-Term Care

Psychiatric Consultation in Long-Term Care

A Guide for Healthcare Professionals

Abhilash K. Desai, M.D., F.A.P.A.
Idaho Memory & Aging Center, Boise, ID
George T. Grossberg, M.D., F.A.P.A.
St. Louis University School of Medicine

CAMBRIDGE
UNIVERSITY PRESS

CAMBRIDGE
UNIVERSITY PRESS

University Printing House, Cambridge CB2 8BS, United Kingdom

One Liberty Plaza, 20th Floor, New York, NY 10006, USA

477 Williamstown Road, Port Melbourne, VIC 3207, Australia

4843/24, 2nd Floor, Ansari Road, Daryaganj, Delhi – 110002, India

79 Anson Road, #06–04/06, Singapore 079906

Cambridge University Press is part of the University of Cambridge.

It furthers the University's mission by disseminating knowledge in the pursuit of education, learning, and research at the highest international levels of excellence.

www.cambridge.org
Information on this title: www.cambridge.org/9781107164222
DOI: 10.1017/9781316687024

First published 2017
Reprinted 2018

Printed in the United States of America by Sheridan Books, Inc

A catalogue record for this publication is available from the British Library.

Library of Congress Cataloging-in-Publication Data
Names: Desai, Abhilash K., author. | Grossberg, George T., author.
Title: Psychiatric consultation in long-term care : a guide for healthcare professionals / Abhilash Desai, George Grossberg.
Description: Second edition. | Cambridge ; New York, NY : Cambridge University Press, 2017. | Includes bibliographical references and index.
Identifiers: LCCN 2017024711 | ISBN 9781107164222 (hardback)
Subjects: | MESH: Aged – psychology | Long-Term Care – psychology | Mental Disorders – therapy | Assisted Living Facilities | Nursing Homes | Homes for the Aged
Classification: LCC RC451.4.A5 | NLM WT 150 | DDC 618.97/689–dc23
LC record available at https://lccn.loc.gov/2017024711

ISBN 978-1-107-16422-2 Hardback

Contents

Preface

A coauthored text such as this, unlike edited texts, gives the authors a unique opportunity to present state-of-the-art information regarding biopsychosocial spiritual and environmental approaches in long-term care (LTC) together with our philosophy of caring for older adults who live in LTC settings. Our philosophy of care is that "there is life in the nursing home" and other LTC facilities and that health care professionals in many disciplines – physicians, physician assistants, nurse practitioners, clinical nurse specialists, nurses, administrators, nursing assistants (nurse aides), social workers, various rehabilitative therapists, pharmacists, psychologists, chaplains, clergy, activity therapists, recreational therapists, music therapists, art therapists, and others – all have a lot to offer in improving the quality of life for LTC residents and their families. Every health care provider has an important role to play as a member of the health care team.

Our philosophy of care places the needs and dignity of the LTC resident at its center. It promotes the notion that, to some degree, we can help every LTC resident and his or her family. A caring attitude on the part of all health care professionals in LTC is vital in meeting this goal. Our philosophy sees the LTC environment as warm, nurturing, and supportive. For residents, it is the source of their extended family or, at times, their only family.

Achieving excellence in the care of LTC residents will require physicians not only to be responsible to each individual resident, but also to promote the well-being of family members and other professional caregivers, as well as to understand the systems of care. This means a team approach – in addition to individual assessments – to determine what person-centered, individualized, strength-based approaches and interventions are most effective, to standardize care where possible, and to eliminate errors.

Our philosophy of care promulgates the use of biological therapies, when appropriate, in the context of robust psychosocial, sensory, spiritual, and environmental approaches. In fact, one of the longest chapters in this text is devoted to proactively promoting psychosocial spiritual wellness of LTC residents.

As part of updating the material for this second edition, we have adopted the *Diagnostic and Statistical Manual of Mental Disorders*, fifth edition (*DSM-5*) of the American Psychiatric Association terminology for all mental disorders. We have also made significant modifications in each of the chapters to incorporate the considerable advances in LTC medicine, mental health, and well-being, as well as the person-centered care movement since the publication of our first edition.

This guide is written to be user-friendly and is targeted at physicians, physician assistants, nurse practitioners, clinical nurse specialists, nurses, social workers, administrators, rehabilitation specialists, and other health care professionals involved or interested in improving the well-being of all LTC residents. It can also be useful for students and trainees who desire to learn more about wellness, aging, and LTC. We hope our book will further education and training regarding LTC by describing compassionate care practices complemented by evidence-based, state-of-the-science health care.

We would like to thank our spouses, children, and families for their support of this project. We also appreciate the superb editorial work of Ms. Wendy Harris. Without her help, this book would not have reached its potential. Lastly, we have learned a great deal from our patients, their families, and the staff of the outstanding LTC facilities with which we have been affiliated.

We hope you enjoy reading this book and find it helpful in your work with LTC residents.

Abbreviations

AAMI	age-associated memory impairment
ACSH	ambulatory care-sensitive hospitalization
AD	Alzheimer's disease
ADE	adverse drug event
ADHD	attention deficit hyperactivity disorder
ADLs	activities of daily living
AIDS	acquired immunodeficiency syndrome
AL	assisted living
ALS	amyotrophic lateral sclerosis
aMCI	amnestic mild cognitive impairment
ANH	artificial nutrition and hydration
APS	Adult Protective Services
BEHAVE-AD	behavioral symptoms in Alzheimer's disease
BIMS	Brief Interview for Mental Status
BMI	body mass index
BMP	basic metabolic panel
BNPS	behavioral, neurocognitive, and psychological symptoms
BPSD	biopsychosocial-spiritual distress
BUN	blood urea nitrogen
bvFTD	behavioral variant frontotemporal dementia
BZD	benzodiazepine
CADASIL	cerebral autosomal dominant arteriopathy with subcortical infarct and leukoencephalopathy
CAM	Confusion Assessment Method
CBC	complete blood count
CBD	corticobasal degeneration
CBT	cognitive behavioral therapy
CBZ	carbamazepine
CCRC	continuing care retirement community
ChEI	cholinesterase inhibitor
CHF	congestive heart failure
CIWA	Clinical Institute Withdrawal Assessment
CJD	Creutzfeldt-Jakob disease
CMAI	Cohen-Mansfield Agitation Inventory
CMS	Centers for Medicare and Medicaid Services
CNA	certified nursing assistant
CNS	central nervous system
COPD	chronic obstructive pulmonary disease
COWAT	Controlled Oral Word Association Test
CPAP	continuous positive airway pressure
CPE	comprehensive psychiatric evaluation
CQI	continuous quality improvement
CR	cognitive rehabilitation
CRP	C-reactive protein
CSDD	Cornell Scale for Depression in Dementia
CSDH	chronic subdural hematoma
CSF	cerebrospinal fluid
CST	cognitive stimulation therapy
CT	computed tomography
CTE	chronic traumatic encephalopathy
CVA	cerebrovascular accident
DAST	Drug Abuse Screening Test
DBS	deep brain stimulation
DIP	drug-induced Parkinsonism
DLB	dementia with Lewy bodies
DNH	Do Not Hospitalize
DNI	Do Not Intubate
DNR	Do Not Resuscitate
DRM	disease-related malnutrition
DS	Diogenes syndrome

DSM	*Diagnostic and Statistical Manual of Mental Disorders*
DWI	diffusion-weighted imaging
ECT	electroconvulsive therapy
ED	emergency department
EDS	excessive daytime sleepiness
EEG	electroencephalogram
EKG	electrocardiogram
EMDR	eye movement desensitization and reprocessing
EMR	electronic medical records
EOL	end of life
EPS	extrapyramidal symptoms
ERP	exposure and response prevention
ESRD	end-stage renal disease
FAQ	Functional Activities Questionnaire
FAST	Functional Assessment Staging for Alzheimer's disease
FDA	Food and Drug Administration
FLAIR	fluid-attenuated inversion recovery
FTA	fluorescent treponemal antibody
FTD	frontotemporal dementia
GABA	gamma amino butyric acid
GAD	generalized anxiety disorder
GDS	Geriatric Depression Scale; Global Deterioration Scale
GERD	gastroesophageal reflux disease
GNA	geriatric nursing assistant
HAART	highly aggressive antiretroviral therapy
HAD	HIV-associated dementia
HAND	HIV-associated neurocognitive disorder
HCP	health care provider
HD	Huntington's disease
HIV	human immunodeficiency virus
HSE	herpes simplex encephalitis
IADLs	instrumental activities of daily living
IBS	irritable bowel syndrome
IDT	interdisciplinary team
IED	intermittent explosive disorder
IEED	involuntary emotional expression disorder
iNPH	idiopathic normal pressure hydrocephalus
IPSRT	interpersonal and social rhythm therapy
LFT	liver function test
LGBT	lesbian, gay, bisexual, and transgender
LPN	licensed practical nurse
LTC	long-term care
MA	multisystem atrophy
MAOI	monoamine oxidase inhibitor
MBSR	mindfulness-based stress reduction
MCI	mild cognitive impairment
MDD	major depressive disorder
MDS	Minimum Data Set
MHN	mental health navigator
MHP	mental health professional
MMSE	Mini-Mental State Examination
MNA	Mini-Nutritional Assessment
MNCD	major neurocognitive disorder
MOCA	Montreal Cognitive Assessment
MRI	magnetic resonance imaging
MRSA	methicillin-resistant *Staphylococcus aureus*
MS	multiple sclerosis
MSA	multiple system atrophy
MVA	motor vehicle accident
NCD	neurocognitive disorder
NDRI	noradrenaline dopamine reuptake inhibitor
NH	nursing home
NMDA	N-methyl D-aspartate
NORC	naturally occurring retirement community
NPH	normal pressure hydrocephalus
NPI-NH	Neuropsychiatric Inventory – Nursing Home
NSAID	nonsteroidal anti-inflammatory drug
OAB	overactive bladder
OCD	obsessive-compulsive disorder
OSA	obstructive sleep apnea
OSAHS	obstructive sleep apnea / hypopnea syndrome
OTC	over the counter
PAS	Pittsburgh Agitation Scale
PBA	pseudobulbar affect
PCC	person-centered care
PCLTCC	person-centered long-term care community
PCP	primary care physician / primary care provider
PCT	palliative care team
PD	Parkinson's disease

PDD	Parkinson's disease dementia
PEG	percutaneous endoscopic gastrostomy
PET	positron emission tomography
PHQ	Patient Health Questionnaire
PIM	potentially inappropriate medication
PIP	potentially inappropriate prescription
PLMD	periodic limb movement disorder
PM	psychotropic medication
PMT	psychotropic medication therapy
PNFA	progressive nonfluent aphasia
POLST	Physician Orders for Life-Sustaining Treatment
PPI	proton pump inhibitor
PPN	peripheral parenteral nutrition
PSMS	Physical Self-Maintenance Scale
PSP	progressive supranuclear palsy
PTSD	post-traumatic stress disorder
RAI	Resident Assessment Instrument
RBD	REM sleep behavior disorder
REM	rapid eye movement
RLS	restless leg syndrome
RN	registered nurse
RPD	rapidly progressive dementia
rTMS	repetitive transcranial magnetic stimulation
SCI	subjective cognitive impairment
SD	semantic dementia
SLE	systemic lupus erythematosus
SLUMS	Saint Louis University Mental State Exam
SNRI	serotonin and norepinephrine reuptake inhibitor
SPMI	severe and persistent mental illness
SPPEICE	strength-based, personalized, psychosocial sensory spiritual environmental initiatives and creative engagement
SSRD	somatic symptom and related disorder
SSRI	selective serotonin reuptake inhibitor
SUD	substance use disorder
TBI	traumatic brain injury
TCA	tricyclic antidepressant
TD	tardive dyskinesia
TENS	transcutaneous electrical nerve stimulation
TIA	transient ischemic attack
TMS	transcranial magnetic stimulation
TMT	Trail Making Test
TPN	total parenteral nutrition
TSH	thyroid-stimulating hormone
UTF	universal transfer form
UTI	urinary tract infection
VaD	vascular dementia
VNS	vagal nerve stimulation
WMH	white matter hyperintensities

Commonly Used Psychotropic Drugs

Generic Names: Brand Names

Acamprosate: Campral
Alprazolam: Xanax
Amitriptyline: Elavil
Armodafinil: Nuvigil
Aripiprazole: Abilify, Aripiprazole Lauroxil
Asenapine: Saphris
Bupropion: Wellbutrin, Zyban
Buspirone: Buspar
Cariprazine: Vraylar
Carbamazepine: Tegretol
Chlordiazepoxide: Librium
Citalopram: Celexa
Clomipramine: Anafranil
Clonazepam: Klonopin
Clozapine: Clozaril, Fazaclo
Desipramine: Norpramin
Desvenlafaxine: Pristiq
Diazepam: Valium
Disulfiram: Antabuse
Doxepin: Sinequan, Silenor
Duloxetine: Cymbalta
Escitalopram: Lexapro
Eszopiclone: Lunesta
Flunitrazepam: Rohypnol
Fluoxetine: Prozac
Fluphenazine: Prolixin
Flurazepam: Dalmane
Fluvoxamine: Luvox
Haloperidol: Haldol
Iloperidone: Fanapt
Imipramine: Tofranil
Lamotrigine: Lamictal
Levomilnacipran: Fetzima
Lithium: Eskalith, Lithobid
Lorazepam: Ativan
Lurasidone: Latuda
Mesoridazine: Serentil
Methylphenidate: Ritalin
Milnacipran: Savella
Mirtazapine: Remeron, Remeron Sol
Modafinil: Provigil
Naltrexone: Revia
Nortriptyline: Pamelor
Olanzapine: Zyprexa, Zydis Zyprexa
Oxazepam: Serax
Oxcarbazepine: Trileptal
Paliperidone: Invega, Invega Sustenna, Invega Trinza
Paroxetine: Paxil
Perphenazine: Trilafon
Pimavanserin: Nuplazid
Quetiapine: Seroquel, Seroquel XR
Ramelteon: Rozerem
Risperidone: Risperdal
Selegiline: EMSAM, Eldepryl
Suvorexant: Belsomra
Tasimelteon: Hetlioz
Temazepam: Restoril
Thioridazine: Mellaril
Thiothixene: Navane
Topiramate: Topamax
Trazodone: Desyrel
Triazolam: Halcion
Trimipramine: Surmontil
Valproate, Valproic acid: Depakote, Depakote DR, Depakote ER, Depakene, Depakote sprinkles
Venlafaxine, Venlafaxine ER: Effexor, Effexor XR
Vilazodone: Viibryd
Vortioxetine: Trintellix
Zaleplon: Sonata
Ziprasidone: Geodon
Zolpidem: Ambien, Ambien CR, Zolpimist, Intermezzo

Chapter 1

The Need for High-Quality Comprehensive Mental Health Services in Long-Term Care

Long-term care is simply a means to ensure that older people with a significant loss of capacity can still experience *Healthy Ageing.*
World Health Organization, World Ageing and Health Report *(2015; emphasis added).*

Conservative estimates are that one in four older adults (age 65 or older) is currently receiving long-term care (LTC) (World Health Organization 2015). This means that millions of older adults around the world are currently receiving LTC. More than 15 percent of adults receiving LTC are younger than age 65. Adults receiving LTC are typically severely disabled due to advanced physical health problems and/or major neurocognitive disorders (MNCD), primarily dementias (Rosenblatt and Samus 2011). They require 24-hour functional support and assistance with basic activities of daily living (ADLs) and instrumental activities of daily living (IADLs) and/or have advanced MNCD with significant behavioral and psychological symptoms. With the aging of the population, the number of adults in LTC is expected to triple in the next two decades.

LTC is typically provided in a facility staffed with health care professionals (Sanford et al. 2015). For the majority of residents, this becomes their home for the rest of their life. Often, a section of the facility provides skilled rehabilitation to promote recovery of function after acute hospitalization so that individuals can be discharged back home. Such rehabilitation typically involves intensive physical, occupational, and/or speech therapy and/or complex medical initiatives (e.g. intravenous antibiotics, total parenteral nutrition, management of pressure ulcers). Although admissions to LTC are usually from home or another LTC facility, a substantial proportion of admissions are from the rehabilitation section, where the resident has made insufficient progress in recovering function to live safely on his or her own and has insufficient resources to be cared for safely at home.

The Spectrum of Long-Term Care

LTC primarily includes nursing homes (NHs) and assisted living (AL) (in the United States), long-term care homes (in Canada), residential aged care homes (in Australia), and similar facilities in other countries (Sanford et al. 2015). The spectrum of residents in LTC ranges from very disabled individuals living in NHs, AL homes, special care units, and hospice, to less-disabled individuals living in community-based residential facilities, small foster care homes, board-and-care or personal care homes, or congregate housing, as well as people in retirement communities who receive assistance with ADLs or whose medications are monitored.

LTC settings are making efforts to adopt a more person-centered approach that emphasizes independence, dignity, privacy, decision-making, autonomy, and aging in place (Morley 2012). Besides providing complex physical-health-related services, the majority of LTC facilities also provide oversight of personal and supportive services, social services, recreational activities, meals, housekeeping and laundry, and transportation. Although the public perception is that no one likes living in a LTC facility, many residents prefer the reassurance of medical care, socialization, and a safe environment, and they find the experience to be positive. Many family members of the residents also find some relief in knowing that their loved one is safe and receiving the complex care they are unable to provide at home.

The Epidemiology of Psychiatric Disorders among Residents in Long-Term Care

At least one in three residents in LTC at any given time has a treatable serious psychiatric disorder, and one in five has two or more treatable psychiatric disorders (Commission on Long-Term Care 2013; Steiz, Purandare, and Conn 2010). If we include the management of MNCD (dementias), then four out of five residents in LTC at any given time would benefit from psychiatric treatment (Desai and Grossberg 2017). This, combined with high point prevalence of use of multiple psychotropic medications (15–30 percent) (psychotropic medications are medications used to treat psychiatric disorders) and psychiatric mismanagement, results in substantial psychological and functional morbidity (Jacquin-Piques et al. 2015; Kotlyar et al. 2011; Vasudev et al. 2015; Wei et al. 2014). (See Tables 1.1 and 1.2.) In addition, psychiatric disorders have a substantial negative effect on

Table 1.1 Prevalence, Key Concerns, and Evidence-Based Approaches by Mental Health Team for Common Psychiatric Disorders in Long-Term Care Populations

Psychiatric Disorder (Point Prevalence [%])	Key Concerns and Common Examples of Psychiatric Mistreatment or Undertreatment	Evidence-Based Approaches and Therapeutic Pearls
Major neurocognitive disorders (MNCD) / Dementias (40–90)	– Undertreatment of reversible causes of cognitive impairment – Inappropriate use / nonuse of cholinesterase inhibitors and/or memantine	– Work-up to identify potentially reversible cause(s) of cognitive impairment – Appropriate use of cholinesterase inhibitors and/or memantine based on APA Practice Guidelines
Agitation and/or aggression as part of behavioral symptoms of MNCD (BPSD) (20–50)	– Overtreatment with psychotropic medication – Lack of knowledge, skill, and practice of nonpsychotropic approaches	– Discontinue antipsychotics and, if necessary, replace them with safer alternatives such as citalopram or dextromethorphan-quinidine (both off-label) – Staff training in person-centered care, communication skills, dementia care mapping, and SPPEICE (strength-based, personalized, psychosocial sensory spiritual environmental initiatives and creative engagement)
Depressive Disorders (include depression due to a MNCD) (10–30)	– Use of antidepressant to treat adjustment disorder – Suboptimal use of antidepressant for moderate to severe major depression and failure to recommend electroconvulsive therapy for severe/psychotic depression	– Discontinue antidepressants and institute SPPEICE (e.g. individualized pleasant activity schedule, individual psychotherapy) – Optimize appropriate antidepressant treatment based on APA Practice Guidelines for treatment of major depressive disorders
Prevalence of delirium (2–5; may be up to 50% in newly admitted residents receiving rehabilitation after hospitalization)	– Hypoactive delirium often mistaken for depression or diagnosis missed. – Underdiagnosis of medication-induced delirium	– Comprehensive psychiatric evaluation (CPE) to accurately differentiate depression from delirium – High index of suspicion for medication-induced delirium (especially medications on Beers list)

Table 1.1 (cont.)

Psychiatric Disorder (Point Prevalence [%])	Key Concerns and Common Examples of Psychiatric Mistreatment or Undertreatment	Evidence-Based Approaches and Therapeutic Pearls
Depression due to undertreated chronic pain (5–15)	– Underuse of nondrug approaches to manage chronic pain – Underuse of antidepressant to treat chronic pain	– Educate staff regarding nondrug approaches to manage chronic pain (e.g. relaxation strategies, cognitive strategies, hot and cold compresses, physical therapy, music, distraction) – Improve use of appropriate antidepressants to treat chronic pain
Psychotic symptoms due to MNCD and/or due to a general medical condition or to medication (5–15)	– Inadequate work-up to clarify etiology of psychotic symptoms – Overuse of antipsychotics for management – Failure to recognize psychosis triggering severe agitation	– CPE to clarify etiology of psychotic symptoms and institute appropriate treatment – Implement SPPEICE and limit use of antipsychotics for severe symptoms – Use antipsychotics judiciously and promptly when necessary
Schizophrenia, bipolar disorder, and schizoaffective disorders (0–5)	– Suboptimal psychotropic medication therapy leading to poor symptom control and high frequency of adverse effects – Inadequate staff knowledge about the illness leading to countertherapeutic approach	– Optimize appropriate psychotropic medication therapy (PMT) for improved control of symptoms and lowered adverse effects – Educate and train staff
Anxiety disorders (5–10)	– Overuse of benzodiazepines for management – Inadequate use of relaxation, mindfulness-based, and distraction strategies	– Minimize use of benzodiazepines and replace them with safer approaches when appropriate (e.g. antidepressants, buspirone) – Case-based staff education and training regarding relaxation and distraction strategies they can help resident use
Post-traumatic stress disorder and other trauma-related disorders (0–5)	– Underdiagnosis of PTSD and related disorders – Suboptimal PMT	– Routine screening for PTSD and other trauma-related disorders among residents who have persistent anxiety, depressive symptoms, and/or resistance to care – Optimize appropriate PMT
Substance use disorder (addiction) and misuse of medications (2–10)	– Overuse of benzodiazepines and opioids in this population – Many staff see these problems as character flaws	– Taper and discontinue benzodiazepines and opioids and replace them with safer alternatives and SPPEICE – Case-based staff education
Mild to moderate agitation and aggressive behaviors, including resident-to-resident	– Under-recognition by staff that these behaviors usually are a reaction to one or more unmet	– Educate and train staff (e.g. train with *Bathing without a Battle* DVD)

Table 1.1 (cont.)

Psychiatric Disorder (Point Prevalence [%])	Key Concerns and Common Examples of Psychiatric Mistreatment or Undertreatment	Evidence-Based Approaches and Therapeutic Pearls
aggression and sexually inappropriate behavior in the context of MNCD (10–30)	needs (e.g. experiences and perspectives of residents being heard and understood, boredom, loneliness, pain, constipation) – Inappropriate use of PMT	and institute SPPEICE to better meet resident's needs – Taper and discontinue PMT
Severe and persistent agitation and aggressive behaviors in the context of MNCD (5–10)	– Undertreatment of multiple reversible factors contributing to these behaviors – Inappropriate and suboptimal PMT	– Identify and treat reversible contributing causes of these behaviors (e.g. pain, countertherapeutic staff approach) – Optimize appropriate PMT
Sleep disorders (5–15)	– Inappropriate use of hypnotics – Underuse of nondrug approaches	– Discontinue inappropriate hypnotics and optimize use of appropriate hypnotics – Institute sleep hygiene and other nondrug approaches
Personality disorders and personality change due to a neurological condition (1–10)	– Inadequate staff knowledge leading to countertherapeutic interactions with the resident – Staff stress and burnout while caring for these residents	– Case-based staff education and training and institute SPPEICE – Support and guide staff, educate and train staff in mindfulness-based strategies to prevent burnout
Psychiatric symptoms due to use of psychotropic medication (5–15)	– Apathy, anxiety, insomnia due to antidepressants and/or antipsychotics – Cognitive impairment due to anticholinergic effects of many commonly used psychotropic medications (e.g. amitriptyline, paroxetine)	– Taper and discontinue offending medications – Minimize use of psychotropic medications that have anticholinergic activity
Psychiatric symptoms due to inappropriate use of nonpsychotropic medication (5–15)	– Steroid- and opioid-induced mood, cognitive and psychotic symptoms – Psychotic symptoms and impulse control problems due to dopaminergic therapy used to treat Parkinson's disease and Parkinsonism	– Educate staff and primary care clinician and taper and discontinue steroids as soon as is feasible – Educate staff and primary care clinician and reduce dopaminergic therapy whenever feasible
Difficulty recognizing need for palliative and end-of-life care, especially for residents who have advanced MNCD	– Futile and burdensome care for residents in last phase of life, causing further decline in quality of life – Inappropriate/suboptimal PMT for treatment of depression, agitation, and pain	– Institute palliative and hospice care that is in keeping with resident's values and wishes – Optimal appropriate PMT to treat depression, agitation, and pain

APA: American Psychiatric Association

Table 1.2 Prevalence of Use of Common Psychoactive Medications in Long-Term Care Populations and Risks Associated with Their Use

Psychoactive Medications (commonly used) (Point Prevalence)	Key Serious Adverse Risks for Physical Health	Key Serious Adverse Risks for Mental Health
Antipsychotics (e.g. risperidone, haloperidol, olanzapine, quetiapine, aripiprazole, ziprasidone, paliperidone, iloperidone, lurasidone, brexpiprazole, asenapine, cariprazine) (5–20)	Decline in ADLs, falls, increased mortality and stroke risk among residents who have MNCD, drug-induced Parkinsonism	Cognitive slowing, apathy, restlessness, dysphoria
Antidepressants (e.g. citalopram, escitalopram, sertraline, mirtazapine, duloxetine, venlafaxine, paroxetine, trazodone, desvenlafaxine, vilazodone, vortioxetine, levomilnacipran) (10–30)	Falls, risk of bleeding if used concomitantly with blood thinners (e.g. NSAIDs, aspirin, clopidrogel, warfarin), hyponatremia	Apathy, insomnia, agitation
Benzodiazepines (e.g. lorazepam, alprazolam, diazepam, clonazepam) (5–20)	Falls, decline in ADLs	Cognitive impairment, delirium, daytime sleepiness, dependence
Opioids (e.g. hydrocodone, oxycodone) and tramadol (10–40)	Falls, decline in ADLs	Cognitive impairment, daytime sleepiness, delirium, dependence
Anticonvulsants (e.g. valproate, gabapentin) (5–15)	Falls, decline in ADLs	Daytime sleepiness, delirium
Hypnotics (e.g. zolpidem, zaleplon, eszopiclone) (5–20)	Falls	Daytime sleepiness, dependence

residents' quality of life, disability, mortality, care needs, and cost of care.

MNCD and delirium are two of the most common neurocognitive disorders seen among LTC residents. Behavioral and psychological symptoms of MNCD are the most common reason for psychiatric consultation. Between 70 and 90 percent of all people who have MNCD eventually develop one or more clinically significant behavioral and psychological symptoms. The lifetime prevalence of delirium (or acute confusional state) among LTC residents is more than 50 percent. LTC residents who are transferred to a LTC facility from a hospital have a high point prevalence of delirium (20–50 percent), especially after surgery to repair a hip fracture (American Geriatrics Society 2012).

Depression (both mild and moderate to severe) is the second category of psychiatric disorder prevalent in LTC populations. Moderate to severe depression among LTC residents occurs in 6–10 percent of the population with MNCD and 20–25 percent of those without MNCD, and 4.3 percent of residents develop new-onset depression within one year of admission to a LTC facility (Hui and Sultzer 2013). Mild depression is even more prevalent, and more than 20 percent of residents may have mild depression escalate to moderate to severe depression within one year. More than one-third of newly admitted residents may develop depressive symptoms by day 14, and the majority of these (66 percent) will continue to experience depressive symptoms on day 60. Less than half of the residents who do not improve have changes in their treatment. More than half of the residents who have moderate to severe depression continue to have moderate to severe depression, and almost one-third of those who have mild depression still have mild depression one year later. Thus, depression is undertreated in LTC populations. Although we have made strides in recognizing depression in LTC populations, it is under-recognized in many subgroups, especially among the oldest residents and residents who have neurocognitive impairment.

Psychotic disorders affect 5–15 percent of LTC residents, compared with 2–5 percent of community-dwelling older adults. More than 40 percent of residents who have MNCD due to probable Alzheimer's disease (AD) have some form of psychotic symptoms (e.g. delusion, hallucination) at some point during the course of that illness. The lifetime prevalence of psychotic symptoms in MNCD with Lewy bodies and with Parkinson's disease is even higher, reaching 90 percent. The prevalence of severe and persistent mental illness (e.g. schizophrenia, schizoaffective disorder, bipolar disorder, recurrent major depression, post-traumatic stress disorder) ranges from 0.2 to 2.5 percent in LTC. Older persons who have schizophrenia or schizoaffective disorder make up the majority of these residents, although among veterans of war, post-traumatic stress disorder (PTSD) also makes up a substantial proportion.

Insomnia as a symptom and sleep disorders are prevalent in LTC populations and are associated with inappropriate use of hypnotics and other inappropriate and potentially dangerous pharmacological agents (e.g. sedating atypical antipsychotics, such as quetiapine) and inadequate use of sleep hygiene and other nondrug approaches (Gindin et al. 2014).

Resident-to-resident aggression is ubiquitous in LTC. Self-injurious behaviors (e.g. pinching or scratching oneself, banging one's fist against an object) are often seen among residents who are immobile. Sexually inappropriate behaviors are also common in LTC populations, especially among male residents who have frontal lobe damage or cerebrovascular disease.

The prevalence of psychotropic medication use is high in LTC populations (Jacquin-Piques et al. 2015; Vasudev et al. 2015; Wei et al. 2014). (See Table 1.2.) The point prevalence of the use of two antidepressants is high (5–15 percent) and of two or more psychotropic medications is even higher (15–30 percent). The use of antipsychotics especially is worrying because of the significant risk of stroke and mortality associated with its use by individuals who have MNCD. On average, more than 10 percent of LTC residents are taking an antipsychotic at any given time; additionally, more than half are receiving an antipsychotic at a dose exceeding the maximum level, are receiving duplicative therapy, and/or have inappropriate indications. More than 25 percent of residents who have dementia and spend more than 100 days in a LTC facility are prescribed an antipsychotic. Antipsychotics and hypnotics are often prescribed in the hospital, and these medications are continued after admission to a LTC facility, especially when staffing levels are low. In addition, there are considerable gaps between the psychotropic medications that clinical evidence recommends and the psychotropic medications that clinical practice delivers. The use of antidepressants and antipsychotics by LTC residents who have MNCD has risen dramatically, and these medications are primarily administered to manage behavioral and psychological symptoms associated with MNCD.

The proportion of LTC residents who have serious behavioral problems (especially aggressive behavior toward staff and/or other residents) ranges from 30 to 50 percent and typically is part of behavioral symptoms accompanying MNCD.

Psychosocial and Medical Complexity of Long-Term Care Residents

In demographics, residents of LTC facilities are typically older than 75, and female residents are older than male residents (mean age 83 versus 76) (Rosenblatt and Samus 2011). The majority are women (70 percent), and more than 40 percent of all residents are 85 years of age or older (Erol, Brooker, and Peel 2015; Commission on Long-Term Care 2013). Most residents are not living with a marital partner, and more than 50 percent are widowed. More than 50 percent of admissions to LTC are unplanned and/or the resident has not been involved in the decision. Most LTC facilities are located in a metropolitan area, where mental health professionals are more available than in rural areas. Admission to LTC is strongly associated with age and the presence of advanced MNCD, even after adjusting for disability (Brodaty et al. 2014). The majority of LTC residents have multiple treatable comorbid physical health problems that are often undertreated (Table 1.3). At least one in five residents needs assistance with three to four ADLs. Additionally, the functional status of most residents usually declines with time.

Physical health conditions are typically in advanced stages and more disabling among LTC populations than among community-dwelling age- and gender-matched adults (Table 1.4) (Rosenblatt and Samus 2011). Almost 80 percent of the patients hospitalized for a stroke and 65 percent of the patients hospitalized for a hip fracture are discharged to skilled nursing facilities for rehabilitation services. The psychosocial well-being of LTC residents is also significantly influenced by comorbid physical conditions. Sensory deficit, urinary tract infection, dehydration, constipation, musculoskeletal pain, electrolyte imbalance, falls, and the mood- and mind-altering effects of commonly prescribed drugs are some of the most common treatable physical conditions encountered among LTC populations. Significant hearing impairment and vision impairment

Table 1.3 Common Untreated or Undercorrected Physical Health Problems among Long-Term Care Residents Who Have Psychiatric Disorders

Physical Health Problem	Point Prevalence (%)	Key Mental Health Concern Associated with the Physical Health Problem
Hearing deficit	20–50	Depression or paranoia
Vision deficit	10–30	Depression, visual hallucination or illusion
Pain (acute, acute over chronic, chronic)	10–25	Depression, agitation, aggression
Constipation	20–60	Depression, agitation, aggression, delirium
Dehydration	5–15	Depression, fatigue, delirium
Urinary incontinence	5–20	Agitation, aggression
Pressure ulcer	5–20	Depression, agitation
Moderate to severe obesity	15–30	Depression, anxiety, sleep disturbance
Inappropriate medication	10–50	Cognitive impairment, agitation
Frailty	20–40	Cognitive impairment, depression
Malnutrition (including vitamin deficiency, especially vitamins B_{12} and D)	30–60	Depression, agitation, cognitive impairment
Obstructive sleep apnea	5–15	Cognitive impairment, insomnia
Hypoglycemic episodes due to overtreatment of diabetes	5–10	Anxiety, cognitive impairment, delirium
Hyponatremia	5–10	Cognitive impairment, agitation
Under- or overcorrection of hypothyroidism	5–10	Depression, anxiety, agitation, insomnia

are underdetected in a substantial number of LTC residents, especially residents who have MNCD (Koch et al. 2005). Arthritis and osteoporosis are also often undetected and undertreated. Frequently, the work-up for infection is inadequate, and in 25–75 percent of the cases, the antibiotic chosen is inappropriate. Asymptomatic bacteriuria and pyuria are often inappropriately treated with antibiotics.

A substantial proportion of LTC residents are being prescribed medications that are inappropriate and are responsible for considerable excess physical and mental health morbidity (American Geriatrics Society 2015; Kotlyar et al. 2011). Routine use of opioids to manage chronic noncancer pain is common among LTC residents (point prevalence 20–40 percent) and as-needed use of opioids for chronic noncancer pain management is even higher (40–70 percent). The use of multiple opioid medications is also prevalent (5–15 percent). Opioid use to manage chronic noncancer pain is often inappropriate and carries substantial risks of delirium, falls, daytime sedation, decline in ADLs, irritability, severe constipation, and memory impairment. Use of more than one drug with significant anticholinergic activity is also high (point prevalence 30–60 percent) and carries risks of memory impairment, delirium, and falls.

Nearly 25 percent of older adults will spend some time in a nursing facility, typically for rehabilitation after a hospitalization (Sanford et al. 2015). The majority will subsequently return home, but a significant number (5–7 percent) are likely to require continued care in a LTC facility. Many LTC residents develop acute physical health problems requiring hospitalization and typically return to the LTC facility for rehabilitation. Delirium and depression are even more prevalent among residents receiving rehabilitation than among LTC residents (Hui and Sultzer 2013).

More than 20 percent of older adults die in LTC facilities (Institute of Medicine 2014; Teno et al. 2013). Palliative and end-of-life care for LTC residents is inadequate, and many residents spend their last days or weeks in substantial suffering due to poorly managed agitation, depression, and/or pain. LTC facilities must be able to provide excellent palliative and end-of-life care for all residents, and addressing mental health is an essential component of such care (Desai and Grossberg 2011).

Table 1.4 Common Advanced Physical Health Problems among Long-Term Care Residents and Associated Mental Health Concerns

Common Advanced Physical Health Problem (point prevalence)	Key Associated Mental Health Concern	Key Commonly Used Psychotropic Medication to Avoid or Use with Extra Caution
Cerebrovascular accident(s) (10–30)	Cognitive impairment, depression	Antipsychotics
Coronary heart disease (20–40)	Depression	Tricyclic antidepressants
Heart disease with prolonged QTc interval	Depression	Citalopram, ziprasidone
Congestive heart failure (10–30)	Depression	Tricyclic antidepressants
Chronic obstructive pulmonary disease (10–30)	Anxiety, depression	Benzodiazepines
Stage 4 or higher chronic kidney disease (10–30)	Depression, chronic pain	Lithium, gabapentin
Morbid obesity (10–20)	Depression	Olanzapine, quetiapine, valproate, mirtazapine
Obstructive sleep apnea (5–20)	Depression, insomnia	Benzodiazepines
Diabetes (10–30)	Depression, cognitive impairment	Olanzapine, quetiapine
Hip fracture(s) (10–20)	Depression, chronic pain	Benzodiazepines
Epilepsy (5–15)	Cognitive impairment, depression	Bupropion

Family caregivers' reasons for admitting someone to a LTC facility include the resident's MNCD-related behavior (most common); the caregivers' health; and the resident's incontinence, need for more skilled care, and need for more assistance (Balestreri, Grossberg, and Grossberg 2000; Brodaty et al. 2014). These factors are usually evident in the year before admission. The number of people who have MNCD is increasing, and physicians have recommended that they move into a LTC facility for one or more of the following reasons: safety (administration of medications, regular intake of meals, safe wandering areas), medical problems (incontinence), and psychosocial issues (socialization to address loneliness, meaningful activities to address boredom, insomnia, and agitation). Many other older adults move to a LTC facility because of frailty, a stroke, or other serious medical condition.

Most LTC facilities are not designed to allow plenty of natural light to come in, nor do they have safe areas for wandering. Excessive nighttime noise, poor lighting, and limited exposure to plants and nature pose significant harm to residents' emotional and spiritual well-being. Most LTC staff members do not have adequate education and training in understanding and managing behavioral and psychological symptoms associated with MNCD, nor do they receive adequate support from administrative leadership. Stress and burnout are ubiquitous among LTC staff, and staff turnover in LTC is among the highest in all health care institutions. This is primarily because staff members are often underpaid, overworked, and underappreciated.

Given the complexity and frailty of LTC residents and the enormous psychosocial and environmental issues, meeting the mental health needs of these residents presents enormous challenges for the already strained LTC health systems.

Evidence-Based Psychiatric Approaches

Our health care system is currently failing to meet the mental health needs of LTC populations (Institute of Medicine 2014; Prince, Prina, and Guerchet 2013; World Health Organization 2015). Primary reasons for this are underdetection, undertreatment, and mistreatment of psychiatric disorders (Desai and Grossberg 2017). This is happening despite increasing evidence from randomized-controlled trials and outcomes from real-life treatment that residents who receive appropriate treatment for psychiatric disorders have improved daily functioning and quality of life (American Geriatrics Society 2011; Cummings et al. 2015; Kales, Gitlin, and Lyketsos 2014; Kopke et al. 2012; Porteinsson et al. 2014; Poudel et al. 2015; Testad et al. 2014; Mulsant and Pollock 2015). (See Tables 1.1, 1.5, and 1.6.) Strength-based, personalized, psychosocial sensory spiritual environmental initiatives and creative engagement (SPPEICE) are sufficient to treat mild to moderately severe mental health problems, and judicious use of evidence-based psychotropic medication may be necessary in addition for severe mental health problems and for chronic mental illness (Kales, Gitlin, and Lyketsos 2014). It is time we champion changes in mental health care services so that LTC facilities can provide integrated care that uses evidence-based psychiatric approaches to prevent and treat psychiatric disorders with close collaboration between the primary care team and mental health professionals.

Making a Case for Routine Availability of High-Quality Comprehensive On-Site Mental Health Services

LTC populations must be able to receive excellent mental health care as an integral part of overall care (Desai and Grossberg 2017; Streim 2015). Primary care clinicians often find the diagnosis and management of psychiatric disorders in LTC populations daunting even with all the practice guidelines available from various organizations regarding evidence-based psychiatric approaches (American Geriatrics Society 2011; Canadian Coalition for Seniors' Mental Health 2014). This is not surprising, given the complexity of psychiatric disorders among residents who are already severely compromised by advanced physical health problems, cognitive deficits, sensory deficits, and limitations in performing ADLs. Hence, the availability of a team of mental health professionals who have expertise to provide such complex care is essential. Additionally, psychiatric mismanagement is prevalent and often catastrophic for residents and medico-legally expensive for the facility. (See Table 1.1.) Input from mental health professionals who have expertise in LTC psychiatry often changes understanding of the resident's emotional distress, mental health diagnosis, treatment, and outcome (Poudel et al. 2015; Desai and Grossberg 2017; Streim 2015). Psychiatric disorders are often chronic and disabling, and on-site mental health professional services can improve care. Last but not least, residents and family members might insist that residents deserve treatment on site by experts in the condition because of the considerable burdens posed by transportation of severely disabled and frail residents to an outpatient mental health clinic. Hence, on-site availability of mental health professionals who have expertise in LTC psychiatry is essential to meet the mental health needs of vulnerable LTC populations.

Mental health professionals include geriatric psychiatrists, adult psychiatrists, psychiatric nurse practitioners and psychiatric physician assistants, neuropsychologists, gerontologists, psychologists, and social workers. See Box 1.1 for common reasons for seeking help from a mental health professional who has expertise in LTC psychiatry. Only geriatric psychiatrists receive comprehensive training in LTC psychiatry. Other mental health professionals need to have training in LTC psychiatry before working in LTC.

Residents in LTC facilities live with each other in close settings 24 hours a day, seven days a week. They have their own rooms (often shared with another resident) but come together for meals, socializing, activities, and entertainment. These are small, intense communities, and LTC staff will need to manage the associated conflicts and disputes by conflict resolution in order to maintain the residents' autonomy yet keep control of the situation. Mental health professionals can guide LTC staff in creative ways of addressing conflict (between residents, between resident and family, and between resident/family and staff) to prevent unnecessary or excessive emotional distress of residents and staff burnout. This is especially important in conflict situations involving residents who have personality disorder.

It is not uncommon to find a married couple residing in a facility, and this situation comes with its unique set of psychosocial challenges. Typically, one spouse is cognitively impaired and the other is healthier but has chosen to live in the facility so as to continue to live with the spouse. For the cognitively impaired spouse, psychosocial approaches focus on how to prevent further decline, and for the healthier spouse, professional caregivers should help the person cope with loss, grief, stress, and situational depression. Mental health professionals can guide LTC staff in the prevention of mental health problems between spouses living in LTC.

The psychosocial well-being of many LTC residents depends considerably on the well-being of

BOX 1.1 Mental Health Team Members and Key Reasons for Seeking Their Help

Mental Health Team Member	Key Reasons for Seeking Help
Psychiatrist	Assess and manage risk for suicide Assess and manage risk for violence Consult regarding psychiatric emergencies Assess and manage psychiatric symptoms* Assess capacity to make health care decisions Assess need for palliative care Consult regarding optimizing brain function Educate and train staff** Guide facility leadership toward person-centered care (PCC) culture Consult for gradual dose reduction of psychotropic medication (PM) Consult for addressing high-risk PMT Consult for reducing use of antipsychotic medication Design programs to diminish caregiver burnout
Neuropsychologist	Clarify severity and etiology of cognitive decline Assess capacity to make health care decisions Consult regarding optimizing brain function
Gerontologist/psychologist	Provide individual psychotherapy Provide group psychotherapy Aid staff-resident conflict resolution Educate and train staff Design programs to diminish caregiver burnout
Social worker	Provide individual psychotherapy Provide family therapy and conflict resolution Provide group psychotherapy Aid staff-resident conflict resolution Educate and train staff Design programs to diminish caregiver burnout
Psychiatric nurse	Educate and train staff Teach relaxation strategies to residents and staff Design programs to diminish caregiver burnout

* Psychiatric symptoms include but are not limited to the following: cognitive decline, depression, anxiety, insomnia, hypersomnia, psychotic symptoms, suicidal ideas, self-harmful behavior, homicidal ideas, agitation, verbal and/or physical aggression, sexually inappropriate behavior, addiction problems, and pain.

** Topics for staff education and training include: importance of validating residents' experiences and inquiring about and routinely incorporating their perspectives into care plans; psychosocial environmental approaches to manage behavioral symptoms of MNCD; nondrug management of pain; nondrug management of sexually inappropriate behavior; sleep hygiene and other nondrug approaches for management of insomnia/sleep disorder; relaxation strategies, mindfulness-based approaches; monitoring adverse effects of PMT; Beers list of drugs that are inappropriate for LTC populations; assessment of risk for suicide; assessment of risk for violence; strategies to de-escalate resident aggression and prevent resident-to-resident aggression.

family and professional caregivers. Family members (especially a spouse) may not be able to spend enough time with the resident, adding to the resident's losses. Family members may themselves be stressed, experience guilt and anxiety, and be depressed. These negative emotions can have a negative effect on the resident, either directly (e.g. resident feels guilty and feels a burden) or indirectly (e.g. family spends less time with the resident). Many family caregivers continue to carry a substantial burden of caregiving even after the loved one enters LTC. Caring for a loved one who resides in an LTC facility can be rewarding, but also overwhelming at times. Factors that are stressful for family caregivers of LTC residents are different in many ways from those for family caregivers of older adults living in the community. The job of LTC staff is also uniquely challenging and stressful, due to their daily exposure to verbal and physical aggression, the burden of caring for many residents, and low salary. Nursing assistants in LTC facilities – who often experience harassment, threats, and assaults from residents – have the highest incidence of workplace assault of all workers. A substantial proportion (60–80 percent) of aggressive incidents in LTC facilities go unreported. One of the major problems adversely affecting emotional and spiritual well-being for LTC residents is the high rate of staff turnover. Hence, the emotional well-being of family and LTC staff needs to be routinely inquired into and addressed, along with the psychosocial well-being of residents. This goal creates not only challenges for those working in LTC but also opportunities to enhance the quality of life for both residents and caregivers. Mental health professionals are in a unique position to understand all these complex determinants of residents' psychosocial and spiritual well-being and have the skills and expertise to address them. Additionally, mental health professionals are best equipped to design and participate in programs to diminish workplace triggers for burnout among caregivers in LTC facilities.

Residents' emotional and spiritual well-being also depends to a considerable extent on their functional abilities and medical comorbidity. Improving or maintaining function, or slowing functional decline, rather than curing disease, is the major goal for LTC residents. Untreated medical comorbidity often manifests in behavioral and psychological symptoms, contributes to decreased psychosocial functional capacity, and interferes with the resident's ability to age in place (Morley 2012). Mental health professionals are in an ideal position to help the primary care team differentiate behavioral and psychological symptoms due to untreated medical comorbidity from those related to environmental stressors and/or psychiatric disorder.

Trends in the Characteristics of Long-Term Care Residents

Over the past 20 years, financing changes, policy changes, and innovation in the private sector and the government have fundamentally altered the system of LTC supports. Today's LTC residents are much sicker, have more disabilities, and have shorter life expectancy than those admitted just 10 years ago. The number of residents in LTC facilities who use a wheelchair or who have contracture has increased over the last 10 years and is expected to continue to increase. So have rates of moderate to severe obesity. However, the single characteristic that evidences the greatest shift is the increasing prevalence of residents who have MNCDs with secondary behavioral and psychological issues and the notion that LTC facilities are becoming like psychiatric hospitals. This is in addition to the growing use of psychotropic medications in LTC populations. This is alarming, as the majority of psychotropic medication prescribed for LTC residents is not evidence-based, is often inappropriate, and causes more harm than good, especially for residents who have MNCD. The number of residents who have MNCD has also dramatically increased in the last two decades, primarily due to an increase in the prevalence of MNCD in older adults in general. Ostomy care has also risen significantly in LTC, as has bowel and bladder incontinence. The number of dedicated long-term beds has increased for dialysis, MNCD ("memory care"), and ventilator needs. The gender ratio has risen toward more women residents than men (3 to 1 currently), although there is a growing number of men in LTC and they adapt differently from women.

The population of middle-aged adults who have advanced MNCD (especially related to stroke, traumatic brain injury, chronic traumatic encephalopathy, Huntington's disease, multiple sclerosis, alcohol-related MNCD) needing LTC has slowly increased to more than 15 percent in the last decade and is expected to continue to rise in the next decade. In contrast, the use of LTC by the oldest old, those age 85 or older, declined sharply over the last decade. Possible reasons include more government-supported home-based services for disabled older adults, new and cheaper alternatives to traditional LTC, less disability, improved financial resources of the oldest old (especially long-term care insurance), and alterations in the patterns of LTC.

The newest trend is for couples to become residents of LTC facilities when one spouse's health has been compromised and the other spouse can no longer provide the needed care. Some of these couples have been married for 40, 50, or more years and have never been without each other.

LTC populations and their health care providers are changing in race and ethnicity (increase in ethnic minority elders) and sexual orientation (increase in residents self-identifying as belonging to the LGBTQ community) (American Geriatrics Society Ethics Committee 2015; World Health Organization 2015). The first step is to recognize that the cultures of both the resident and the health care provider influence clinical care. Additionally, psychosocial needs of these minority groups are considerably different from those of others.

While the number of LTC residents will invariably increase as a result of the aging of the population in general, the use rate of LTC facilities (especially nursing homes, but also assisted living) may continue to decline as innovative strategies are implemented to keep the elderly disabled population at home, corresponding with development of naturally occurring retirement communities (NORCs) and continuing care retirement communities (CCRCs). This means that the need for mental health professionals who have expertise in LTC psychiatry to meet the needs of older adults receiving LTC at home will also increase and may need to be met in innovative ways (e.g. telepsychiatry).

With longevity increasing, a growing emphasis on strategies to promote healthy aging, and an exponential growth in medical advances, the identity of LTC has changed and will continue to change. The current population shift is undoubtedly not the last. Population and its driving forces are not static, and the skills of health care providers should not be, either. More residents will be divorced, have stepchildren, come from different cultural backgrounds, and believe in active aging. Also, the children and spouses of residents may be more active, assertive, and involved, want to micromanage, and be more vigilant. There may be more choices and more frequent changes in LTC due to family dissatisfaction.

Health care professionals working in LTC need to keep pace with all these changes in LTC populations, understand the unique psychosocial needs of various populations, and ensure that the care delivered is culturally sensitive.

Priorities for Future Research and Funding Mental Health Services

The residents' characteristics (acuity, prevalence of MNCD, etc.) and the services provided vary considerably from one LTC facility to another, from one region to another, and from one country to another. On the whole, LTC facilities are more different than similar. Thus, across all community and facility settings, more consistency is needed in the information collected on the characteristics of the settings and the services offered, as well as on the characteristics of residents, so that analyses (big data research analytics) can identify factors associated with the choice of setting, transitions between settings, and outcomes. Increased funding for research to investigate which mental health services are most effective in improving outcomes cost effectively is needed. Future research needs to include input from residents, their family, and LTC staff into the study design and seek their experiences and perspectives to better understand and meet residents' psychological and social needs. For mental health professionals, training in long-term care psychiatry should be standardized and scaled up. Government and private payers and LTC facilities should cover the comprehensive mental health services that integrate mental health, physical health, and social services for residents. Professional organizations and academic institutions should establish standards of practice that payers and LTC facilities can adopt. Government should fund health care innovation awards specifically geared toward mental health care in LTC populations. If successful innovative models are identified, we will then have the ability to extend or expand them. Such broad-based approaches are vital to overcoming three key barriers to LTC residents receiving consistent, high-quality mental health care: physicians' dearth of training in LTC psychiatry, inadequate reimbursement for mental health care in LTC populations, and a definition of mental health care that does not include prevention and limits its use until residents develop severe mental health problems. See Table 1.7 for a list of evidence-based mental health prevention and wellness strategies for LTC residents (Livingston et al. 2014; Streim 2015; Desai and Grossberg 2017). It is time medicine's successes in prevention, chronic disease management, and palliative care for LTC residents is extended to include comprehensive high-quality mental health care for prevention, psychosocial and spiritual wellness, and optimal management of psychiatric disorders.

Table 1.5 Examples of Individualized Strength-Based Psychosocial Environmental Approaches

Therapeutic Approach (professional delivering the approach)	Common Indication	Strength of the Resident
Individual psychotherapy (licensed therapist)	– Depression and/or anxiety – Stress management	Relatively preserved cognitive function
Group psychotherapy (licensed therapist)	– Depression and/or anxiety – Stress management	Relatively preserved cognitive function
Individualized pleasant activity schedule (facility staff with guidance by mental health professional)	Prevent and treat boredom, loneliness, and depression	Applicable to all residents irrespective of level of cognitive function
Bright light therapy (nursing staff with education and guidance by mental health professional)	Prevent and treat seasonal affective disorder, insomnia, and behavioral symptoms associated with MNCD	Capacity to sit in one place for 15 minutes or more at a time
TimeSlips (www.timeslips.org) (facility staff trained in TimeSlips)	Prevent and treat boredom, loneliness, and agitation	Relatively good vision and language functions
Cognitive Stimulation Therapy (CST) (www.cstdementia.com) (facility staff trained in CST)	Prevent and treat boredom, cognitive decline, and agitation	Relatively good language functions
Music therapy (music therapist) and music-based activities (recreational therapist, nursing staff)	Prevent and treat depression, anxiety, insomnia, and agitation	Relatively good auditory function
Drawing, coloring, and other art-based activities (recreational therapist, activity therapist, nursing staff)	Prevent and treat depression, anxiety, and agitation	Some ability to draw and/or color
Aromatherapy (recreational therapist, activity therapist, nursing staff)	Prevent and treat depression, anxiety, insomnia, and agitation	Reasonably good olfactory function
Massage therapy (nursing staff)	Prevent and treat insomnia, anxiety, depression, and agitation	Useful to almost all residents (extra caution with residents who have neuropathy and allodynia [experience touch as pain])
Pet- / animal-assisted therapy	Prevent and treat anxiety, depression, and agitation	Useful for all residents, especially residents who have history of having pets
Gardening / Eden experiment	Prevent and treat anxiety, depression, and agitation	Useful for all residents, especially residents who have history of engaging in gardening
Physical activity / Exercise program (includes Tai Chi, yoga, walking program) (nursing staff)	Prevent and treat depression, anxiety, insomnia, agitation, and chronic pain	Reasonably good upper and/or lower limb movement functions
Online brain training programs (nursing staff with guidance from mental health professional)	Optimize cognitive well-being and slow cognitive decline	At least some motivation and relatively good cognitive functioning
Support groups (early-stage dementia, stroke) (any LTC staff with guidance from mental health professional)	Reduce emotional toll dementia/MNCD/stroke can take on the resident and improve emotional well-being	Willing residents
Dignity therapy	Prevent and treat depression during last phase of life	Relatively good cognitive functioning

Table 1.6 Evidence-Based Psychotropic Medication Therapy to Manage Commonly Occurring Psychiatric Disorders

Psychiatric Disorder	First-Line Psychotropic Medication(s)	Psychotropic Alternative(s) to Consider in Certain Situations
Major neurocognitive disorder (Alzheimer's disease, Lewy bodies, Parkinson's disease, cerebrovascular disease)	Cholinesterase inhibitors and/or memantine	No other evidence-based option
Delirium associated with severe agitation	Antipsychotics per 2010 National Institute for Health and Care Excellence (NICE) guidelines for the prevention and treatment of delirium	Benzodiazepines to manage severe anxiety in end-of-life delirium
Major depression	Antidepressants and, for nonresponsive or partially responsive residents, or residents who have psychotic symptoms, atypical antipsychotics per 2010 APA practice guidelines for treatment of major depression	Electroconvulsive therapy (ECT) for life-threatening depression
Schizophrenia and schizoaffective disorders	Atypical antipsychotics per 2010 APA guidelines for the treatment of schizophrenia	Typical antipsychotics in refractory situations
Bipolar disorder	Valproate, lamotrigine, atypical antipsychotics per 2013 International Society for Bipolar Disorder guidelines for the management of bipolar disorder	Lithium in refractory situations
Post-traumatic stress disorder	Antidepressants and prazosin per 2010 Department of Veterans Affairs, United States guidelines for the treatment of post-traumatic stress	Low-dose atypical antipsychotics in refractory situations
Pseudobulbar affect	Dextromethorphan and quinidine combination (Nuedexta)	Antidepressants if Nuedexta not tolerated, not available, or not effective
Persistent agitation and/or aggression associated with MNCD not responding to SPPEICE and not due to any treatable medical comorbidity	Citalopram and escitalopram per 2011 American Geriatrics Society (AGS) guidelines for treatment of psychotic symptoms and neuropsychiatric symptoms of dementia in older adults	Antipsychotics for severe and persistent aggressive behaviors not responding to SPPEICE and antidepressants per 2016 APA guidelines for the treatment of agitation in persons with dementia
Panic disorder	Antidepressants per the 2011 NICE guidelines for the treatment of panic disorder	Low-dose short-term use of short-acting benzodiazepines
Generalized anxiety disorder	Antidepressants per the 2011 NICE guidelines for the treatment of generalized anxiety disorder	Low-dose short-term use of short-acting benzodiazepines
Obsessive compulsive disorder	Antidepressants per 2013 APA guidelines for the treatment of obsessive compulsive disorder	Low-dose atypical antipsychotics in refractory situations
Insomnia disorder	Ramelteon, suvorexant	Short-term use of trazodone
Hypersomnia in residents who have obstructive sleep apnea	Modafinil, armodafinil	Low-dose stimulants if first-line therapy not tolerated, not available, or not effective

Table 1.7 Mental Health Prevention and Wellness in Long-Term Care

Prevention and Wellness Condition	Evidence-Based Strategies	Potential Outcome
Cognitive aging (aging-associated changes in cognitive function)	Exercise program, Mediterranean diet, online brain training programs, discontinuation of drugs with anticholinergic properties	Improve cognitive well-being
Mild neurocognitive disorder	Exercise program, Mediterranean diet, online brain training programs, discontinuation of drugs with anticholinergic properties	Prevent or delay progression of cognitive decline
Adjustment disorder with depressed mood	Individual psychotherapy, individualized pleasant activity schedule	Prevent progression to major depression
Recurrent major depression	Mindfulness-based cognitive behavior therapy	Prevent relapse of major depression
Adjustment disorder with anxious mood	Relaxation strategies, stress management strategies, meditation, individual psychotherapy	Prevent progression to generalized anxiety disorder
Insomnia	Sleep hygiene, discontinuation of medications that cause/worsen insomnia, minimizing caffeinated drinks	Prevent progression to chronic insomnia and complication of major depression
Chronic pain	Hot and cold compress therapies, cognitive behavior therapy, relaxation strategies, physical therapy, exercise program	Prevent depression related to suboptimal control of chronic pain
Subsyndromal delirium	Multicomponent approaches, discontinuation of all unnecessary medication	Prevent progression to delirium
Subsyndromal frailty (frequently associated with depressed mood)	Physical therapy, strength-training programs, nutrition therapy	Prevent progression to frailty and improve mood
Sarcopenia (frequently associated with depressed mood)	Physical therapy, strength-training programs, nutrition therapy	Prevent falls and improve mood
Boredom and loneliness	Continuous activities programming	Prevent agitation and aggression
Helplessness and existential angst	Individual psychotherapy (especially meaning-centered psychotherapy), regular interaction with a member of the clergy	Prevent progression to major depression
Fear of falls and related refusal to ambulate	Individual psychotherapy, relaxation strategies	Prevent progression to disabling phobia and dependence on wheelchair
Tobacco use disorder	Motivational interviewing, nicotine replacement therapy, bupropion, varenicline	Prevent development and worsening of chronic obstructive pulmonary disorder, lung cancer, anxiety disorder related to hypoxia and hypercapnia, and neurocognitive disorder due to cerebrovascular disease

Table 1.7 (cont.)

Prevention and Wellness Condition	Evidence-Based Strategies	Potential Outcome
Opioid pain medication-seeking behavior for chronic noncancer pain	Comprehensive psychiatric assessment to evaluate unrecognized depression, anxiety, or addiction issues	Prevent opioid use to manage chronic noncancer pain
Medically unexplained symptoms	Comprehensive psychiatric evaluation and staff education regarding management of atypical depression, anxiety, and somatoform disorders	Prevent unnecessary and repeated medical testing
Wish for assisted dying and/or euthanasia	Palliative care, meaning-centered psychotherapy	Prevent suicide and attempted suicide

> Psychiatric consultation provides insight into residents with dementia and mental illness and how to improve their quality of life by implementing non-pharmacological interventions before adding medication. We have had several successful dose reductions and completely eliminated psychotropic medications on some residents with positive results. Also, we are completely restraint free on our behavioral care unit. Our psychiatrist provides valuable education to staff regarding the benefits of fewer medications and increased activity involvement such as increased physical activity, periods of time outside for the benefits of sunshine/bright light therapy and Individual Pleasant Activity Schedule (IPAS) to improve psychosocial wellbeing of residents.
>
> Desert View Care Center of Buhl, Buhl, Idaho

Summary

Long-term care populations must be able to receive excellent mental health care as an integral part of overall care. Neglect of treatable serious psychiatric disorders and inappropriate use of psychotropic medication are seen in one in three adults receiving long-term care and severely compromise their quality of life. Our health care system is currently failing to meet the mental health needs of long-term care populations. Primary reasons for this are underdetection, undertreatment, and mistreatment of psychiatric disorders. This is happening despite increasing evidence from randomized controlled trials and outcomes from real-life treatment that residents who receive appropriate treatment for mental health problems have improved daily functioning and quality of life. Providing evidence-based mental health care is challenging for primary care teams due to the high complexity of psychiatric disorders among residents who are already severely compromised by advanced physical health problems, sensory deficits, and limitations in performing basic activities of daily living. Hence, the availability of a team of mental health care professionals who have expertise to provide such complex care is essential. Staff education and training, reduction of inappropriate use of psychotropic and other medications, routine use of SPPEICE, and optimal use of appropriate psychotropic and nonpsychotropic medications are key evidence-based approaches to prevent and treat psychiatric disorders in long-term care populations.

Key Clinical Points

1. Treatable serious psychiatric disorders and inappropriate use of psychotropic medication are seen in one in three residents receiving long-term care and severely compromise residents' quality of life.
2. Providing evidence-based mental health care is challenging for the primary care team due to the complexity of psychiatric disorders among residents who are already severely compromised by advanced physical health problems, sensory deficits, and limitations in performing basic activities of daily living.
3. Routine provision of evidence-based treatment by a mental health care team that has expertise in long-term care psychiatry is essential for maintaining dignity, reducing suffering, and improving quality of life for all residents receiving long-term care.
4. Staff education and training, discontinuation of inappropriate medications, strength-based, personalized, psychosocial sensory spiritual

environmental initiatives and creative engagement, and optimal appropriate psychotropic and nonpsychotropic medication interventions are evidence-based strategies to improve mental health and well-being in long-term care populations.

References

American Geriatric Society. 2011. *Guide to the Management of Psychotic Disorders and Neuropsychiatric Symptoms Associated with Dementia in Older Adults*. dementia .americangeriatrics.org/GeriPsych_index.php (accessed September 29, 2016).

American Geriatric Society. 2012. *Postoperative Delirium in Older Adults. Best Practice Statement from the American Geriatrics Society*. www.journalacs.org/article/S1072-7515%2814%2901793-1/pdf (accessed September 30, 2016).

American Geriatrics Society. 2015. 2015 Updated Beers Criteria for Potentially Inappropriate Medication Use in Older Adults. American Geriatrics Society Beers Criteria Update Expert Panel. *Journal of the American Geriatrics Society* **63**:2227–2246.

American Geriatrics Society Ethics Committee. 2015. American Geriatrics Society Care of Lesbian, Gay, Bisexual, and Transgender Older Adults Position Statement. *Journal of the American Geriatrics Society* **63**:423–426.

Balestreri, L.A., A. Grossberg, and G.T. Grossberg. 2000. Behavioral and Psychological Symptoms of Dementia as a Risk Factor for Nursing Home Placement. *International Psychogeriatrics* **12**(1):7–16.

Brodaty H., M.H. Connors, J. Xu, et al. 2014. Predictors of Institutionalization in Dementia: A Three-Year Longitudinal Study. *Journal of Alzheimers Disease* **40**:221–226.

Canadian Coalition for Seniors' Mental Health. 2014. *National Guidelines for Seniors' Mental Health. The Assessment and Treatment of Mental Health Issues in Long-Term Care Homes (Focus on Mood and Behavior Symptoms)*. www.ccsmh.ca (accessed October 1, 2016).

Commission on Long-Term Care. 2013. *Report to United States Congress*. www.medicareadvocacy.org/wp-content/uploads/2014/01/Commission-on-Long-Term-Care-Final-Report-9-18-13-00042470.pdf (accessed October 1, 2016).

Cummings, J.L., C.G. Lyketsos, E.R. Peskind, et al. 2015. Effect of Dextromethorphan-Quinidine on Agitation in Patients with Alzheimer Disease Dementia: A Randomized Clinical Trial. *Journal of the American Medical Association* **314**(12):1242–1254.

Desai, A.K., and G.T. Grossberg. 2011. Palliative and End-Of-Life Care in Psychogeriatric Patients. *Aging Health* 7:395–408.

Desai, A.K. and G.T. Grossberg. 2017. Psychiatric Aspects of Long-Term Care. In B.J. Saddock, V.A. Saddock, and P. Ruiz (eds.), *Comprehensive Textbook of Psychiatry*, 10th ed., pp. 4221–4232. Virginia: American Psychiatric Press Inc.

Erol, R., D. Brooker, and E. Peel. 2015. *Women and Dementia: A Global Research Review*. London: Alzheimer's Disease International. www.alz.co.uk/sites/default/files/pdfs/Women-and-Dementia.pdf (accessed October 1, 2016).

Gindin, J., T. Shochat, A. Chetrit, et al. 2014. Insomnia in Long-Term Care Facilities: A Comparison of Seven European Countries and Israel: The Services and Health for Elderly in Long-Term Care Study. *Journal of the American Geriatrics Society* **62**:2033–2039.

Hui, C., and D. Sultzer. 2013. Depression in Long-Term Care. In H. Laveretsky, M. Sajatovic, C.F. Reynolds III (eds.), *Late-Life Mood Disorders*, pp. 477–499. Oxford: Oxford University Press.

Institute of Medicine. 2014. *Dying in America: Improving Quality and Honoring Individual Preferences Near the End Of Life*. Washington, DC: National Academies Press. www.nationalacademies.org/hmd/Reports/2014/Dying-In-America-Improving-Quality-and-Honoring-Individual-Preferences-Near-the-End-of-Life.aspx (accessed October 1, 2016).

Jacquin-Piques, A., G. Sacco, N. Tavassoli, et al. 2015. Psychotropic Drug Prescription in Patients with Dementia: Nursing Home Residents versus Patients Living at Home. *Journal of Alzheimer's Disease* **49**(3):671–680.

Kales, H.C., L.N. Gitlin, and C.G. Lyketsos; Detroit Expert Panel on Assessment and Management of Neuropsychiatric Symptoms of Dementia. 2014. Management of Neuropsychiatric Symptoms of Dementia in Clinical Settings: Recommendations from a Multidisciplinary Expert Panel. *Journal of the American Geriatric Society* **62**:762–769.

Koch, J.M., G. Datta, S. Makhdoom, and G.T. Grossberg. 2005. Unmet Visual Needs of Alzheimer's Disease Patients in Long-Term Care Facilities. *Journal of the American Medical Directors Association* **6**(4):233–237.

Kopke, S., I. Muhlhauser, A. Gerlach, et al. 2012. Effect of a Guideline-Based Multicomponent Intervention on Use of Physical Restraints in Nursing Homes: A Randomized Controlled Trial. *Journal of the American Medical Association* **307**(20):2177–2184.

Kotlyar, M., S.L. Gray, R.L. Maher Jr., and J.T. Hanlon. 2011. Psychiatric Manifestations of Medications in the Elderly. In M.E. Agronin and G.J. Maletta (eds.), *Principles and Practice of Geriatric Psychiatry*, 2nd ed., pp. 721–733. Philadelphia: Lippincott, Williams & Wilkins.

Livingston, G., L. Kelly, E. Lewis-Holmes, et al. 2014. Non-Pharmacological Interventions for Agitation in Dementia: Systematic Review of Randomized Controlled Trials. *British Journal of Psychiatry* **205**:436–442.

Morley, J.E. 2012. Aging in Place. *Journal of the American Medical Directors Association* **13**(6):489–492.

Mulsant, B.H., and B.G. Pollock. 2015. Psychopharmacology. In D.C. Steffens, D.G. Blazer, M.E. Thakur (eds.), *The Textbook of Geriatric Psychiatry*, 5th ed., pp. 527–588. Arlington, VA: American Psychiatric Publishing.

Porteinsson, A.P., L.T. Drye, B.G. Pollock, et al. 2014. CITAD Research Group. Effect of Citalopram on Agitation in Alzheimer Disease: The CitAD Randomized Clinical Trial. *Journal of the American Medical Association* **311**(7):682–691.

Poudel, A., N.M. Peel, C.A. Mitchell, et al. 2015. Geriatrician Interventions on Medication Prescribing for Frail Older People in Residential Aged Care Facilities. *Clinical Interventions in Aging* **10**:1043–1051.

Prince, M., M. Prina, and M. Guerchet. 2013. *World Alzheimer Report 2013. Journey of Caring: An Analysis of Long-Term Care for Dementia.* London: Alzheimer's Disease International. https://www.alz.co.uk/research/worldAlzheimerReport2013.pdf, (accessed January 28, 2016).

Rosenblatt A., and Q.M. Samus 2011. The Aging Patient and Long-Term Care. In M.E. Agronin and G.J. Maletta (eds.), *Principles and Practice of Geriatric Psychiatry*, 2nd ed., pp. 31–36. Philadelphia: Lippincott, Williams & Wilkins.

Sanford, A.M., M. Orrell, D. Tolson, et al. 2015. An International Definition for "Nursing Home." *Journal of the American Medical Directors Association* **16**:181–184.

Steiz, D., N. Purandare, and D. Conn. 2010. Prevalence of Psychiatric Disorders among Older Adults in Long-Term Care Homes: A Systematic Review. *International Psychogeriatrics* **22**:1025–1039.

Streim, J. 2015. Clinical Psychiatry in the Nursing Home. In D.C. Steffens, D.G. Blazer, M.E. Thakur (eds.), *The Textbook of Geriatric Psychiatry*, 5th ed., pp. 689–748. Arlington, VA: American Psychiatric Publishing.

Teno, J.M., P.L. Gozalo, J.P. Bynum, et al. 2013. Change in End-of-Life Care for Medicare Beneficiaries: Site of Death, Place of Care, and Health Care Transitions in 2000, 2005, and 2009. *Journal of the American Medical Association* **309**:470–477.

Testad, I., A. Corbett, D. Aarsland, et al. 2014. The Value of Personalized Psychosocial Interventions to Address Behavioral and Psychological Symptoms in People with Dementia Living in Care Home Settings: A Systematic Review. *International Psychogeriatrics* **26**(7):1083–1098.

Wei, Y., L. Simoni-Wastila, I. H. Zuckerman, et al. 2014. Quality of Psychopharmacological Medication Prescribing and Mortality in Medicare Beneficiaries in Nursing Homes. *Journal of the American Geriatrics Society* **62**:1490–1504.

World Health Organization. 2015. *World Report on Ageing and Health.* www.who.int/ageing/publications/world-report-2015/en/ (accessed October 1, 2016)

Vasudev, A., S. Z. Shariff, K. Liu, et al. 2015. Trends in Psychotropic Dispensing among Older Adults with Dementia Living in Long-Term Care Facilities: 2004–2013. *American Journal of Geriatric Psychiatry* **23**(12):1259–1269.

Chapter 2

Comprehensive Psychiatric Assessment Process

Regular screening, comprehensive assessment, and evidence-based, state-of-the-science treatment of mental disorders are central to high-quality care for residents in long-term care (LTC) (Canadian Coalition for Seniors' Mental Health 2014). A comprehensive psychiatric assessment process for initial evaluation involves a thorough history (from the resident, family, professional caregivers, and previous records), pertinent physical and neurological examination, detailed mental status examination, use of standardized assessment scales, pertinent laboratory tests and/or brain imaging if indicated, and good documentation (American Psychiatric Association 2016). A good follow-up assessment involves pertinent information from the resident, staff, and family, focused mental status examination, assessment of response to treatment, and modification of the treatment plan as necessary. (See Figure 2.1.) The mental health professional (MHP) should ask all residents screening questions to identify abuse and uncontrolled pain (Dong 2015), and should ask at least one screening question during each visit. (See Box 2.1.)

The initial interview focuses on gathering data to help the MHP understand the etiology of a resident's behavioral, neurocognitive, and psychological symptoms (BNPS), arrive at an accurate diagnosis, and formulate a treatment plan. Other equally important goals of the assessment process are to build a therapeutic relationship, instill hope in the resident and/or family, restore the resident's sense of self-worth, emphasize strengths at the end of the interview, and review past coping skills and successes

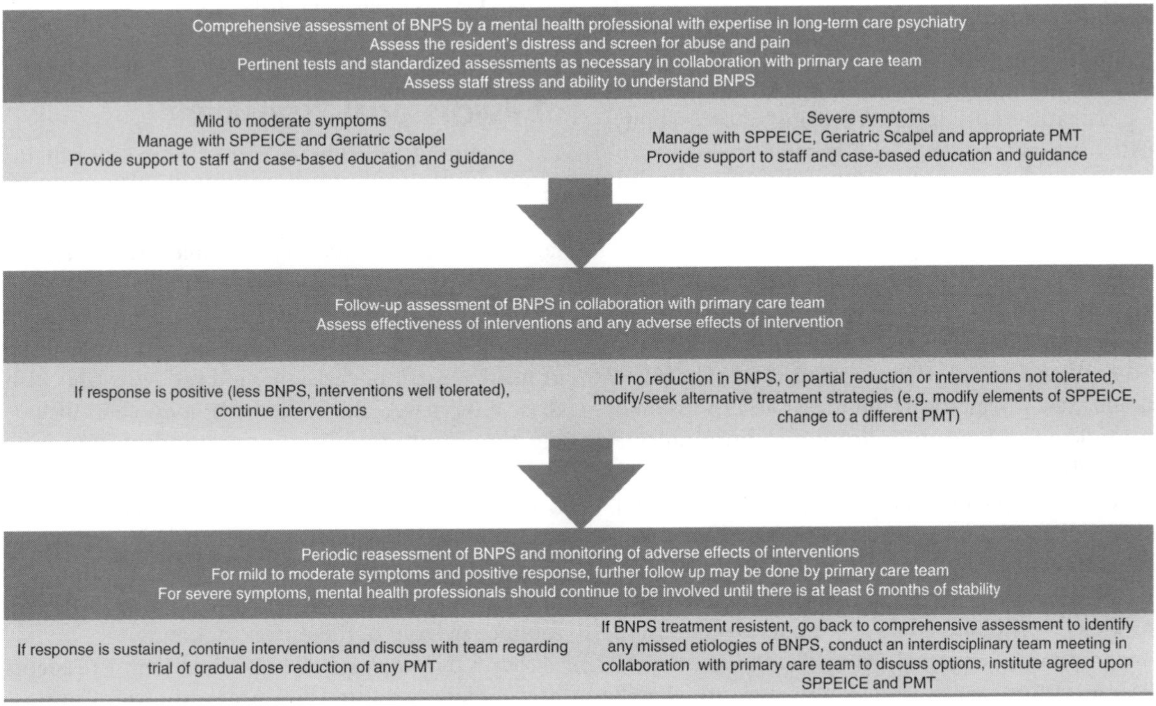

Figure 2.1 Comprehensive assessment of BNPS by a mental health care professional with expertise in long-term care psychiatry

BOX 2.1 Screening Questions to Assess Abuse and Pain

Abuse
- "Is the staff treating you well?"
- "Is anyone bothering you?"
- "Are your needs being addressed?"
- "Is anyone trying to hurt you?"
- "Has anyone hurt you physically?"
- "Has anyone mistreated you?"

Pain
- "Are you in pain?"
- "Are you hurting anywhere?"
- "Do you have any aches or pains?"

(Carlat 2011; Blazer 2015). (See Box 2.2.) While the primary reason for psychiatric consultation is to reduce BNPS, the MHP uses this opportunity not only to address the BNPS that triggered the assessment but also to screen for potential abuse and identify excess disability (listed in Box 2.2). The MHP also has the opportunity to address the needs of the family and the needs and concerns of the staff. Thus, the assessment process should incorporate the well-being of the resident, the family, and staff. In addition, the MHP uses each consultation as an opportunity to educate staff on environmental (e.g. adequate lighting of the facility) and cultural issues (e.g. negative attitude toward aging and disability, myths such as residents who have advanced neurocognitive disorder [dementia] do not experience pain) that commonly impose additional psychosocial stress on residents.

Etiology of BNPS involves identifying predisposing, precipitating, perpetuating, and protective factors (Galik 2016; Galvin 2016; O'Rourke et al. 2015; Taylor 2014; Winkelman 2015). (See Box 2.3.) The MHP should view psychiatric symptoms as an expression of the resident's unmet biopsychosocial-environmental needs (listed in Box 2.3). Any of these unmet needs could serve as predisposing, precipitating, or perpetuating. For the majority of residents, BNPS are multifactorial. Thus, even when one factor (such as uncontrolled pain) is identified, the MHP should look for other contributing factors (such as depression, inappropriate medication, untreated neurocognitive disorder). Assessment should also seek to identify factors that may reduce the potential for BNPS.

BOX 2.2 Excess Disability

- Undercorrected vision or hearing impairment
- Undercorrected pain
- Untreated dementia/major neurocognitive disorder (MNCD)
- Potentially inappropriate prescription
- Unnecessary medication (such as statin for a resident who has advanced MNCD, aspirin for a resident on hospice, proton pump inhibitor for a resident who does not have gastroesophageal reflux disease or other justifying medical condition)
- Undercorrected medical problem (e.g. anemia, pressure ulcer, diabetes mellitus, congestive heart failure, obstructive sleep apnea)
- Overcorrected medical problem (e.g. overcorrected hypothyroidism, diabetes mellitus)
- Limited mobility
- Ill-fitting dentures

(See Box 2.4.) BNPS and risk factors for BNPS are prevalent in LTC populations, so an assessment of BNPS should occur regularly; for example, on admission, at each quarterly review, when there is significant change in condition, and whenever BNPS are suspected.

Improving the Resident's Experience of Psychosocial Assessment

For the initial and subsequent interviews and therapeutic sessions, we recommend finding a quiet, private place free from distraction, including a trusted family member or staff when possible, using the same place for each encounter, and remaining sensitive to the need for confidentiality. For residents receiving individual psychotherapy, residents who are capable of making medical decisions, and residents who wish to be interviewed alone, the MHP may avoid including family or staff. For many residents (such as a resident who becomes agitated when moved to a different place or a resident who has lost the ability to communicate verbally), it may be appropriate for the follow-up assessment to take place where the resident is at the time of the visit (such as in the TV room or in front of the nurses' station).

For a thorough initial assessment, most residents need far more time and patience than a typical evaluation of a young adult in the office. The MHP should sit

BOX 2.3 The Resident's Biopsychosocial-Environmental Needs

Biological needs

- Food and water
- Clothing (to protect from cold, heat, sun, insects)
- Comfortable positioning (in chair, in bed, etc.)
- Sexual needs
- Optimal vision and hearing
- Freedom from physical pain
- Treatment of medical conditions and medication-induced BNPS
- Treatment of BNPS of MNCD
- Treatment of BNPS due to pre-existing severe and persistent mental illness (schizophrenia, bipolar disorder, other psychotic disorder)
- Treatment of psychiatric symptoms due to pre-existing other psychiatric disorder (major depression [single episode or recurrent], obsessive compulsive disorder, panic disorder, social phobia, generalized anxiety disorder, personality disorder, etc.)

Psychosocial needs

- To be treated with dignity (to be respected, honored, valued, acknowledged)
- To be useful
- To engage in meaningful (purposeful) activities
- Freedom from boredom
- Companionship
- Creative expression
- Spiritual expression (includes religious rituals)
- To be appreciated
- To be found attractive
- To be liked
- To be part of the community
- To be able to have pets
- To be able to interact with children regularly
- To be close to nature
- Cultural needs (language, ethnic food, ethnic clothing, celebration of ethnic festivals)

Environmental needs (physical environment and caregiving environment)

Physical environment

- Adequate natural light and artificial lighting
- Freedom from excessive noise
- Clean and well-smelling environment
- Esthetics (paintings, sculpture, well-designed architecture that addresses residents' unique cognitive, emotional, and spiritual needs, etc.)
- Ability to walk and wander safely
- Nature and natural surroundings
- Other safety needs (carpeting, etc.)

Caregiving environment (includes professional caregivers [staff-resident interaction], family caregivers [family-resident interaction], residents [resident-resident interaction], and volunteers [volunteer-resident interaction])

- Caregiver is argumentative with resident or frequently corrects resident's impaired memory

BOX 2.3 (cont.)

- Caregiver ignores resident's nonverbal communication (e.g. caregiver is "too busy" to realize that resident has decreased social interaction dramatically in the last few days)
- Caregiver ignores resident's verbal communication (e.g. staff walk past a resident who is calling out, "Help me, help me")
- Caregiver's expectations are beyond resident's capacity (due to cognitive and functional deficits)
- Caregiver does the functional activity (such as bathing) that resident can do on his or her own (if given time, props, and other help)
- Caregiver provides too much stimulation / too many activities for the resident
- Fewer supervisory staff at mealtime
- Lack of consistent care from the same caregiver (high staff turnover)
- Two residents arguing with each other
- The resident (who has severe hearing impairment) next door keeps the volume of the TV too loud
- A volunteer is becoming overly involved and excessively attached to the resident who has BNPS
- Abuse of the resident by staff, family, another resident, volunteer, or visitor

BOX 2.4 Key Factors That May Protect the Resident from Severe BNPS

- Well-trained staff
- Adequate number of staff
- High staff satisfaction
- Low staff turnover
- Well-educated family members
- Good social support
- Planned admission to LTC facility
- Experience with adult day program before moving to LTC facility
- Antidementia drugs for residents who have dementia/MNCD (Alzheimer's type, Lewy body type, MNCD due to Parkinson's disease)
- Small, homelike setting
- Clean environment with lots of natural light
- Path to allow safe wandering or pacing
- Person-centered care strategies (e.g. using dementia care mapping)
- Use of technology to reduce medication error and inappropriate prescription
- Palliative care programs
- Availability of mental health care providers who have geriatric expertise for routine rounds and consultation
- Continuous activity program
- Robust opportunity to socialize and interact with peers, staff, family, and pets
- Easy access to outdoors and nature, and opportunities for gardening

down for the initial assessment. If the resident is being treated for certain infections (such as infection due to methicillin-resistant *Staphylococcus aureus* [MRSA] or *Clostridium difficile* [C. diff]), the MHP should avoid sitting on the resident's bed. It is important to try to be at the same eye level as the resident, with the MHP's face in clear view of the resident. The MHP may need to repeat information and ask the resident to verify what he or she has heard the MHP say. If the MHP suspects an uncorrected or undercorrected hearing or vision deficit, he or she should consider referral to an audiologist or ophthalmologist before the next visit. For some residents (for example, those who become easily tired, frustrated, or agitated), it may take two visits (either on the same day or on separate days) to complete the initial assessment.

We recommend making sure the resident who has vision impairment has eyeglasses and uses them, and the resident who has hearing impairment has hearing aids and is wearing them (adjusted properly with batteries in working condition). The MHP should sit close to a resident who has significant hearing impairment, speak into the preferred ear, and speak in a slow, clear voice with a low pitch. Some residents read lips to help them understand what is being said, so the MHP should sit where they can see the MHP's face. For residents who have visual impairment, verbal and physical (touch) communication may be more important than visual communication (such as facial expression, gestures). If the MHP needs to speak loudly, he or she should bear in mind confidentiality and the possibility of disturbing nearby residents. A resident who has neurocognitive disorder may become discouraged if the questions force the resident to acknowledge the cognitive deficit again and again. In such a situation, it is prudent to avoid detailed cognitive testing, at least until rapport is established over time. Alternatively, the MHP can ask another staff member to perform standardized cognitive testing.

A resident who has difficulty walking may have trouble meeting the MHP in a room far away from the resident's room. It may be necessary for the MHP to arrange for staff to bring the resident in a wheelchair, or the MHP can wheel the resident. A resident who has chronic pain may find it difficult to sit comfortably during the interview, so the MHP should offer breaks for repositioning. A resident who needs to use the restroom is likely to have difficulty concentrating during the interview, so the MHP should be aware of this need as well. The MHP should also pay attention to the temperature of the interview room if it is different from the resident's room, as it may be warmer or cooler than the resident finds comfortable; this needs to be addressed at the onset of the interview. Providing a comfortable chair for the resident, having a beverage available, keeping a box of tissues at hand, and commenting on memorabilia or pictures of family/friends in the room may enhance the resident's comfort level for the interview.

Changes in the body with aging can leave residents feeling unattractive and "untouchable." Thus, holding a hand, touching the arm gently, rubbing the back, commenting on nice clothes, or giving a hug may be a rare and welcome connection for many residents, and the MHP should integrate touch and praise into the initial and follow-up encounters as and when appropriate (culturally and based on the individual's personal characteristics). Many residents may view mental illness as a personal defect or something shameful and may not comply with the interview. It might be worthwhile for the MHP to anticipate this, have a friendly attitude, and consider sharing something from his or her own life to gain the resident's trust and put the resident at ease, so that the interview can proceed. In fact, older adults may benefit from (indeed, may expect) a higher degree of personal disclosure than younger adults, especially in the LTC setting. For a resident who is skeptical about mental health treatment, sharing information about the MHP's training and experience, quoting research and support from reputable organizations, and requesting that the resident give the MHP a chance may help overcome the barrier to mental health assessment.

Understanding the resident's values, beliefs, interactional styles, and expectations of diverse cultures is also important for establishing therapeutic alliance. Some other strategies to enhance the resident's experience and the quality of the assessment include: limiting or eliminating extraneous noise (TV/radio, trolleys), using short simple sentences, speaking slowly and clearly, giving time for each sentence to be understood, writing down simple questions if hearing is severely impaired (or using pre-printed cards with routine questions in large print), writing down simple questions if the resident has difficulty comprehending spoken language but not written language, pointing to objects or people as you mention them, being literal and avoiding the use of metaphors, breaking down commands into a series of individual steps (task segmentation), having staff or family members repeat questions if necessary (especially if the MHP is from a different cultural and/or ethnic heritage), and coming back at a later time if the resident is agitated, eating, or sleeping.

For residents who speak limited or no English, the MHP should include a family member or staff member who speaks the resident's language. The MHP should also recognize that many cultures may lack an understanding of neurocognitive disorders and potential benefits of psychiatric treatment. Thus, the MHP may need to educate the resident and/or family members before starting the assessment process.

The Assessment Process

The assessment process includes how psychiatric consultation is initiated, initial evaluation, follow-up assessment, and documentation.

Who Initiates Psychiatric Consultation for Residents in LTC?

Most commonly, the staff recognizes the need for psychiatric consultation because they suspect the resident is depressed (for example, is frequently tearful, losing weight), agitated (persistent yelling, sexually inappropriate behavior), or aggressive (verbal and physical aggression), and the staff is unable to manage the behavior with psychosocial environmental approaches. Often, the resident's family requests a psychiatric consultation because they suspect the loved one is depressed or anxious, especially if the loved one has a past history of psychiatric illness or there is a family history of psychiatric illness. Occasionally, the primary care provider (PCP, whether physician, nurse practitioner, or physician assistant) initiates psychiatric consultation because the resident continues to be psychiatrically ill (has treatment-resistant depression, persistent aggression) despite treatment with psychiatric medication or because the PCP is reluctant to prescribe antipsychotic medication due to the recent warnings by governmental regulatory authorities (of increased mortality and cerebrovascular events associated with the use of antipsychotics). For residents in LTC facilities that receive governmental funding, the presence of pre-existing severe and persistent mental illness requires evaluation by a psychiatrist. An ombudsman may recommend psychiatric assessment if he or she suspects abuse or neglect and the resident gives consent. Any other team member (e.g. pharmacist, dietician) may also initiate psychiatric consultation.

We recommend that managers (e.g. directors of nursing, assistant directors of nursing, unit managers) empower all staff members to initiate psychiatric consultation with the help of the resident's primary nurse. Referral to a pharmacist to review the resident's medications before a psychiatric consultation (especially if the resident is taking several medications) is a good practice, as the pharmacist can play a crucial role in identifying drug-induced neurocognitive and other psychiatric symptoms, identifying correct dosages of psychotropic medication because of liver and/or kidney impairment, identifying potentially inappropriate medication (based on Beers list) (American Geriatrics Society 2015), and identifying potential adverse drug–drug interactions between psychotropic and nonpsychotropic medications. Documented consent from the resident or surrogate health care decision-maker (or both) for the interview to assess BNPS is a necessary first step. A formal order from the resident's PCP for psychiatric consultation should be in the resident's record before the assessment.

Enhancing the Efficiency of "Psychiatric Rounds" in LTC

We recommend assigning a staff person (such as a nurse or social worker) the task of improving the efficiency of "psychiatric rounds" by the MHP. Such a person can be called a "mental health navigator" (MHN). The MHN is available for 2–6 hours during rounds days, maintains a "mailbox" for the MHP for staff to leave messages (a notebook for writing specific resident concerns), and is responsible for preparing a list of residents to be seen, involving family in the assessment and treatment process (informing family about the visit and results of assessment, and encouraging active participation), keeping charts and documentation ready on the day of the rounds, locating residents and having them ready when they are to be seen (if necessary, with the help of a nursing assistant and/or nurse), and acting as a liaison among team members and consultants. The MHN could also become the facility mental health expert through "hands-on" coaching (on assessment of BNPS and problem solving) provided by the MHP during rounds. Larger LTC facilities may need two MHNs, each for a certain section of the facility (e.g. one for the LTC section and one for the skilled rehabilitation services section). Having a second MHN also allows psychiatric rounds to remain efficient when one MHN is on leave. The MHN can become the MHP's "eyes and ears" and be able to think like the MHP and help the facility solve problems even before the MHP does the assessment.

In complex or treatment-resistant cases, we recommend a "mini-huddle" in which different team members gather for a few minutes to problem solve, identify potential etiological factors for BNPS, and discuss treatment strategies that have been tried and have failed and those that need to be tried. We recommend that the team adopt the BEST approach during such a "huddle": identifying the biological, environmental, social and psychological, and treatment-related factors contributing to continued BNPS. For example, the "mini-huddle" can quickly identify biological factors (medications, medical condition), environmental factors (overstimulation of resident, new caregiver who needs more training), social and psychological factors (lack of companionship, boredom), and treatment factors (which of the previous recommendations were carried out, barriers to implementation of previous treatment [e.g. lack of confidence of staff or family regarding aromatherapy as an effective treatment; over-expectation from staff or family that medication will "fix" the problem], identifying treatment recommendations that are impractical or unsustainable [such as staff staying one to one with the resident]).

History

Taking a thorough history is the critical first step in the assessment process. History is obtained from family and staff (typically the nursing assistant and the nurse primarily assigned to the resident) most familiar with the resident, because in many situations the resident may not be able to give a reliable history due to neurocognitive or other impairment (such as aphasia, dysarthria, severe hearing deficit). Consultation with family members and significant others may be useful in establishing a family history of psychiatric illness (such as neurocognitive disorder, depression, psychosis) and prior psychotic or affective episodes. It is also important to assess the context in which the resident's psychiatric problems are arising. For example, a resident may be agitated because of a "roommate" problem. Although this concern needs to be addressed specifically, it might be worthwhile inquiring whether the resident has had difficulty interacting with others in a constructive way in the past.

History of Present Illness

Whether the history is obtained primarily from the resident, the family, or a professional caregiver should be mentioned at the start. The history of the present illness should elicit details about the chief complaint (description, frequency, intensity, context in which it occurs, triggers, relieving factors), other symptoms accompanying the chief complaint, and review of psychiatric symptoms (anxiety, depression, psychotic, cognitive, sleep, impulse control [aggressive, sexual], appetite). The MHP should look for predisposing and precipitating factors. Is excessive demand or stress placed on the resident? Is there a balance between sensory-stimulating and sensory-calming activities? Is there sufficient human interaction for this particular resident?

How the resident, family, and staff rate the resident's quality of life can give valuable insights into the severity and nature of the problem. A poor rating by the resident of quality of life usually indicates symptoms of depression, anxiety, or pain. Poor ratings by the staff of a resident's quality of life usually indicate that the resident has behavioral problems.

It is important to inquire into the reason for admission to LTC and whether it was planned or not. Planned admission usually helps reduce agitation and depression after admission. Also, admission to a LTC facility due to BNPS related to dementia/major neurocognitive disorder (MNCD) or stroke gives some indication of the seriousness and chronicity of the BNPS. A resident's BNPS in the context of being admitted only a few days or a few weeks to the LTC facility may indicate that the resident is adjusting to the loss of the previous home and living with "strangers."

It is important to inquire for potential triggers of "agitated" behaviors. Caregivers may report that a problem behavior occurred out of the blue. Detailed analysis of problematic behavior often indicates a specific trigger. Analysis of the event in which a resident is resisting bathing and becoming physically aggressive may indicate that the behavior followed a specific event, such as a Hoyer lift moving upward, a whirlpool motor being turned on, the shock of the skin first touching water, or being unable to see the caregiver who is helping with bathing.

Withdrawal, restlessness, procrastination, and escapism (such as watching TV all day) may suggest depression. Many residents are unlikely to express feelings of sadness or hopelessness. Grumbling about headache, backache, or other physical complaints may be a sign of depression and a reaction to multiple losses (such as loss of independence, loss of purpose to live, loss of spouse, loss of home, loss of driving, lack of adequate help for sexual expression [masculinity or femininity] and sexual intimacy).

The symptom analysis (anxiety, depression, pain, etc.) should be detailed, but it can also be short. In addition to documenting symptoms, the initial assessment should include the effectiveness of previous efforts to relieve symptoms; the resident's, family's, and staff's satisfaction with the current management of symptoms; and other diagnoses or comorbidity that may contribute to the symptoms. This helps the MHP develop and implement an individualized care plan.

It is important to ask about BNPS in different ways to encourage reporting. For example, the MHP could ask: "Are you feeling down?" "Are you feeling 'blah'?" "Are you happy?" "If you had one wish, what would it be?" The response to the last question may often give a glimpse of what losses the resident is dealing with currently. Some common responses include "I want to go home," "I wish I could walk," or "I wish I could remember." BNPS are often nonspecific. Many residents, including some who do not have cognitive impairment, cannot readily report or describe BNPS regarding duration, severity, onset, precipitating and perpetuating factors, factors that relieve BNPS, and response to previous treatment. It is thus necessary to seek as much objective information as possible to distinguish various causes, as the treatment varies with the cause.

Agitation (verbal or physical [such as repetitive questioning, pacing]) should be differentiated from resistance to care (resistance to assistance with activities of daily living [ADLs], such as bathing, eating, taking medication), as they are two distinct behavioral problems that require different management strategies.

Assessment of Specific BNPS

Assessment of specific BNPS includes assessment of suicidality and violence, sexually inappropriate behavior, and sleep disturbance.

Assessment of Suicidality and Violence. Suicidality is one of the most serious clinical concerns among residents. Demographic factors (older age, male gender, white race), presence of mood disorder (most notably depression), cognitive issues (e.g. hopelessness, demoralization), physical health factors (e.g. persistent pain, high medical comorbidity), and social factors (e.g. recent loss of a loved one, stressful life events, low social interaction) increase the risk of suicidality (Bolton, Gunnell, and Turecki 2015). A past history of suicide attempts is one of the most important risk factors for future suicidality. Most studies have not associated neurocognitive disorder (especially dementia) with suicidality.

Among cognitively intact residents, it is important to elicit a history of the resident's expressing suicidal or self-harming thoughts, plans, behaviors, and intent; whether the resident has considered specific methods for suicide, their lethality, and the resident's expectation about lethality, as well as accessibility to means (firearm, hoarding medication, use of a cord round the neck, etc.); evidence of hopelessness, demoralization, impulsiveness, agitation, anxiety, or aggression; reasons for living and plans for the future; current alcohol use; thoughts, plans, or intentions of violence toward others; overt behaviors indicating suicidal gestures, attempts, intentional aggression toward others (staff, residents, visitors) outside the context of personal care. The MHP also needs to assess previous suicide attempts, other self-harming behavior, family history of suicide, previous or current medical diagnoses (especially severe pain, visual impairment, neurological disorder, malignancy), and psychosocial situation (acute crises/losses, chronic stressors [financial, interpersonal conflicts, etc.], support system; cultural and religious beliefs about death or suicide). Finally, the MHP should also inquire into individual strengths and vulnerabilities (coping skills, personality traits [high rigidity, low openness to experience], past responses to stress, capacity for reality testing, ability to tolerate psychological pain and satisfy psychological needs).

For assessment of physical aggression, the MHP should look into various predisposing factors (Stahl et al. 2014). The severity of cognitive impairment (especially executive impairment) is the most significant predisposing factor for aggressive behavior among older adults in LTC facilities. Physical or chemical restraint is also associated with aggressive behavior. Orbitofrontal injury due to stroke, head injury, etc., is strongly correlated with impulsive aggression.

Assessment of Sexually Inappropriate Behavior. The MHP should inquire about details of "sexually inappropriate behavior" (setting, context, exact description of the behavior, frequency, staff approach, outcome of staff approach) so that he or she can differentiate between true sexually inappropriate behavior (e.g. resident masturbates during personal care) and pseudo-sexually inappropriate behavior (e.g. resident disrobes due to feeling "hot"). With residents who exhibit sexually aggressive behavior (repeated grabbing of the private parts of staff), the MHP should inquire about past history of sexually inappropriate behavior, past history of sexually abusive behavior toward spouse or partner, and legal history (e.g. for pedophilia). Is the staff approach therapeutic? Does the staff support appropriate expression of resident's sexual needs (e.g. give the resident opportunity to masturbate in his or her room with the door closed)? Does the staff "ignore" inappropriate behavior and thereby inadvertently give a wrong message that the behavior is "okay"? Are all staff members approaching the problem in a consistent, mutually agreed on, and professional manner? To understand and treat sexually inappropriate behavior, the MHP needs to ask all these questions.

Assessment of Sleep Disturbance. For residents who have insomnia, the MHP should inquire about excessive daytime sleepiness, nighttime snoring, leg discomfort, crossing legs repeatedly, rubbing legs, pacing, flexing legs, general restlessness, constant movement of legs at night, and presence of any "strange" behavior in the middle of the night to identify a variety of sleep disorders such as obstructive sleep apnea (OSA), restless leg syndrome (RLS), periodic limb movement disorder (PLMD), and REM sleep behavior disorder (RBD). Does the resident get enough daytime exercise (such as a program of walking)? Is the resident exposed to natural sunlight or enough bright light during the day? At night, is there any loud noise or bright light that disturbs the resident? Is the resident taking naps during the daytime? Does the resident go to bed at the same time and wake up at the same time? Could any medication or food item (such as caffeine-containing drink or food item) be causing sleep problems? These questions usually help the MHP identify causes of sleep problems and potential remedies. We recommend evaluation for sleep disorders among treated depressed residents who have residual symptoms of depression that include insomnia.

Allergy

The MHP should note any allergy to medication and differentiate it from adverse effects. Many adverse effects can be managed, but a true allergic reaction means that drug should not be prescribed.

Current Medications

We recommend a thorough review of all medications the resident is currently taking on a routine basis and on an as-needed basis. The MHP should routinely inquire into the frequency of use of as-needed medication and the response to the medication. To clarify the possibility of medication-induced (or medication withdrawal–related) BNPS, the MHP should ask about any recent reduction or discontinuation of psychoactive drug. The MHP should specifically inquire into the use of over-the-counter medications, vitamins, herbal remedies, and nonherbal supplements because some cognitively intact residents and some family members may administer such medications without the knowledge of the staff. The MHP should also look for any correlation between onset of BNPS and start of a new medication (for example, onset of BNPS after starting an antibiotic or steroid).

Past Psychiatric History

The MHP should routinely ask about any past history of clinically significant psychiatric symptoms (depression [may be expressed as "nervous breakdown," postpartum "nervous breakdown," etc.], longstanding anxiety [expressed as "I have always been a worrier," "He/She has always been hyper, easily stressed"], psychotic or manic symptoms [expressed as "nervous breakdown"]), suicide attempt, violence, being a victim of a traumatic event, trauma-related symptoms (e.g. nightmares, flashbacks) and the treatment (with psychotropic medication, counseling, electroconvulsive therapy ["shock treatment"], hospitalization in an inpatient psychiatric unit), and response to treatment.

Use of Street Drugs, Tobacco, Prescription Drugs, and Alcohol

The MHP should routinely ask about alcohol use, as many residents continue to drink alcohol on a daily basis after moving into a LTC facility. One or two drinks of alcohol may not have been a problem for most of the resident's life, but with the development of a neurocognitive disorder or other serious medical condition, the same amount of alcohol may be toxic and sufficient to cause significant cognitive, behavioral, affective, psychotic symptoms, or symptoms of anxiety. The MHP should also inquire into the use and abuse of prescription drugs (such as benzodiazepines, opiates), caffeinated drinks, tobacco (smoking, chewing), and street drugs (marijuana, cocaine, etc.). The MHP should ask about recent cessation or resumption of cigarette smoking because of the potential for chronic smoking (using nicotine) to induce cytochrome P450 1A2 isoenzymes, which in turn may affect drug levels of certain psychotropic medications (such as clozapine, olanzapine, fluvoxamine) metabolized by 1A2 isoenzymes.

Medical History

Assessment of BNPS includes inquiring for potentially undiagnosed current medical conditions as well as review of pre-existing medical conditions. (See Table 2.1.) Table 2.1 lists common medical conditions that are often the primary cause or exacerbation of BNPS in LTC populations. Among residents who have severe cognitive/intellectual impairment (such as advanced neurocognitive disorder, aphasia, severe intellectual disability), psychiatric symptoms such as agitation may be the only or first manifestation of an underlying medical disease. The MHP should consider nonverbal behaviors, vocalizations,

Table 2.1 Common Under-Recognized or Undercorrected Physical Health Problems Causing or Contributing to BNPS among LTC Residents

Physical Health Problem	Point Prevalence (%)	BNPS that May Be the Initial or Only Manifestation of Physical Health Problem
Hearing deficit	20–50	Depression and paranoia
Vision deficit	10–30	Depression, visual hallucination or illusion
Pain (acute, acute over chronic, chronic)	10–25	Depression, agitation, aggression
Constipation (including fecal impaction)	20–60	Depression, agitation, aggression
Dehydration and electrolyte imbalance	10–20	Depression, fatigue, anxiety, paranoia
Urinary problem (incontinence, retention, urinary tract infection)	10–25	Agitation, aggression, delirium
Skin condition (pressure ulcer, dry skin)	5–20	Depression, agitation, skin-picking behavior
Moderate to severe obesity	15–30	Depression, anxiety, sleep disturbance
Inappropriate medication or adverse effect of appropriate medication	10–50	Cognitive impairment and delirium, agitation, depression, anxiety, insomnia, psychosis, mania, impulse control problem (including sexually inappropriate behavior), skin-picking behavior
Frailty	20–40	Cognitive impairment, depression
Malnutrition (including vitamin deficiency [especially vitamins B_{12} and D])	30–60	Depression, agitation, cognitive impairment
Obstructive Sleep Apnea	5–15	Cognitive impairment, insomnia
Hypoglycemic episodes due to overtreatment of diabetes	5–10	Anxiety, cognitive impairment including delirium
Hyponatremia	5–10	Cognitive impairment including delirium, agitation
Under- or overcorrection of hypothyroidism	5–10	Cognitive impairment, depression, anxiety, agitation, insomnia
Gastrointestinal problem (gastritis, GERD)	3–8	Agitation, anxiety
Hyperammonemia	2–5	Delirium, psychosis
Seizure (especially complex partial seizure)	2–5	Delirium, agitation, psychosis
Acute pulmonary, cardiovascular, or cerebrovascular event (includes pneumonia, myocardial infarction, heart failure, stroke)	2–5	Delirium, agitation
Other acute event (includes acute renal failure, gallstone, kidney stone, intestinal obstruction, acute blood loss)	2–5	Delirium, agitation

changes in function, and caregiver reports to assess pain among residents who are unable to report pain due to severe cognitive impairment. Aggressiveness and resistance to care, for example, may be attempts to guard against pain with movement. Auditory behaviors that suggest pain include moaning, growling, and increased loudness of vocalizations. Resistance to mobility may be due to arthritic pain rather than depression. Failure to recognize toxic-metabolic-structural causes may result in inappropriate administration of psychiatric medication, which may further obscure an underlying medical condition, sometimes with fatal consequences. If a resident needs an antipsychotic, we recommend assessing cerebrovascular risk so that the MHP can compare the individualized risk of stroke and mortality associated with antipsychotic use to potential benefits before initiating long-term administration of an antipsychotic. A resident who has a history of incontinence may show problem behaviors as a consequence of incontinence, and the MHP should inquire whether a toileting schedule and prompted voiding has been implemented.

Residents who have vision problems that require eyeglasses may not be actively using eyeglasses for a variety of reasons: the resident is too cognitively impaired to request them, glasses are broken or misplaced, staff are not aware that the resident uses eyewear, or the prescription is no longer sufficient to correct the vision. The MHP should inquire whether the eyewear is labeled, whether there is an extra pair, and whether the resident is having an annual or biannual eye exam. Residents who have hearing problems and need hearing aids may not be actively using hearing aids for reasons similar to those mentioned above. In addition, the hearing aids may need new batteries, the resident is too cognitively impaired to know how to use them and often misplaces them, the hearing aid does not fit well or hurts, or it is not functioning well. Furthermore, the staff may not have been trained in the use or maintenance of hearing aids. Also, there is often lack of delegation of responsibility for the management of hearing, and family members are often asked to maintain hearing aids.

Is the resident dehydrated? Because of the decrease in the sensation of thirst with normal aging, the resident may deny thirst when asked "Are you thirsty?" Typical symptoms of gastroesophageal reflux disease (GERD), such as heartburn, abdominal pain, and indigestion, may be absent in residents who have GERD. In contrast, other symptoms, such as weight loss, anorexia, or anemia, may be the only manifestation. Although the typical features of obstructive sleep apnea (OSA) are snoring and daytime sleepiness, its presentation with neuropsychiatric symptoms (such as confusion in the daytime and hallucination at night in a resident who is overweight and has hypertension) is not uncommon.

Social, Spiritual, and Developmental History

We recommend asking questions to elucidate premorbid personality (personality characteristics before the onset of neurocognitive disorder). For example, "agreeableness" as a personality trait is associated with less agitation after one develops a MNCD. Hostile, antisocial, or paranoid characteristics can make it difficult to establish a therapeutic alliance. A resident who has always been timid and passive with a dependent personality may have difficulty being assertive with staff or may find it difficult to express ideas or concerns. It is important to distinguish between characterological features that are part of the resident's premorbid nature and those that emerge as a consequence of neurocognitive disorder, stroke, traumatic brain injury, Parkinson's disease, multiple sclerosis, Huntington's disease, or other neurological disorders. Statements from family such as "He was never as short tempered as he is now" or "Ever since I've known him, he has been pessimistic" help the MHP understand the resident's personality problem.

Because a person's spiritual beliefs may provide an important source of strength and comfort, the MHP should assess the degree to which the resident relies on spiritual beliefs to cope with life's difficulties. Assessment of spirituality may include questions such as: Is spirituality important for the resident? How does the resident express and experience spirituality? Has the resident been actively religious throughout life? What are the spiritual/religious rituals the resident engaged in before living in LTC?

Obtaining information regarding the resident's occupational history, extent of education, previous traumatic event (if any and residents' ability to cope with the event), previous losses, hobbies and interests, and what the resident has been passionate about is also recommended. Some inquiry into whether the resident had an abusive or exceptionally difficult childhood may help the MHP and staff develop compassion for the resident who is behaving in an abusive manner.

Legal History

A past history of felony due to violence, incarceration due to sexually abusive behavior toward children, and driving under the influence of drugs or alcohol are some of the many situations that the MHP should inquire into if indicated from the resident's current behavioral problems or other historical information. Although most residents who exhibit sexually inappropriate touching do not have a past history of pedophilia, residents who exhibit sexually violent behavior may have a past history of pedophilia and family members may have not been forthcoming with this information but may acknowledge it if specifically inquired into.

Caregiver's Assessment

Residents' behavior can be influenced to a substantial degree by caregivers' (family and staff) attitudes, emotions, and behavior. Assessment of family and staff's beliefs about aging, disability, life in LTC, and death is an important part of the assessment process. This is especially important in assessment of a resident during end-of-life care. Family and/or staff who feel uncomfortable about issues of loss of control, are anxious about physical illness or death, or are anxious about "losing one's mind" in the context of advanced neurocognitive disorder may see suffering and depression as an unavoidable part of aging. Family and/or staff may believe that residents are not interested in sexual activity or are not interested in expressing sexuality. Thus, they may neglect residents' sexual needs and fail to understand residents' suffering in relation to this. Family and/or staff may doubt that mental health treatment can be of any benefit for advanced MNCD and may not be forthcoming with input during the assessment process. Family and/or staff may be reinforcing dependency by doing things for the resident that he or she is capable of doing. Family relationships that have been poor for many years may inhibit progress by dredging up old conflicts that undo gains mental health treatment may make in the resident's mood and attitude. Also, if the caregiver (family or staff) is overburdened, he or she may have little motivation to cooperate with the MHP's recommendations, which may further increase stress and the risk of caregiver burnout.

Family members and staff can be an important resource in implementing the treatment plan. Assessing and acknowledging strengths of family and staff in the initial and subsequent encounters is important. Building a therapeutic bond with the family is important not only in achieving family members' well-being but also in partnering with them to improve the resident's quality of life.

Examination of Previous Records (Psychiatric and Medical)

Because of diagnostic complexities, the MHP should review all previous diagnostic evaluations. This is especially helpful with residents who have a psychiatric illness that existed before the disability caused by MNCD, stroke, or other disabling condition that precipitated functional decline and admission to LTC. We strongly recommend examination of previous psychiatric records, which will greatly help in the differential diagnosis, and getting direct input from previous mental health care providers. In complex cases, it may be worthwhile to review all previous diagnostic evaluations and consider consulting with the resident's nonpsychiatric care providers. The MHP should bear in mind that many elderly persons carry "labels" of problems and take medications for years, only later to realize they never had the problem or perhaps no one thought to discontinue the medication. It is important for the MHP to recognize that valuable information is often omitted during the transition from hospital to LTC facilities (and vice versa). We recommend using the Universal Transfer Form (UTF) to facilitate the transfer of necessary patient information between care settings. The form is available at www.aafp.org/afp/2010/0515/afp20100515p1219-f1.pdf.

Reviewing the Minimum Data Set

The Minimum Data Set (MDS) is part of the federally mandated Resident Assessment Instrument (RAI) developed as a primary assessment tool for residents in skilled nursing facilities in the United States. Other countries usually have a similar instrument. Items in the MDS include demographics and patient history, functional capabilities, cognitive and mood/behavior patterns, psychosocial well-being, medication use, continence, nutritional and dental status, activity patterns, and potential for discharge. The MDS helps LTC staff identify health problems on admission, and quarterly thereafter, to create a comprehensive care plan for each resident. The MDS can give the MHP significant information and thus make further information gathering and assessment easier.

Elucidating the Resident's Existing Strengths and Skills

Inquiring about the resident's current strengths and skills is as important as inquiring about the etiology of current BNPS (Anderson and Heyne 2013). (See Box 2.5.) Residents, even in moderate stages of MNCD, retain the ability to learn new images. Appropriate social behavior in a one-to-one interaction may be maintained in the face of extreme cognitive difficulties, suggesting that basic response to social cues is retained throughout the course of the illness.

BOX 2.5 Assessment of Strengths and Skills

1. Attitude (e.g. optimistic)
2. Drive (e.g. highly self-motivated, high energy)
3. Language (e.g. retained comprehension of spoken language, capacity to read, capacity to have a conversation)
4. Cognition (e.g. retained social cognition, capacity to empathize)
5. Social/interpersonal (e.g. easily makes friends, initiates conversations)
6. Ambulation (e.g. can ambulate on his or her own, participate in walking programs)
7. Physical strength (e.g. can transfer on his or her own, can use and enjoy strength-training equipment)
8. Sense of humor (e.g. great capacity to laugh at self or situation and not take life too seriously)
9. Cooking (e.g. great interest in all aspects of cooking)
10. Musical abilities (e.g. able to play a musical instrument)
11. Vision (e.g. can see well)
12. Hearing (e.g. can hear well)
13. Gardening (e.g. has a green thumb)
14. Spirituality (e.g. involved in church activities, regularly prays)
15. Self-care (e.g. able to do activities of daily living with only minimal assistance)
16. Altruism (e.g. often expresses compassion, tries to help others)
17. Social support (e.g. lots of family and friends come to visit and are supportive)
18. Financial assets (e.g. can afford weekly or twice-weekly massage therapist, can afford a professional caregiver to give one-to-one support and activities for several hours a day)

Pertinent Physical and Neurological Examination

We recommend measurement of vital signs as part of routine assessment, especially if the MHP suspects delirium, infection, or exacerbation of underlying medical condition (congestive heart failure, COPD, etc.). If the resident is complaining of pain, we recommend a brief examination of the site during initial psychiatric evaluation. If the resident grimaces, moans, and/or pulls away when the limbs are moved, the resident could be experiencing pain. The MHP should use physical examination to focus on the potential etiology of pain among residents experiencing pain. The MHP should pay specific attention to the neurologic examination for paresthesia, hyperesthesia, numbness, or allodynia, and to the muscular system for tenderness, inflammation, deformity, or trigger points. If the resident is not moving any limb, the MHP should assess whether this is part of resident's baseline deficit or a new problem.

We recommend routine assessment of posture and movement for all residents who may need antipsychotic medication. Does the resident have stooped posture, unsteady gait, involuntary movement (tremor, akathisia, tardive dyskinesia, myoclonic jerks)? If the MHP suspects abuse, we recommend looking for lesions that do not appear to be organically caused (e.g. bruising under the breast, in the armpits, or behind the knees) and for patterns of injury (e.g. two black eyes without scratches or injury to the nose, indicating that black eyes were not due to a fall).

We recommend physical exam to assess signs of dehydration. Poor central skin turgor ("tenting" of skin over the forehead, sternum, thigh, or subclavian area) is a better indicator of hydration status than peripheral skin turgor ("tenting" of the skin over the dorsum of the hand, which may occur with normal age-related loss of subcutaneous tissue). Some residents who deny thirst may enthusiastically drink an entire glass or two of water or other liquid (all at once or in frequent small sips) when it is offered to them.

Detailed Mental Status Examination

Detailed mental status examination is an essential part of a comprehensive psychiatric evaluation. It involves the following:

Alertness: Is the resident awake and alert, or drowsy, sleepy, overly sedated?

Orientation: Is the resident oriented to time, place, and person?

Attention: Is the resident attentive, inattentive, or distractible?

Appearance: Is the resident well groomed or unkempt, disheveled; does the resident look the stated age or older or younger?

Eye contact: Does the resident make eye contact or look down during interview (taking into account vision impairment or hearing impairment)?

Attitude: Is the resident cooperative, defensive, taciturn, distrustful, or hostile?

Behavior: Does the resident show normal psychomotor activity, or is restless (increased psychomotor activity) or has psychomotor retardation? Is the resident calm or yelling or showing other signs of agitation?

Mood (subjective emotional state): Does the resident voice depressed or anxious mood, fearful mood, and/or apathetic mood?

Affect (objective emotional state at the time of the interview): Does the resident look sad or depressed? Is the resident tearful, anxious, fearful, perplexed? Does the resident have bright and cheerful affect or euthymic and broad affect?

Speech: Does the resident have oral, written, or reading (or global) language deficits (deficits in comprehension [receptive aphasia], or expression [expressive aphasia] or both [global aphasia])? Does the resident have difficulty finding words? Does the resident have slurred speech or other form of dysarthria? Is the speech normal in tone and volume or loud, or is the flow of speech rapid and difficult to interrupt (pressure of speech) or slow (slowness in thinking or bradyphrenia)?

Thought processes: Are the resident's thought processes coherent and logical or incoherent, illogical, difficult to follow, tangential? Does the resident show perseveration (giving the same answer to a different question)? Does the resident show flight of ideas (jumping from one topic to another rapidly and topics are somehow related)?

Thought content: Does the resident have paranoid ideas/delusions, other delusions (grandiosity, jealousy, infidelity, persecutory, somatic, delusional misidentification)? Does the resident have ideas of hopelessness, helplessness, guilt, and worthlessness? Does the resident have suicidal or homicidal ideas, intentions, or plans?

Memory: Does the resident have short-term memory impairment? Does the resident have long-term memory impairment?

Insight: Does the resident have good insight into his or her illness and disability? Does the resident have intellectual but not emotional insight? Is the resident in denial?

Judgment: Test judgment is assessed by asking the resident what the resident would do if he or she found a stamped and addressed envelope on a road. Most residents may not need formal testing of judgment because of obvious signs of significant cognitive impairment. Social judgment is assessed by observing the resident's verbal and physical behavior during social interaction and in social settings. Does the resident show normal test and social judgment? Does the resident show impaired social judgment (for example, as shown by sexually disinhibited behavior)?

Standardized Assessment Scales

Table 2.2 lists recommended scales for standardized assessment of cognition, function, BNPS, pain, and caregiver grief. Although standardized assessment scales may require an additional 2–10 minutes to complete, we recommend their routine use (at least in complicated or treatment-resistant cases) to avoid (or discontinue) futile treatment and measure response to new treatment. Staff training to administer most of the standardized assessment scales can greatly improve the assessment process and may improve the staff's understanding of the problems.

Cognitive Assessment Scales

Cognitive scales to assess global cognitive function include the Mini-Mental State Examination, the Veterans Affairs Saint Louis University Mental State, the Montreal Cognitive Assessment, and the Brief Interview for Mental State (Scott, Ostermeyer, and Shah 2016). All of these scales have some bias associated with age, education, race, and socioeconomic status.

The Mini-Mental State Examination (MMSE) is commonly used as a screening tool for cognitive function in LTC. With MMSE, residents are asked to respond to a 10-minute, 30-point questionnaire that assesses memory, orientation skills (e.g. time, place, naming), reading/writing, and ability to follow a three-stage command. The MMSE is scored from 0 to 30 points – the lower the score, the greater the cognitive impairment. Individuals who have MNCD usually score no higher than 24 points. MMSE scores on average may decline by three to four points per year among individuals who have Alzheimer's disease (AD). The MMSE is a highly sensitive screening tool for moderate to severe MNCD, and thus ideally suitable for residents in LTC, because most residents have moderate to severe neurocognitive deficit. Many residents (especially highly educated

Table 2.2 Recommended Standardized Assessment Scales

Assessment Scale	Key Benefits	Key Limitations
Cognitive Assessment Scales		
Mini-Mental State Exam (MMSE)	Excellent tool to assess global cognitive function	(1) May miss executive dysfunction (2) Copyright issues limit its routine use
Saint Louis University Mental State (SLUMS)	Excellent tool to assess global cognitive function	Not as well validated as MMSE and MOCA
Montreal Cognitive Assessment (MOCA)	(1) Excellent tool to assess global cognitive function (2) Is translated into multiple languages	Not as commonly used in research studies as MMSE
Brief Interview of Mental Status (BIMS)	Easy-to-use tool to assess global cognitive function that is part of the MDS 3.0	Low sensitivity in identifying residents who have Mild Neurocognitive Disorder or Mild MNCD
Trail Making Test–oral (TMT-oral)	Easy to use at bedside to measure executive function	Cannot be used as the only test to assess executive function, as it can be normal in some individuals who have significant executive dysfunction
Controlled Oral Word Association Test (COWAT)	Easy to use at bedside to measure executive function	Cannot be used as the only test to assess executive function, as it can be normal in some individuals who have significant executive dysfunction
Confusion Assessment Method (CAM)	Excellent screening tool to diagnose delirium	Professional administering the test needs some training in its appropriate use
Functional Assessment Scales		
Functional Activities Questionnaire (FAQ)	Excellent tool to assess IADLs	With individuals who have impaired insight, needs a knowledgeable informant for accurate assessment
Physical Self-Maintenance Scale (PSMS)	Excellent tool to assess ADLs	With individuals who have impaired insight, needs a knowledgeable informant for accurate assessment
Katz Index of Activities of Daily Living	Excellent tool to assess ADLs	With individuals who have impaired insight, needs a knowledgeable informant for accurate assessment
Barthel Inventory	Excellent tool to assess ADLs	With individuals who have impaired insight, needs a knowledgeable informant for accurate assessment
Behavioral and Psychological Symptoms Assessment Scales		
Patient Health Questionnaire–9 (PHQ-9)	(1) Excellent tool to screen for depression (2) Well known in primary care and easy to use	Not useful with individuals who have moderate to severe neurocognitive deficit
Geriatric Depression Scale – 15 (GDS-15)	Excellent tool to screen for depression	Not useful with individuals who have moderate to severe neurocognitive deficit

Table 2.2 (cont.)

Assessment Scale	Key Benefits	Key Limitations
Cornell Scale for Depression in Dementia (CSDD)	Excellent tool to screen for depression in individuals who have moderate to severe cognitive deficits	Professional administering the test needs some training in its appropriate use
Saint Louis University AM SAD (SLU AM SAD)	Easy-to-use tool to screen for MDD in LTC populations and monitor response to treatment	Not as well studied as PHQ-9, GDS, and CSDD
Cohen Mansfield Agitation Inventory (CMAI)	Excellent tool to screen for agitation and monitor response to treatment	Professional administering the test needs some training in its appropriate use
Pittsburgh Agitation Scale (PAS)	Excellent tool to measure severity of distress expressed as agitation in LTC populations with moderate to severe MNCD and monitor response to treatment	Requires staff training for reliable use
Neuropsychiatric Inventory–Nursing Home versions (NPI-NH)	Excellent tool to assess behavioral and psychological symptoms and monitor response to treatment	Professional administering the test needs some training in its appropriate use
Behavioral symptoms in Alzheimer's Disease (BEHAVE-AD)	Excellent tool to screen for agitation and monitor response to treatment	Professional administering the test needs some training in its appropriate use
Pain Assessment Scales		
Visual Analog Scale	Excellent tool to assess severity of pain and easy to use	Not useful with individuals who have moderate to severe neurocognitive deficit, as they may not comprehend what is asked of them
Numerical Rating Scale (Likert Scale)	Excellent tool to assess severity of pain and easy to use	Not useful with individuals who have moderate to severe neurocognitive deficit, as they may not comprehend what is asked of them
Pain in Alzheimer's Disease (PAIN-AD)	Excellent tool to assess and manage pain in individuals who have moderate to severe AD or other MNCD	Professional administering the test needs some training in its appropriate use

residents) who have mild MNCD do not score below 24 (the generally accepted cutoff score). If the MHP has a high Index of suspicion based on history, we recommend neuropsychological testing to confirm the diagnosis of MNCD.

The MMSE can also be used to stage MNCD in AD (Perneczky et al. 2006). The MMSE ranges are 21–24 for mild, 11–20 for moderate, and 0–10 for severe MNCD. Clinical use of the MMSE has become more expensive since its copyright was purchased by Psychological Assessment Resources, and photocopying and Internet download of the form without permission are no longer allowed. To purchase and print a copy of the MMSE, go to www.minimental.com.

The Saint Louis University Mental State Exam (SLUMS) is another tool that can be used to screen for MNCD in LTC populations. It is similar in format to the MMSE but includes some additional cognitive tasks (e.g. paragraph recall). A score of 27–30 is normal, 21–26 is mild neurocognitive disorder, 1–20 is

MNCD for individuals who have high school education or higher. Its advantage over the MMSE includes the lack of copyright (i.e. it is freely available) and that it may be a better tool to detect mild MNCD and mild neurocognitive disorder (mild cognitive impairment [MCI]) (Cummings-Vaughn et al. 2014).

The Montreal Cognitive Assessment (MOCA) is another tool that can be used to screen for MNCD in LTC populations. Its advantage over the MMSE includes the lack of copyright (i.e. it is freely available) and that it may be a better tool to detect mild MNCD and mild neurocognitive disorder/MCI (Nasreddine et al. 2005). Results are compiled into a summary score (maximum is 30). The higher the score, the better the cognitive function.

The Brief Interview for Mental Status (BIMS) is part of the MDS 3.0 and helps assess cognitive function at the time of admission to a nursing facility and periodically thereafter. It consists of three components: repetition of three words, temporal orientation, and recall. Results are compiled into a summary score (maximum is 15). The higher the score, the better the cognitive function. It lacks sensitivity in identifying mild neurocognitive disorder or mild MNCD.

Assessment of Executive Dysfunction. "Executive dysfunction" refers to deficits in initiating, planning, and modifying goal-directed behavior (Elliot 2003). Assessing executive function can help the MHP determine a resident's capacity to execute health care decisions and discharge planning decisions. With impaired executive functioning, the resident's capacity to exercise command and self-control, and to direct others to provide care, becomes diminished. Trail Making Test, oral version (TMT-oral), is a simple bedside screening test for executive dysfunction. This test elicits mental flexibility, which is impaired among residents who have executive dysfunction. TMT-oral requires the subject to count from 1 to 26 and then recite the 26 letters of the alphabet. For testing, the resident is asked to pair numbers with letters in sequence (e.g. 1-A, 2-B, 3-C, etc.) until the pair 13-M is reached. More than two errors in 13 pairings is considered impairment (Ricker and Axelrod 1994). The Controlled Oral Word Association Test (COWAT) is another simple test to assess working memory (attention-concentration), which is impaired in residents who have executive dysfunction. With categories beginning with the letter "F," then "A," then "S," the COWAT asks residents to fill the category by providing words of 3 or more letters. For example, correct responses to the category cue "F" would include "fish, foul, fact," etc. Residents free of executive dysfunction will produce 10 words in each category within one minute. We also recommend assessment of executive dysfunction for residents who are significantly impaired in ADLs but have minimal or mild impairment in MMSE.

Tests to Detect Delirium. One effective instrument for diagnosing delirium is the Confusion Assessment Method (CAM) (Inouye et al. 1990). The CAM is primarily used to detect delirium in the hospital setting but may be used for LTC populations, especially residents who have just been transferred from the hospital.

Functional Assessment Scales

Functional impairment is a key criterion for a diagnosis of MNCD. A functional assessment helps determine a resident's ability to perform the activities of daily living (ADLs) needed for personal care as well as the more complex tasks required for independent living (instrumental activities of daily living [IADLs]). We recommend the Functional Activity Questionnaire (FAQ) (Pfeffer et al. 1992) to assess IADLs and Physical Self-Maintenance Scale (PSMS) (Lawton and Brody 1969), Katz Index of independence in activities of daily living (Katz et al. 1970), or Barthel Index (Mahoney and Barthel 1965) to assess ADLs. The severity of MNCD correlates closely with the progressive loss of function. The least complex ADL is eating and the most complex is bathing. Hence, it is not surprising that bathing is the ADL most commonly associated with severe behavioral consequences.

Behavioral and Psychological Symptoms Assessment Scales

For assessment of depression among LTC residents, we recommend the Geriatric Depression Scale (GDS) for residents who have MMSE above 15 and the Cornell Scale for Depression in Dementia (CSDD) for residents who have MMSE below 15 (Alexopoulos et al. 1988; Yesavage et al. 1983). Saint Louis University scale for depression assessment (SLU AM SAD) and the Patient Health Questionnaire–9 (PHQ-9) are also good tools to assess depression in LTC populations (Chakkamparambil et al. 2015;

Saliba et al. 2012). For assessment of behavioral and psychological symptoms, we recommend one the following measurement tools: Behavioral symptoms in Alzheimer's disease (BEHAVE-AD) (Reisberg et al. 1987), Cohen-Mansfield Agitation Inventory (CMAI) (Cohen-Mansfield. Marx, and Rosenthal 1989), Pittsburgh Agitation Scale (PAS) (Rosen et al. 1994), and Neuropsychiatric Inventory–Nursing Home version (NPI-NH version) (Wood et al. 2000). These measures establish a baseline documenting the behaviors that can be monitored to assess response to treatment. These measures also help the MHP decide which resident should have antipsychotic medications not reduced or discontinued (residents continuing to have moderate scores on these measures) and which residents should receive a trial of antipsychotic dose reduction or discontinuation (for example, residents who have low scores on these measures).

The BEHAVE-AD test involves asking the resident questions covering behaviors over the most recent two weeks in seven domains: paranoid and delusional ideation, hallucination, activity disturbance, aggressiveness, diurnal rhythm disturbance, affective disturbance, and anxiety and phobia. There are 25 questions with answers rated from 0 to 3, and then a global rating from 0 (not at all troubling to the caregiver or dangerous to the resident) to 3 (severely troubling or dangerous) is assigned.

The CMAI rates 14 areas of distressed behavior, including hitting, verbal aggression, grabbing, constant requests for attention, repetitive sentences, weird laughter, and hiding or hoarding things. The frequency of these behaviors is tabulated on a five-point scale, from never to a few times per hour.

The PAS is a four-item scale that measures intensity of behaviors (aberrant vocalization, motor agitation, aggressiveness, resisting care) during a particular period (e.g. each shift). The intensity is tabulated on a five-point scale (0–4) corresponding to no agitation to most severe forms of agitation.

The NPI-NH version is a 12-item scale that measures the frequency and severity of behavioral and psychological symptoms such as agitation, anxiety, apathy, irritability, and disinhibition over the preceding four weeks. Information is provided by staff regarding the resident's behavior and associated caregiver stress. If the symptom has been present, the rater answers yes and rates the frequency and severity on a four-point scale and caregiver distress on a 0–5 scale. Scores range from 0 to 144, with higher scores indicating greater disturbance. Certain subsections of these scales (e.g. agitation and aggression section of NPI-NH) may also be used to monitor baseline scores and response to treatment with antipsychotics.

Pain Assessment Scales

For residents whose cognition is relatively intact and residents who have mild to moderate MNCD, we recommend a numerical rating scale (Likert scale) because it is quick and reliable. It is a simple scale to document the intensity of pain on a scale of 0 to 10 (0 being no pain and 10 being the worst pain). For residents who have advanced neurocognitive disorder, we recommend using the Pain Assessment in Advanced Dementia (PAINAD) scale (Warden, Hurley, and Volicer 2003). Facial expression scales are useful for residents who have impaired communication (Herr et al. 1998).

Laboratory Tests

We recommend that tests for liver function (serum bilirubin, liver enzymes, and serum albumin) and kidney function (serum blood urea nitrogen [BUN] and serum creatinine) be done before prescribing psychiatric medications if these tests have not been done in the last three months (Wang, Thakur, and Doraiswamy 2015). More recent tests may be needed if there has been a significant change in the resident's physical functioning recently. For residents on hospice or in terminal stages of dementia, these baseline blood tests may not be needed. We recommend additional tests, such as basic metabolic panel (serum levels of sodium, potassium, BUN, creatinine), to detect electrolyte imbalance and renal insufficiency, urine analysis and culture and sensitivity if indicated to detect urinary tract infection, thyroid stimulating hormone (TSH) level to detect thyroid disorder, and vitamins B_{12} and D levels for some residents to assess etiology of new-onset or resistant BNPS. If the MHP suspects infection such as pneumonia, complete blood count may be added, although frail residents may not have elevated white blood cell count seen typically among community-dwelling healthy adults who have pneumonia. We recommend an electrocardiogram (EKG/ECG) if the MHP decides to prescribe psychotropic medication that may prolong corrected QT (QTc) interval (e.g. citalopram). For residents who have prolonged QTc interval, checking potassium and magnesium levels may detect reversible causes of prolonged QTc. The MHP should also consider subtle seizure disorder in the differential diagnosis of new-onset or atypical psychiatric syndrome, which may require electroencephalogram (EEG) test and referral to a neurologist. The MHP may consider free testosterone for male residents who have suspected androgen deficiency syndrome manifesting as fatigue, depression, weight loss, cognitive impairment, and sarcopenia (muscle cell loss). In some situations, the MHP may need to order a polysomnogram or nocturnal pulse oximetry to evaluate for sleep disorders such as OSA, RLS, PLMD, and RBD.

Neuroimaging

For residents who have suspected new stroke or fall with head injury and residents who have MNCD that has not been evaluated to identify the cause of neurocognitive deficit, the MHP should consider neuroimaging unless the resident is in severe or terminal stage of MNCD or terminal stage of another condition or is on hospice. Computerized tomography (CT) of the brain is the neuroimaging of choice for residents who have advanced MNCD and residents requiring urgent neuroimaging, as it takes much less time than magnetic resonance imaging (MRI) and is less affected by motion artifacts. MRI of the brain is preferred if the resident can tolerate the test, as it detects commonly occurring neuropathology (e.g. ischemic cerebrovascular disorder related brain abnormality) better than CT scan.

Assessment of Residents Who Have Severe and Persistent Mental Illness

Residents who have severe and persistent mental illness (SPMI) may have schizophrenia, schizoaffective disorder, or bipolar disorder. MDS is not a suitable rating instrument to evaluate the symptoms and functional characteristics of residents who have SPMI. We recommend a thorough assessment by a mental health professional and review of previous records for all residents who have SPMI.

Screening Tests

No screening test should be used in isolation. Screening should not be based on chronological age but should be targeted to a high-risk group. We recommend screening all residents for neurocognitive disorder on admission (if not formally diagnosed) and every six months after that. Screening tests for neurocognitive disorder include MMSE, MOCA, and SLUMS. Mandatory depression screening in LTC facilities can improve treatment rates. We recommend screening for depression using GDS or CSDD. A recent study found that PHQ-9 was more reliable and efficient than GDS and took less time to complete (Saliba et al. 2012). The PHQ-9 is a nine-item depression scale that has been validated for depression screening in primary care (Spitzer, Kroenke, and Williams 1999). MDS 3.0 scale is not reliable in detecting depression among NH residents. We recommend screening for depression two to four weeks after admission to a LTC facility and at least every six months (Consensus Statement on Improving Quality of Mental Health Care in US Nursing Homes 2003). New onset or worsening of symptoms should prompt an assessment that includes psychological, situational, and medical evaluations. Residents who have suicidal ideas should be referred to a MHP. Residents who have psychotic symptoms and have not responded to six or more weeks of treatment should be referred to a MHP.

We recommend screening for pressure ulcers using the Braden Risk Assessment Scale, ideally within eight hours of admission, and implementing preventive action within 24 hours for those identified as at risk (Braden and Bergstrom 1989). We also recommend screening for hospice care any resident who has limited life expectancy (such as severe and terminal-stage MNCD, end-stage CHF or COPD, dependent on staff for basic ADLs). Although no specific screening tools have been devised to identify residents in need of hospice care, the MHP should refer to hospice for evaluation any resident who has MMSE of 5 or less, is dependent on caregivers for all ADLs, is unable to recognize family, and has an acute decline in health. We also recommend screening residents for pain on admission and every one to four weeks. Screening guidelines should take into account potential benefit and, most important, the resident's preferences. Futile medical screening tests such as colonoscopy, breast self-exam and clinical exam, mammography, and tests for lipid levels may be discontinued for residents who have limited (e.g. less than five years) life expectancy (which would be the majority of residents). Futile testing may cause considerable psychosocial stress.

The Individualized Care Plan

The MHP should work with the resident, family, and staff to develop and implement an individualized care plan for BNPS. We recommend figuring out which approaches are realistic and monitoring (and documenting) the response to the treatment. We also recommend trying to anticipate adverse events (such as constipation with pain medication) and including treatment for adverse events in the care plan. It is not enough for the MHP to be ready to assess and manage BNPS among LTC residents. The rest of the staff has to be trained to assess BNPS, monitor treatment, and document the findings. Training should also be aimed at overcoming any bias or misconception about BNPS. For example, regarding opiates for pain management, some of the nursing assistants may not understand differences among tolerance, physical dependence, and addiction. Educating staff will improve resident care as well as performance on surveys. Coordinating care with hospice when the resident is receiving hospice care is also important, as the LTC facility is still responsible for any uncontrolled BNPS.

While the self-report is important information, additional direct examination is needed to help identify characteristics and possible causes of BNPS. Therefore, a self-report should not be the sole basis for discussing BNPS with a MHP or for initiating treatment. It is important to seek the cause of BNPS. However, it is reasonable to try to address BNPS even if the cause is unknown – although this should be done carefully.

BNPS needs to be managed one step at a time. Often a serial trial of different approaches is needed before the final group of approaches (psychosocial environmental and pharmacological) that are effective have been identified.

During the development of the treatment plan, the first concern to be addressed is whether the BNPS the resident is experiencing are so severe that they cannot be safely managed in the LTC facility; if so, the resident may need to be transferred to an inpatient psychiatric unit (preferably a geropsychiatric unit) in a hospital.

BOX 2.6 **Some Routine Questions to Ask during Follow-up with Residents Who Have Moderate to Severe Major Neurocognitive Disorder (MNCD / Dementia)**

Moderate MNCD (some open-ended questions are okay)

- How are you doing?
- Do you have any complaints?
- Are you hurting anywhere?
- Did you sleep well last night?
- Did you like the food?
- Are you nervous?
- Are you tired?
- If you had one wish, what would it be?

Severe MNCD (primarily yes or no questions, simple questions)

- Are you hurting?
- Are you in pain?
- Are you hungry?
- Are you thirsty?

Follow-Up Assessments

Follow-up assessments are usually much shorter than the initial assessments, although in complicated cases or when new problems emerge, follow-up assessments may take considerable time. Family meetings to address palliative care and other treatment concerns also require a longer time for follow-up encounters. During follow-up, the MHP should routinely assess all residents for pain management, abuse, sleep pattern, nutritional status (Are they eating well? Are they losing weight?), and, if ambulatory, whether they have been experiencing falls or unsteady gait. At some point during follow-up for all residents (and during initial assessment for residents in terminal stages of MNCD or of other medical conditions), we recommend that the MHP in collaboration with the primary care team discuss with the resident and/or family palliative care goals, when to forego life-prolonging treatment, and when to consider hospice. For residents who have advanced cognitive impairment, we recommend some simple questions mentioned in Box 2.6. Even if a resident who has moderate MNCD may not accurately report whether he or she slept well or is eating well, the answers to these questions may reflect the current subjective emotional state (positive answers indicating subjective well-being and negative answers indicating lack of well-being at that moment).

Assessment Pearls

The assessment process for LTC populations is as much an art as a science, especially for residents who have severe cognitive impairment. The MHP should routinely seek the opinion and input of primary care providers (primary care physician, nurse practitioner,

BOX 2.7 Some Assessment Pearls

Depression among residents who have moderate cognitive impairment may manifest with atypical symptoms:

- Multiple somatic complaints
- Irritability and verbally abusive behavior
- Procrastination
- Escapism (watching TV all the time)
- Avoiding socialization
- Pain not improving with standard treatment

Depression among residents who have severe cognitive impairment may manifest with

- Depressed affect (tearfulness, looks "sad")
- "Help me, help me" statements
- Persistent yelling
- Restlessness
- Verbal and or physical aggression
- Resistance to ADL care

Delirium is often missed, and diagnosis can be improved by looking for

- Acute (1–5 days) change in mental status (staff reports that the resident "is not acting like herself")
- Acute onset of disorientation (in a resident who is usually oriented at least partially to time and place), distractibility, disorganization in thinking and/or speech
- Acute onset (over 1–5 days) of "depression"
- Acute onset (over 1–5 days) of "not eating"
- Acute onset (over 1–5 days) of "agitation"
- Sudden exacerbation of previously well-controlled BNPS
- Frequent napping but can be aroused
- Inability of resident to repeat 5-digit number

Psychosis is often missed, and diagnosis can be improved by

- Asking if the resident feels "safe" in the LTC facility
- Asking if the resident feels the food is poisoned
- Asking if the resident feels people are talking about him or her
- Yelling at imaginary people
- Verbal and or physical aggression
- Sexually aggressive behavior
- Complains of "strange smell" in the room or food

physician assistant), as they may often identify changes in the treatment of physical health issues (e.g. plan to reduce opioids) that can directly affect the resident's BNPS. The typical questions to assess depression (for example, "Over the past two weeks, have you / has the resident felt down, depressed, or hopeless?" "Over the past two weeks, have you / has the resident felt little interest or pleasure in doing things?") are still useful (especially for cognitively intact residents), but often such questions do not identify the resident's depression due to cognitive impairment and/or cultural issues (many aged residents associate feeling "depressed" with lack of inner strength [or personal failure] and thus say "No" to feeling depressed). Statements such as "I am a burden," "I wish I were dead," and suicidal ideas, plans, and attempt are obvious signs of depression. Box 2.7 lists some assessment pearls that we have found useful in our clinical practice (Desai and Grossberg 2017; Desai, Lo, and Grossberg 2013).

Documentation

The goal of good documentation is to record what was done, the findings of the assessment, the diagnosis, and the treatment plan. Such a document helps all treatment team members have access to and understand the outcome of the assessment. Thorough and accurate documentation is crucial to a high-quality assessment process and for medico-legal purposes. It can also serve as a good teaching tool for new staff. The documentation can be handwritten (if writing is legible), dictated (especially initial evaluation and if handwriting is not legible, even follow-up notes), or typed. Some LTC facilities have implemented electronic medical records (EMR), and the MHP may directly document the assessment in the EMR. Templates for pre-printed history and physical exam and follow-up notes may be used, but adequate individualized information is necessary for documentation to be clinically useful. Figure 2.2 shows a sample preprinted follow-up progress note. This note is a modified version of the SOAP progress note used in common practice.

LTC facilities should have a system in place for formally carrying out the recommendations of a MHP. Usually this involves informing the primary care physician, who then authorizes the recommendations after the resident or surrogate decision-maker expresses agreement with the recommendations. In some situations, the MHP is given the privilege

Name of resident:______________________ Room number: __________

Gender:__________ Date of birth:__________ Place of assessment:__________

Subjective complaints and staff input:______________________________

____

____

____

Is the resident in pain? Yes___No___

Is the resident having sleep impairment? Yes____No____

Is the resident having appetite impairment? Yes___No___

Psychosocial environmental approaches found effective so far: ______________

Allergies:__________________

Current psychotropic medications:______________________________

____

New non-psychotropic medication(s) prescription since last visit:______________

____

Laboratory data and other test results since last visit: ______________________

____

(Staff may document in the progress note up to this point)

HCP confirmed information documented by staff:__________

Objective evaluation / Exam (pertinent physical, neurological and mental status exam)______________

____

____

Assessment / Response to treatment:______________________________

Diagnosis:______________________________

Plan / Treatment recommendations:______________________________

____

____

____

____

Name and signature of the HCP:______________________

Figure 2.2 Sample of Pre-Printed Follow-Up Progress Note

(or is expected to take responsibility for direct management of the BNPS) to write the recommendations as orders directly in the resident's chart, and the primary care physician and resident or surrogate legal decision-maker is informed about the orders. Such privileges, expectations, and roles of the MHP should be clarified before routine rounds for psychiatric care of residents begin. The original copy of the document usually is kept in the resident's chart in the LTC facility. Any changes to the treatment plan or any specific test result that is not being addressed should be documented and the reason for what is done or not done should be stated.

Summary

Behavioral, neurocognitive, and psychological symptoms (BNPS) are among the most challenging for even the best practitioner to assess and manage with residents living in long-term care facilities. No known approach – psychosocial, environmental, or pharmacologic – is invariably effective. Therefore, it is essential to follow a systematic process to evaluate, understand, and manage BNPS. Good intentions must be combined with clinical knowledge, skill, and creativity. A comprehensive psychiatric assessment process for initial evaluation involves a thorough history, pertinent physical and neurological exam, detailed mental status examination, use of standardized assessment scales, pertinent laboratory tests and/or brain imaging if indicated, and good documentation. A good follow-up assessment involves pertinent information from the resident, staff, and resident's family, focused mental status exam, assessment of response to treatment, and modification of the treatment plan as necessary. Other equally important goals of the assessment process should include building a therapeutic relationship, instilling hope in the resident and/or family, restoring the resident's sense of self-worth, and emphasizing the resident's strengths at the end of each interview. Assessment should routinely include screening for potential abuse, identifying excess disability, and addressing the needs of the family and the needs and concerns of staff. Last but not least, the mental health professional also uses each encounter as an opportunity to address environmental and cultural issues that commonly impose additional psychosocial stress on residents through mini-staff education sessions during the assessment process.

Key Clinical Points

1. Regular screening and comprehensive psychiatric assessment are essential to arriving at an accurate diagnosis (or diagnoses) and initiating evidence-based state-of-the-science interventions.
2. Other equally important goals of the assessment process should include building a therapeutic relationship, instilling hope in the resident and/or family, restoring the resident's sense of self-worth, and emphasizing the resident's strengths at the end of each interview.
3. Assessment should routinely include screening for potential abuse, identifying excess disability, and addressing the needs of the family and the needs and concerns of staff.

References

Alexopoulos, G.S., R.C. Abrams, R.C. Young, and C.A. Shamoian. 1988. Cornell Scale for Depression in Dementia. *Biological Psychiatry* **23**:271–284.

American Geriatrics Society. 2015. 2015 Updated Beers Criteria for Potentially Inappropriate Medication Use in Older Adults. American Geriatrics Society Beers Criteria Update Expert Panel. *Journal of the American Geriatrics Society* **63**:2227–2246.

American Psychiatric Association. 2016. *Practice Guidelines for the Psychiatric Evaluation of Adults*, 3rd ed. Arlington, VA: American Psychiatric Association Press.

Anderson, L., and L. Heyne. 2013. A Strengths Approach to Assessment in Therapeutic Recreation: Tools for Positive Change. *Therapeutic Recreation Journal* **46**(2):89–108.

Blazer, D. 2015. The Psychiatric Interview of Older Adults. In D.C. Steffens, D.G. Blazer, M.E. Thakur (eds.), *The Textbook of Geriatric Psychiatry*, 5th ed., pp. 89–106. Arlington, VA: American Psychiatric Publishing.

Bolton, J.M., D. Gunnell, and G. Turecki. 2015. Suicide Risk Assessment and Intervention in People with Mental Illness. *British Medical Journal* **351**:h4978 doi: 10.1136/bmj.h4978

Braden, B.I., and N. Bergstrom. 1989. Clinical Utility of the Braden Scale for Predicting Pressure Sore Risk. *Decubitus* **2**:44–51.

Canadian Coalition for Seniors' Mental Health. 2014. National Guidelines for Seniors' Mental Health. The Assessment and Treatment of Mental Health Issues in Long-Term Care Homes (Focus on Mood and Behavior Symptoms). www.ccsmh.ca (accessed December 12, 2015).

Carlat, D. 2011. The Psychiatric Interview of the Older Patient. In M.E. Agronin ands G.J. Maletta (eds.) *Geriatric Psychiatry*, 2nd ed., pp. 59–66. Philadelphia PA: Lippincott Williams & Wilkins.

Chakkamparambil, B, J.T. Chibnall, E.A. Graypel, et al. 2015. Development of a Brief Validated Geriatric Depression Screening Tool: The SLU "AM SAD." *American Journal of Geriatric Psychiatry* **23**(8):780–783.

Cohen-Mansfield, J., M.S. Marx, and A.S. Rosenthal. 1989. A Description of Agitation in a Nursing Home. *Journal of Gerontology* **44**:M77–M84.

Consensus Statement on Improving the Quality of Mental Health Care in US Nursing Homes. 2003. Management of Depression and Behavioral Symptoms Associated with Dementia, American Geriatrics Society and American Association for Geriatric Psychiatry. *Journal of the American Geriatrics Society* **51**:1287–1298.

Cummings-Vaughn, L.A., N. Chavakula, T.K. Malmstrom, et al. 2014. Veterans Affairs Saint Louis University Mental Status Examination Compared with the Montreal Cognitive Assessment and the Short Test of Mental Status. *Journal of the American Geriatrics Society* **62**:1341–1346.

Desai, A.K., and G.T. Grossberg. 2017. Psychiatric Aspects of Long-Term Care. In B.J. Saddock, V.A. Saddock, and P. Ruiz (eds.), *Comprehensive Textbook of Psychiatry*, 10th ed., pp. 4221–4232. Virginia: American Psychiatric Press Inc.

Desai, A.K., D. Lo, and G.T. Grossberg. 2013. Depression in Older Adults Receiving Hospice Care. In M. Sajatovic and H. Laveretsky (eds.), *Late-Life Mood Disorders*, pp. 516–531. Oxford: Oxford University Press.

Dong, X.Q. 2015. Elder Abuse: Systematic Review and Implications for Practice. *Journal of the American Geriatrics Society* **63**:1214–1218.

Elliot, R. 2003. Executive Functions and Their Disorders. *British Medical Bulletin* **65**:49–59.

Galvin, J.E. 2016. Detection of Dementia. In Marie Boltz and James Galvin (eds.), *Dementia Care: An Evidence-Based Approach*, pp. 33–44. New York, NY. Springer Publishing.

Galik, E. 2016. Treatment of Dementia: Non-Pharmacological Approaches. In Marie Boltz and

James Galvin (eds.), *Dementia Care: An Evidence-Based Approach*, pp. 97–112. New York, NY. Springer Publishing.

Herr, K.A., P.R. Mobily, F.J. Kohout, et al. 1998. Evaluation of the Faces Pain Scale for Use with the Elderly. *Clinical Journal of Pain* **14**:29–38.

Inouye, S.K., C.H. van Dyck, C.A. Alessi, et al. 1990. Clarifying Confusion: The Confusion Assessment Method. A New Method for Detection of Delirium. *Annals of Internal Medicine* **113**:941–948.

Katz, S., T.D. Down, H.R. Cash, and R.C. Grotz. 1970. Progress in the Development of Index of ADL. *The Gerontologist* **10**:20–30.

Lawton, M.P., and E.M. Brody. 1969. Assessment of Older People: Self Maintain and Instrumental Activities of Daily Living. *The Gerontologist* **9**:179–186.

Mahoney, F.I., and D.W. Barthel. 1965. Functional Evaluation. The BARTHEL Index. *Maryland State Medical Journal* **14**:61–65.

Nasreddine, Z.S., N.A. Phillips, V. Badirian et al. 2005. The Montreal Cognitive Assessment, MoCA: A Brief Screening Tool for Mild Cognitive Impairment. *Journal of the American Geriatrics Society* **53**: 695–699.

O'Rourke, H.M., W. Duggleby, K.D. Fraser, and L. Jerke. 2015. Factors that Affect Quality from the Perspective of People with Dementia: A Metasynthesis. *Journal of the American Geriatrics Society* **63**:24–38.

Perneczky, R., S. Wagenpfeil, K. Komossa, et al. 2006. Mapping Scores onto Stages: Mini-Mental State Examination and Clinical Dementia Rating. *American Journal of Geriatric Psychiatry* **14**(2):139–144.

Pfeffer, R.I., T.T. Kurosaki, C.H. Harrah, et al. 1992. Measurement of Functional Activities in Older Adults in the Community. *Journal of Gerontology* **37**:323–329.

Reisberg, B., J. Borenstein, S.P. Salob, et al. 1987. Behavioral Symptoms in Alzheimer's Disease: Phenomenology and Treatment. *Journal of Clinical Psychiatry* **48** (suppl 5):9–15.

Ricker, J.H., and B.N. Axelrod. 1994. Analysis of an Oral Paradigm for the Trail Making Test. *Assessment* **1**(1): 47–51.

Rosen, J., L. Burgio, M. Kollar, et al. 1994. A User Friendly Instrument for Rating Agitation in Dementia Patients. *American Journal of Geriatric Psychiatry* **2**(1):52–59.

Scott, J.G., B. Ostermeyer, and A.A. Shah. 2016. Neuropsychological Assessment in Neurocognitive Disorders. *Psychiatric Annals* **46**(12):118–126.

Saliba, D., S. DiFilippo, M.O. Edelen et al. 2012. Testing the PHQ-9 Interview and Observational Versions (PHQ-OV) for MDS 3.0. *Journal of the American Medical Director's Association* **13**(7):618–625.

Spitzer, R., K. Kroenke, and J. Williams. 1999. Validation and Utility of a Self-Report Version of PRIME-MD: The PHQ Primary Care Study. *Journal of the American Medical Association* **282**: 1737–1744.

Stahl, S.M., D.A. Morrissette, M. Cummings, et al. 2014. California State Hospital Violence Assessment and Treatment (Cal-VAT) Guidelines. *CNS Spectrums* **19**:449–465 doi:10.1017/S1092852914000376

Taylor, W.D. 2014. Depression in the Elderly. *New England Journal of Medicine* **371**:1228–1236.

Wang, S., M.E. Thakur, and P. M. Doraiswamy. 2015. Use of the Laboratory in the Diagnostic Workup of Older Adults. In D.C. Steffens, D.G. Blazer, M.E. Thakur (eds.), *The Textbook of Geriatric Psychiatry*, 5th ed., pp. 107–126. Arlington, VA: American Psychiatric Publishing.

Warden, V., A.C. Hurley, and L. Volicer. 2003. Development and Psychometric Evaluation of the Pain Assessment in Advanced Dementia. *Journal of the American Medical Directors Association* **4**:9–15.

Winkelman, J.W. 2015. Insomnia Disorder. *New England Journal of Medicine* **373**:1437–1444.

Wood, S., J.L. Cummings, M. Hsu, et al. 2000. The Use of the Neuropsychiatric Inventory in Nursing Home Residents. *American Journal of Geriatric Psychiatry* **8**:75–83.

Yesavage, J.A., T.L. Brink, T.L. Rose, et al. 1983. Development and Validation of a Geriatric Depression Scale: A Preliminary Report. *Journal of Psychiatric Research* **17**:37–49.

Chapter 3

Major Neurocognitive Disorders

Cognition is a combination of skills including attention, learning, memory, language, praxis, gnosis, social cognition, and executive functions (such as decision-making, goal setting, planning, and judgment) (Grossberg and Desai 2006). Major neurocognitive disorders (MNCDs) are neuropsychiatric disorders characterized by significant decline from the previous level of cognitive functioning in at least two out of six domains (complex attention, social cognition, perceptual-motor, executive function, language, and learning and memory) which substantially interferes with the ability to perform daily activities (such as paying bills, managing medications) and live independently (American Psychiatric Association 2013). Decline by two or more standard deviations from appropriate norms as tested by formal cognitive testing (third percentile or below) is necessary for a diagnosis of MNCD. For the diagnosis of MNCD, cognitive deficits cannot occur exclusively in the context of a delirium and cannot be better explained by another mental disorder (e.g. major depressive disorder, schizophrenia). MNCD is thus a clinical diagnosis. There are many causes of MNCD (Kimchi and Lyketsos 2015). (See Table 3.1.) Progressive, irreversible MNCDs account for more than 90 percent of all causes of MNCD in long-term care (LTC) populations (Galvin 2016).

Most recent estimates from the Alzheimer's Association indicate that more than 5.6 million Americans have Alzheimer's disease (AD) or related MNCD (Alzheimer's Association 2015). Worldwide, more than 44 million people are living with AD or related MNCD (Alzheimer's Disease International 2015). These numbers are expected to double by 2030 and more than triple by 2050. Onset of MNCD after age 60 accounts for more than 95 percent of individuals who have MNCD. Five percent of those who have MNCD experience onset before age 60 (often in their 30s or 40s) and are said to have young or early-onset dementia.

Approximately one-third of those who have MNCD live in a LTC facility; the other two-thirds live in their homes in the community. A high proportion of people who have MNCD (80–90 percent) eventually enter a LTC facility. Approximately 75–80 percent of LTC residents have MNCD. Some assisted living (AL) homes and nursing homes (NHs) are designed for and care exclusively for people who have MNCD. The average length of stay in a NH for someone who has MNCD is two to three years. This is because many people who have MNCD enter AL first and by the time they move to NH are in a more advanced stage of MNCD. With the availability of hospice, many AL residents who have advanced MNCD spend their last years in AL. Understanding clinical manifestations of different MNCDs, accurate diagnosis, finding the cause(s), instituting appropriate evidence-based treatment, and meeting psychosocial, environmental, and spiritual needs are critical for improving residents' quality of life and helping them live the best life possible.

Alzheimer's Disease

Alzheimer's disease (AD) is a progressive neurodegenerative disorder that has a long (more than two decades) asymptomatic phase and leads to irreversible MNCD (Apostolova 2016). The neuropathology consists of accumulation of abnormal proteins (amyloid and tau) that are thought to cause neuronal death and loss of synapses. AD is the most common cause of MNCD in people age 65 or older, accounting for 60–75 percent of all causes of MNCD (Alzheimer's Association 2015). Insidious onset and a slow but relentless decline in cognition that impairs the ability to perform daily activities is the most striking feature of AD. There is no cure for AD. It is estimated that 5 percent of people over 65 years of age and up to 33 percent of those over 85 are living with AD. Some 98 percent of AD is sporadic and 2 percent is familial

Table 3.1 Common Causes of Major Neurocognitive Disorder in Long-Term Care Populations

Common Causes of Major Neurocognitive Disorder (MNCD)	Clinical Pearls	Evidence-Based Approaches and Therapeutic Pearls
Alzheimer's disease (AD)	AD is a progressive neurodegenerative disease and is the most common cause of MNCD Reversible causes of cognitive impairment (especially depression, medication-induced cognitive impairment, vitamin B_{12} deficiency) are also commonly present	AD is incurable Work-up to identify potentially reversible cause(s) of cognitive impairment Consider cholinesterase inhibitors and/or memantine for all residents (unless in terminal stages)
MNCD due to Lewy bodies (Dementia with Lewy bodies [DLB])	DLB is a progressive neurodegenerative MNCD People who have DLB have high sensitivity to adverse effects of antipsychotics (especially high-potency antipsychotics [e.g. haloperidol, risperidone, paliperidone]) with even fatal outcomes	DLB is incurable Avoid antipsychotics (especially high-potency antipsychotics) Cholinesterase inhibitors may be more effective in DLB than in AD
MNCD due to Parkinson's disease (Parkinson's disease dementia [PDD])	PD is a progressive neurodegenerative disease Average duration of Parkinson's disease is about 8 years before development of MNCD People who have PDD are more prone to severe psychotic symptoms due to levodopa	PD and PDD are incurable Consider cholinesterase inhibitors to treat cognitive decline, but may worsen tremor Consider reducing or discontinuing levodopa before initiating pimavanserin or antipsychotic medication (such as quetiapine or clozapine) to manage severe psychotic symptoms
Major vascular neurocognitive disorder (Vascular dementia [VaD])	VaD is irreversible MNCD due to cerebrovascular disease Two types: poststroke VaD and nonstroke VaD (typically due to cerebral small vessel disease) Nonstroke VaD may mimic AD with insidious onset and gradual progression of cognitive and functional decline	Neuroimaging (especially magnetic resonance imaging of the brain) evidence of significant brain parenchymal injury is essential for diagnosis Optimal control of vascular factors (especially hypertension, diabetes) may delay progression to more severe stages Cholinesterase inhibitors may be appropriate for some residents who have VaD
Major frontotemporal neurocognitive disorder (Frontotemporal dementias [FTDs])	FTDs are progressive neurodegenerative disorders Often misdiagnosed as depression, personality disorder, bipolar disorder, obsessive compulsive disorder, substance use disorder, or a psychotic disorder	FTDs are incurable Cholinesterase inhibitors are not recommended Selective serotonin reuptake inhibitors may be necessary for severe behavioral disturbances not responding to psychosocial environmental intervention

Table 3.1 (cont.)

Common Causes of Major Neurocognitive Disorder (MNCD)	Clinical Pearls	Evidence-Based Approaches and Therapeutic Pearls
	People who have FTD are much younger than people who have MNCD due to AD or DLB	
Alcohol-induced major neurocognitive disorder	People who have alcohol-induced MNCD are much younger than people who have neurodegenerative MNCD and typically have concomitant Korsakoff syndrome (amnestic-confabulatory syndrome) Executive impairment seen early in the course due to neurotoxic effects of alcohol on frontocerebellar networks	Stable abstinence from alcohol and correction of nutritional deficiencies may stabilize cognitive decline in some residents who have low medical comorbidity Cholinesterase inhibitors are not recommended unless HCP suspects coexisting AD
Major neurocognitive disorder due to traumatic brain injury (TBI)	MNCD due to TBI is irreversible Moderate to severe head injury can increase risk of MNCD by two to four times Multiple mild TBIs can lead to chronic traumatic encephalopathy (CTE) that can mimic AD	Cholinesterase inhibitors are not recommended Post-traumatic stress disorder like symptoms may emerge in the context of TBI due to motor vehicular accident or military trauma and need to be anticipated and addressed
Major neurocognitive disorder due to HIV infection (HIV-associated neurocognitive disorder [HAND])	HAND may be the first manifestation of HIV infection in older adults Mild neurocognitive disorder due to HIV infection precedes HAND and gives opportunity for prevention of HAND	Highly aggressive antiretroviral therapy (HAART) with drugs having high central nervous system penetration recommended for treatment Opportunistic infection (e.g. neurosyphilis) may also cause neurocognitive impairment; HCP needs to look for and treat it
Major neurocognitive disorder due to Huntington's disease (HD-associated dementia)	HD is an autosomal dominant progressive neurodegenerative disorder Residents who have HD are some of the youngest in LTC LTC residents who have HD are in advanced stages and usually have severe chorea, gait disturbance, and dysarthria along with MNCD	HD is incurable Cholinesterase inhibitors are not recommended Low-dose, high-potency antipsychotics (e.g. risperidone) may help chorea as well as severe mood and psychotic symptoms that often accompany HD
Major neurocognitive disorder due to multiple sclerosis (MS-associated dementia)	MS is a progressive demyelinating disorder of the brain Residents who have MS are some of the youngest in LTC LTC residents who have MS are in advanced stages and usually have severe motor disability along with MNCD	MS is incurable Cholinesterase inhibitors are not recommended Vigorous efforts to involve retained cognitive functions (reading comprehension, conversational skills, reminiscing past positive events) is recommended

Table 3.1 (cont.)

Common Causes of Major Neurocognitive Disorder (MNCD)	Clinical Pearls	Evidence-Based Approaches and Therapeutic Pearls
Major neurocognitive disorder due to chronic subdural hematoma (CSDH)	LTC populations have multiple risk factors for CSDH (especially fall proneness, taking antiplatelets and anticoagulants, cortical atrophy) Subacute cognitive decline may be the only clinical manifestation	CSDH can spontaneously resolve over time Watchful waiting and symptomatic nonsurgical treatment may be preferred treatment option, as risks of surgical evacuation of hematoma are high in LTC populations
Rapidly progressive neurocognitive disorder (RPD)	Residents may have MNCD that is progressing rapidly (over months rather than years) and LTC team may be the first to recognize it Prion diseases (especially Creutzfeldt-Jakob disease [CJD]) are the prototype RPDs, fortunately rare, as they are incurable	Urgent evaluation and thorough work-up with a team of neurologist, psychiatrist, and primary care physician is recommended, as some causes (e.g. autoimmune encephalopathy) are eminently treatable In majority of situations, death occurs within weeks to months, so HCP needs to discuss palliative care goals with the resident and family as soon as possible after diagnosis
Major neurocognitive disorder due to anoxic brain injury	People who have survived cardiac arrest and/or severe hypotension and hypoxia may develop delirium leading to irreversible MNCD due to anoxic brain injury People who have underlying MNCD develop accelerated cognitive and functional decline after anoxic brain injury	Cholinesterase inhibitors are not recommended For some people who have anoxic brain injury, cognitive and functional impairment may not progressively worsen after the initial insult.
Major neurocognitive disorder due to other medical condition	Reversible MNCDs are rare in LTC populations, but reversible causes of neurocognitive impairment in residents who have irreversible MNCD are common (Box 3.1)	Work-up to identify and treat reversible contributing causes of cognitive decline is recommended for all residents who have MNCD Idiopathic normal pressure hydrocephalus (iNPH) often coexists with AD in LTC populations, and shunt surgery for iNPH may not be as effective in this population as in younger populations in the community
Mixed major neurocognitive disorder	Common in older residents (typically AD with VaD)	HCP may consider prescribing cholinesterase inhibitors if AD or DLB is thought to be one of the etiologies

(autosomal dominant). Age is the biggest risk factor for sporadic AD, although old age by itself is not sufficient to cause AD. Two-thirds of those diagnosed with AD are women (Erol et al. 2015). The longer life span of women than men may be the key factor in the preponderance of women who have AD. A definitive diagnosis of AD can be made only after death, during brain autopsy, when the amyloid plaques and neurofibrillary tangles can be seen under the microscope and correlated with clinical manifestations. In cases of familial AD, genetic testing (identifying mutations in one of the three genes: Amyloid Precursor Protein [chromosome 21], Presenilin 1 [chromosome 14], and Presenilin 2 [chromosome 1]) can also provide accurate diagnosis. The presence of the gene for apolipoprotein E4 (ApoeE4) increases the risk for and decreases the age of onset of AD, with a single copy increasing the risk threefold and two copies increasing the risk fifteenfold.

There is substantial heterogeneity in the clinical presentation of AD. The typical clinical syndrome of AD includes an amnestic type of memory defect with difficulty learning and recalling new information, progressive language disorder beginning with anomia and progressing to fluent aphasia. Short-term memory deficits are classic, with remote memory remaining intact until the advanced stages. Some individuals who have incipient memory loss are aware of their declining abilities, but most individuals who have evolving AD are unaware that they have significant memory dysfunction. Behind the forgetfulness that appears benign may be more serious mistakes, such as forgotten bills, missed appointments, improperly taken medication, and misdirected travel. Disturbances of visual-spatial skills manifested by environmental disorientation are usually absent or mild in early stages but become evident in more advanced stages. Sometimes anomia or visual agnosia can be nearly as prominent as the anterograde amnesia. Individuals who have Down syndrome (trisomy 21) have a high risk of developing AD by the time they are in their 40s or 50s. Ideally, the health care provider (HCP) should interview a knowledgeable informant because genuine memory failure should be evident to those who are close to the individual who has Down syndrome.

Rapidly progressive AD, posterior cortical atrophy, frontal lobe variant AD, and logopenic variant primary progressive aphasia due to AD are atypical presentations of AD (Apostolova 2016). Some 10–30 percent of individuals diagnosed clinically with major frontotemporal neurocognitive disorder (frontotemporal dementia [FTD]) are found to have AD (frontal lobe variant AD) on autopsy.

Criteria for Probable Alzheimer's Disease

Diagnosis of probable AD can be made by using criteria established by the *Diagnostic and Statistical Manual of Mental Disorders*, fifth edition (*DSM-5*) (American Psychiatric Association 2013). Probable AD is determined when a person has

- MNCD confirmed by clinical and/or neuropsychological examination
- Insidious onset and steadily progressive gradual decline
- Obvious evidence of decline in memory and learning.

Diagnostic Testing

Evidence of a genetic cause of AD (based on family history and/or genetic testing) is helpful in the diagnosis of familial AD. The presence of biomarkers for AD (e.g. cerebrospinal fluid [CSF] amyloid beta-42 [abeta-42] and tau protein ratio [decline in abeta-42 by itself or accompanied by elevation in total tau and phosphorylated tau] and positive amyloid positron emission tomography [PET]) provides supporting evidence for underlying AD pathology and thus improves diagnostic accuracy if the presentation is atypical or historical information is insufficient. We do not recommend routine testing for ApoeE4 for diagnostic purposes, as some individuals who are ApoeE4 carriers may never develop AD and some individuals who do not have ApoeE4 may develop AD. Signs of hippocampal and temporoparietal cortical atrophy on a magnetic resonance imaging (MRI) scan and temporoparietal hypometabolism on a fluorodeoxyglucose PET scan support a diagnosis of AD but are less sensitive and specific than amyloid PET and CSF amyloid/tau ratio.

Other Areas of Cognitive Impairment besides Memory

Aphasia. Aphasia (called "dysphasia" if mild) is loss of language ability. Expressive aphasia is loss of the ability to convey oral or written information to others. Anomia, or difficulty finding words, is a common form of expressive aphasia in mild AD. Loss of verbal fluency is profound in moderate and severe stages of AD, although, unlike individuals who have some major frontotemporal neurocognitive disorder (frontotemporal dementias [FTDs], especially progressive nonfluent aphasia [PNFA]), mutism is rare in AD. Receptive aphasia is loss of the ability to understand the meaning of oral (spoken) and written language. Comprehension breaks down in moderate to severe stages of AD, and paraphrases both literal and semantic are prominent. Examples include not understanding questions or instructions and not being able to express what one wants to say. The HCP may consider referral to a speech therapist for residents who have mild AD and significant expressive aphasia.

Agnosia. Agnosia is the inability to recognize familiar objects by sight (visual agnosia), touch (tactile agnosia), sound (auditory agnosia), smell (olfactory agnosia), or taste (gustatory agnosia). Examples include not recognizing a favorite chair (hence one should avoid rearranging the furniture in the resident's room), not recognizing home, and eventually not recognizing family and friends. Frequent if brief visits may help delay the loss of recognition of family and friends.

Apraxia. Apraxia (called "dyspraxia" if mild) is characterized by loss of the ability to execute or carry out skilled movements and gestures, despite having the desire and the physical ability to perform them. Apraxia results from dysfunction of the parietal lobe. Examples of apraxia often seen among residents who have MNCD include ideational apraxia (the inability to coordinate activities with multiple, sequential movements, such as dressing, bathing, and eating) and constructional apraxia (the inability to copy, draw, or construct simple figures).

Executive Dysfunction. Executive function is an interrelated set of abilities that includes cognitive flexibility, concept formation, and self-monitoring (Elliot 2003). Executive dysfunction results in impaired decision-making, goal setting, planning, and exercising good judgment. Assessing executive function can help determine a person's capacity to execute health care decisions. Executive dysfunction is one element in the *DSM-5* criteria for the diagnosis of MNCD and sooner or later occurs in all MNCD diseases. It is seen early in FTDs, among some people who have major depression (clinical depression), and in advanced stages of other degenerative MNCDs (AD, major neurocognitive disorders with Lewy bodies [dementia with Lewy bodies {DLB}]). It is also seen among people who have a stroke involving the frontal lobe (especially dorsolateral prefrontal area) and its projections to and from the basal ganglia.

Stages of Alzheimer's Disease

AD progresses through several stages before the stages of MNCD. (See Table 3.2.) The traditional description of stages helps with accurate diagnosis (with AD biomarkers improving diagnostic accuracy [useful when historical data of cognitive decline are inadequate and/or atypical presentation]) and prognosis and strength-based description of stages helps with efforts to maintain quality of life and highest level of functioning. The MNCD stages (mild, moderate, severe, and terminal) of AD usually span five to eight years on average (range two to 20 years) after diagnosis. The length of survival depends on the age at onset of symptoms (the younger the age, the longer the survival) and comorbid conditions (especially cerebrovascular disease). Younger people who have AD are more likely to survive the full course of the disease process, while older people are more likely to die earlier based on medical comorbidities. For people over age 85, survival after the onset of MNCD may be much shorter (average three years). The Global Deterioration Scale (GDS), with seven stages and substages, provides descriptions of stages of progression of AD that are particularly meaningful for families and caregivers (Reisberg et al. 1982).

The Grossberg-Desai Staging Scale: Retained Strengths by Stage of AD

Pre-MNCD Stages. AD begins in the entorhinal cortex, which is near the hippocampus and has direct connections to it. It then proceeds to the hippocampus, the structure that is essential to the formation of short-term memories. Affected regions begin to atrophy and show synaptic loss. These brain changes start at least 20 years before any visible sign or symptom appears. Subjective memory and other cognitive complaints have been shown to precede MNCD by more than 10 years. Subjective cognitive complaints precede the stage in which objective memory loss develops. Memory loss, the first visible sign, is the main feature of amnestic type of mild neurocognitive disorder (mild NCD [amnestic mild cognitive impairment {aMCI}]). Amnestic mild NCD is usually an initial, transitional phase between normal brain

Table 3.2 Stages of Alzheimer's Disease

Stage	Traditional Description	Strengths-Based Description
1	Presymptomatic (asymptomatic) stage with positive AD biomarkers*	Normal cognitive functions and capacity to live independently
2	Subjective memory and other cognitive complaints may or may not be accompanied by transient mild symptoms of depression, anxiety, and/or apathy; positive AD biomarkers	Normal cognitive functioning on objective cognitive testing and retained capacity to live independently
3	Mild neurocognitive disorder with objective evidence of cognitive decline (two or more standard deviation) accompanied by varying severity of depression, anxiety, and/or apathy; positive AD biomarkers	Retained capacity to live independently and to drive
4	Mild major neurocognitive disorder with difficulties in living independently due to significant cognitive decline accompanied by varying severity of depression, anxiety, and/or apathy; positive AD biomarkers	In general, retained general intellect and capacity to eloquently express one's experience of living with MNCD; retained capacity to live in one's own home with some help; retained capacity to make medical decisions in one's own best interest in most situations; may be able to drive short distances on familiar routes
5	Moderate major neurocognitive disorder with inability to live independently without substantial help accompanied by moderate to severe depression, anxiety, psychotic symptoms; positive AD biomarkers and neuroimaging evidence of obvious temporoparietal cortical atrophy	In general, retained long-term memory and capacity to reminisce past positive experiences; retained conversation skills and capacity for sense of humor; retained capacity to recognize family and friends; retained procedural memory (e.g. dancing, playing a musical instrument); retained reading comprehension, retained capacity for social interactions, engage in creative activities and enjoy music, being with pets, spending time in nature, and spiritual rituals
6	Severe major neurocognitive disorder with need for 24/7 supervision for safety, difficulty recognizing family and friends; difficulty expressing basic needs; severe apathy, psychotic symptoms, and/or distress expressed as agitation, aggression common; positive AD biomarkers and neuroimaging evidence of extensive diffuse cortical atrophy	In general, retained capacity to show affection and enjoy touch and social activities and interactions; retained capacity to dance, enjoy music, being with pets, spending time in nature, and spiritual rituals; retained capacity to show empathy toward others and express gratitude
7	Terminal-stage major neurocognitive disorder with very limited language functions, loss of narrative self; often bed bound and completely dependent on others for all activities, including feeding; distress expressed as agitation is common	In general, retained capacity to enjoy touch, music, show affection, and respond to spiritual rituals

* Alzheimer's disease biomarkers include positive amyloid positron emission tomography (amyloid PET) imaging, cerebrospinal fluid (CSF) abeta/tau ratio (decreased abeta and increased tau in CSF), temporoparietal hypometabolism seen in fluorodeoxyglucose positron emission tomography (FDG PET) and hippocampal atrophy on neuroimaging.

aging and AD (diagnosed as mild NCD due to AD). Change in mood (irritability, depression) and personality (passivity) may predate cognitive symptoms by years in people who have AD (Jost and Grossberg 1996). The MCI stage typically lasts two to 10 years before progressing to MNCD stage. Testing for the presence of diagnostic biomarkers is usually needed for an accurate diagnosis of AD in pre-MNCD stages.

Mild Alzheimer's Disease. As the disease begins to affect the cerebral cortex, memory loss continues and changes emerge in other cognitive abilities (such as language, praxis). The clinical diagnosis of AD is usually made during this stage. Signs of mild AD can include: memory loss, taking longer to accomplish normal daily tasks, trouble handling money and paying bills, poor judgment leading to bad decisions, loss of spontaneity and sense of initiative, confusion about the location of familiar places (getting lost begins to occur), mood and personality changes, and increased anxiety. In mild AD, physical abilities do not decline. At casual glance, these early symptoms can be confused with changes that accompany normal aging. With systematic inquiry, the HCP can reliably diagnose early-stage AD. In general, mild AD does not result in need for LTC unless there is serious disability due to other medical conditions, such as stroke or end-organ failure. The prevalence of major depression in this stage may be up to 20 percent. The prevalence of depressed mood and sadness may be seen in 50–60 percent of individuals in this stage. This stage can last for two to 10 years.

Moderate Alzheimer's Disease. By the moderate stage, AD-induced cell death has spread to the areas of the cerebral cortex that control language, reasoning, sensory processing, and conscious thought. More intensive supervision and care become necessary, and many individuals enter LTC in the latter part of this stage. The symptoms of this stage include: increasing memory loss and confusion, shortened attention span, problems recognizing some friends and distant family members, difficulty with language; problems with reading, writing, working with numbers, difficulty organizing thoughts and thinking logically, inability to learn new things or to cope with new or unexpected situations, repetitive statements, occasional muscle twitches, loss of impulse control (shown through sloppy table manners, undressing at inappropriate times or places, or vulgar language), perceptual-motor problems (such as trouble getting out of a chair or setting the table). Stored long-term memories may be relatively spared early in this stage, prompting family members to make comments such as, "She remembers what happened a long time ago better than I do."

In keeping with the basic tenets of person-centered care, we are replacing the term behavioral and psychological symptoms of dementia with biopsychosocial-spiritual distress (BPSD) (Dementia Action Alliance 2016). People who have moderate-state AD commonly experience anxiety, depression, restlessness, and other expressions of BPSD. People who have AD evidence more severe BPSD in the moderate stage than in the mild stage. BPSD in this stage is often related to delusions and depression and may manifest as tearfulness, anxiety, irritability, and agitation (restlessness, pacing, wandering). Delusions and hallucinations are much more likely in this stage than in the mild or terminal stage. The incidence of delusions in this stage is reported as 37 percent and of hallucinations as high as 24 percent. Paranoid delusions in AD are the most common type of false belief, with commonly occurring delusions including "Someone is stealing my belongings" and "My spouse is having an affair." Psychotic symptoms frequently contribute to agitation and aggression. Depression is also seen in this stage and may contribute to physical aggression. The prevalence of major depression is 10 percent in this stage, whereas the prevalence of depressed mood and sadness is approximately 58 percent. In moderate-stage AD, depression often coexists with prominent anxiety symptoms. The leading features of depression in the later part of this stage may be an inversion of day and night, agitation, and aggression. BPSD expressed as aggression occurs in 20 to 30 percent of people in this stage and appears to vary with severity, correlating with frontal lobe dysfunction, pain and other medical comorbidity, decline in activities of daily living (ADLs), and greater cognitive impairment. The frequency of BPSD expressed as agitation is 40–55 percent in this stage and increases in prevalence from the early part of this stage to the later part. Expression of BPSD can take the form of shouting, pacing, restlessness, and wandering. Problems of gait and movement in this stage contribute significantly to functional decline. Some 30–60 percent of residents who have moderate-stage AD may develop mild extrapyramidal symptoms (EPS) such as amimia, bradykinesia, gait impairment, Parkinsonism, or paratonic rigidity. Gait apraxia, ascribed to impaired frontal lobe function, occurs with increasing frequency in moderate-stage AD. It includes a constellation of impaired trunk and leg movements as well as impaired postural reflexes, disequilibrium, dyskinetic movements, and problems with locomotion. Falls are associated with the severity of AD; more than one-third of individuals who have moderate-stage AD experience this problem. Ability to move themselves and the other objects about is impaired in moderate to severe stages of AD. For example, a person who has AD kneels on a chair instead of sitting or does not sit all the way down (lowers self part of the way and then gets back up). Breaking the task down to small steps by giving verbal and tactile clues (guiding the person with one's hands) helps address this problem. This stage can last for one to eight years.

Severe Alzheimer's Disease. The hallmark of severe-stage AD is profound cognitive impairment. In this stage, the person may not even know his or her own name or recognize a spouse or children. Verbal ability is restricted to answering yes or no to simple questions. Except for some ability to feed self, a resident in this stage is completely dependent on others for all basic activities of daily living (such as dressing, toileting). Many residents even in advanced stages of AD can ambulate and will still have some fleeting memory of their loved ones, which can surprise family and staff. A resident who has not spoken for months may suddenly respond to the spouse's voice. A resident who has not responded to the spouse's presence may suddenly pick up the spouse's hand, kiss the hand, and say "love you." These moments of explicit residual continuity with the resident's past may be most evident in the morning after the resident has had a good night's rest. Such moments are extremely meaningful to the family. One of the authors remembers a resident who, over a six-month period, had never spoken to him or staff suddenly blurted out, "You know, I have Alzheimer's" during his visit with her. The staff person who was with the author was equally surprised. Both urinary and fecal incontinence frequently develop in severe stages of AD. This stage can last for one to four years.

Terminal-Stage Alzheimer's Disease. In the last stage of AD, plaques and tangles are widespread throughout the brain, and large areas of the brain have atrophied further. Individuals in this stage have lost all ability to communicate verbally and are completely dependent on others for care. All sense of narrative self seems to vanish, and self is expressed in nonverbal preferences. Other symptoms can include: weight loss; seizure; skin infection; difficulty swallowing; distress expressed as groaning, moaning, or grunting; increased sleep; lack of bladder and bowel control. At the end, individuals may be in bed much or all of the time. As bedridden status develops, contractures occur commonly. Myoclonus, either focal or multifocal, transient or recurrent, may also occur. Even in such advanced stages, some individuals may have emotional moments of relational recollection. But by now all of these individuals are extremely feeble, have limited mobility, and will begin the dying process by such things as sepsis related to incontinence or aspiration pneumonia or skin ulcer, cardiac arrest or secondary to inanition. At this stage, individuals are in effect dying and may be appropriate for referral to hospice, especially after a superimposed new medical problem, weight loss, or sudden decline. Death typically results from aspiration pneumonia. This stage can last for two months to up to two years.

Major Neurocognitive Disorder due to Lewy Bodies

Dementia with Lewy bodies (DLB) and Parkinson's disease dementia (PDD) are two causes of MNCD with Lewy bodies that are prevalent in LTC populations. Multiple system atrophy (MSA) is a rare cause of MNCD with Lewy bodies. All three MNCDs having Lewy bodies are progressive and incurable neurodegenerative disorders (Gomperts 2016). PDD and DLB are more common in males than females. The neuropathology consists of accumulation of abnormal protein alpha synuclein in the form of round Lewy bodies, which are thought to cause neuronal death and loss of synapses. Lewy bodies are considered a pathological hallmark of DLB and Parkinson's disease (PD). Lewy bodies are never found in a healthy normal brain. In DLB, Lewy bodies are found in the cortex as well as in an area of the brain stem called the substantia nigra, whereas in PD, Lewy bodies first accumulate in the substantia nigra and later spread to the cortex. DLB is differentiated from PDD primarily in the onset of motor symptoms. In PDD, Parkinsonian symptoms have to be present for at least a year (typically for eight or more years) before the onset of cognitive decline, whereas in DLB, the onset of motor symptoms coincides with cognitive decline. Similar to AD, DLB and PDD have a long preclinical period progressing to the MCI stage (mild neurocognitive disorder due to Lewy bodies) before developing MNCD.

DLB is the second most common neurodegenerative disorder (after AD) to cause MNCD, and the second most common MNCD (after AD) in older adults. The cognitive disorder in DLB may be characterized by prominent anterograde amnesia and may be indistinguishable from AD. However, the most common patterns of cognitive deficits in DLB are distinct from those in AD. (See Table 3.3.) In AD the first loss in thinking skills is in memory; in DLB the earliest loss appears to be with attention and

Table 3.3 Differentiating Major Neurocognitive Disorder due to Alzheimer's Disease, Major Frontotemporal Neurocognitive Disorder, and Major Neurocognitive Disorder with Lewy Bodies

Major Neurocognitive Disorder due to Alzheimer's Disease	Major Frontotemporal Neurocognitive Disorder	Major Neurocognitive Disorder with Lewy Bodies
Short-term memory impaired early on	Short-term memory intact early on	Short-term memory impaired early on
New learning impaired from early on	New learning intact early on	New learning impaired from early on
Prominent attentional problems absent	Prominent attentional problems often present	Prominent attentional problems usually present
Executive dysfunction mild early on	Executive dysfunction prominent early on	Executive dysfunction mild early on
Apraxia and agnosia often present from early on	Apraxia and agnosia absent in mild to moderate stages	Apraxia and agnosia often present from early on
Psychomotor slowing absent in mild to moderate stages	Psychomotor slowing absent in mild to moderate stages	Psychomotor slowing often present from early on
Mutism rare	Mutism not uncommon	Mutism rare
Daily fluctuation in cognition with dramatic variations in attention and alertness absent in mild to moderate stages	Daily fluctuation in cognition with dramatic variations in attention and alertness absent	Daily fluctuation in cognition with dramatic variations in attention and alertness are common from early on
Recurrent falls seen in later stages	Recurrent falls seen in later stages	Recurrent falls seen from early on
Spontaneous features of Parkinsonism (slow shuffling gait, hypokinesia, muscle rigidity, rest tremor) absent or minimal	Spontaneous features of Parkinsonism absent (except in rare cases of corticobasal degeneration and progressive supranuclear palsy)	Spontaneous features of Parkinsonism prominent from early on
Visual hallucinations rare in mild stages	Visual hallucinations rare in mild stages	Visual hallucinations common from early on
REM sleep behavior disorder (RBD) absent	RBD absent	RBD may even predate cognitive decline and often present from early on
Social misconduct/behavioral disinhibition absent in mild stages (frontal variant AD is exception)	Social misconduct/behavioral disinhibition common from early on	Social misconduct/behavioral disinhibition absent
Loss of sympathy or empathy absent	Loss of sympathy or empathy often present	Loss of sympathy or empathy absent
Perseverative, stereotyped, or compulsive/ritualistic behaviors absent in mild to moderate stages	Perseverative, stereotyped, or compulsive/ritualistic behaviors often present from early on	Perseverative, stereotyped, or compulsive/ritualistic behaviors absent in mild to moderate stages

Table 3.3 (cont.)

Major Neurocognitive Disorder due to Alzheimer's Disease	Major Frontotemporal Neurocognitive Disorder	Major Neurocognitive Disorder with Lewy Bodies
Hyperorality and dietary changes absent	Hyperorality and dietary changes often present from early on	Hyperorality and dietary changes absent
Capacity for empathy is retained	Capacity for empathy often impaired from early on	Capacity for empathy retained
Severe sensitivity to high potency antipsychotics absent	Severe sensitivity to high-potency antipsychotics is absent or occasional	Severe sensitivity to high-potency antipsychotics is often seen from early on
Initially often misdiagnosed as normal age-related memory loss	Initially often misdiagnosed as primary non-MNCD mental disorder (such as major depression, bipolar disorder, schizophrenia)	Initially often misdiagnosed as Parkinson's disease
Family history of AD often present	Family history of FTDs present in 40% of individuals who have FTD and 10% have an autosomal dominant inheritance pattern	Family history of DLB rare
More common in females than males	Behavioral variant FTD more common in males than females	More common in males than females
Neuroimaging often shows marked disproportionate hippocampal atrophy and temporoparietal cortical atrophy	Neuroimaging often shows frontal and/or temporal cortical atrophy	Neuroimaging may show occipital atrophy
Fluorodeoxyglucose positron emission tomography (FDG PET) often shows temporoparietal hypometabolism	FDG PET often shows frontotemporal hypometabolism	FDG PET may show occipital hypometabolism
Normal striatal dopamine transporter reuptake on SPECT/PET scan	Normal striatal dopamine transporter reuptake on SPECT/PET scan	Reduced striatal dopamine transporter reuptake on SPECT/PET scan
Response to cholinesterase inhibitors is modest	Lack of response to cholinesterase inhibitors	Response to cholinesterase inhibitors may be better than among residents who have Alzheimer's disease
Autopsy shows characteristic amyloid neuritic plaques and tau neurofibrillary tangles	Autopsy shows tau or ubiquitin-associated characteristic neuropathological findings	Autopsy shows characteristic pathological lesions – alpha synuclein Lewy bodies

Note: None of these characteristics can differentiate among AD, FTDs, and DLB with certainty. Definitive diagnosis of each can be made only after death through autopsy and correlating findings with clinical presentation and, when available, biomarker findings.

visual perception. Hence, DLB has also been described as a visual-perceptual and attentional-executive dementia. Individuals who have DLB may have slightly better confrontational naming and verbal memory function than do typical individuals who have AD but have worse executive function and visuospatial functions. Symptoms vary a great deal more from one day to the next than do symptoms of AD. In addition, up to 81 percent of individuals who have DLB have unexplained periods of markedly increased confusion that lasts days to weeks and closely mimics delirium. Individuals who have DLB are typically more apathetic than are individuals who have AD. Diagnosis and treatment of DLB is often complicated by a lack of information about the disease. The HCP should consider DLB if the HCP sees spontaneous features of Parkinsonism, fully formed visual hallucinations, and fluctuating cognition with pronounced variation in attention and alertness early in the course of MNCD. When fluctuating cognition occurs, family or caregivers often describe the individual as "zoned out" or "not with us." Such fluctuation is often mistaken for delirium superimposed on AD. Other symptoms that may help differentiate DLB from AD include daytime drowsiness and lethargy despite getting enough sleep the night before; falling asleep two or more hours during the day; staring into space for long periods and episodes of disorganized speech; REM sleep behavior disorder (RBD) (dream enactment behavior occurring during REM sleep phase with loss of normal muscular atonia); recurrent falls; and change in personality early in the course of MNCD (especially passivity). RBD is often a precursor to DLB, occurring years before the onset of MNCD, and is present in about half of individuals who have DLB. Cholinergic deficits in DLB occur early and are more widespread than in AD. This may explain some of the clinical differences and somewhat better response to cholinesterase inhibitors (ChEIs) than with AD. Individuals who have DLB are more functionally impaired (due to extrapyramidal motor symptoms) and have more neuropsychiatric difficulties (such as visual hallucinations seen in 80 percent of people who have DLB) than individuals who have AD and similar cognitive scores.

The cognitive deficits of individuals who have PDD are similar to those of DLB. Resting tremor, usually of the upper extremities, hypokinesia (slowed movement), masked facial expression, soft voice (hypophonia), tiny handwriting (micrographia), cogwheel rigidity of the limbs, and gait problems, including asymmetrical or decreased arm swing and abnormal postural reflexes, may be found on neurological examination. Approximately 1.5 million Americans have PD. Up to 80 percent of individuals who have PD eventually develop MNCD.

MSA presents with a heterogeneity of symptoms, including: ataxia (MSA-cerebellar type) or tremor and rigidity (MSA-Parkinsonian type) along with symptoms of autonomic failure (recurrent fainting spells, bladder dysfunction, irregular heart rate) and cognitive decline. In advanced stages, muscle contractures, Pisa syndrome (leaning toward one side, resembling the Leaning Tower of Pisa), antecollis (neck bending forward and head dropping down), and involuntary and uncontrollable sighing and gasping may also be seen. MSA includes rare neurodegenerative disorders previously termed Shy-Drager syndrome, olivopontocerebellar atrophy, and striatonigral degeneration.

Clinical Case 1: "I am tired all the time"

Ms. S, a 79-year-old woman residing in a nursing home, was referred to us for evaluation of suspected depression. She had a history of memory problems, disorientation at times, recurrent falls, and sleep disturbances beginning two to three years prior and had been progressively getting worse. The most recent fall was a week ago and caused her to have a bruise on her face but no fracture. Over the last two weeks, she was increasingly withdrawn, staying in her room with mild impairment in appetite. On evaluation, the resident's main complaint was fatigue; she stated, "I am tired all the time." Her past medical history was positive for hypertension, peripheral vascular disease, osteoarthritis of the knees, and carpal tunnel syndrome. A review of systems revealed dysuria. She presented mentally slowed, with flat affect and moderately disoriented to time and place. Her Montreal Cognitive Assessment (MOCA) score was 12. Physical examination revealed a low-frequency tremor of the arms and slow gait. Laboratory results were within normal range and urinalysis revealed a bladder infection, which was treated with antibiotics. Ms. S was currently taking amlodipine, acetaminophen, and lorazepam 0.5 mg three times a day. To rule out a chronic subdural hematoma, the HCP recommended an emergency CT scan of the head, which showed old diffuse ischemic white matter changes and mild cortical atrophy. The lorazepam was gradually tapered and discontinued over two weeks. Ms. S was started on donepezil 5 mg once daily. Family and staff were counseled to have her walk regularly, as she had always enjoyed walking. After one month, she was sleeping better and her dysuria had cleared up, but she still complained of fatigue. She had tolerated donepezil well so far without developing any nausea or vomiting. Her tremor was no worse. The donepezil was increased to 10 mg daily. Water painting was added to her activity schedule, as Ms. S had shown interest in this activity when she was in an adult day program. After another month, she appeared to be doing much better. She still complained of fatigue, but less often. Her family felt she was more alert and interactive. Her repeat MOCA score was 15. Final diagnosis of probable DLB was given.

Teaching Points

It is important to note that adverse effects of benzodiazepines, such as fatigue, may take several weeks to improve after the drug is discontinued. Also, a urinary tract infection (UTI) may manifest as fatigue, depression, and/or increased confusion. Often, there are multiple causes of symptoms and disability, with untreated MNCD being one of them. In this case, treatment of UTI, discontinuation of lorazepam, institution of cholinesterase inhibitor (ChEI) therapy, and aggressive use of strength-based personalized psychosocial sensory spiritual environmental initiatives with creative engagement (SPPEICE) helped improve the resident's quality of life.

Major Vascular Neurocognitive Disorder

Major vascular neurocognitive disorder (vascular dementia [VaD]) is the second most common cause of irreversible MNCD if mixed MNCDs are considered, with the majority of VaD occurring along with other degenerative neuropathology (especially AD) (Smith 2016). The MCI stage (mild vascular neurocognitive disorder) of VaD has also been described. VaD can be further classified into poststroke VaD and nonstroke VaD (typically due to small vessel cerebrovascular disease), and neuroimaging evidence of significant cerebrovascular disease is essential for its diagnosis. With poststroke VaD, cognitive impairment can be abrupt in onset followed by stepwise deterioration, as opposed to the insidious onset and slow and steady decline seen in AD. Physical exam reveals neurological signs typical of stroke (focal neurological deficit, motor and reflex asymmetry). Neurocognitive change exhibited by individuals who have VaD is characterized by problems with decision-making, poor organizational ability, difficulty adjusting to change (due to impaired executive functions), difficulty sustaining attention, and the appearance of apathy. Memory function, while impaired in VaD, is not the principal and devastating feature that it is with AD. Impaired judgment, mood changes including depression, emotional lability, personality changes, frank aphasia, abulia, or visuospatial disturbances may predominate either alone or in combination correlating with networks damaged by cerebrovascular disease. Many individuals who have VaD also demonstrate Parkinsonian symptoms (retropulsion, shuffling gait, loss of postural reflexes) and early urinary incontinence. As many as 30 percent of stroke survivors may develop VaD by 6 months after the stroke. The risk of MNCD increases ninefold over that of individuals of the same age and sex who do not have a new stroke. There is a remarkably high rate of silent infarct on imaging, maybe as high as 20 percent. Silent infarct increases the risk of subsequent MNCD by 2.26. Neuroimaging in individuals who have poststroke VaD may show one or more large vessel infarcts, a strategically placed single infarct or hemorrhage, two or more lacunar infarcts outside the brain stem.

Besides stroke, VaD is also caused by small-vessel cerebrovascular disease caused by either arteriolosclerosis or amyloid angiopathy. Individuals who have this type of VaD usually have a subcortical pattern of MNCD with psychomotor slowing (bradyphrenia) and relative preservation of naming and other language skills, although amnestic syndrome indistinguishable clinically from AD is also seen. Vascular depression is a term used to describe older adults who have symptoms of major depressive disorder along with psychomotor slowing and executive impairment with neuroimaging evidence of significant small-vessel ischemia (extensive and confluent white matter lesions). For many individuals, vascular depression may be a prodrome of VaD. MRI of the brain is the neuroimaging method of choice and shows obvious evidence of severe small-vessel cerebrovascular disease. White matter hyperintensities (WMH) (leukoariosis) if severe are associated with 3 times the risk of subsequent MNCD. WMH are an independent predictor of cognitive decline, even more powerfully than the presence of lacunar infarcts.

Infarcts may involve the hippocampus directly, and subcortical ischemic vascular disease can also affect hippocampal volume. Thus, although the presence of hippocampal atrophy is highly indicative of AD, it cannot be taken as proof that AD is the cause of MNCD to the exclusion of VaD. Thus, differentiating VaD from AD through neuropsychological testing or neuroimaging is not as useful as determining the cerebrovascular disease burden for all individuals who have AD. Pure VaD in individuals who have MNCD and are older than 70 is rare. In younger individuals who have significant cerebrovascular disease, the possibility of pure VaD is more likely.

Major Frontotemporal Neurocognitive Disorder

Frontotemporal MNCDs (frontotemporal dementias [FTDs]) are a group of diseases characterized by neuronal degeneration involving primarily the frontal and temporal lobes. The neuropathology consists of accumulation of abnormal proteins (tau or ubiquitin) that are thought to cause neuronal death and loss of synapses. Individuals who have FTD are approximately evenly divided between tau and ubiquitin inclusions. There are no reliable clinical differences between FTD with tau and FTD with ubiquitin inclusions. Up to 15 percent of individuals who have FTD have clinical and electromyographic findings consistent with amytrophic lateral sclerosis (ALS, or Lou Gehrig's disease).

FTDs are the fifth most common cause of progressive irreversible MNCDs, ranking behind AD, DLB, VaD, and PDD (Finger 2016). The incidence is probably higher due to problems in recognition and diagnosis. Symptoms of FTD typically appear between the ages of 40 and 65, with mean age of onset between approximately 52 and 58 years. In young-onset MNCD (onset before age 60), FTD may be at least as common as AD if not more so. Up to 25 percent of cases have onset after the age of 65 years. Up to 40 percent of cases have a positive family history, and approximately 10 percent of cases have autosomal dominant pattern of inheritance. Six clinical groups of FTDs have been identified: behavioral variant FTD [bvFTD]; two speech and language conditions, termed progressive nonfluent aphasia (PNFA; also called progressive nonfluent variant primary progressive aphasia) and semantic dementia (SD; also called semantic variant primary progressive aphasia); and three FTDs associated with prominent motor features, termed corticobasal degeneration (CBD), progressive supranuclear palsy (PSP), and FTD with motor neuron disease (ALS). Individuals who have PSP will have vertical supranuclear gaze palsy, symmetrical axial-predominant Parkinsonism causing early postural instability, and retropulsion that will help differentiate them from PD and PDD. Individuals who have CBD have asymmetric rigidity, limb apraxia, postural instability, myoclonus, alien limb phenomenon, and cortical sensory loss. Similar to AD, DLB, and PDD, all FTDs have a long preclinical phase progressing to MCI (mild frontotemporal neurocognitive disorder, typically nonamnestic type) before developing MNCD.

The bvFTD is characterized by insidious onset of behavioral and personality changes, and typically initial presentation lacks clear neurological signs or symptoms. Core diagnostic criteria for bvFTD include personality changes, such as emotional blunting and lack of insight. The clinical manifestations of bvFTD are variable but may include poor judgment (neglecting normal responsibilities), disinhibition (impolite behavior), loss of empathy and sympathy for others, compulsive or socially inappropriate behaviors, excessive eating and weight gain, apathy, substance abuse, or aggression early in the course of MNCD. Social misconduct in the form of theft or offensive language may occur in nearly half of individuals who have bvFTD. Symptoms such as rigidity, stubbornness, self-centeredness, and adoption of compulsive rituals typically occur with disease progression. Individuals who have bvFTD may exhibit dramatic alterations in the self as defined by changes in political, social, or religious values. Stereotyped behaviors, such as compulsive cleaning, pacing, and collecting, are also common in bvFTD. In later stages, hyperorality, repetitive movement, and mutism may occur. Memory loss is not prominent until later in the disease. Initially individuals who have bvFTD are typically misdiagnosed as having a psychiatric disorder (such as major depression, bipolar disorder, schizophrenia, personality disorder, obsessive compulsive disorder, addiction disorders) and may have been under the care of a psychiatrist for years (Ducharme et al. 2015). Only when symptoms advance to the point of obvious cognitive (loss of speech, memory deficits) and physical (stiffness and balance problems) deficits is the correct diagnosis made. Up to one-third of people who have bvFTD exhibit euphoria, which can take the form of elevated mood, inappropriate jocularity, and exaggerated self-esteem that can be indistinguishable from hypomania or mania. Gluttonous overeating and an exaggerated craving for carbohydrates are also common in bvFTD.

Cognitive dysfunction (specifically executive deficits) may precede other neurocognitive deficits (e.g. memory and new learning, language) by decades in bvFTD. Another key clinical element of bvFTD is the relative preservation of verbal and visual memory (unlike AD). (See Table 3.3.) Also, individuals who have bvFTD typically have preservation of visuospatial functions (unlike individuals who have DLB). On formal testing of delayed recall, individuals who have bvFTD may score in the normal range. People in the earlier stages of bvFTD, as compared to AD, often achieve higher scores on bedside tests assessing global cognitive functioning. (See Table 3.4.) Bedside cognitive tests thus are often insensitive to detecting the early and isolated executive function deficits of people who have bvFTD. Individuals who have bvFTD often display echolalia and echopraxia (repeating whatever the other person says), perseveration (giving the same answer to a new question), and motor impersistence. By the time of the diagnosis, most people who have bvFTD perform poorly on psychometric tests of executive function. Individuals who have bvFTD

Table 3.4 Standardized Bedside Assessment Tools for Evaluating and Managing Major Neurocognitive Disorder in Long-Term Care Populations

Standardized Assessment Tools	Key Benefits	Key Limitations
Mini-Mental State Exam (MMSE)	Excellent tool to assess global cognitive function	Copyright issues limit routine use MMSE may miss executive dysfunction
Montreal Cognitive Assessment (MOCA)	Excellent tool to assess global cognitive function Available in 35 languages Reliably assesses executive function	Requires staff training for reliable use Not as commonly used in research studies as MMSE
Saint Louis University Mental State (SLUMS)	Excellent tool to assess global cognitive function Reliably assesses executive function	Requires staff training for reliable use Not as well validated as MMSE and MOCA
Brief Interview of Mental Status (BIMS)	Easy to use tool to assess global cognitive function that is a part of the Minimum Data Set (MDS) 3.0 used in nursing homes in the United States	Low sensitivity in identifying residents who have mild neurocognitive disorder and mild stage major neurocognitive disorder
Trail Making Test–Oral (TMT-Oral)	Easy to use tool to measure executive function quickly	Cannot be used as the only test to assess executive function, as it can be normal in some individuals who have significant executive dysfunction
Controlled Oral Word Association Test (COWAT)	Easy to use tool to measure executive function quickly	Cannot be used as the only test to assess executive function, as it can be normal in some individuals who have significant executive dysfunction
Confusion Assessment Method (CAM)	Excellent screening tool for diagnosis of delirium, especially among residents who have MNCD	Requires staff training for reliable use
Functional Activities Questionnaire (FAQ)	Excellent tool to assess functioning in instrumental activities of daily living (such as keeping appointments, managing money)	With residents who have impaired insight, this tool requires a knowledgeable informant for accurate assessment
Physical Self-Maintenance Scale (PSMS)	Excellent tool to assess functioning in basic activities of daily living (such as grooming, toileting, bathing, feeding)	With residents who have impaired insight, this tool requires a knowledgeable informant for accurate assessment
Katz Index of Activities of Daily Living	Excellent tool to assess functioning in basic activities of daily living (such as grooming, toileting, bathing, feeding)	With residents who have impaired insight, this tool requires a knowledgeable informant for accurate assessment

Table 3.4 (cont.)

Standardized Assessment Tools	Key Benefits	Key Limitations
Barthel Inventory	Excellent tool to assess functioning in basic activities of daily living (such as grooming, toileting, bathing, feeding)	With residents who have impaired insight, this tool requires a knowledgeable informant for accurate assessment
Patient Health Questionnaire–9 (PHQ-9)	Excellent tool to screen for depression in LTC population with mild MNCD and monitor response to treatment Easy to use Well known in primary care	Not reliable with residents who have more advanced MNCD
Geriatric Depression Scale–15 (GDS)	Excellent tool to screen for depression in LTC population with mild MNCD and monitor response to treatment Easy to use Also available in 5-, 10-, and 30-item versions	Not reliable with residents who have more advanced MNCD Requires some staff training for reliable use Not as easy to use as PHQ-9
Cornell Scale for Depression in Dementia (CSDD)	Excellent tool to screen for depression in LTC populations with moderate to severe MNCD and monitor response to treatment	Requires staff training for reliable use
Saint Louis University AM SAD (SLU AM SAD)	Easy-to-use tool to screen for MDD in LTC populations and monitor response to treatment	Not as well studied as PHQ-9, GDS, and CSDD
Cohen-Mansfield Agitation Inventory (CMAI)	Excellent tool to measure severity of distress expressed as agitation in LTC populations with moderate to severe MNCD and monitor response to treatment	Requires staff training for reliable use
Pittsburgh Agitation Scale (PAS)	Excellent tool to measure severity of distress expressed as agitation in LTC populations with moderate to severe MNCD and monitor response to treatment	Requires staff training for reliable use
Neuropsychiatric Inventory–Nursing Home Version (NPI-NH)	Excellent tool to screen for behavioral and psychological symptoms in LTC populations with MNCD and monitor response to treatment	Requires staff training for reliable use
Behavioral symptoms in Alzheimer's Disease (BEHAVE-AD)	Excellent tool to screen for behavioral and psychological symptoms in LTC populations with MNCD and monitor response to treatment	Requires staff training for reliable use
Numerical Rating Scale (Likert scale)	Excellent tool to assess severity of pain among residents who have mild to moderate AD and monitor response to treatment Easy to use	Not reliable with residents who have severe MNCD and residents who have significant receptive language impairment
Pain in Alzheimer's Disease (PAIN-AD)	Excellent tool to assess severity of pain and monitor response to treatment among residents who have severe AD	Requires staff training for reliable use

make more concrete, literal interpretations and have severe impairment in social cognition (interpret social situations and ascribe mental states to others). Neuropsychological testing is highly valuable when bvFTD is being considered because bedside testing of executive function is inadequate. Normal performance on neuropsychological testing does not rule out bvFTD, especially early in its course. Some individuals who have bvFTD and present with predominantly behavioral and personality manifestations may have only equivocal deficits on neuropsychological tests of executive function. Having a high index of suspicion with individuals who have onset of personality change and/or other atypical psychiatric syndrome in their 40s is key to diagnosing bvFTD early.

Behavioral symptoms usually emerge later in the two language subgroups. Individuals who have PNFA demonstrate expressive aphasia with prominent word-finding difficulty, diminished ability to produce speech, and progressive difficulty with writing and reading. Mutism eventually occurs. PNFA typically starts in the 40s or 50s. Individuals who have PNFA remain more functionally intact than individuals who have other subtypes. Changes in behavior and personality do not occur until later stages (after several years). Many people who have PNFA are independent in IADLs, despite profound aphasia. Individuals who have SD exhibit a loss of knowledge of the meaning of words and objects. Individuals who have SD have a fluent dysphasia with severe difficulty in naming and understanding words and difficulty in stating or demonstrating the function of tools or utensils. The average age for first symptoms of FTD is 50–56 years. Survival is typically shorter with the FTD subgroups than with AD, with the possible exception of SD, in which the duration of illness is similar to that of AD. Despite the higher cognitive scores, those who have FTD demonstrate profound deficits in the ability to manage day-to-day activities. These functional losses are secondary to judgment problems and behavioral symptoms, in contrast to the memory deficits of AD. Most people who have FTD, especially when behavioral symptoms exist, have difficulty engaging in occupational or family pursuits. There may be financial problems due to the affected person's job loss, bad investment, or overspending.

FTD has a strong genetic component, with up to 10 percent of cases showing a highly penetrant, autosomal dominant pattern of disease transmission. Progranulin mutations linked to chromosome 17q21 account for 10 percent of cases of FTD and approximately 20 percent of cases with family history. There is great clinical variability, even within families sharing the same progranulin mutation. The motor difficulties experienced by individuals who have FTD with progranulin mutations frequently take the form of mild Parkinsonism. In some cases, familial FTD is linked to a mutation in the tau gene also found in chromosome 17. This disorder, called frontotemporal dementia with Parkinsonism linked to chromosome 17 (FTDP-17), is much like other types of FTD but often includes psychiatric symptoms such as delusions and hallucinations. FTDP-17 is relatively uncommon, even in familial forms of FTD.

Clinical Case 2: "I am okay"

Mr. C, a 55-year-old male, became socially withdrawn, developed poor decision-making ability, and had a significant weight gain over two years. He entered a LTC facility for rehabilitation after surgery for a hip fracture. Mr. C seemed not to be bothered by the hip fracture and needed encouragement during physical therapy. He was diagnosed with depression and tried various antidepressants without success. He was referred to a psychiatrist for a trial of electroconvulsive therapy (ECT). Mr. C told the psychiatrist during the interview, "I am okay" and did not endorse depressive symptoms. The psychiatrist felt this was a new-onset apathy syndrome. The psychiatrist ordered an MRI of the brain to rule out any neurological cause of new-onset apathy. Mr. C had no past history of depression before the two-year period of weight gain, no family history of depression, and there was vague history of possible transient ischemic attack (TIA). The MRI revealed right temporal, frontal, and parietal atrophy. The psychiatrist referred Mr. C to a neurologist at a local memory and aging disorder clinic at an academic institution for evaluation of possible FTD. Mr. C underwent a comprehensive evaluation, including neuropsychological testing, and was diagnosed with probable FTD (behavioral variant). Mr. C's socially withdrawn behavior was thought to reflect apathy more than depression. All antidepressants were discontinued without any worsening of clinical symptoms. The family and staff at the LTC facility were educated about the diagnosis. SPPEICE were identified and initiated to address apathy. Mr. C passed away six years after the diagnosis of FTD due to complications related to advanced stages of FTD. A brain autopsy was performed and the pathological diagnosis of FTD (ubiquitin positive) was given.

Teaching Points

The initial presentation of FTD is often mistaken for depression. Accurate diagnosis requires a high index of suspicion. A history of insidious onset of apathy and lack of concern for self should raise the possibility of FTD. We strongly recommend referral to a geriatric psychiatrist or a neurologist for early accurate diagnosis.

Mixed Major Neurocognitive Disorders

Mixed MNCDs (typically degenerative MNCDs coexisting with each other [AD and DLB, AD and PDD] or with VaD [AD with VaD, DLB with VaD, PDD with VaD]) are more common than is usually recognized and should be considered in the differential diagnosis. Concomitant AD is present in 66 percent of people who have DLB and 77 percent of people who have VaD. Most people who have clinical VaD have low to moderate AD coexisting. Even older adults who have high burdens of CVD may still have some AD. More clinical evidence of CVD implies greater likelihood of VaD as the dominant etiologic factor in people who have MNCD. AD can never be ruled out on clinical or imaging grounds. At autopsy, people who have PDD will frequently have pathologic findings of AD as well. Diagnosing mixed MNCDs has implications for treatment (e.g. trial of ChEIs in individuals who have mixed AD and VaD) and prognosis (e.g. more rapid decline in cognition and function, more adverse effects associated with use of antipsychotics).

Alcohol-Induced and Other Substance/Medication-Induced Major Neurocognitive Disorder

Substance/medication-induced MNCD involves cognitive and functional decline that persists long after the period of acute intoxication and withdrawal is over. Alcohol-induced MNCD (alcohol-induced neurotoxicity) is by far the most common cause of substance-induced MNCD in LTC populations. It is characterized by a decline in visuospatial and executive functions (Rao and Draper 2015). Although regular modest consumption of alcohol may be neuroprotective, heavy drinking is harmful to cortical as well as subcortical areas of the brain. Heavy consumption also damages cerebellum and frontocerebellar circuits, leading to executive dysfunction. It is prevalent in LTC populations and often coexists with other conditions causing neurocognitive disorders (especially Wernicke-Korsakoff syndrome [due to thiamine deficiency {vitamin B_1}], other nutritional deficiencies, alcohol-related advanced liver disease, chronic subdural hematoma, Traumatic Brain Injury, AD, cerebrovascular disease, depression), which results in substantial heterogeneity in presentation. Accurate history is key to accurate diagnosis. Relatively better performance on semantic tasks and verbal memory recognition tests and poor performance on visuospatial and executive functioning early on can help the HCP differentiate it from AD. In the absence of neurodegenerative disorders, abstaining from further alcohol use and correction of underlying nutritional deficiencies may result in stabilization of cognitive deficits with minimal progression over subsequent years.

Methamphetamine use disorder is associated with microhemorrhages and large areas of cerebral infarction that can lead to MNCDs. Chronic use of inhalants or barbiturates can also lead to MNCD. There are conflicting studies (one positive and one negative) about chronic use of benzodiazepines leading to MNCD. Benzodiazepines can exacerbate pre-existing cognitive impairment.

Major Neurocognitive Disorder due to Traumatic Brain Injury

Falls are the most common cause of traumatic brain injury (TBI) among LTC residents. Mild neurocognitive disorder due to TBI is often seen in residents after a fall and head injury. If the resident has underlying MNCD, the TBI may result in accelerated cognitive decline. Individuals who have moderate to severe TBI (loss of consciousness of 30 minutes or more and/or post-traumatic amnesia of 24 hours or more) due to motor vehicle accident (MVA) are often left with severe cognitive impairment, motor deficit, and seizure disorder (especially in the first year) and eventually need LTC. Military veterans who have blast neurotrauma are another group at risk for MNCD due to TBI. The nature of cognitive deficits will depend on the location of brain damage caused by TBI (coup-contrecoup injuries). Executive impairment is most common, but damage to the hippocampus can lead to cognitive impairment that may mimic AD. Moderate to severe TBI increases the risk of MNCD by two- to fourfold (Shively et al.

2012). Multiple mild brain injuries (loss of consciousness of less than 30 minutes and/or posttraumatic amnesia less than 24 hours and/or confusion and disorientation after head injury) as experienced by professional boxers, football players, and hockey players can lead to chronic traumatic encephalopathy (CTE) that has distinct neuropathology (specifically, accumulation of hyperphosphorylated tau neurofibrillary and glial tangles) leading to progressive brain atrophy. CTE typically progresses slowly from mild neurocognitive disorder to MNCD. Moderate to severe TBI is also a risk factor for future development of AD, Parkinson's disease, and motor neuron disease. Changes in mood (e.g. irritability, hostility) or personality (e.g. impulsivity, disinhibition, apathy) and complaints of headache, photosensitivity, sleep disturbance, fatigue, or dizziness often accompany MNCD due to TBI. Post-traumatic stress disorder may emerge in the context of TBI due to MVA or military trauma, and the HCP should anticipate and address it. Residents who have TBI often have reduced tolerance of psychotropic medications. For some residents who have TBI, the cognitive impairment and functional loss may not progressively worsen after the initial insult.

Major Neurocognitive Disorder due to HIV Infection

HIV disease is caused by human immunodeficiency virus type 1 (HIV-1). More than 50 percent of people who have HIV are 50 years old or older. Cognitive impairment is twice as common in older adults who have HIV than in younger adults. The HCP should consider HIV-associated dementia (HAD) in any resident who has cognitive decline and is HIV positive or at high risk of being HIV positive. It occurs even in individuals who have HIV infection and are treated with highly active antiretroviral therapy (HAART) (Elbirt et al. 2015). HAD is more frequently the first presenting sign of HIV infection in older adults than in younger adults. HAD is associated with executive dysfunction, psychomotor slowing, abnormal gait, and hypertonia. Individuals who have HAD have fewer problems with recall than do those who have AD. For all residents who have suspected HAD (except those in terminal stages), we recommend referral to an infectious disease specialist and neurologist to rule out reversible causes of cognitive decline (such as opportunistic infections related to HIV/AIDS [autoimmune deficiency syndrome], such as cryptococcosis, toxoplasmosis, or herpes simplex encephalitis). In older adults, cardiovascular disease and AD may be comorbid with HAD. All residents who have MNCD should be adequately screened for HIV infection risk factors. Mild neurocognitive disorder due to HIV infection is typically a precursor for later development of HAD. Serum HIV testing and CSF testing (disproportionate viral load in CSF versus in the plasma) can confirm the diagnosis. MRI and CSF testing can help exclude opportunistic infections and other medical conditions (CNS lymphoma) as etiological agents of MNCD. HAART (especially with drugs that have high central nervous system penetration) is currently the only treatment recommended for HAD.

Major Neurocognitive Disorder due to Huntington's Disease

Huntington's disease (HD) is one of the most common hereditary disorders (autosomal dominant with 100 percent penetrance caused by the abnormality in the Huntington's gene on chromosome 4) and typically presents with involuntary movements (Johnson and Paulsen 2014). HD causes chorea – involuntary jerky, arrhythmic movements of the body – as well as muscle weakness, clumsiness, and gait disturbances. The children of people who have the disorder have a 50 percent chance of inheriting it. The disease causes degeneration in many regions of the brain (especially the basal ganglia [caudate nucleus and putamen]) and spinal cord. Like AD, MNCD due to HD has a long preclinical phase leading to mild neurocognitive disorder and then progressing to MNCD. Symptoms of HD begin usually when people are in the 30s or 40s. Executive dysfunction and psychomotor slowing are key cognitive deficits. Cognitive symptoms of HD typically begin with mild personality changes, such as irritability, accompanied by anxiety and depression, and progress to severe MNCD. Neuroimaging shows atrophy of the caudate and putamen. Genetic testing confirms the diagnosis. There is no cure for HD. Tetrabenazine is often given for symptomatic treatment of chorea, but its use carries risk of depression. Most residents who have HD have severe chorea that substantially interferes with ambulation and provision of personal care (e.g. feeding, bathing, dressing). The HCP may consider prescribing high-potency atypical antipsychotics (such as risperidone) to treat chorea. Symptomatic treatment of anxiety and depression with psychosocial (such as counseling in early stages) and pharmacological interventions (such as antidepressants) may be appropriate. The majority of LTC residents who have HD are in advanced stages, with severe disability in ambulation and speech, malnutrition, and severe BPSD. Management follows similar principles to that of advanced AD and related neurocognitive disorders.

Major Neurocognitive Disorder due to Multiple Sclerosis

Multiple sclerosis (MS) is an autoimmune-mediated demyelinating disorder of the central nervous system (brain and spinal cord) that affects more women than men. MS is incurable. The average age of individuals living with MS is 55 years and number of older adults who have MS-related disability is rising due to the aging of the population at large. Residents who have MS in LTC are typically in advanced stages with severe motor disability accompanied by significant cognitive impairment in multiple domains. Cognitive impairment often involves impairment in coding leading to short-term memory problems. Attentional impairment, executive dysfunction, word-finding difficulty, and visuospatial impairment has been described in addition to memory impairment in individuals who have MS. Individuals who have MS retain long-term memory, general intellect, conversation skills, and reading comprehension until late stages of MNCD.

Major Neurocognitive Disorder due to Chronic Subdural Hematoma

Chronic subdural hematoma (CSDH) is due to rupture of bridging veins crossing the subdural space due to head injury, resulting in collection of liquefied blood between the arachnoid and the dura mater of the brain. As the blood liquefies, the hematoma enlarges over weeks. Thus, CSDH often presents weeks after the head injury. We recommend that the HCP have a high index of suspicion in LTC populations, as a history of head injury may not always be available. The incidence of CSDH increases with age (Shapey, Glanez, and Brennan 2016). LTC residents are at significant risk of CSDH as they are prone to falls and head injury in the context of cerebral atrophy (age-related and/or related to pre-existing MNCD). People who have a history of alcohol use disorder and people taking antiplatelet and/or anticoagulant medication are at even higher risk of CSDH. Although motor symptoms (e.g. limb weakness, ataxia), headache, and mild reduction in the level of consciousness may be present, CSDH (including residents who have bilateral CSDH) may manifest primarily with subacute onset of cognitive impairment that may progress slowly (resembling AD) or rapidly (resembling rapidly progressive MNCDs). We recommend collaboration among the primary care physician, neurologist, and psychiatrist to clarify the potential benefits of surgical evacuation of hematoma versus watchful waiting due to high risks of surgery in LTC populations. Spontaneous resolution of CSDH has been reported in literature. We recommend treating symptoms (e.g. acetaminophen for headaches) and watchful waiting for frail residents who have CSDH.

Rapidly Progressive Major Neurocognitive Disorders

Rapidly progressive MNCDs (rapidly progressive dementias [RPDs]) typically have a subacute onset (weeks to months) and rapid decline (over three to six months). The LTC team may be the first to diagnose RPD in a resident. Differential diagnosis of RPDs should include prion disease, autoimmune encephalopathy, atypical forms of degenerative MNCD, VaD, brain neoplasm, some infections, dural arteriovenous fistula, and CSDH (Geschwind 2016). All RPDs require urgent evaluation, preferably by a team of primary care physician, neurologist, and psychiatrist. Prion diseases are the prototype RPDs and are fortunately rare. They are clinically fairly distinct from more common forms of neurodegenerative MNCD. Creutzfeldt-Jakob disease (CJD) is the most common prion disease, and the HCP should suspect it in all residents who have RPD. Most residents who have CJD die within one year. Although the cognitive profile of CJD is not particularly distinct from those of other MNCDs, typically residents who have CJD may initially experience problems with ataxia, myoclonus, startle reflex, personality change, and impaired vision along with cognitive impairment. Other symptoms may include insomnia and depression. As the illness progresses, cognitive impairment becomes severe and blindness may develop. Eventually individuals lose the ability to move and speak and go into a coma. Pneumonia and other infections often occur in these residents and can lead to death. Triphasic wave pattern in electroencephalography (EEG) in the context of a RPD is strongly suggestive of CJD. Other biomarkers of CJD include characteristic lesions (multifocal gray matter hyperintensities in subcortical and cortical regions) on MRI with diffusion-weighted imaging (DWI) or fluid-attenuated inversion recovery (FLAIR) and tau or 14-3-3 protein in the CSF. Definitive diagnosis of CJD requires brain biopsy. There is no specific treatment or cure for CJD. Drugs such as clonazepam may help myoclonus.

Major Neurocognitive Disorder due to Anoxic Brain Injury

Residents who have survived cardiopulmonary resuscitation and residents who received care in an intensive care unit for severe hypotension and/or hypoxia often develop delirium that leads to MNCD (due to anoxic/hypoxic brain injury) over weeks to months. Residents who have pre-existing MNCD may develop accelerated cognitive and functional decline after experiencing anoxic brain injury. In residents who have anoxic encephalopathy and low comorbidity, the cognitive impairment and functional loss may not progressively worsen after the initial insult.

Major Neurocognitive Disorder due to Another Medical Condition

Reversible causes of MNCD are rare in LTC populations. Nevertheless, case reports of reversible MNCDs in these populations are periodically seen in the literature. However, reversible causes of cognitive impairment in residents who have pre-existing MNCD are common and are listed in Box 3.1 (Geschwind 2016; Williams and Malm 2016). Some of these conditions may cause MNCD on their own. In the latter case, the MNCD may be reversible (partially or completely) with treatment of the cause. Vitamin B_{12} deficiency is estimated to affect 10 to 15 percent of older adults. Hematologic abnormalities may not occur with vitamin B_{12} deficiency, particularly if the nervous system is involved. Vitamin B_{12} supplementation/injections to treat B_{12} deficiency should improve cognition and prevent disability associated with progressive myelopathy and peripheral neuropathy. Vitamin B_{12} levels that are close to the lower limit of the normal range may also be treated with oral B_{12} 1000 mcg daily. Acute thiamine (vitamin B_1) deficiency causes Wernicke encephalopathy (characterized by delirium, ophthalmoplegia, lateral gaze palsy, and ataxia), and chronic thiamine deficiency causes Korsakoff syndrome (severe impairment of short-term memory with confabulation). Older adults who have alcohol use disorder and poor nutrition often develop thiamine deficiency. Treatment involves parenteral thiamine administration to treat Wernicke encephalopathy and thiamine oral supplementation (100 mg thiamine daily) for Korsakoff syndrome. The HCP may consider other vitamin deficiencies, such as folate deficiency and pellagra (niacin deficiency), for residents who were severely malnourished before entering LTC. Thyroid disease, especially hypothyroidism, is common in LTC populations. However, apathetic hyperthyroidism (i.e. paradoxical presentation of hyperthyroidism with fatigue, attentional impairments, psychomotor retardation, and weight gain) also occurs in this population. A history of hypothyroidism (loss of appetite and weight gain, decreased tolerance of cold) or hyperthyroidism (increased appetite with weight loss, decreased tolerance of heat), physical examination (to look for signs of hypothyroidism, such as bradycardia, skin cold to touch, presence of goiter, dry skin, or hyperthyroidism, such as tachycardia, exophthalmos),

BOX 3.1 Common Reversible Causes of Cognitive Impairment Co-occurring with Major Neurocognitive Disorder (Acronym DEMENTIAS)

- D: Dehydration, depressive disorder, diabetes (severe hyperglycemia and hypoglycemia episodes), dyscontrol of blood pressure (very high or very low blood pressure affecting cerebral blood flow)
- E: Electrolyte imbalance (e.g. hyponatremia, hypernatremia, hypercalcemia)
- M: Medication-induced cognitive impairment (especially anticholinergic drugs, benzodiazepines)
- E: Epilepsy/seizures (especially complex partial seizures and postictal cognitive impairment)
- N: Normal pressure hydrocephalus, nutritional deficiencies (especially vitamin B_{12})
- T: Thyroid disorder (hypothyroidism, hyperthyroidism), testosterone deficiency
- I: Infection (especially urinary tract infection, pneumonia)
- A: Apnea (obstructive sleep apnea) and hypoxia (especially due to advanced chronic obstructive pulmonary disease, chronic heart failure)
- S: Sedentary lifestyle (prolonged sitting is considered the "new smoking"), substance abuse (especially alcohol, nicotine)

and testing for thyroid-stimulating hormone (TSH) and free thyroxine levels (T4) are indicated to evaluate the cause of reversible MNCD. New-onset epilepsy in LTC residents often presents as complex partial seizures that can resemble rapid-onset MNCD. Postictal confusion and cognitive impairment may last longer in residents who have pre-existing MNCD.

For residents who have cognitive decline and unexplained focal findings, the HCP should consider atypical presentations, including urinary incontinence, stumbling gait, seizures, or severe headache early in the course of MNCD, the so-called surgically treatable causes – idiopathic normal pressure hydrocephalus (iNPH), CSDH, and brain tumor – but these typically do not present as isolated MNCD. NPH manifests initially with gait apraxia (leading to falls) followed by urinary incontinence and MCI progressing to MNCD. Neuroimaging shows dilated ventricles, and diagnosis can be confirmed by demonstrating improvement in gait after removal of some amount of CSF through lumbar puncture. Treatment of iNPH involves insertion of a ventriculoperitoneal shunt. Primary gastrointestinal disorders such as Whipple disease may involve the CNS without gastrointestinal symptoms. CNS symptoms of Whipple disease may manifest as Parkinson's disease – plus syndrome that resembles PSP. Tumors involving the parietal cortex may mimic AD. The parietal cortex is not directly connected with motor output systems, and paralysis and abnormal reflexes may be absent despite significant mass effect. Although other abnormalities (i.e. sensory, complex behavioral, and visual-focal deficits) may occur, residents who have tumor involving the parietal lobe are usually unaware of these deficits (anosognosia), and they may be missed on a cursory examination. Neoplasms in the frontal lobe may present with apathy and executive dysfunction, mimicking bvFTD. In general, residents who have MNCD due to brain tumor are younger (less than 70 years) than the typical residents who have AD (more than 70 years). Neuroimaging (especially MRI with and without contrast) confirms the diagnosis of brain tumor.

Amnesia and changes in mood or personality, delirium, or seizures can indicate paraneoplastic limbic encephalitis, a rare remote effect of cancer associated with non-small-cell lung cancer but also with thymoma, Hodgkin's disease, and cancer of the breast, colon, bladder, and testicle. Most people who have limbic encephalitis are not known to have cancer until their mental status changes. Most commonly, limbic encephalitis occurs rapidly, over days to weeks, and may be accompanied by other neurologic symptoms (e.g. ataxia, visual changes, neuropathy). Treatment of the primary tumor may produce substantial cognitive improvement for a substantial number of individuals. The HCP should consider paretic neurosyphilis, although rare in the general population, with residents who have a past history of sexually transmitted disease and/or HIV infection acquired through sexual transmission. Clinical presentation is that of disinhibited bvFTD. If the clinical picture strongly suggests paretic neurosyphilis, we recommend fluorescent treponemal antibody absorption (FTA-ABS) test. The treatment of paretic neurosyphilis is antibiotics (such as penicillin). Other medical conditions associated with MNCDs in LTC populations include chronic heart failure (leading to cerebral hypoperfusion), autoimmune disorders (e.g. systemic lupus erythematosus [SLE]), chronic hepatic and/or chronic renal failure, advanced chronic obstructive pulmonary disease, and intracranial radiation therapy. Many people who have potentially reversible MNCD may not fully recover the premorbid cognitive abilities after starting appropriate therapy. However, the symptoms may stabilize for long periods and they may be protected from other significant consequences of the disorder.

Differential Diagnosis of Major Neurocognitive Disorder

MNCDs should be differentiated from age-associated memory impairment, mild neurocognitive disorder (mild cognitive impairment), delirium, depression, and schizophrenia.

Age-Associated Memory Impairment

A hallmark of normal cognitive aging is slowed speed of processing (Blazer, Yaffe, and Liverman 2015). Particularly after age 70 but most marked in the population over 85 is a tendency to have increasing difficulty accessing names of people and objects, difficulty processing information rapidly, and the need for additional time to learn things/skills (such as using technology), grasp new ideas (particularly complicated skills or ideas), and think through problems. Age-associated memory impairment (AAMI, also called benign senescent forgetfulness or benign forgetfulness) involves forgetting the name of someone, particularly someone whom one has not seen in a while, finding it difficult to recall the right word to express oneself, or even not remembering the name of an event or object, particularly something that is not familiar. None of these problems is sufficient to cause impairment in daily activities or the ability to live independently. Memory function as measured by delayed recall of newly learned material is not substantially decreased in older adults. People experiencing AAMI complain of memory loss but usually have normal scores on psychometric testing for their age group. Results of office-based memory testing are usually in the normal range. Although most people who have subjective memory complaints do not experience significant decline in memory or functioning over time (months to years), subjective memory difficulties may be the earliest symptom of future MNCD among highly educated people. Subjective cognitive impairment (SCI) is a term that has been introduced in the literature to describe older adults who have subjective complaints of cognitive impairment (e.g. forgetfulness) but no objective evidence of cognitive decline. SCI is often accompanied by emotional distress and fear that SCI could be a sign of beginnings of AD. Although biomarkers for AD may help differentiate individuals who have SCI due to AD from those who have SCI related to AAMI, its use in this context is controversial, as positive biomarker studies may cause additional emotional distress to the individual (Colijn and Grossberg 2015). Clinically, it is best to reassure individuals who have SCI that objective testing was normal, that there is currently no evidence of AD, and to provide counseling regarding comprehensive brain and wellness programs (see Boxes 3.2, 3.3, and 3.4). Although the cognitive impairments associated with normal aging may impair quality of life, cognitive decline with aging is not inevitable, and many older adults, including some centenarians, appear to avoid cognitive decline even into the eleventh decade of life.

BOX 3.2 **A Comprehensive Brain and Memory Wellness Plan**

Nutrition: Mediterranean diet
Physical Activity: Aerobic exercise (e.g. brisk walking), strength training, balance training, exercises to promote flexibility, yoga, Tai-Chi, leading a physically active lifestyle
Intellectual Activity and Cognitive Training: Engaging in stimulating and challenging intellectual activities (e.g. puzzles, computer-based games, rekindling hobbies and passions), cognitive training (see Box 3.3)
Social and Spiritual Activities: Engaging in daily meaningful social activities (especially intergenerational) and spiritual activities and rituals
Sleep: Strategies to promote optimal sleep (not too little, not too much) through sleep hygiene and sleep diary
Stress Management: Relaxation strategies, identifying and correcting cognitive distortion, mindfulness-based stress reduction, meditation and mindfulness exercises, spending time in nature, music-based activities
Treatment of Reversible Causes of Cognitive Impairment: Evaluation and treatment of reversible causes of cognitive impairment (see Box 3.1)
Treatment of Cardiovascular Risk Factors (e.g. hypertension)
Medications: Low-dose acetylsalicylic acid (aspirin), omega 3 fatty acids, and cholinesterase inhibitors as appropriate
Resources: Education about brain and memory wellness (see Box 3.4)

Note: Intensity matters, as the brain is neuroplastic but needs engagement in a daily and fairly rigorous manner for optimal benefit.

Mild Neurocognitive Disorder/Mild Cognitive Impairment

Mild Cognitive Impairment (MCI) is a syndrome characterized by impairment in a single cognitive domain, usually memory (amnestic MCI), or moderate impairment in several cognitive domains, but people who have MCI do not have significant impairment in the ability to perform activities of daily living and do not meet the criteria for MNCD (Petersen 2016). Accurate diagnosis (and differentiation from AAMI and MNCD) usually requires neuropsychological testing. Decline in cognitive functioning from baseline on neuropsychological cognitive testing is in the 1–2 standard deviation range (between the 3rd and 16th percentiles). The prevalence of MCI among LTC residents varies from 5 to 10 percent in many NHs to up to 30 percent in some AL homes. The most frequently encountered form of MCI is the amnestic type. Less-common variants of MCI present with localized impairment of

BOX 3.3 The ART of Cognitive Training Strategies

Attention Training: Attention is the gateway to all cognitive functions. Attention and concentration skills can be improved through simple strategies, such as focused breathing (bringing one's attention repeatedly to one's breath for 5–20 minutes one or more times a day), mindfulness in daily living (e.g. mindful eating, mindful walking), and computerized attention-training exercises.

Repetition and Relaxation: Repetition is a key strategy to improve memory. Repetition can be done by repeating in one's mind, repeating aloud, rehearsing, and visualizing. Adding emotional value and context to the information being repeated can enhance consolidation of memory through repetition. Computerized memory-training programs are also useful. It is important to relax by taking some slow deep breaths and making some self-soothing statements if one finds oneself becoming tense in an effort to remember. Spaced retrieval training, in which one repeats information after gradually increasing intervals (10 seconds, 30 seconds, 1 minute, 5 minutes, 15 minutes, 30 minutes, once a day) is useful for remembering information that is important and not likely to change (e.g. one's new telephone number, new grandchild's name).

Tricks and Tools: Tricks include but are not limited to: mnemonics, acronyms, using cues, verbal elaboration, visual elaboration, and "chunking." ART is an example of using mnemonics to remember different cognitive training strategies. If one has to remember a new number, 3145778000, it can be remembered in three chunks: 314 577 8000. Tools to aid memory and planning (executive function) include use of smart phones, written lists, electronic pill dispensers, and sticky notes as reminders.

Note: The effectiveness of cognitive training is enhanced by leading a physically, socially, intellectually, and spiritually active life, consuming brain-healthy nutrition, and correcting reversible factors causing cognitive impairment.

other cognitive domains (such as executive dysfunction in FTDs). Individuals who have amnestic MCI commonly progress to AD, converting from one diagnosis to the other at a rate of approximately 10–15 percent per year on average. Thus, for many people who have MCI, MCI represents the earliest

BOX 3.4 Resources for a Brain and Wellness Program

Peer-reviewed journal article

Anderson, K., and G. T. Grossberg. 2014. Brain Games to Slow Cognitive Decline in Alzheimer's Disease. *Journal of the American Medical Directors Association* 15:536–537. This article has an excellent list of apps for games that can enhance brain function.

Books

- Small, G., and G. Vorgan. 2012. *The Alzheimer's Prevention Program*. New York: Workman Publishing Company.
- Hartman-Stein, P.E., and A. La Rue. 2011. *Enhancing Cognitive Fitness in Adults: A Guide to the Use and Development of Community-Based Programs*. New York: Springer Publication.
- Doidge, N. 2007. *The Brain That Changes Itself*. New York: Penguin Books.

Audio CD

Weil, A., and G. Small. 2007. The Healthy Brain Kit. Audio CDs, brain-training cards, and workbook. Boulder, Co: Sound True.

Internet resources

- www.lumosity.com (computerized brain exercises)
- www.cdc.gov/aging/healthybrain/index.htm (Healthy Brain Initiative by the CDC)
- Apps for tablet PC and smart phones (e.g. Brainyapp)

manifestation of AD. Not everyone who has MCI will convert to AD or other MNCD. Although most people who convert from MCI to a MNCD have AD, many others may convert to VaD, FTD, DLB, and other less-common MNCDs. Major depressive disorder is common in people who have MCI, and its presence increases the chances of people who have MCI converting to a MNCD in the next few years. Although recollection is impaired in MCI, familiarity-based recognition is intact compared to impaired familiarity-based recognition in AD. Reversible causes of cognitive impairment (see Box 3.1) are more prevalent in MCI than in MNCD, and work-up to identify and treat them is a key component of management of MCI. We recommend discussing the option of treating residents who have amnestic MCI with a ChEI as part of a comprehensive plan to prevent or delay progression to MNCD. Such a plan should include physical activity/exercise, intellectually challenging activities, nutritional strategies, cognitive training, and stress-management strategies. (See Boxes 3.2, 3.3, and 3.4.) The HCP should strongly consider prescribing a trial of ChEI for MCI if there is a family history of AD, if the person is young (less than 70 years of age), has comorbid mild depression or subtle change in personality (passivity), a history suggestive of RBD (indicating that the individual may develop DLB in the future), a history of falls or weight loss accompanying memory deficit, family members mention mild impairment in complex activities (not sufficient to be diagnosed with MNCD), memory deficits have insidious onset and are progressive, there is no history of stroke, and MRI shows hippocampal atrophy but mild or minimal cerebrovascular disease. Individuals who have amnestic MCI and positive AD biomarkers such as CSF amyloid/tau ratio or amyloid PET have mild neurocognitive disorder due to AD and are candidates for a trial of ChEI.

Delirium

Among LTC residents, cognitive impairment due to delirium may be confused with a MNCD, especially if the staff are not familiar with the resident's baseline functioning. Delirium typically has an acute, dateable onset, fluctuating levels of alertness in which the resident may appear drowsy, hyperalert, etc., and difficulty with concentration or attention and in maintaining attention (Saczynski and Inouye 2015). As well, delirium may be accompanied by behavior changes such as agitation or psychotic symptoms such as visual hallucinations. Often called acute confusion, the quiet/apathetic subtype is often missed. Depending on the cause, in some cases the onset of delirium may be subacute. This is in contrast to typical insidious onset in degenerative MNCDs. Impairment in awareness (hyperalert, drowsy, stuporous), attention, and diurnal dramatic fluctuation in symptoms (especially cognition but also behavior) are three key clinical features of delirium that help differentiate it from MNCD (except in people who have DLB). Orientation is usually impaired and memory deficits are also seen. Thinking is disorganized. The HCP should always assume delirium to be treatable or reversible until proven otherwise. By identifying and removing the cause, the HCP can help the resident return to the premorbid cognitive and functional baseline. People who have MNCD (especially in advanced stages) are at high risk of delirium, which often manifests as acute onset of psychotic symptoms and/or agitation/aggression. The Confusion Assessment Method (CAM) is a formal delirium assessment tool that may help the HCP accurately diagnose delirium in residents who have MNCD (Inouye et al. 1990).

Major Depressive Disorder

Major depressive disorder (MDD) may be associated with complaints of memory impairment, difficulty thinking and concentrating, difficulty finding words, and an overall reduction in intellectual abilities (Trivedi and Greer 2014). This condition used to be called "depressive pseudodementia," but is more properly termed "the dementia syndrome of depression." This is a recognition that older adults who have MDD may look like and even believe they have AD because MDD can impair cognition. However, if only MDD is causing cognitive changes, once it is effectively treated, the person should return to the premorbid cognitive baseline. Unfortunately, MDD may be an early marker as well as a risk factor for AD. Also, MDD can coexist with AD in 30–50 percent of people who have AD and can lead to accelerated cognitive and functional decline. In people who have MNCD and exhibit acute cognitive or behavioral decline, the HCP should suspect comorbid MDD (besides delirium) and aggressively treat it.

Some people are unaware of their mood state (alexithymia) and deny sadness, guilt, and the other usual symptoms of MDD. Changes in self-attitude (such as helplessness, hopelessness, worthlessness, guilt), frequent crying spells, and the presence of suicidal ideas usually indicates the presence of MDD, especially if these symptoms are persisting for two or more weeks. If there is a past history of a MDD episode, less than two-week duration of symptoms is to be treated as recurrence of MDD. Although apathy (lack of motivation), psychomotor retardation, weight loss, and impaired concentration may be present in MDD and AD, it is possible to reliably differentiate MDD from AD in most clinical situations. (See Table 3.5.) Many people who have AD may also have comorbid depression. A history of gradual cognitive decline predating depressive symptoms may help the HCP diagnose AD with depression. To clarify the diagnosis, it is sometimes helpful to use an assessment tool, such as the Patient Health Questionnaire-9 (PHQ-9) (for individuals who have early MNCD)

Table 3.5 Differentiating Major Depression from Major Neurocognitive Disorder due to Alzheimer's Disease

Clinical Symptom	Major Depressive Disorder	Major Neurocognitive Disorder due to Alzheimer's Disease
Onset of symptoms	Over weeks (subacute)	Over years (insidious)
Temporal sequence of symptoms	Depressive symptoms and cognitive symptoms start at the same time	Usually cognitive decline starts months to years before significant depressive symptoms
Diurnal mood variation	Often present	Usually absent
Family history of depression	Often present	Usually absent
Family history of Alzheimer's disease	Usually absent	Often present
Persistent tearfulness	Often present	Usually absent
Insomnia	Usually present and persistent	Usually transient
Early-morning awakening	Often present	Usually absent
Decreased appetite	Frequently present	Usually absent in mild stages
Weight loss	Frequently pronounced	Usually mild if present
Nature of cognitive impairment	Executive dysfunction and attentional and motivational impairment typically present and performance on objective cognitive tests is variable	Memory and language impairment typically present and performance on cognitive tests is consistently impaired
Subjective memory complaints and wish to receive help for memory difficulty	Often present	Typically absent
Language impairment	Absent	Often present
Apraxia	Absent	Often present
Agnosia	Absent	Often present
Performance in clock drawing test	Normal	Often abnormal
Inability to copy drawing	Absent	Often present
Left/right disorientation	Absent	Often present
Hopelessness	Often present	Absent
Helplessness	Often present	Absent
Worthlessness	Often present	Absent
Guilt feelings	Often present	Absent
Multiple somatic complaints	Often present	Absent
Suicidal ideas	Often present	Absent
Severity of depression	Correlated with cognitive impairment	Cognitive impairment much worse than depression
Response to treatment of depression	Dramatic reduction in depressive symptoms and corresponding improvement in cognitive functioning	Continued cognitive impairment

or the Cornell Scale for Depression in Dementia (most useful for individuals who have advanced MNCD) (Alexopoulos et al. 1988; Spitzer, Kroenke, and Williams 1999). In difficult cases, close follow-up after aggressive and successful treatment of MDD clarifies the diagnosis by eliciting continued cognitive decline in the absence of significant depressive symptoms. People who have late-life MDD (MDD after age 65 with no past history of depression) and cognitive impairment may experience improvement in specific domains following antidepressant treatment but may not necessarily reach normal levels of performance, particularly in memory and executive function. This subgroup of people who have late-life MDD is likely at high risk of developing a progressive MNCD and thus the HCP should follow them every three to six months to detect MNCD at the earliest signs. Depression in MCI and in early MNCD must also be distinguished from late-onset MDD and the cognitive impairment that may accompany mood disorder. In the latter group of individuals, cognitive impairment often resolves partially or even fully with successful treatment of the depression. However, because as many as one-half of such individuals may develop MNCD within five years, we recommend close follow-up to diagnose MNCD as early as possible. Neuropsychological testing is one of the best ways to reliably differentiate between cognitive deficits related to depression from MCI with MDD and early MNCD with depression. Neuropsychological testing may show executive dysfunction, but the typical neuropsychological profile of AD is absent in people who have MDD but no MNCD.

Schizophrenia

Cognitive impairment is a core feature of schizophrenia, and older adults who have schizophrenia are living longer and are thus at risk of other age-related disorders that cause neurocognitive impairment (Jeste and Maglione 2013). Usually, residents who have schizophrenia have a long history of psychotic symptoms and psychiatric treatment extending back to age 20 or 30 with one or more psychiatric hospitalizations. Cognitive deficits usually involve problems with attention and executive dysfunction and are not progressive. A subset of chronic, institutionalized residents who have schizophrenia may show some intellectual and functional decline. Older adults who have schizophrenia may be more susceptible to develop common MNCDs such as AD and VaD because of the high prevalence of vascular risk factors (e.g. hypertension, diabetes mellitus, obesity, metabolic syndrome, hyperlipidemia, OSA, sedentary lifestyle, cigarette smoking, and substance abuse). We recommend neuropsychological testing to help differentiate people who have schizophrenia with cognitive deficit from those who have schizophrenia and superimposed MNCD.

Differential Diagnosis of Major Neurocognitive Disorder and Its Cause

Current tools for diagnosing MNCD include:

- Detailed history from the individual and from family or other reliable informant
- Physical and neurological examination and laboratory tests
- Neuroimaging
- Office-based standardized tests to assess cognition, function, and mood (depression) (see Table 3.4) (Folstein, Folstein, and McHugh 1975; Yesavage et al. 1983; Reisberg et al. 1987; Inouye et al. 1990; Ricker and Axelrod 1994; Rosen et al. 1994; Cohen-Mansfield 1996; Alexopoulos et al. 1988; Spitzer, Kroenke, and Williams 1999; Wood et al. 2000; Elliot 2003; Warden, Hurley, and Volicer 2003; Nasreddine et al. 2005; Saliba et al. 2012a, 2012b; Cummings-Vaughn et al. 2014; Gitlin et al. 2014; Chakamparambil et al. 2015; Herr et al. 1998).
- Neuropsychological testing by a neuropsychologist for staging, to establish a cognitive baseline, and when the diagnosis or etiology is unclear (Scott, Ostermeyer, and Shah 2016).

Tests to Clarify Diagnosis

To date, there is no antemortem test to definitively diagnose degenerative MNCD (Galvin 2016). We recommend blood tests, such as complete blood count (CBC), basic metabolic panel (BMP), liver function tests (LFT), calcium, vitamin B_{12} and folate levels, and thyroid-stimulating hormone (TSH) level, to detect potentially reversible causes of cognitive impairment, such as severe anemia, hyponatremia, severe renal disease, hypercalcemia, vitamin deficiency, and thyroid disorder. These conditions are usually comorbid with irreversible MNCD, but correcting them may improve cognition and may slow future cognitive decline. Structural neuroimaging is also usually recommended, at least during initial diagnosis (MRI preferred over computed tomography [CT] scan of the brain, usually without contrast) to detect vascular lesions, NPH, tumors, subdural hematoma, etc. Neuroimaging is not recommended for residents who have MNCD in advanced stages because obtaining a brain scan may be too burdensome for these residents and any findings on neuroimaging may not influence treatment decisions.

The prevalence of reversible MNCDs has been decreasing over the last few decades. Some HCPs may order plasma homocysteine and C-reactive protein (CRP) levels. High plasma homocysteine level is considered a risk factor for AD, and treatment with folate may reduce homocysteine level (even for people who have normal folate levels). CRP is a biomarker for inflammation, and chronic inflammation is implicated in the pathophysiology of AD. Elevated CRP levels may be treated with low-dose aspirin. In select cases (such as a history of sexually transmitted disease or intravenous drug abuse), a fluorescent treponemal antibody (FTA-ABS) test for neurosyphilis or HIV testing for CNS manifestations of AIDS may be warranted. A urine analysis, electrocardiogram (EKG), and chest X-ray may be useful to detect comorbid urinary tract infection or lung infection if the HCP suspects that the resident has delirium superimposed on MNCD. The HCP may consider ordering an FDG PET scan for an occasional resident to help differentiate between AD and FTD (this scenario is the only one in which Medicare will cover an FDG-PET scan). Neither a CT nor an MRI scan can diagnose AD, but looking for the degree of atrophy or focal atrophy and hippocampal atrophy may be useful in differentiating between FTD and AD. Atrophy out of proportion to age is also important in diagnosing degenerative MNCD. MNCD diagnoses may be inaccurate for many LTC residents. The HCP may consider ordering neuropsychological testing, if available, to diagnose MNCD more accurately. Neuropsychological testing is a useful tool for clarifying the diagnosis in people who have MDD and MNCD, to differentiate between MCI and MNCD, and to differentiate between AD and other neurodegenerative MNCD. Neuropsychological testing is also an important tool to diagnose AD among people who, at baseline, had extremely high or relatively low levels of cognitive/intellectual function (such as those who have intellectual disability due to Down syndrome and developed insidious onset and progress cognitive and functional decline from the baseline).

The HCP should consider referral to a neurologist for evaluation of uncommon causes of MNCD if the resident is very young, if signs of Parkinsonism are present, if there is a history of seizure, or when neurosurgical intervention needs to be considered (as in the case of brain tumor, NPH, subdural hematoma, etc.). The HCP should refer residents who have unusually rapid progression of symptoms of MNCD and presence of myoclonus, or other atypical presentation, to a neurologist for spinal fluid examination to evaluate for CJD and infectious etiologies of MNCD (such as neurosyphilis, herpes simplex encephalitis [HSE]) (Schmahmann 2014).

We recommend genetic testing in cases of familial AD (AD with autosomal dominant pattern of inheritance for people who typically have onset of MNCD in their 30s or 40s), some cases of FTD that have an autosomal dominant pattern of inheritance, people who have suspected Huntington's disease, and people who have suspected cerebral autosomal dominant arteriopathy with subcortical infarct and leukoencephalopathy (CADASIL). The HCP may also consider genetic testing for people who have onset of AD or FTD in their 40s to detect mutations in certain genes (e.g. Presenilin 1, Presenilin 2). We strongly recommend genetic counseling by a professional genetic counselor or clinical geneticist or other expert at an academic center before any genetic testing. Testing for APOE-4 genotype is usually not recommended for use in diagnosis.

Biopsychosocial-Spiritual Distress

In keeping with the basic tenets of person-centered care, we are replacing the term "behavioral and psychological symptoms of dementia" with "biopsychosocial-spiritual distress (BPSD)" (Dementia Action Alliance 2016). "Behavioral disturbances" and "behavioral and psychological symptoms of dementia" should be seen as personal expressions of biopsychosocial-spiritual distress. Essentially, this means that distress is due to a mix of unmet biological, psychological, social, and spiritual needs, with one or more domains predominating in a particular individual at a particular time (Cohen-Mansfield 2000; Desai and Grossberg 2017). Personal expression of distress may be through agitation and aggression besides expressions of worries, tearfulness, or fear. The perspective needs to change to prevention and reduction of distress through person-centered approaches, and the perspective of "fixing behaviors" with "interventions" should be abandoned. Words matter, and it is important to replace stigmatizing words with words that reflect compassion and respect.

Mild BPSD is nearly universal in all stages and all etiologies of MNCD (Geda et al. 2013). Moderate to severe BPSD is also common in people who have MNCD, with point prevalence of around 60 percent and lifetime prevalence of more than 90 percent.

Among the most neurobiologically validated syndromes causing BPSD are apathy, depression, psychosis, and sleep disturbance of AD (Geda et al. 2013; Marano, Rosenberg, and Lyketsos 2013; Vitalta-Franch et al. 2013). The prevalence of BPSD does not vary by setting, but the prevalence of specific expressions of BPSD does vary by setting (higher prevalence of BPSD expressed as aggression among LTC residents than among people who have MNCD in the community) and by stage. Apathy is seen in all types of MNCD and across all stages (Vilalta-Franch et al. 2013). Apathy is characterized by decreased motivation and goal-directed behavior (pursue daily activities or hobbies) along with reduced emotional responsiveness (constricted or flat affect). Its prevalence increases with advancing cognitive impairment. BPSD expressed as agitation is seen more commonly as the MNCD progresses to moderate and severe stages. Agitation (such as wandering, verbal outburst, physical threat/violence, agitation/restlessness, and sundowning) predicts cognitive decline, functional decline, and institutionalization (Thakur and Gwyther 2015). The prevalence of BPSD expressed as agitation and aggression is approximately 25 percent in people who have MNCD residing at home and 45 percent in those residing in LTC. The prevalence of clinically significant depression is approximately 32 percent in mild stage, 23 percent in moderate stage, and 18 percent in severe stage. We recommend mandatory screening of depression for all residents who have MNCD because this improves the implementation of person-centered approaches to relieve it.

Psychotic symptoms such as delusions and hallucinations are also prevalent in people who have MNCD. Sleep disturbance and anxiety symptoms are also common in people who have MNCD and often occur along with depression, psychosis, and agitation. BPSD, especially related to psychosis and expressed as agitation and problem wandering (safety issue), are the leading triggers for admission of a person who has MNCD to LTC.

BPSD can be a risk factor for MNCD as well as a risk factor for more rapid progression of MNCD, a symptom of MNCD due to neurobiological change, and an expression of unmet need (Kimchi and Lyketsos 2015). In addition, BPSD are the most common reason for caregiver stress, caregiver burnout, and entering LTC (Balestreri, Grossberg, and Grossberg 2000).

Biological Factors

Neural networks for cognition and emotion have extensive and reciprocal connections. Hence, it is not surprising that BPSD are universal in all stages and all etiologies of MNCD (van der Linde et al. 2016). Several neuroanatomic and neurochemical correlates for depression, psychotic symptoms, sleep disturbance, and apathy in people who have MNCD have been identified. Monoamine changes are robust findings in AD and may account for many observed symptoms of depression. The risk of psychosis of AD appears to be increased by several genes also implicated in schizophrenia. The circadian breakdown in the sleep-wake cycle commonly seen in AD may be due to degeneration of the suprachiasmatic nucleus (or circadian pacemaker or "body clock"). Psychosis in DLB appears to be related to cholinergic deficit. RBD is intricately related to synucleinopathies, such as DLB and PDD. Frontal lobe damage is associated with apathy and socially inappropriate behavior. Neurochemical alterations in the cholinergic and dopaminergic systems have also been implicated as cause of apathy in people who have MNCD. The presence of cerebrovascular disease correlates with depression in those who have MNCD. Low CSF 5-hydroxyindoleacetic acid and diminished orbitofrontal and caudate metabolism occur in depression associated with AD and PD. In AD, depression correlates with frontal hypometabolism. Depression in VaD is most common when the ischemic injury involves the deep white matter or there are multiple lacunes in the basal ganglia. Dysfunction of a related set of frontal-subcortical structures appears to be a common underlying feature of depression in MNCD. Delusions and agitation/aggression are more common and severe among homozygous APOE epsilon4 carriers than among heterozygous or APOE-epsilon4-negative individuals who have probable AD. Psychotic symptoms and other BPSD in mild AD have been linked to accelerated progression to severe AD, indicating that efforts to prevent and relieve BPSD in mild AD have the potential to slow the progression to more disabling cognitive and functional decline (Kimchi and Lyketsos 2015).

Biological factors also include hunger, thirst, sexual needs, comorbid physical health conditions (e.g. pain, adverse effects of medication, infection, constipation, dehydration), delirium, pre-existing chronic mental illness (e.g. schizophrenia, bipolar disorder),

Table 3.6 Prevalence of Use of Common Psychoactive Medications in Long-Term Care Populations and Risks Associated with Their Use

Psychoactive Medications (Commonly Used) (Point Prevalence)	Key Serious Adverse Risks for Physical Health	Key Serious Adverse Risks for Behavioral Health
Antipsychotics (e.g. risperidone, paliperidone, haloperidol, olanzapine, quetiapine, aripiprazole, ziprasidone, iloperidone, lurasidone, brexpiprazole, cariprazine, asenapine) (15–35)	Decline in ADLs, falls, increased mortality and stroke risk among residents who have MNCD, drug-induced Parkinsonism	Cognitive slowing, apathy, restlessness, dysphoria
Antidepressants (e.g. citalopram, escitalopram, sertraline, mirtazapine, duloxetine, venlafaxine, paroxetine, trazodone, desvenlafaxine, vilazodone, vortioxetine, levomilnacipran) (30–50)	Falls, risk of bleeding if used concomitantly with blood thinner (e.g. NSAID, aspirin, clopidrogel, warfarin), hyponatremia	Apathy, insomnia, agitation
Benzodiazepines (e.g. lorazepam, alprazolam, diazepam, clonazepam) (10–25)	Falls, decline in ADLs	Cognitive impairment, delirium, daytime sleepiness, dependence
Opioids (e.g. hydrocodone, oxycodone) and tramadol (20–50)	Falls, decline in ADLs	Cognitive impairment, daytime sleepiness, delirium, dependence
Anticonvulsants (e.g. valproate, gabapentin) (10–20)	Falls, decline in ADLs	Daytime sleepiness, delirium
Hypnotics (e.g. zolpidem, zaleplon, eszopiclone) (10–25)	Falls	Daytime sleepiness, dependence
Anticholinergic drugs (e.g. oxybutynin, tolterodine, diphenhydramine, hydroxyzine) (10–25)	Urinary retention, dry mouth, blurred vision	Cognitive impairment, visual hallucinations
Dopaminergic agents (e.g. levodopa, ropinirole, pramipexole, rotigotine) (5–10)	Dyskinesia	Delusions and hallucinations, delirium, daytime sleepiness, impulse dyscontrol (such as compulsive sexual behavior)
Corticosteroids (5–10)	Easy bruising, falls	Delirium, hypomania, mania, insomnia

and impaired hearing and/or vision. People who have MNCD are often given inappropriate medication (Table 3.6) that can cause BPSD. Undertreatment, overtreatment, and mistreatment of treatable medical and psychiatric conditions is also prevalent among people who have MNCD and often manifest as BPSD (see Tables 3.7 and 3.8).

Environmental Factors

Countertherapeutic staff approaches (e.g. impatience), excessive noise and stimulation, lack of structure and routine in daily life, inadequate lighting, lack of safe areas to pace and wander, inadequate exposure to nature, and confusing surroundings are some of the common environmental factors that often cause BPSD. The HCP should inquire into them and, if present, correct them.

Psychosocial Factors

Residents who have MNCD, even in advanced stages, are much more aware of the environment than is usually recognized (Desai et al. 2016). BPSD are often a response to the staff's not taking the resident's experiences and perspectives into account in the effort to understand what is distressing the resident. Caregivers' responses vary considerably and have the power to alter the trajectory of BPSD. Many residents experience significant periods of boredom and loneliness and because of MNCD are unable to address it themselves. In such situations, "agitation" and/or

Table 3.7 Common Untreated or Undercorrected Physical Health Problems among Residents Who Have Neurocognitive Disorder

Physical Health Problem	Point Prevalence (%)	Key Behavioral Health Concern Associated with Physical Health Problem
Hearing deficit	20–50	Depression or paranoia
Vision deficit	15–35	Depression, visual hallucination or illusion
Pain (acute, acute over chronic, chronic)	15–30	Depression, agitation, aggression
Constipation	20–60	Depression, agitation, aggression, delirium
Dehydration	10–20	Depression, fatigue, delirium
Urinary incontinence	10–30	Agitation, aggression
Pressure ulcer	5–20	Depression, agitation
Moderate to severe obesity	10–20	Depression, anxiety, sleep disturbance
Inappropriate medication	30–75	Cognitive impairment, agitation
Frailty	20–40	Cognitive impairment, depression
Undernutrition (including vitamin deficiency, especially vitamins B_{12} and D)	30–60	Depression, agitation, cognitive impairment
Obstructive sleep apnea	5–15	Cognitive impairment, insomnia
Hypoglycemic episodes due to overtreatment of diabetes	5–10	Anxiety, cognitive impairment, delirium
Hyponatremia	5–10	Cognitive impairment, agitation
Under- or overcorrection of hypothyroidism	5–10	Depression, anxiety, agitation, insomnia

Table 3.8 Prevalence, Key Concerns, and Evidence-Based Approaches for Common Psychiatric Disorders among Residents Who Have Major Neurocognitive Disorder

Psychiatric Disorder (Point Prevalence [%])	Key Concerns and Common Examples of Psychiatric Mistreatment or Undertreatment	Evidence-Based Approaches and Therapeutic Pearls
Major neurocognitive disorder (MNCD)/dementia (40–90)	– Undertreatment of reversible causes of cognitive impairment – Inappropriate use/nonuse of cholinesterase inhibitors and/or memantine	– Work-up to identify potentially reversible cause(s) of cognitive impairment – Appropriate use of cholinesterase inhibitors and/or memantine based on APA Practice Guidelines
Agitation and/or aggression as part of behavioral symptoms of MNCD (BPSD) (20–50)	– Overtreatment with psychotropic medication – Lack of knowledge, skill, and practice of psychosocial spiritual approaches	– Discontinue antipsychotics and, if necessary, replace them with safer alternatives, such as citalopram or dextromethorphan-quinidine (both off-label) – Staff training in person-centered care, communication skills, dementia care mapping, and SPPEICE
Depression due to a MNCD (10–30)	– Use of antidepressant to treat adjustment disorder	– Discontinue antidepressants and institute SPPEICE (e.g. individualized pleasant activity

Table 3.8 (cont.)

Psychiatric Disorder (Point Prevalence [%])	Key Concerns and Common Examples of Psychiatric Mistreatment or Undertreatment	Evidence-Based Approaches and Therapeutic Pearls
	– Suboptimal use of antidepressant for moderate to severe major depressive disorder and failure to recommend electroconvulsive therapy for severe/psychotic depression	schedule, individual psychotherapy) – Optimize appropriate antidepressant treatment based on APA Practice Guidelines for treatment of major depressive disorders
Prevalence of delirium (5–10; may be up to 80% among newly admitted residents receiving rehabilitation after hospitalization)	– Hypoactive delirium often mistaken for depression or missed – Underdiagnosis of medication-induced delirium	– CPE to accurately differentiate depression from delirium – High index of suspicion for medication-induced delirium (especially medications on Beers list)
Depression and/or distress (expressed as agitation) due to undertreated chronic pain among residents who have MNCD (10–20)	– Underuse of nondrug approaches to manage chronic pain – Underuse of antidepressant to treat chronic pain – Overuse of opioids for management of chronic noncancer pain	– Educate staff regarding nondrug approaches to manage chronic pain (e.g. relaxation strategies, cognitive strategies, hot and cold compresses, physical therapy, music, distraction) – Improve use of appropriate antidepressants to treat chronic pain and reduce use of opioids to treat noncancer pain
Psychotic symptoms due to MNCD and/or to a general medical condition or to medication among residents who have MNCD (20–40)	– Inadequate work-up to clarify etiology of psychotic symptoms – Overuse of antipsychotics for management – Failure to recognize psychosis triggering severe agitation	– CPE to clarify etiology of psychotic symptoms and institute appropriate treatment – Implement SPPEICE and limit use of antipsychotics for severe symptoms – Use antipsychotics judiciously and promptly when necessary – Use of pimavanserin to treat Parkinson's disease psychosis
Anxiety symptoms (persistent worries, panic attacks, seeking repeated reassurances) (15–30)	– Overuse of benzodiazepines for management – Inadequate use of relaxation, mindfulness-based, and distraction strategies	– Minimize use of benzodiazepines and replace with safer approaches when appropriate (e.g. antidepressant, buspirone) – Case-based staff education and training regarding relaxation and distraction strategies they can help resident use
Mild to moderate agitation and aggressive behaviors, including resident-to-resident aggression and sexually inappropriate	– Underrecognition by staff that these behaviors usually are a reaction to one or more unmet needs (e.g. experiences and perspectives of residents not being heard and understood,	– Educate and train staff (e.g. train with *Bathing without a Battle* DVD; *Hand in Hand* DVD, a nursing home training tool kit by the CMS) and institute SPPEICE to better meet resident's needs

Table 3.8 (cont.)

Psychiatric Disorder (Point Prevalence [%])	Key Concerns and Common Examples of Psychiatric Mistreatment or Undertreatment	Evidence-Based Approaches and Therapeutic Pearls
behavior in the context of MNCD (10–30)	boredom, loneliness, pain, constipation) – Inappropriate use of PMT	– Taper and discontinue PMT
Severe and persistent agitation and aggressive behaviors in the context of MNCD (5–15)	– Undertreatment of multiple reversible factors contributing to these behaviors – Inappropriate and suboptimal PMT	– Identify and treat reversible contributing causes of these behaviors (e.g. pain, countertherapeutic staff approach) – Optimize appropriate PMT
Sleep disorder (15–30)	– Inappropriate use of hypnotics – Underuse of nondrug approaches	– Discontinue inappropriate hypnotics and optimize use of appropriate hypnotics – Institute sleep hygiene and other nondrug approaches
Behavioral symptoms due to use of psychotropic medication (10–20)	– Apathy, anxiety, insomnia due to antidepressants and/or antipsychotics – Cognitive impairment due to anticholinergic effects of many commonly used psychotropic medications (e.g. amitriptyline, paroxetine)	– Taper and discontinue offending medications – Minimize use of psychotropic medications that have anticholinergic activity
Behavioral symptoms due to inappropriate use of nonpsychotropic medication (10–20)	– Steroid- and opioid-induced mood, cognitive, and psychotic symptoms – Psychotic symptoms and impulse control problems due to Dopaminergic therapy used to treat Parkinson's disease and Parkinsonism	– Educate staff and primary care clinician and taper and discontinue steroids and or opioids as soon as feasible – Educate staff and primary care clinician and reduce dopaminergic therapy whenever feasible
Difficulty recognizing need for palliative and end-of-life care for residents who have advanced MNCD	– Futile and burdensome care for residents in last phase of life, causing further decline in quality of life – Inappropriate/suboptimal PMT to treat depression, agitation, and pain	– Institute palliative and hospice care that is in keeping with resident's values and wishes – Optimal appropriate PMT to treat depression, agitation, and pain

APA: American Psychiatric Association

"aggressive behaviors" are an expression of unmet psychosocial needs. MNCD can have a tremendous negative effect on a resident's self-esteem and feelings of security, especially if the resident has insight (partial or full) into the cognitive and functional limitations. Many behaviors labeled disturbing are personal expressions of the individual's way of coping with feelings of fragmentation and emptiness when the ability to self-soothe is diminished. In such situations, the resident needs empathic, mirroring responses from caregivers who can understand the symbolic meaning of such behaviors. Another example is a resident who has MNCD and constantly follows a family or professional caregiver (such a behavior is often called "shadowing") and frets when the person is out of sight. To this resident, who cannot remember the past or anticipate the future, the world can be strange and frightening. Staying close to a trusted and familiar caregiver may be the only thing that makes sense and provides security. Besides dependency, other personality factors also influence BPSD. Lower premorbid agreeableness (a personality factor) is associated with BPSD expressed as agitation and irritability.

Agitation is a generic term that includes verbally aggressive behaviors (e.g. swearing, threats), verbally nonaggressive behaviors (e.g. repetitive vocalization, pleas for help), physically aggressive behaviors (e.g. hitting, biting, scratching, kicking, pushing), and physically nonaggressive behaviors (e.g. pacing, wandering) (Cohen-Mansfield et al. 1996). The HCP should consider agitation and aggressive behaviors the resident's attempt to communicate or respond to an unmet need, such as hunger, thirst, need for affection, intimacy, or comfort. For example, taking clothes off may seem reasonable to a resident who has MNCD who feels hot and doesn't understand or remember that undressing in public is not a socially acceptable behavior. Aggressive behavior is often associated with invasion of the individual's personal sphere (for example, during toileting or dressing). Labeling resistance to help with personal activities as a behavioral disturbance seems inappropriate, as the resident often does not recognize the caregiver or understand the meaning of his or her actions. The resident may also be pushing staff away during personal care because she has neuropathic pain and hot water or touch may be causing distress. The resident's anger and aggressiveness is thus an appropriate response to a strange situation. A resident who screams frequently may be trying to communicate that he is lonely or experiencing some discomfort (e.g. irritating urinary catheter, arthritis pain, uncomfortable position while sitting or lying down). Some behaviors labeled "disturbing" (such as persistent yelling) may be the resident's trying to assert the right to be heard and to have needs met promptly. Whenever a staff notes "violent behavior," "inappropriate motor activity," "demanding behavior," etc., obtaining a more detailed account of the behavior, the context in which it occurs, and staff's approach will clarify that the behavior is a form of communication of an unmet need rather than a "medical or psychiatric problem." Spending time with the resident and addressing the discomfort are better interventions than labeling the resident's behavior as dysfunctional and prescribing a psychotropic medication.

Many behaviors are an attempt by the resident who has MNCD to feel connected to the surroundings. Looking for one's parent or wanting to go home, for example, may be a way of expressing the need to feel safe and secure in a strange environment. For the resident, being with her parents or at home calmed her and helped her feel connected to herself, others, objects, events, time, and place. Looking for one's small children (when all the children are middle-aged adults) may be the resident's way of expressing the need to be needed, to have responsibility, to be useful, to feel like a responsible adult rather than an invalid. Blaming someone for stealing one's belongings may be a mechanism to protect one's self-esteem from the blow of knowing one is slowly losing one's cognitive faculties. Blaming a spouse for infidelity may be an expression of insecurity and fear of being abandoned by the spouse or fear of being sent away (institutionalized). Repeatedly asking the same questions may be an expression of a need to be reassured that everything will be okay, that the resident will be not left to fend for herself.

Often, the resident's reality is different from the caregiver's. The resident and caregiver could dwell in different times and places. Residents who have MNCD can be seen as "displaced persons, refugees without a past, occupying the present but unconnected to it." Reminiscence work may greatly alleviate emotional distress in such situations. Catastrophic reaction is an acute expression of overwhelming anxiety and fearfulness some residents who have MNCD experience, usually triggered by a frustrating experience (e.g. difficulty dressing self) or anticipation of one. These spells are typically brief, lasting less than 30 minutes, and self-limited. Behaviors labeled "sexually inappropriate" (e.g. patting the knee of another resident, attempting to kiss another resident) are usually the resident's efforts to meet the needs of intimacy, affection, and sexual expression.

Spiritual Factors

Many people have been attending religious services regularly all their lives but lose this ritual to spiritual expression after entering LTC. Spirituality encompasses organized religion (and rituals associated with it) as well as love for nature, volunteer activities, and all activities that involve making the world a better place. Lack of meaningful activities, feeling that one is not in touch with God, and infrequent opportunities to participate in religious rituals are just some common examples of unmet spiritual needs that often are expressed as sadness, anxiety, agitation, and even aggressive behaviors.

Wandering

Wandering is one of the most common expressions of BPSD among people who have MNCD, often resulting in their entering a LTC facility that offers a secured unit or other safeguard (e.g. use of wanderguard alarm system). Wandering manifests as aimless or purposeful motor activity that involves leaving a safe place, getting lost, or intruding into inappropriate places or situations. Residents who have MNCD often wander, with rates of 35–40 percent per year of reported elopement from facilities. Residents who have MNCD and remain ambulatory and in relatively good physical health are at higher risk for expressing BPSD through wandering behaviors. Wandering often leads to early admission to LTC. Addressing the distress expressed as wandering primarily involves person-centered approaches that adapt the environment (biological, psychological, social, spiritual). For example, some residents may wander due to a need for socialization or stimulation and may benefit from a structured individualized activity schedule (such as a daily walking plan). The availability of safe and esthetically pleasing areas (for example, therapeutic gardens with walking paths) to wander may allow residents to walk without risk of elopement. There are no "antiwandering" drugs. For residents who wander but also have untreated moderate to severe depression and/or anxiety, a trial of antidepressants may be appropriate. We do not recommend prescribing antipsychotics to treat wandering. Other aberrant motor behaviors, such as restlessness and pacing, are also common expressions of BPSD in residents who have MNCD. The HCP should monitor residents who pace a lot for weight loss due to excessive caloric expenditure and for sores on their feet. Proper footwear is critical for all residents who ambulate, especially for residents who pace or wander and residents at high risk of pressure ulcer (e.g. residents who have diabetes mellitus, peripheral vascular disease). The HCP should consider referral to an orthopedic surgeon for evaluation of foot, knee, or hip joint problems, need for orthotics, and pain management for residents who pace and/or wander. We do not recommend restraining residents from pacing or wandering.

Pain

Undertreatment and inappropriate treatment of pain in residents who have MNCD is prevalent and one of the most common causes of BPSD. It is a myth that residents who have MNCD are less sensitive to pain. They may fail to interpret sensations as painful, may often be less able to recall pain, and may not be able to communicate it verbally to caregivers (Hallenbeck 2015). A label of MNCD/dementia may bias the interpretation of pain cues, and thus may contribute to lower use of as-needed analgesics by residents who have MNCD than by cognitively intact residents. Residents who have MNCD, like those who do not have MNCD, are at risk for multiple sources and types of pain, including chronic pain from conditions such as osteoarthritis and acute pain. (See Box 3.5.) Untreated pain in individuals who have MNCD can reduce quality of life; cause depression, agitation, or aggression; delay healing; disturb sleep and activity patterns; reduce function; and prolong hospitalization. Pain influences behavioral disturbances among residents in severe stages of MNCD more often than those in moderate or mild stages of MNCD, and residents who have chronic pain and severe MNCD are more likely to express distress by agitation/aggression than residents who have chronic pain and earlier stages of MNCD. Terminal stages of all MNCDs are often associated with pressure ulcers, limb contracture, and pain that can be much more difficult to assess (Mitchell 2015). There is no evidence that surgery for hip fracture improves pain. The primary reason to consider a surgical approach for hip fracture over a palliative care approach is when gain in function (especially ambulation) is the aim. We recommend palliative care (pain control, skin care, bed rest, DVT prophylaxis, personal care) to treat hip fracture for residents in severe or terminal stages of a MNCD because of their limited life expectancy and inability to participate in postoperative physical therapy (necessary to achieve gain in function). Scheduled analgesics are preferred over as-needed pain medication for residents who have MNCD because they typically forget to ask for pain medication. Regular (scheduled) administration of acetaminophen has been found to raise the levels of general activity, social interaction, and engagement with television or magazines among LTC residents who have moderate to severe MNCD, indicating undertreated musculoskeletal pain in this population. Pain assessment should also clarify acute versus chronic pain, one or more

BOX 3.5 Common Causes of Pain with Major Neurocognitive Disorder

Type of Pain	Common Cause
Acute pain	Fall with bruise and/or muscle sprain
	Fracture
	Urinary tract infection
	Postoperative
	Toothache
	Migraine and other headaches
	Muscle spasm
	Pressure ulcer
	Acute gout and other arthritic conditions or flare-ups
	Cancer with bone metastasis
	Polymyalgia rheumatic
	Acute ischemia/infarction (e.g. cardiac, mesentery)
	Deep vein thrombosis (e.g. in calf)
	Acute intestinal obstruction
Chronic pain	Arthritis (especially osteoarthritis, rheumatoid arthritis)
	Degenerative disc disease
	Spinal stenosis
	Diabetic neuropathy
	Fibromyalgia
	Chronic migraine and other chronic headaches
	Muscle contracture
	Compression fracture of the vertebrae
	Polymyalgia rheumatica
	Cancer with bone metastasis
	Intermittent claudication
	Parkinson's disease with muscle stiffness
	Irritable bowel syndrome
	Chronic constipation

causes of pain, and whether pain is nociceptive, neuropathic, or both, as the treatments of different pain syndromes are different.

Abrupt Decline

Over the course of MNCD, many residents may develop an abrupt decline in cognition. They may suddenly become more confused, with slurred speech, somnolence, agitation, tremulousness, unsteadiness, falls, and worsened incontinence. Often, this is due to a superimposed delirium often due to an infection such as a UTI, stroke, medication side effects, etc. Many older adults develop cognitive decline for the first time after a major surgery. Several perioperative factors, such as hypoxia and anesthetics, can cause postoperative cognitive decline, in some cases via triggering AD neuropathogenesis. At first glance, many of the people who have postoperative cognitive decline may present with delirium that seems to develop into MNCD, but on further detailed inquiry, a history of subtle cognitive and functional decline for months to years before surgery is usually obtained, indicating that the MNCD processes had started before the surgery.

Treatment of Major Neurocognitive Disorder

Comprehensive, multidisciplinary state-of-the-science treatment of MNCD has the potential to dramatically improve quality of life for residents living with MNCD (Brandt and Mansour 2016). See Box 3.6 for the role of various health care professionals in caring for residents who have MNCD. Treatment of a MNCD is treatment of its cause. Thus, treatment of a reversible MNCD is to treat the cause (correcting vitamin and nutritional deficiencies, treating depression, etc.). For all residents who have MNCD, the HCP should consider reducing and discontinuing all medications that are on the Beers list and/or have anticholinergic effects (American Geriatrics Society 2015). Box 3.7 lists the goals of treatment of irreversible MNCD. Early and comprehensive management of irreversible MNCD can delay the progression of symptoms and help maintain the quality of life of both the resident and the caregiver. Individualized and multimodal treatment plans are required to address the broad range of cognitive, behavioral, and psychological symptoms associated with all MNCDs (American Geriatrics Society 2011). Specialized care units for MNCD (dementia care units) may offer optimal care for residents who have advanced MNCD. When making any treatment decision for a resident who has a MNCD, the HCP must take into account both the resident's current level of functioning and the potential effect on quality of life. Parkinsonian symptoms often accompany some MNCDs (DLB, PDD, MSA, VaD, advanced stages of AD) and may benefit from speech, physical,

BOX 3.6 Health Care Team Members and Key Reasons for Seeking Their Help

Health Care Team Member	Key Reasons for Seeking Help
Primary care provider*	Accurate diagnosis of major neurocognitive disorder
	Assess appropriateness of use of ChEIs** and/or memantine
	Discontinuation of anticholinergic medication
	Discontinuation of medications on Beers list
	Optimal management of comorbid medical conditions
	Discussion with resident and family about goals of care
	Ongoing discussion regarding life-sustaining treatment
	Referral to psychiatrist for management of complex cases
Psychiatrist	Accurate diagnosis of major neurocognitive disorder
	Assess appropriateness of use of ChEIs** and/or memantine
	Prevention and relief of BPSD***
	Assess appropriateness of PMT****
	Assess capacity to make health care decisions
	Assess need for palliative care
	Consult regarding optimizing brain function
	Educate and train staff*****
	Guide facility leadership toward PCC culture
	Consult for gradual dose reduction of psychotropic meds
	Consult for addressing high-risk PMT***
	Consult for reducing use of antipsychotic medication
	Design programs to prevent staff burnout
Neuropsychologist	Clarify severity and etiology of cognitive decline
	Assess capacity to make health care decisions
	Consult regarding optimizing brain function
Gerontologist/psychologist	Provide individual psychotherapy
	Provide group psychotherapy
	Aid resolution of staff-resident conflict
	Educate and train staff
	Design programs to diminish caregiver burnout
Social worker	Provide individual psychotherapy
	Provide family therapy and conflict resolution
	Provide group psychotherapy
	Aid staff-resident conflict resolution
	Educate and train staff
	Design programs to diminish caregiver burnout
Nurse	Educate and train staff
	Teach relaxation strategies to residents and staff
	Design programs to diminish caregiver burnout
Speech language therapist	Therapy for hypophonia in Parkinson's disease
	Therapy for aphasia in early stages of MNCD
	Therapy for cognitive impairment in early stages of MNCD
Physical therapist	Therapy for Parkinsonism
Occupational therapist	Therapy for tremor-related disability

* Primary care providers: primary care physician, nurse practitioner, physician assistant

** ChEIs: cholinesterase inhibitors

*** BPSD: biopsychosocial spiritual distress

**** PMT: psychotropic medication therapy

***** Topics for staff education and training include: importance of validating residents' experiences and inquiring about and routinely incorporating residents' perspectives into care plans; psychosocial environmental approaches to manage BPSD in residents who have major neurocognitive disorder; nondrug management of pain; nondrug management of sexually inappropriate behavior; sleep hygiene and other nondrug approaches to manage insomnia/sleep disorder; relaxation strategies, mindfulness-based approaches; monitoring adverse effects of PMT; Beers list of drugs that are inappropriate for LTC populations; strategies to de-escalate resident aggression and prevent resident-to-resident aggression.

BOX 3.7 Goals of Treatment of Major Neurocognitive Disorders in Long-Term Care

Individual	Goal
Resident who has MNCD	Maintain dignity Slow cognitive decline Slow functional decline Improve quality of life Establish advance care directives early Establish research-specific advance directives early Prevent BPSD* Diagnose and promptly treat BPSD* Optimally treat excess disability Preserve strengths for as long as possible Achieve aging in place Ensure better transitions to and from hospitals/facilities Avoid futile or unnecessary medical care Achieve a timely, peaceful, and dignified death
Family of resident	Prevent and treat caregiver depression Address caregiver grief Reduce caregiver stress and burden Improve confidence and comfort level to make decisions Minimize the impact of caregiver stress on caregiver health

* BPSD: Biopsychosocial spiritual distress

and occupational therapy. Except for Parkinsonian symptoms in residents who have PDD, benefits of levodopa for Parkinsonian symptoms in other MNCDs may not outweigh risks (e.g. agitation, psychotic symptoms).

Treatment for Cognitive and Functional Deficits

Five MNCDs (AD, VaD, DLB, PDD, and FTD) account for 95 percent of all MNCDs in LTC populations. At present, no therapy has been shown to prevent, cure, or arrest the progression of cognitive and functional decline associated with these MNCDs (Small and Greenfield 2015). We recommend a trial of one of the ChEIs, such as donepezil, rivastigmine, or galantamine, for people who have a mild, moderate, or severe stage of AD, DLB, or PDD. ChEIs are not recommended for treatment of FTDs. We recommend a trial of memantine (N-methyl-D-aspartate [NMDA] receptor agonist), usually with a ChEI, for residents who have AD in moderate to severe stages. Residents who have MNCD may be more at risk of adverse effects and may have less beneficial effects from ChEIs and memantine than community-dwelling people who have MNCD because of the higher prevalence of frailty, medical comorbidity, and polypharmacy (especially anticholinergic medications) in LTC residents. Thus, ChEIs and memantine should be used with extra caution in LTC populations and we strongly recommend close monitoring of adverse effects and optimal staff education about adverse effects of these drugs. At the same time, residents who have MNCD should not be routinely denied a trial of a ChEI and/or memantine just because they are frail and have multiple medical comorbidities. Treatment with a ChEI and/or memantine has the potential for a small but clinically meaningful effect in slowing cognitive and functional decline, reducing the risk of BPSD in the future, and reducing the need for psychotropics in the future for many residents who have commonly occurring MNCDs.

Staging of AD through the application of cognitive scales such as the MOCA, SLUMS, or MMSE inherently limits the applied benefit to the drug's cognitive effects at the exclusion of behavioral and functional benefits. A relatively high proportion of LTC residents taking ChEIs may not be benefiting enough from these medications to warrant continuation. ChEIs should be tapered gradually rather than withdrawn abruptly to avoid a withdrawal effect. For residents in severe stages of MNCD, gradual tapering may not result in adverse clinical outcomes or sudden deterioration, although the HCP should monitor for such outcomes. Common adverse effects of ChEIs are nausea, vomiting, diarrhea, dizziness, vivid nighttime dreams, and insomnia. These adverse effects tend to be mild to moderate in severity but in frail residents who have MNCD, even mild adverse effects are burdensome and can significantly impair quality of life. In general, these adverse effects tend to wane within two to four days, so if residents can tolerate unpleasant effects in the early days of treatment, they may be more comfortable later on. Use of rivastigmine transdermal patch is associated with much lower gastrointestinal adverse effects than oral rivastigmine and hence is preferred over oral rivastigmine. Mild itching and redness at the site of the patch and mild rash at the site of the patch can occur. Changing the site of the patch every day and not using the same site for at least two weeks can usually reduce the risk of skin rash. Topical steroids can be used to treat the rash. With residents who have PDD, ChEIs may worsen tremor. Uncommon adverse effects of ChEIs include muscle cramp, bradycardia (which can be dangerous in residents who have cardiac conduction problems and/or residents taking beta blockers), syncope, decrease in appetite, and weight loss. ChEIs increase the production of gastric acid, a particular concern for those who have a history of peptic ulcer. Pre-existing bradycardia, sick sinus syndrome or conduction defects, undiagnosed nausea, vomiting, and diarrhea, gastritis, and ulcerative disease should be considered a relative contraindication for ChEIs. Finally, ChEIs may induce or exacerbate urinary obstruction, worsen asthma and chronic obstructive pulmonary disease (COPD), cause seizures, and exaggerate the effects of some muscle relaxants during anesthesia. Thus, the HCP should use extra precaution when prescribing ChEIs for residents who have cerebrovascular disease, seizure, or COPD. Residents taking anticholinergic medications may not benefit from ChEIs, and we strongly recommend that the HCP make an effort to discontinue anticholinergic medication before initiating ChEI therapy. Residents taking beta-blockers may have higher risks of dizziness and syncope with concomitant use of ChEIs. Table 3.9 shows the dosing and dosages of ChEIs. ChEIs should be given in the morning on a full stomach. If the person tolerates the starting dose, the dose of ChEIs should be increased after a minimum of four weeks. For frail residents and residents who are sensitive to medication adverse effects, the starting dose of ChEI can be half the standard starting dose (for example, donepezil can be given as 2.5 mg and then increased by 2.5 mg increments, galantamine can be given as 4 mg once a day and then increased by 4 mg increments, rivastigmine can be given as 1.5 mg once a day with food and then increased by 1.5 mg increments). When the resident who has AD gets to the terminal stages where there is no specific function that is being preserved (ability to recognize family, ability to answer simple questions, ability to eat with assistance), we recommend taking individuals off

Table 3.9 Cholinesterase Inhibitors and Memantine

Medication	Starting Dose and Dosing Schedule	Therapeutic Daily Dose (Range)
Donepezil	5 mg once a day after meals, may increase every 4 weeks by 5 mg to highest tolerated therapeutic daily dose	5–23 mg
Rivastigmine transdermal patch	4.6 mg/24 hours patch applied on a clean, dry, hairless part (upper back usually), may be increased every 4 weeks to the highest tolerated therapeutic daily dose	9.5–13.3 mg
Rivastigmine	1.5 mg twice daily after meals, may increase every 4 weeks by 3 mg/day to the highest tolerated therapeutic daily dose	6–12 mg
Galantamine extended release	8 mg once daily after meals, may increase every 4 weeks by 8 mg to the highest tolerated therapeutic daily dose	16–24 mg
Memantine extended release	7 mg once daily, may increase by 7 mg every 7 days to the highest tolerated therapeutic daily dose	14–28 mg (7–14 mg for residents who have creatine clearance less than 30)
Memantine	5 mg once a day, may increase by 5 mg per week to the highest tolerated therapeutic daily dose	20 mg in two divided doses (5–10 mg for residents who have creatine clearance less than 30)

Note: We recommend using a lower final dose for frail residents.

ChEIs and memantine treatment as well as other medications not necessary to maintain comfort (e.g. statins, vitamins, medications for osteoporosis, etc.).

The HCP should recognize the potential for cognitive rehabilitation for motivated residents in early stages of MNCD. An individualized comprehensive brain and memory wellness plan may help highly motivated residents in the early stages of MNCD to achieve highest levels of cognitive function and slow cognitive and functional decline (Anderson and Grossberg 2014; Haynes, Seifan, and Isaacson 2016). (See Boxes 3.2, 3.3, and Box 3.4 and Table 3.10.)

Memantine is an N-methyl D-aspartate (NMDA) receptor antagonist. The HCP should consider treatment with memantine for all residents who have moderate to severe AD. Adding memantine for a resident who is already taking a ChEI may provide added benefits. Expectations from memantine are similar to those from ChEIs in that 30–40 percent of residents taking memantine may have modest benefit. Benefit involves some slowing of cognitive and functional decline. In addition, residents who have AD and are taking memantine may have less agitation in the future. Memantine is started at 5 mg given at

Table 3.10 Mental Health Prevention and Wellness for Residents Who Have Major Neurocognitive Disorder and Residents at Risk for Major Neurocognitive Disorder

Prevention and Wellness Condition	Evidence-Based Strategies	Potential Outcome
Cognitive aging (aging-associated changes in cognitive function)	Exercise program, Mediterranean diet, online brain-training programs, discontinuation of drugs with anticholinergic properties	Improve cognitive well-being
Mild neurocognitive disorder	Exercise program, Mediterranean diet, online brain-training programs, discontinuation of drugs with anticholinergic properties	Prevent or delay progression of cognitive decline
Insomnia	Sleep hygiene, discontinuation of medications that cause/worsen insomnia, minimizing caffeinated drinks	Prevent progression to chronic insomnia and complication of major depressive disorder
Chronic pain	Hot and cold compress therapies, cognitive behavior therapy, relaxation strategies, physical therapy, exercise program	Prevent depression and cognitive dysfunction related to suboptimal control of chronic pain
Subsyndromal delirium	Multicomponent approaches, discontinuation of all unnecessary medication	Prevent progression to delirium
Boredom and loneliness	Continuous activities programming	Prevent agitation and aggression
Helplessness and existential angst	Individual psychotherapy (especially meaning-centered psychotherapy), regular interaction with a member of the clergy	Prevent progression to major depressive disorder
Fear of falls and related refusal to ambulate	Individual psychotherapy, relaxation strategies	Prevent progression to disabling phobia and dependence on wheelchair
Wish for assisted dying and/or euthanasia	Palliative care, meaning-centered psychotherapy	Prevent suicide and attempted suicide

Note: Multicomponent approaches: Frequent reorientation, involvement in cognitively stimulating activities, promotion of sleep with sleep-inducing stimuli (e.g. relaxation tapes, warm milk) and a sleep-promoting environment (e.g. noise reduction), encouragement of physical activity, use of visual and auditory aids, early treatment of dehydration

bedtime and increased at 5 mg a week interval to the therapeutic dose of 10 mg in the morning and 10 mg at bedtime. Alternatively, (and preferably), long-acting memantine formulation (extended release) can be given once a day starting at 7 mg daily for 7 days and increasing by 7 mg/week to reach 28 mg daily. Residents taking 10 mg of memantine twice daily can switch to memantine ER 28 mg once daily without titration. For residents who have severe kidney disease, frail residents, and residents who cannot tolerate 20 mg/day of memantine or 28 mg/day of once-a-day formulation, we recommend a final dose of 10 mg/day given at bedtime for memantine with close monitoring for adverse effects. Adverse effects of memantine include constipation, dizziness, agitation, headache, and transient hallucinations. Memantine may interact with other NMDA receptor antagonists, such as methadone, dextromethorphan (often used to treat cough in LTC populations and, in combination with quinidine, used for treatment of pseudobulbar affect). Such combinations should be avoided. Memantine has 5HT3-blocking effects and may theoretically protect against some gastrointestinal side effects of ChEIs.

The cholinergic system in FTD appears to be relatively intact. Thus, we do not recommend prescribing ChEIs for residents who have FTD. Memantine also has not been found to be useful for managing DLB, PDD, and FTDs, although preliminary data suggest that glutamate may play a role in FTD.

Person-Centered Approaches to Prevent and Reduce Biopsychosocial-Spiritual Distress

The goal of person-centered approaches is to promote the dignity, safety, and well-being of the resident (Galik 2016). It includes efforts to prevent BPSD, reduce the severity of BPSD, and reduce caregiver distress (Brasure et al. 2016; British Columbia, Canada, Department of Health 2012). Person-centered approaches include staff education and training to create an environment that supports the resident's capacity to live the best life possible by routinely and proactively addressing biological, psychological, social, spiritual, and environmental needs of residents who have MNCD (Livingston et al. 2014). Such approaches include discontinuing harmful medication, optimal treatment of comorbid physical and mental health conditions, architectural approaches to make the physical environment more soothing and accommodating to residents' disabilities, and strength-based personalized psychosocial sensory spiritual environmental initiatives and creative engagement (SPPEICE) (Desai and Grossberg 2017). See Table 3.11 (Morley and Cruz-Oliver 2014; Brasure et al. 2016). SPPEICE are the primary mode (first line) of person-centered approaches for helping residents live the best life possible, preventing BPSD, and reducing BPSD. Commonly employed SPPEICE include structured and unstructured activities, exercise, music, dance, reminiscence, massage therapy, aromatherapy, pet therapy (animal-assisted therapy), therapeutic gardens, simulated presence therapy (e. g. hearing family members' taped recordings), painting, other activities that allow creative expression, and spirituality (Brasure et al. 2016). Although research support for these approaches is modest, lack of robust effect is because the activities are not sufficiently individualized, not done as regularly and consistently, nor given sufficient time to show benefits. Daily exercises (walking, resistance training, flexion, and stretch exercises) improve "functional fitness" and are critical for maintaining muscle mass and slowing cognitive and functional decline. Music-based activities should also be routinely offered, as the effects can be remarkable, as shown wonderfully by the movie *Alive Inside* (www.aliveinside.us). Viewing this movie should be mandatory for all staff working in LTC.

There is growing consensus that spirituality is of great importance for not only those who have MNCD but also for their caregivers. Often it is at the later stages (and even in terminal stages) that the spiritual experiences of those who have MNCD are most profound. Accordingly, the decline in cognitive functioning does not reflect a loss of spiritual capacity, and those who have advanced MNCD remain capable of high levels of spiritual well-being and engagement in spiritual activities, rituals, and interactions. Helping a resident who has MNCD continue to observe faith can be beneficial and rewarding for both the resident and family caregivers. Songs and prayers from childhood often stay firmly rooted in the memory long after MNCD takes its toll.

Environmental approaches, such as bright light therapy, also have the potential to prevent and reduce BPSD (especially insomnia, depression, and agitation). Bright light has a modest benefit in improving

Table 3.11 Examples of Strength-Based Personalized Psychosocial Sensory Spiritual Environmental Initiatives and Creative Engagement (SPPEICE) for Residents Who Have Major Neurocognitive Disorder

Therapeutic Initiative/Approach (professional delivering the approach)	Common Indication	Strength of the Resident
Individual psychotherapy (licensed therapist)	Depression and/or anxiety Stress management	Relatively preserved cognitive function
Group psychotherapy (licensed therapist)	Depression and/or anxiety Stress management	Relatively preserved cognitive function
Individualized pleasant activity schedule (facility staff with guidance by mental health professional)	Prevent and treat boredom, loneliness, and depression	Applicable to all residents irrespective of level of cognitive function
Bright light therapy (nursing staff with education and guidance by mental health professional)	Prevent and treat seasonal affective disorder, insomnia, and some behavioral symptoms associated with MNCD	Capacity to sit in one place for 15 minutes or more at a time
TimeSlips (www.timeslips.org) (facility staff trained in TimeSlips)	Prevent and treat boredom, loneliness, and agitation	Relatively good vision and language functions
Cognitive Stimulation Therapy (CST) (www.cstdementia.com) (facility staff trained in CST)	Prevent and treat boredom, cognitive decline, and agitation	Relatively good language functions
Music therapy (music therapist) and music-based activities (recreational therapist, nursing staff)	Prevent and treat depression, anxiety, insomnia, and agitation	Relatively good auditory function
Drawing, coloring, and other art-based activities (recreational activity therapist, nursing staff)	Prevent and treat depression, anxiety, and agitation	Reasonably good ability to draw and/or color
Aromatherapy (recreational activity therapist, nursing staff)	Prevent and treat depression, anxiety, insomnia, and agitation	Reasonably good olfactory function
Massage therapy (nursing staff)	Prevent and treat insomnia, anxiety, depression, and agitation	Useful to almost all residents (extra caution with residents who have neuropathy and allodynia [experience touch as pain])
Pet-/animal-assisted therapy	Prevent and treat anxiety, depression, and agitation	Useful for all residents, especially residents who have history of having pets
Gardening/Eden experiment	Prevent and treat anxiety, depression, and agitation	Useful for all residents, especially residents who have history of engaging in gardening
Montessori-based activities	Prevent and treat eating difficulties, anxiety, depression, and agitation	Useful for all residents
Physical activity/Exercise program (includes Tai Chi, yoga, walking program) (nursing staff)	Prevent and treat depression, anxiety, insomnia, agitation, and chronic pain	Reasonably good upper and/or lower limb movement functions
Online brain-training program (nursing staff with guidance from mental health professional)	Optimize cognitive well-being and slow cognitive decline	At least some motivation and relatively preserved cognitive functioning

Table 3.11 (cont.)

Therapeutic Initiative/Approach (professional delivering the approach)	Common Indication	Strength of the Resident
Support group (early-stage MNCD, stroke) (any LTC staff with guidance from mental health professional)	Reduce emotional toll MNCD/ stroke can take on the resident and improve emotional well-being	Willing residents
Dignity therapy	Prevent and treat depression during last phase of life	Relatively preserved cognitive functioning

some cognitive and noncognitive (e.g. mood, sleep) symptoms of MNCD.

The health care team should make every effort to inquire into and understand the experiences and perspectives of residents who have MNCD, even in advanced stages (Desai et al. 2016). Research has shown that individuals who have MNCD retain a remarkable level of awareness even in advanced stages (Clare 2010). Residents who have MNCD should be considered expert in what will make their lives more meaningful and happy. Professional and family caregivers need to develop the skill to follow their lead (expressed verbally and nonverbally).

STAR Approach to Assessment and Treatment of Biopsychosocial-Spiritual Distress

We recommend the STAR approach for understanding, preventing, and reducing BPSD.

S: Safety and security of self and others should be assessed and addressed first. This includes discussion of need for inpatient psychiatric treatment for behavioral emergencies.

T: Team approach is recommended to identify triggers and modifiable causes of BPSD.

A: Action plan (individualized treatment plan with SPPEICE and, when appropriate, pharmacological approaches) should be devised and implemented.

R: Reassessment of the response to treatment and appropriate modification of person-centered approaches if the response is inadequate.

Ensuring safety and security is crucial, as often BPSD may be severe and can be expressed in a potentially life-threatening manner (such as attempted suicide) or as behaviors that pose risk to other residents (such as pushing another resident, causing a fatal head injury) and to staff (such as punching staff in the face). Ensuring safety is also crucial, as agitation in residents may put them or others at risk for serious injury (such as falls and fracture). If safety cannot be ensured, alternative placement of the resident may be necessary (such as an acute inpatient psychiatric unit for a resident who made a serious attempt at suicide). In situations of behavioral emergency (severe agitation or aggression), emergency administration of psychotropic medication (e.g. lorazepam or haloperidol) may be necessary (orally or intramuscularly) to stabilize the resident before team-based assessment can be undertaken or transfer to an emergency department of a local hospital can be safely initiated. Identifying triggers is important, as modifying triggers often ameliorates BPSD. Medical disorders (such as untreated pain, UTI) and psychiatric disorders (MDD, generalized anxiety disorder) are common causes of agitation in residents who have MNCD and are eminently treatable. A typical psychosocial-environmental approach can involve continuous activity programming tailored to the unique needs, strengths, and interests of each resident that can prevent and abort many agitated behaviors in residents who have MNCD. Not all agitation needs intervention. If the resident does not seem to be distressed (e.g. pacing without any distressed facial expression), then it is best to tolerate the agitation and leave the resident alone, as efforts to evaluate and intervene may paradoxically cause distress in some residents. Although SPPEICE is thought to have virtually no reports of adverse effect in research, some residents may experience adverse effects (Brasure et al. 2016). For example, some music-based approaches may increase distress. Although such negative reactions are usually mild, they add to distress and need to be addressed.

Clinical Case 3: "Leave me alone"

Over the last several weeks, Mrs. L, who has MNCD due to probable AD in moderate stage, had been growing agitated in the afternoon and evening, attempting to leave, and would become physically aggressive when prevented from leaving. Mrs. L often yelled, "Leave me alone, let me go." Mrs. L was taking citalopram 40 mg daily, donepezil 10 mg daily in the morning, and memantine 10 mg twice daily for MNCD and anxiety symptoms. These medications had helped decrease Mrs. L's agitation to some extent, but she continued to have at least one incident a week of physical aggression toward staff. Mrs. L was referred to a consultant psychiatrist for more medication to "control her aggression." After comprehensive psychiatric evaluation with team discussion, the psychiatrist ruled out easily correctable causes (e.g. anticholinergic medication, medical conditions). The psychiatrist met with the team members (Mrs. L's family, certified nursing assistant, licensed practical nurse, social worker) and discussed various potential SPPEICE that could be instituted. Mrs. L's daughter mentioned that her mother had always loved to work in the house rather than watch TV or play games. Mrs. L had never had pets and did not like them and had never been a regular listener of music. The team decided to give Mrs. L simple tasks, such as setting the table, folding napkins, putting letters in envelopes. Other interventions, such as pets or music group, were not selected. After two weeks of implementing these person-centered approaches, Mrs. L had become significantly less distressed, as shown by reduction in agitated behaviors, and was more easily reassured and redirected.

Teaching Points

Knowing the resident well (including the resident's role in life before entering LTC, the resident's daily interests, and what activities give the resident meaning in life [life history]) is key to significantly improving the success rate of SPPEICE. If the team had not tried to address Mrs. L's underlying need to feel useful and engage in activities that gave meaning to her life, her agitation and aggression could have continued and she may even have been prescribed antipsychotic medication, putting her at risk for accelerated cognitive and functional decline.

Psychotropic Medication

The Food and Drug Administration (FDA) has not approved any medication (including antipsychotics) for the management of BPSD in people who have MNCD. The FDA has approved dextromethorphan-quinidine for the treatment of pseudobulbar affect typically seen among individuals who have ALS but also seen among individuals who have MNCD. The FDA has approved pimavanserin for the treatment of PD psychosis. Psychotropic medications may be appropriate in a variety of clinical situations. (See Table 3.12.) Citalopram, dextromethorphan-quinidine, and atypical antipsychotics (risperidone, olanzapine, and aripiprazole, in particular) have been found to have modest benefit in reducing severe and persistent BPSD in AD, but the latter carry substantial risks (Porteinsson et al. 2014; Cummings et al. 2015). Risperidone is the only antipsychotic approved for short-term (6 weeks) treatment of severe behavioral and psychological symptoms of MNCD (symptoms are unresponsive to psychosocial interventions or there is severe and complex risk of harm) in Australia, Canada, Great Britain, and New Zealand (The Royal Australian and New Zealand College of Psychiatrists 2016; National Institute of Health and Clinical Excellence 2012). Hence, the use of antipsychotics should be restricted to residents who have severe and persistent BPSD that is posing significant danger to self and others (emergency situations) or in the presence of severe, disabling psychotic symptoms and/or severe agitation and aggressive behaviors (American Psychiatric Association 2016). Before initiating antipsychotics, the HCP should rule out treatable medical comorbidity (including medication induced BPSD), and it is important to ensure that no environmental factors are directly responsible for the severe BPSD (e.g. countertherapeutic staff approach that escalates distress expressed as mild agitation to severe agitation) (Kales, Gitlin, and Lyketsos 2014). Citalopram, olanzapine, and risperidone do not appear to be effective in managing BPSD in individuals who have DLB, but there is some support for the use of clozapine, clonazepam, and ramelteon (Stinton et al. 2015). Also, individuals who have DLB have extreme sensitivity to high-potency antipsychotic medications (e.g. haloperidol, fluphenazine, risperidone, paliperidone) and thus the HCP should avoid these medications due to increased risk of morbidity and mortality. Pimavanserin (first-line agent), clozapine (second-line agent), and quetiapine (third-line agent) are appropriate for treatment of severe psychotic symptoms in residents who have PD and PDD if reduction of dopaminergic agents is not

Table 3.12 Evidence-Based Psychotropic Medication Therapy to Manage Commonly Occurring Mental Health Disorders among Residents Who Have Major Neurocognitive Disorder

Mental Health Disorder	First-Line Psychotropic Medication(s)	Psychotropic Alternative(s) to Consider in Certain Situations
Major neurocognitive disorder (Alzheimer's disease, Lewy bodies, Parkinson's disease, cerebrovascular disease)	Cholinesterase inhibitors and/or memantine	No other evidence-based option
Delirium associated with severe agitation	Antipsychotics per 2010 NICE guidelines for prevention and treatment of delirium	Benzodiazepines to manage severe anxiety in end-of-life delirium
Major depressive disorder	Antidepressants and, for nonresponsive or partially responsive residents, or residents who have psychotic symptoms, atypical antipsychotics per 2010 APA practice guidelines for treatment of major depressive disorder	Electroconvulsive therapy (ECT) for life-threatening depression
Severe apathy due to MNCD not responding to SPPEICE and not due to any treatable medical comorbidity	Methylphenidate	Sertraline, bupropion
Pseudobulbar affect	Dextromethorphan and quinidine combination	Antidepressants if dextromethorphan-quinidine not tolerated, not available, or not effective
Persistent agitation and/or aggression associated with MNCD not responding to SPPEICE and not due to any treatable medical comorbidity	Citalopram and escitalopram per 2011 AGS guidelines for treatment of psychotic symptoms and neuropsychiatric symptoms of MNCD in older adults	Antipsychotics for severe and persistent aggressive behaviors not responding to SPPEICE and antidepressants
Psychotic symptoms among residents who have MNCD due to Parkinson's disease	Pimavanserin	Clozapine
Generalized anxiety disorder	Antidepressants per 2011 NICE guidelines for treatment of generalized anxiety disorder	Low-dose short-term use of short-acting benzodiazepines
Insomnia disorder	Ramelteon, suvorexant, melatonin	Short-term use of low-dose trazodone
REM sleep behavior disorder	Melatonin	Low-dose clonazepam
Hypersomnia among residents who have obstructive sleep apnea	Modafinil, armodafinil	Low-dose stimulants if first-line therapy not tolerated, not available, or not effective

effective or clinically contraindicated or not tolerated. SSRIs (selective serotonin reuptake inhibitors) are usually given to treat anxiety, depression, obsessive-compulsive symptoms, and agitation in residents who have FTD based on well-described serotonergic deficits in FTD. Residents who have FTD are particularly prone to developing extrapyramidal side effects with use of antipsychotics because of dopaminergic deficits seen in the brain of people who have FTD.

Inappropriate prescription of psychotropic medication (including psychotropic polypharmacy) is prevalent among LTC residents who have MNCD and may be the primary cause of resident distress expressed as agitation, aggressive behaviors, anxiety, insomnia, and apathy (see Table 3.7) (Jacquin-Piques et al. 2015). In addition, inappropriate psychotropic medication causes substantial additional morbidity and functional decline in this vulnerable population. For all residents who have MNCD, the HCP should routinely initiate periodic gradual dose reduction of all appropriate psychotropic medications (not just antipsychotics) and discontinue inappropriate psychotropic medications. Use of antipsychotics by residents who have MNCD carries a risk of increased mortality, cerebrovascular accident, hospitalization, dysphagia, pneumonia, Parkinsonism, tardive dyskinesia, and hip fracture. Despite these risks, antipsychotics have a role in the management of severe BPSD in residents who have MNCD (Jennings and Grossberg 2013). Atypical antipsychotics (such as risperidone, olanzapine) are preferred over typical (conventional) antipsychotics (such as haloperidol). SSRIs carry increased risk of bleeding, especially in residents also taking NSAIDs (e.g. ibuprofen, naproxen, diclofenac), antiplatelet therapies (acetylsalicylic acid [aspirin], clopidrogel, dipyridamole), and/or anticoagulant (e.g. warfarin, dabigatran, rivaroxaban, apixaban). SSRIs also carry increased risk of hyponatremia, especially if used concomitantly with diuretics, such as furosemide and hydrochlorothiazide. The use of antipsychotics by residents who have MNCD should be restricted to situations in which the resident poses an imminent danger to self and/or others due to severe and persistent BPSD and for behavioral emergency. In addition, the HCP should prescribe the lowest effective dose and closely monitor any adverse effects. The use of any psychotropic medication by residents who have MNCD is fraught with serious risks, and hence informed consent from the resident and/or the surrogate decision-maker is crucial before initiating psychotropic medication therapy. It is important for the prescriber to educate the resident, family, and staff that typically benefits are modest and efforts to gain more from medication (by increasing the dose) may cause more harm than benefit. The HCP should recognize that approximately one-third of LTC residents who have MNCD are prescribed antipsychotics, in many instances with inappropriate reason (e.g. wandering) and/or at inappropriately high dose. As a direct result of such excessive use in the context of known severe risks associated with use of antipsychotics by people who have MNCD (especially risk of stroke and mortality), the Centers for Medicare and Medicaid Services (CMS) initiative as mandated by the US Congress to reduce the use of antipsychotic medication has resulted in the Department of Health and Human Services expanding the efforts to reduce the use of antipsychotics by older adults who have MNCD.

Addressing Medical Comorbidity

More than 60 percent of people who have MNCD have three or more advanced physical health conditions. (See Table 3.13.) People who have MNCD have a higher incidence of Parkinsonism, seizures, infections, malnutrition, sensory impairment, hip fractures and other injuries, and pressure sores than residents who do not have MNCD. Lack of treatment, overtreatment, and undertreatment of medical comorbidity is prevalent among residents who have MNCD and often manifests as agitation and aggression. (See Table 3.7.) Optimal diagnosis and treatment of comorbid physical illnesses are essential components of the management of MNCD and are key to sustaining cognition in the resident who has MNCD and to preventing BPSD. The HCP who is treating comorbidity in residents who have MNCD should weigh the potential benefits against the burdens imposed by such treatment. Also, the goals of treating comorbidity should be in keeping with the resident's overall goals of care (palliative [comfort only] versus life-prolonging treatment). For every resident who has MNCD, the HCP should consider discontinuing medication with potential for significant anticholinergic symptoms. Residents who have MNCD are frequently transferred to emergency rooms and hospitalized for medical conditions (such as pneumonia), putting them at high risk for delirium, falls, need for restraint, and functional decline during and after hospitalization despite successful treatment of the medical condition. Hospitalization for residents who have MNCD (especially frail residents and residents in severe and terminal stages of MNCD) is extremely stressful. The HCP should discuss all of these risks of hospitalization before deciding to hospitalize the resident and ideally soon after the resident enters LTC. Many hospitalizations (e.g. due to infection [such as pneumonia]) are eminently preventable by instituting

Table 3.13 Common Advanced Physical Health Problems among Residents Who Have Major Neurocognitive Disorder and Associated Mental Health Concerns

Common Advanced Physical Health Problem (point prevalence)	Key Associated Mental Health Concern	Key Commonly Used Psychotropic Medication to Avoid or Use with Extra Caution
Cerebrovascular accident (20–40)	Cognitive impairment, depression	Antipsychotics
Coronary heart disease (20–40)	Depression	Tricyclic antidepressants
Heart disease with prolonged QTc interval (20–40)	Depression	Citalopram, ziprasidone
Congestive heart failure (10–30)	Depression	Tricyclic antidepressants
Chronic obstructive pulmonary disease (10–30)	Anxiety, depression	Benzodiazepines
Stage 4 or higher chronic kidney disease (10–30)	Depression, chronic pain	Lithium, gabapentin, memantine, paliperidone
Morbid obesity (10–20)	Depression	Olanzapine, quetiapine, valproate, mirtazapine
Obstructive sleep apnea (5–20)	Depression, insomnia	Benzodiazepines
Diabetes (15–35)	Depression, cognitive impairment	Olanzapine, quetiapine
Hip fracture(s) (15–25)	Depression, chronic pain	Benzodiazepines
Epilepsy (10–20)	Cognitive impairment, depression	Bupropion, clozapine

treatment in the facility. Many residents who have advanced stages of MNCD receive medication of questionable benefit but incur substantial associated costs, including hospitalization. For all residents who have advanced MNCD, the HCP should consider discontinuing medication that is of questionable benefit (such as statins, vitamins, medications for osteoporosis). We recommend psychiatric consultation (preferably by a geriatric psychiatrist) to relieve distress typically expressed as agitation by residents who have MNCD and have been hospitalized.

Palliative Care

High-quality palliative care is a key component of comprehensive care of all LTC residents who have MNCD (Desai and Grossberg 2011). MNCDs are the sixth most common cause of death among older adults. Discussion of the wishes of a person who has MNCD regarding life-prolonging treatment during advanced stages (moderate, severe, and terminal stage) should ideally take place when the person is in the mild stages (preferably the first half of the mild stage) because in this stage, the person retains the capacity to make medical decisions, fully participate in the discussion, and express wishes to the family (Brody 2016). In general, as the MNCD progresses, the burdens of life-prolonging treatment (such as hospitalization for pneumonia) increase dramatically and the potential benefits (such as increased duration of survival and improved quality of life) decrease considerably. Families of most residents who are in the terminal stages of MNCD opt for "comfort only" care (indicating no life-prolonging treatment, such as treatment of pneumonia, but want all treatment interventions that improve comfort and reduce pain and discomfort). Some families of residents may not want to wait for terminal stages but even in severe stages may opt for "comfort only" care. Other families of residents in severe stages may want life-prolonging treatment. The family may choose life-prolonging treatment for a person in severe stages of MNCD for several reasons: because they are not sure what the loved one would want and are erring on the "side of caution"; or because they are not ready to "let go" or feel that not providing life-prolonging treatment means they are "giving up" instead of understanding it as "letting go"; or think that this is what their loved one would want even in severe stages. Many family members may not be fully aware of the considerable burdens and limited benefits potentially life-prolonging interventions (e.g. hospitalization for treatment of pneumonia, tube feeding for management of poor food intake and severe weight loss) pose to residents in severe stages of MNCD. The HCP should assure the family that there is no right or wrong answer and help the family understand what the person who has MNCD would want and to keep their promise and respect the wishes of their loved one. The HCP should also understand the tremendous grief (and sometimes guilt) the family may be dealing with at that time, as these can influence decisions. Addressing these complex feelings can help the family make the decision regarding life-prolonging treatment that is in keeping with the wishes and values of the resident who has MNCD.

Other aspects of palliative care – such as when to forgo cardiopulmonary resuscitation ("Do Not Resuscitate" [DNR] order), when to forgo intubation ("Do Not Intubate" [DNI] order), when to forgo hospitalization ("Do Not Hospitalize" [DNH] order), degree of pain control versus adverse effects of pain medications (such as severely compromised awareness), placement of a feeding tube, criteria for palliative sedation, and criteria for referral to hospice – should also be discussed as early in the course of MNCD as is possible and with the involvement of the family (Powers and Herrington 2016). Complications related to a feeding tube account for half of all emergency department visits by residents who have advanced MNCD and are being tube fed. Residents in mild to moderate stages of MNCD who are frail and have advanced physical health conditions (such as severe congestive heart failure with very low ejection fraction, end-stage chronic obstructive pulmonary disease, end-stage renal disease) may also benefit from switching goals of care from life prolonging to palliative if this is in keeping with the resident's values and wishes. It is crucial in all discussions that the HCP focus more on understanding the values of the person who has MNCD, what gives the person meaning in life, and importance that the person places on how strictly his or her wishes are to be carried out by the surrogate decision-maker (i.e. that advance care planning document is more than a document, that it is a family covenant or promise).

Special Populations and Special Issues

Hospitalization for psychiatric emergency, sex and sexuality, aging in place, capacity to make medical decisions, and caregiver well-being are of particular concern if residents who have MNCD are to have high quality of life.

Hospitalization for Psychiatric Emergency

Residents who have MNCD may require admission to a psychiatric unit for treatment of behavioral emergencies and severe persistent and treatment resistant BPSD (often expressed as severe physical aggression, severe depression with suicide attempt or minimal oral intake). Admission to a geriatric psychiatry or medical psychiatric unit is preferable over general psychiatric unit when such option is available. Many state laws prohibit such admission without involvement of law enforcement agencies, which adds additional strain on the resident needing help, their loved ones and the long-term care staff. Although admission to psychiatric units for evaluation and management of behavioral emergencies is necessary in some residents who have MNCD and severe psychiatric symptoms, in many such cases the admission could have been prevented by early recognition and aggressive evidence-based treatment of the psychiatric disorders combined with person-centered approaches either by availability of psychiatric team at the facility, consultation with a geriatric psychiatrist via telepsychiatry, or by an outpatient psychiatric team. Transfers to a psychiatric unit from a LTC facility should be undertaken only after ensuring that such a treatment intervention is in keeping with the resident's goals of care. For many residents in severe or terminal stage of MNCD who have documented "comfort only" measures as goals of care, referral to hospice and sedation with psychiatric medications may be more appropriate than transfer to a psychiatric unit. If the resident is admitted to a psychiatric unit, the HCP should discuss palliative care goals with the resident and the family as soon as possible after admission.

Sex and Sexuality

Sexuality conceptualized in the broadest terms includes affection, romance, companionship, personal grooming, touch, and the need to feel attractive and feminine or masculine. Thus, sexual activity is any activity that portends the sensation of "feeling loved." Sexual expression among residents is a basic human need. Many residents feel sexually unattractive. The major mode of sexual expression as seen by LTC residents is trying to remain physically attractive. Sexual identity is closely interwoven with one's concept of self-worth. Denying a resident's sexuality can deleteriously affect not only the resident's sex life but also self-image, social relationships, and emotional well-being (Agronin 2015). For a LTC facility to provide a nurturing environment that promotes the health and well-being of the person as a whole, sexuality can not be ignored. It is important to recognize that many LTC residents have sexual thoughts and fantasies. Libido persists despite infirmity and institutionalization. Sexual behavior in younger years is a strong predictor of current behavior. For many residents, sexual expression is limited to caressing, kissing, hugging, or mutual manual genital stimulation. However, self-stimulation is not rare, particularly among males. Female residents often find few potential partners, due to increasing demographic gender disparity in the LTC. Also, for the current generation of residents, most male residents have a living spouse, whereas most female residents are widowed.

Physicians, staff, and family should address this need as part of their duty to enhance the quality of life and well-being of the residents. LTC staff should make every reasonable effort to support privacy and sexual needs of residents. Staff and family need to understand that residents (at any age) maintain a significant degree of sexual drive and often wish to be sexually expressive. Residents who have MNCD and are in a romantic or sexual relationship should be assessed carefully for capacity to participate in such a relationship. Implications of the progression of MNCD for the relationship should be anticipated, and contingencies should be developed for evolving needs for supervision and advocacy. The staff should protect residents' rights to homosexual and interracial relationships. Institutional and staff biases against sexual expression of all residents should be addressed through educational and training programs and the creation of clear institutional policies that support residents' rights. The facility should make provisions for staff nonparticipation in direct care when the implications of the sexual activity in care are unavoidable and are morally or religiously offensive to the staff member. At the same time, staff members should not be permitted to refuse to provide care in general for a sexually active resident.

Structured and regimented environments leave residents in a situation where control over most aspects of their lives is eroding. Ensuring privacy is of paramount importance. Residents' personal activities should not be discussed, documented, judged, or gossiped about. Many staff and family members may think that it is not necessary for residents to maintain sexuality. Use of fixed scheduling and treatment priorities as an excuse to deter intimacy among residents should be discouraged. Compromising privacy is not justified even if physical health can be enhanced. Cultural diversity among staff and residents in areas of sexuality is as important to address as in areas of food, clothing, and religion.

Understanding "Sexually Inappropriate Behavior" (SIB). Sexuality is always a difficult and challenging issue for professional and family caregivers to address with residents. This is particularly the case in relation to responding to incidents of hypersexuality or inappropriate sexual expression as a result of MNCD. Inappropriate undressing/disrobing in public or touching their genitals may be occurring because of uncomfortable clothes, clothes that are too hot, or itching or discomfort. This should not be considered inappropriate sexual behavior. Family and staff often see SIBs (such as using explicit sexual language, lewd sexual references, inappropriate sexual acts like exposing genitalia for sexual gratification or inappropriately touching a staff member [groping], masturbating during personal care activities) as a problem to be eliminated or fixed rather than as a compromised expression of need for love and intimacy. Some other SIBs include attempting or having intercourse with another resident, fondling, and exposing private parts to other residents or visitors. These are more serious problems that should be considered behavioral emergencies (and addressed promptly by the team) as safety of other residents (often residents who cannot deter such boundary violations) can potentially be seriously compromised and their emotional well-being be put at risk. SIBs are usually seen in residents who have significant cerebrovascular disease (stroke, VaD, mixed [AD and VaD] MNCDs) and when MNCDs involve the frontal lobes (advanced AD, FTD, TBI involving frontal lobes). All SIBs should be addressed promptly using the "STAR" approach described above.

The Role of Health Care Providers. HCPs should incorporate a discussion of needs for sexual expression into the routine care of residents. HCPs should learn as much as they can about the factors that influence sexual expression in residents. Availability of accurate educational materials for residents and their family, furnishing written materials in areas frequently visited by residents and family so that the materials can be picked up for reading, are a sign that HCPs welcome discussion about residents' sexual concerns and that these needs should be considered. We also recommend asking residents if they are sexually active, correcting any misconceptions and answering any questions they might have about their sexual activities, teaching residents about the physical changes of aging which may affect sexual functioning, and educating residents about the importance of protection from sexually transmitted diseases (STDs), including HIV for sexually active residents. The HCP should provide support for appropriate expression of residents' sexuality and act as a resident advocate with other HCPs and residents who may express discomfort. If a resident who has lost a spouse is feeling that he or she is violating the marriage vows by forming an intimate relationship with another resident/nonresident, the HCP should provide counseling (or make referral to a mental health professional with expertise in geriatrics and LTC) to process this through discussion and also consider involving a member of the clergy the resident has a relationship with and trusts. The HCP should always protect residents unable to make their own decisions about engaging in sexual activity. The HCP should also protect residents from themselves when they are not in control of their own behavior. The HCP should advocate for the healthy expression of sexual behavior. Helping residents feel physically attractive, such as providing beauty salons and cosmetic services can dramatically improve the satisfaction of residents regarding their sexual needs. HCPs should not assume sexual preferences. Many LGBTQ (lesbian, gay, bisexual, transgender, queer/questioning) older adults may be reluctant to identify themselves as such. However, as they enter LTC, many find their previously private lives are now open for scrutiny. HCPs need to challenge their own preconceived notions, explore their own negative attitudes towards the LGBTQ individuals and be an advocate for all residents irrespective of their sexual orientations. HCPs should also evaluate for medication-induced sexually inappropriate behaviors (e.g. hypersexuality caused by dopamine agonists) and psychiatric disorders (hypomania/mania) as cause of sexually inappropriate behaviors. Endocrine causes (e.g. elevated testosterone levels) are rarely implicated in LTC population with SIBs but may need to be considered if presentation is atypical (e.g. presence of other signs and symptoms of an endocrine disorder such as polycythemia).

Approaches and Interventions. (See Box 3.8.) We recommend meeting residents' need for intimacy and affection by allowing appropriate touching, hugging, and handholding. A male resident exhibiting SIB should be seated away from female residents. Male staff should be requested to care for male residents who have SIB during personal care. Choosing clothing that opens in the back, and considering twin beds for husband and wife if one of them is sexually

BOX 3.8 Strategies to Better Meet the Need for Sexual Expression of Residents Who Have Major Neurocognitive Disorder

Staff education and sensitivity training

Detailed sexual history to improve understanding of the resident's sexual needs

Staff openly discuss their attitudes and concerns, pick up cues that may indicate unmet need for intimacy

Promote privacy (no room sharing, "Do Not Disturb" sign outside the door, knocking on the door and calling the resident's name and asking permission to enter)

Allow conjugal visits, home visits

Individualized high-touch care

Encourage alternative forms of sexual expression, such as hugging and kissing

Beauty salons and cosmetic services

Educate residents and family about their rights and resources to meet sexual needs

Encourage friendships and relationships

Transfer care to another staff member if there is conflict between the staff member's duty to address the resident's sexual needs and the staff member's personal value system

Address physical limitations and poor health (better pain management, excess disability)

When appropriate, offer means and encouragement to residents to help them meet their sexual goals

inappropriate are examples of environmental strategies to consider. The facility should provide private space for residents to engage in sexual activity. The facility must strive to maintain privacy of information and association, although difficult within closed monitored quarters. Staff should not infantilize residents who voice interest in sexual expression, and health professionals should routinely consider sexuality in the overall assessment of residents. Two residents may show sexually intimate behaviors (such as kissing, groping) in public. This situation can be addressed by discretely taking the residents to their room, closing the door, and putting a "Do Not Disturb" sign outside the room. Family members should be involved in the discussion of supporting residents' sexual expression if the residents involved have significantly compromised cognitive functioning and capacity to give valid consent. In complicated situations, we recommend involving the facility's ethics committee or seeking guidance from a geriatric psychiatrist (in person or via telepsychiatry).

The staff should be flexible in their actions as advocates and need to evolve their role as conditions warrant. The staff may be obligated to disallow a physically intimate relationship if the resident's interests (however the interests are defined) are not served and/or the integrity of the resident's life is violated. The staff may need to negotiate with the couple (and the family) some limited breaches of privacy in order to assess, over time, the kind of advocacy the resident needs and whether the relationship continues to be in the resident's best interest and in keeping with the resident's values before MNCD. The greater the resident's cognitive capacity, the less paternalistically the staff should behave. Psychiatric and neuropsychological evaluations may clarify the resident's decision-making capacity.

Redirecting behavior verbally or physically, telling the resident in a firm but respectful and kind manner that behavior is inappropriate, improving consistency in staff approach, ignoring unwanted behaviors and encouraging appropriate behaviors, involving family as appropriate, and avoiding inadvertent reinforcement of unwanted behavior (smiling and laughing when redirecting or voicing "You are being naughty again; stop that") are some examples of behavior therapy. Recording the instructions (especially with physician's voice and/or a trusted family member's voice) and spending a few minutes every morning to go over plan for that day with the resident using the recording may help overcome mild executive and memory deficits of the resident and prevent SIBs.

The FDA has not approved any drug for treatment of SIB for individuals who have MNCD. Pharmacotherapy for SIB includes SSRIs as first-line agents for moderate to severe behavior that has not responded to person-centered approaches, including environmental and behavioral initiatives. SSRIs may benefit by their potential to reduce impulsivity or due to adverse sexual effects (such as reduction in libido) or through their antidepressant and anxiolytic effects (depression and anxiety symptoms often are comorbid with SIB). The HCP may consider prescribing an antipsychotic when there is persistent sexual aggression and the HCP suspects that psychotic symptoms underlie the behavior (e.g. a male resident is convinced that a female resident is his wife). The use of hormonal therapies (estrogens, medroxyprogesterone acetate, cyproterone acetate, gonadotropin-releasing hormone analogue) is controversial, but the HCP may consider it if sexually aggressive behavior is severe and persists despite all other interventions and the resident's behavior cannot be managed without control of these symptoms. We recommend thoroughly educating the surrogate decision-maker about the risks and benefits of hormonal interventions before initiating these interventions.

Educating and Counseling Family and Staff. Family (and staff) need to be educated that MNCD may result in inappropriate expression of sexual needs (because of disinhibition) but these needs are real. Staff actions are often misinterpreted. Bending over to do care may be interpreted as an invitation to have a blouse undone or a zipper pulled down. Occasionally, MNCD can cause a seemingly indefatigable desire for sexual gratification. The level of comprehension of the act itself and the emotions involved are not present. The HCP should also address a spouse's guilt over not wanting to be a willing partner and counsel the spouse regarding what is appropriate and acceptable for the spouse as well as the resident. No spouse should feel guilty about the decision to forgo gratifying the partner's sexual needs. We feel that integrity of the resident's and spouse's life journey needs to be protected against the waywardness created by MNCD. HCPs can help negotiate between the duty to respect a spouse's wish for sexual intimacy and preventing sexual abuse of the cognitively impaired resident or cognitively intact spouse. If the resident is unable to recognize the spouse, the potential emotional trauma the resident may feel after the sexual act with the spouse may be a serious enough concern that the resident may be asked to forgo the wish to be sexually intimate. Duty to promote health versus duty to protect from abuse, injury, and neglect can raise ethical conflicts when trying to meet some residents' needs for sexual expression. Conflicts between prevailing social moral values and resident behavior are also a concern. Staff may express confusion, embarrassment, anger, denial, and helplessness when they discover that residents are having sexual relations. Staff is often not sure when to involve the family and feel torn between moral norms and the duty to respect residents' rights. HCPs should improve their own knowledge and skills to enhance sexual expression of residents in LTC and take a leadership role in educating and training the staff to meet the need for optimal sexual expression for all residents. In complex cases, the HCP should promptly seek the help of a LTC mental health expert (such as a geriatric psychiatrist).

Clinical Case 4: "Just one kiss."

Ms. H was a 78-year-old woman who had been living in a nursing home for two years. Since she was admitted, staff had noticed that Ms. H had tried to invite various male residents to her room and had tried to kiss them or would ask for "just one kiss." A consultant psychiatrist was consulted because of the staff's report that Ms. H was "sexually aggressive" toward male residents. After detailed interview and input from various staff members, the psychiatrist found out that the nursing assistants who were involved in caring for Ms. H for the first one and a half years had left. The new nursing assistants had just obtained their certifications and were not sure how to deal with Ms. H's SIB. One nursing assistant felt that the behavior was "cute" and "funny" and even giggled when Ms. H exhibited SIB, while another nursing assistant felt the behavior was "abhorrent" and needed to be stopped. In fact, the latter nursing assistant had told Ms. H that she was not behaving like a "lady" and another staff member found Ms. H was found crying after this exchange. The "sexually aggressive" behavior that precipitated the consult was that Ms. H had succeeded in getting a male resident into her room, and they were found kissing. During the interview, Ms. H was a cheerful woman who asked the psychiatrist to give her "just one kiss." The psychiatrist showed her his wedding ring, but Ms. H responded by stating, "Your wife will not know." The psychiatrist told her that he loved his wife and could not grant Ms. H's wish. The psychiatrist was pleasant and nonjudgmental during the entire interview, and shook Ms. H's hand at the end of the interview. The psychiatrist spent a lot of time educating the staff caring for Ms. H that Ms. H's need for sexual gratification was normal, although expressed inappropriately because of her MNCD, and emphasized the importance of being nonjudgmental and the need for a consistent staff approach. The psychiatrist also discussed the role of damage to the frontal lobe or its connections in predisposing the resident to sexually disinhibited behavior. Over the next eight weeks, with a nonjudgmental approach and firm and consistent redirection by all staff, with encouraging Ms. H to hug and hold hands of male residents who liked it (and whose family was in agreement with such contact), Ms. H's SIB was much more manageable. The psychiatrist also met with the director of nursing and administrator, and they together decided to have a facility-wide in-service training addressing this topic for all staff.

Teaching Points

Nursing assistants often have a high turnover rate. Adequate education of new nursing assistants regarding SIBs (as well as other behaviors) and ongoing training are key to preventing misinterpretation of residents' sexual expressions as something that needs to be "fixed," stopped, or eliminated.

Clinical Case 5: "This is humiliating."

Mr. S was a 58-year-old single male who had chronic paranoid schizophrenia and lived in a community nursing home. He had been moved there several years ago from the state hospital ward/unit for chronically mentally ill patients. Mr. S was stable on his antipsychotic drug regimen of clozapine 100 mg qam and 300 mg qhs. He was mostly reclusive but did leave his room to go to the dining room for meals. Mr. S collected pornographic magazines and videotapes, which he would read and watch in the privacy of his room. One day, on returning from breakfast in the dining room, he found his dresser and other belongings in the hallway. He apparently was not told that his room would be recarpeted. His magazines and tapes were also moved into the hallway. He became angry, agitated, and upset – accusing the staff of messing with his personal belongings. "This is humiliating," he stated. His dormant suspiciousness became blatant, and he required hospitalization after a serious suicide attempt.

Teaching Points

Knowing the resident and taking extra precautions to ensure privacy for residents who are managing their own sexual needs appropriately is crucial not only to support residents' rights of sexual expression but also to prevent serious trauma and humiliation experienced by residents whose privacy is violated due to lack of mindfulness on the part of staff.

Aging in Place

Early comprehensive management of MNCD and BPSD can increase the chance of a resident's aging in place; that is, if the resident is in an AL home, it can delay for a few years having to move to a nursing home (and save money, as the cost of living in a nursing home is much higher than the cost of living in AL home) (Morley 2012). With the availability of hospice and improved understanding of palliative care for people who have MNCD, many residents may live the last years of life entirely in AL without having to transfer to a NH or hospital, and residents in NH can avoid hospitalization.

The Capacity to Make Health Care Decisions

Assessing capacity of a resident who has MNCD to make medical and financial decisions is one of the important skills required by physicians working with LTC populations. Decision-making requires that a person understand information, appreciate the situation and consequences of the decision, manipulate information in a rational manner, and be able to communicate their decisions and choices (Peisah et al. 2013). The communication framework involving three distinct components of decision-making – information exchange, deliberation about treatment options, and responsibility for the choice – may help model the physician-resident encounter.

Decision-making capacity (DMC) is a functional decision that is based on the specific abilities that are relevant to the decision at hand. In general, the higher the risks, the higher the burden on the resident who has MNCD to clearly express understanding of the risks and potential benefits of a choice. The person who has MNCD whose capacity to make decisions is being assessed should be given all the information about the benefits and risks of proposed treatment/recommendation (for example, recommendation to stay in LTC), the implications of not having treatment, what alternatives are available and the practical effects on his/her life of having and not having the treatment. Cognitive ability also may vary from day to day for individuals. Decision-making is not an "all or none" phenomenon. A resident may not have the DMC to make major decisions about health care (e. g. pros and cons of undergoing chemotherapy versus radiation therapy versus surgery for cancer) but may have the capacity to decide whether to take a sleeping pill or express a preference for a particular family member to be the power of attorney for health care. Lack of DMC is not always a permanent condition. For example, residents who have delirium may lack DMC but once the delirium resolves, they may regain the capacity to make their own decisions. Any physician or a licensed psychologist with a doctoral degree can and should be able to assess a resident's DMC. It is important to remember that residents have a right to trust that health care providers and their legal advisors will not divulge confidential information without express permission, even when the resident has diminished capacity. Assessment of capacity for decision-making should be differentiated from competency to make decisions for oneself. Competency to make health care and financial decisions or to delegate the right to make such decisions is a legal conclusion requiring help from an elder law attorney and involvement of the legal system. Western civilization's concept of personal autonomy and self-determination are at the core of health care decision-making, but health care providers must be aware that other cultures do not always share this value system. Sensitivity to multicultural diversity in this context is imperative to maintain individual self-esteem and respect, for both the resident and the resident's family. We recommend the following five principles of care regarding evaluation of capacity in all residents who have MNCD.

Key principles to guide the evaluation of capacity of residents who have MNCD to make decisions include

1. Preserving autonomy should be the guiding principle in exercising professional judgment in relation to a person who has diminished capacity. This requires upholding the values of individual choice, control, privacy, and dignity in the LTC setting.

2. Residents who have MNCD should always be presumed to be capable of making health care decisions, unless a formal evaluation of capacity by two physicians has shown the opposite.
3. Residents who have MNCD are not to be treated as unable to make a decision unless all practicable steps to help them do so have been taken without success.
4. For a resident who has MNCD to give valid consent, he/she must be capable of making decisions in his or her own best interest, acting voluntarily, and provided with enough information to enable decision-making.
5. Help from family, friends, caregivers, and advocates who can help the resident who has MNCD understand the issues (especially in situations of language and cultural barriers) and make decisions should also be considered whenever possible.

The decision to participate in research is becoming increasingly important, and many residents may want to participate in research. Helping residents identify a trusted individual to become a legally appointed representative as a research proxy can increase flexibility and authenticity to the choice. By appointing the proxy early and functioning as "concurrent proxy" (meaning the decisions are being made jointly early in the course of MNCD) can enable the proxy to learn more about the resident's values and wishes. Even after the diagnosis of MNCD, it is often possible to obtain a valid proxy research directive.

Caring for Family Caregivers

Caring for family members of residents who have MNCD is an essential component of comprehensive care of residents living with MNCD (Sanders 2016). Caring for a loved one who has MNCD increases the risk of death for the caregiver. MNCD puts a gradually increasing burden on caregivers as the NCD progresses. Caregivers commonly report poor self-rated health, increased levels of depressive symptoms, and greater use of psychoactive medication. Caregivers often experience a profound sense of loss as the NCD slowly diminishes and disables the loved one. The relationship as it once was gradually ends, and plans for the future must be radically changed. Family caregivers of residents who have MNCD may have experienced many negative effects of caregiving (employment complications, emotional distress, fatigue and poor physical health, social isolation, family conflict, emotional and physical abuse, less time for leisure, self, and other family members), but research has shown that caregiving may also have important positive effects for some caregivers (such as a new sense of purpose or meaning in life, fulfillment of a lifelong commitment to a spouse, an opportunity to give back to a parent some of what the parent has given them, renewal of religious faith, closer ties with people through new relationships or stronger existing relationships) (McGillick and Murphy-White 2016).

Most primary caregivers are family members. Spouses are the largest group of caregivers, and most are older too, and many have their own health problems to deal with. Daughters are the second largest group of primary caregivers. Many daughters are married and raising children of their own. Juggling two sets of responsibilities is often tough for these members of the "sandwich generation." Daughters-in-law (third largest group of family caregivers), sons, brothers, sisters, grandchildren, friends, neighbors, and fellow faith community members constitute the remaining group of caregivers. In general, caregivers who are male spouses, have few breaks from caregiving responsibilities, and have pre-existing medical or psychiatric disorder are most vulnerable to the physical and emotional stresses associated with caregiving. Although physical demands of caregiving dramatically decrease when the person who has MNCD enters LTC, feelings of guilt, loneliness, and efforts to make regular visits to the resident can be exhausting. Depletion of financial resources may cause additional distress to the family caregivers.

It can be emotionally and spiritually draining to watch as neurocognitive disorder diminishes a loved one's memory and sense of self. Caregivers should be supported in their efforts to continue to hold a spiritual perspective on life (i.e. have spiritual beliefs that are incorporated into their philosophy of life). LTC staff can facilitate caregiver well-being by providing peer support programs/caregiver support groups (or information to find one) that link caregivers with trained volunteers who also have been caregivers of people who have MNCDs. Such programs are especially useful for family of residents entering LTC for the first time and the family members with weak social support networks or who are undergoing caregiver burnout. Family caregivers must be reminded that there is no "right" way to help their loved one with MNCD. Even small interventions (referral to support group, expressing support) may translate into improvements in the quality of life or confidence of the family caregiver. We recommend that the HCP educate family members about MNCD, its effects on the resident, how best to respond to symptoms, and how to access and use all available resources (such as involving other willing family members, contacting the local chapter of the Alzheimer's Association or similar local organizations). We also recommend counseling and ongoing support for the family members, including both individual and family counseling, telephone counseling, and encouraging caregivers to join support groups, especially for caregivers with limited social support and caregivers experiencing depression. We also recommend improving social support and reducing family conflict to help the caregiver withstand the hardships of caregiving and to help family members understand the primary caregiver's needs and how best to be helpful. Improving caregiver well-being delays the need for LTC for individuals who have AD. This may help the person entering the LTC facility adjust to the facility better, as he or she may be less aware of entering a "facility" because of advanced MNCD and thus, may make less effort to leave. Ideally, we recommend a structured multicomponent intervention (in-home sessions and telephone sessions over several months to address caregiver depression, burden, self-care, and social support and care recipient problem behaviors) adapted to individual risk profiles to increase the quality of life of ethnically diverse caregivers of residents who have MNCD.

After the death of the resident who has MNCD, it is important for the LTC team members to offer support to family members and help them recognize that it is normal and okay to feel relief that the loved one is suffering no more. Any unresolved feelings may paradoxically increase family members' distress after the resident's death, and the LTC team can guide family members in addressing such feelings and, if necessary, urge them to seek help from a psychotherapist (Rowe, Farias, and Boltz 2016).

Summary

Approximately 75–80 percent of the residents in long-term care have Major Neurocognitive Disorder (MNCD), and some assisted living (AL) homes and nursing homes (NHs) are designed for and care exclusively for people who have MNCD. Residents and their family have a right to receive competent, compassionate, stage-appropriate, and consistent care. Although most MNCDs are incurable, appropriate comprehensive treatment can substantially improve the quality of life of residents, family, and professional caregivers. With appropriate care, we can substantially reduce the number of residents who have MNCD and pain, depression, and/or agitation and reduce the number of residents who have MNCD and receive inappropriate medical treatment (hospitalization, surgery, medication) and futile procedures. Understanding clinical manifestations of different MNCDs, accurate diagnosis, finding the cause(s), instituting appropriate evidence-based treatment, and meeting psychosocial environmental and spiritual needs are critical for improving residents' quality of life and helping them live the best life possible. Staff education and training in person-centered care, discontinuation of inappropriate medication, strengths-based personalized psychosocial sensory spiritual environmental initiatives and creative engagement (SPPEICE), and optimal appropriate use of psychotropic and nonpsychotropic medications are four key initiatives necessary to improve the mental health and well-being of residents who have MNCD.

Key Clinical Points

1. Approximately 75–80 percent of the residents of LTCF have MNCD and some assisted living homes and nursing homes are designed for and care exclusively for people who have MNCD.
2. Progressive, irreversible MNCDs account for more than 95 percent of all causes of MNCDs in LTC populations.
3. Understanding clinical manifestations of different MNCDs, accurate diagnosis, treatment of reversible cause(s) of cognitive impairment, institution of appropriate evidence-based treatment, and meeting psychosocial, environmental, and spiritual needs are critical for improving residents' quality of life and helping them live the best life possible.
4. Staff education and training in person-centered care, discontinuation of medications that are inappropriate or harmful, strengths-based personalized psychosocial sensory spiritual environmental initiatives and creative engagement (SPPEICE), and use of optimal appropriate psychotropic and nonpsychotropic medication are four key initiatives necessary to improve the mental health and well-being of residents who have MNCD in long-term care.

Additional Educational Resources/ Further Reading

1. Dementia Care: An Evidence-Based Approach. Marie Boltz and James E. Galvin, Eds. Springer, NY. 2016.
2. Memory: Your Annual Guide to Prevention, Diagnosis, and Treatment. Peter V. Rabins, Johns Hopkins University 2016 White Papers.
3. Dementia, Friendship and Flourishing Communities. Susan H. McFadden and John T. McFadden. Johns Hopkins University Press. Baltimore, MD. 2010.
   Online free educational resources
4. University of Washington Memory and Brain Wellness Center handbook titled "Living with Memory Loss: A Basic Guide" available for download at: http://depts.washington.edu/MBWC/resources/living-w0th-memory-loss
5. Alzheimer's Disease Education and Referral Center (ADEAR). www.nia.nih.gov/alzheimers
6. Alzheimer's Association. www.alz.org
7. Alzheimer's Society. www.alzheimer.org.uk
8. Lewy Body Dementia Association. www.lbda.org
9. Association of Frontotemporal Degeneration. www.aftd.org
10. Alzheimer's Research Forum. www.alzforum.org

References

Agronin, M.E. 2015. Sexuality and aging. In D.C. Steffens, D.G. Blazer, M.E. Thakur (eds.), *The Textbook of Geriatric Psychiatry*, 5th ed., pp. 389–414. Arlington, VA: American Psychiatric Publishing.

Alexopoulos, G.S., R.C. Abrams, R.C. Young, and C.A. Shamoian. 1988. Cornell Scale for Depression in Dementia. *Biological Psychiatry* **23**:271–284.

Alzheimer's Association. 2015. 2015 Alzheimer's Disease Facts and Figures. *Alzheimers & Dementia* **11**(3):322–384.

Alzheimer's Disease International. 2015. *World Alzheimer's Report 2015.* www.alz.co.uk/worldalzheimerreport-sheet.pdf (accessed December 12, 2015).

American Geriatric Society. 2011. *Guide to the Management of Psychotic Disorders and Neuropsychiatric Symptoms Associated with Dementia in Older Adults.* dementia.americangeriatrics.org/GeriPsych_index.php (accessed September 29, 2016).

American Geriatrics Society. 2015. 2015 Updated Beers Criteria for Potentially Inappropriate Medication Use in Older Adults. American Geriatrics Society Beers Criteria Update Expert Panel. *Journal of the American Geriatrics Society* **63**:2227–2246.

American Psychiatric Association. 2013. Neurocognitive Disorders. In *Diagnostic and Statistical Manual of Mental Disorders*, 5th ed., pp. 591–643. Arlington, VA: American Psychiatric Association Press.

American Psychiatric Association. 2016. *The American Psychiatric Association Practice Guideline on the Use of Antipsychotics to Treat Agitation or Psychosis in Patients with Dementia.* psychiatryonline.org/doi/pdf/10.1176/appi.books.9780890426807 (accessed May 5, 2016).

Anderson, K., and G.T. Grossberg. 2014. Brain Games to Slow Cognitive Decline in Alzheimer's Disease. *Journal of the American Medical Directors Association* **15**:536–537.

Apostolova, L.G. 2016. Alzheimer's Disease. *Continuum* **22**(2):419–434.

Balestreri, L.A., A. Grossberg, G.T. Grossberg. 2000. Behavioral and Psychological Symptoms of Dementia as a Risk Factor for Nursing Home Placement. *International Psychogeriatrics* **12**(1):7–16.

Blazer, D.G., K. Yaffe, and C.T. Liverman (eds.) 2015. Cognitive Aging: Progress in Understanding and Opportunities for Action. Washington, DC: National Academies Press. www.iom.edu/cognitiveaging (accessed February 5, 2016).

Brandt, N.J., and D.Z. Mansour. 2016. Treatment of Dementia: Pharmacological Approaches. M. Boltz and J.E. Galvin (eds.), *Dementia Care*, pp. 73–95. Switzerland: Springer International Publishing.

Brasure, M.E., E. Jutkowitz, E. Fuchs, et al. 2016. Nonpharmacologic Interventions for Agitation and Aggression in Dementia. Comparative Effectiveness Review No. 177. AHRQ Publication No. 16-EHC019-EF. Rockville, MD: Agency for Healthcare Research and Quality. www.effectivehealthcare.ahrq.gov/reports/final.cfm (last accessed November 16, 2016).

British Columbia, Canada, Department of Health. 2012. Best Practice Guideline for Accommodating and Managing Behavioral and Psychological Symptoms of Dementia in Residential Care. www.health.gov.bc.ca/library/publications/year/2012/bpsd-guideline.pdf (last accessed November 16, 2016).

Brody, A. 2016. Dementia Palliative Care. In M. Boltz and J.E. Galvin (eds.), *Dementia Care*, pp. 247–260. Switzerland: Springer International Publishing.

Chakkamparambil, B, J.T. Chibnall, E.A. Graypel, et al. 2015. Development of a Brief Validated Geriatric Depression Screening Tool: The SLU "AM SAD." *American Journal of Geriatric Psychiatry* **23**(8):780–783.

Clare, L. 2010. Awareness in People with Severe Dementia: Review and Integration. *Aging & Mental Health* **14**:20–32.

Cohen-Mansfield, J. 1996. Conceptualization of Agitation: Results Based on the Cohen-Mansfield Agitation Inventory and the Agitation Behavior Mapping Instrument. *International Psychogeriatrics* **8** supplement 3:309–315.

Cohen-Mansfield, J. 2000. Theoretical Frameworks for Behavioral Problems in Dementia. *Alzheimer Care Today* **1**:8–21.

Colijn, M.D., and G.T. Grossberg. 2015. Amyloid and Tau Biomarkers in Subjective Cognitive Impairment. *Journal of Alzheimer's Disease* **14**(1):1–8.

Cummings, J.L., C.G. Lyketsos, E.R. Peskind, et al. 2015. Effect of Dextromethorphan-Quinidine on Agitation in Patients with Alzheimer Disease Dementia: A Randomized Clinical Trial. *Journal of the American Medical Association* **314**(12):1242–1254.

Cummings-Vaughn, L.A., N. Chavakula, T.K. Malmstrom, et al. 2014. Veterans Affairs Saint Louis University Mental Status Examination compared with the Montreal Cognitive Assessment and the Short Test of Mental Status. *Journal of the American Geriatrics Society* **62**:1341–1346.

Dementia Action Alliance. 2016. *Living with Dementia: Changing the Status Quo.* White paper.

Desai, A.K., and G.T. Grossberg. 2011. Palliative and End-of-Life Care in Psychogeriatric Patients. *Aging Health* 7:395–408.

Desai, A.K., and G.T. Grossberg. 2017. Psychiatric Aspects of Long-Term Care. In B.J. Saddock, V.A. Saddock, and P. Ruiz (eds.), *Comprehensive Textbook of Psychiatry*, 10th ed., pp. 4221–4232. Virginia: American Psychiatric Press Inc.

Desai, A.K., F. Galliano Desai, S. McFadden, and G.T. Grossberg. 2016. Experiences and Perspectives of Persons with Dementia. In M. Boltz, J.E. Galvin (eds.), *Dementia Care*, pp. 97–112. Switzerland, Springer International Publishing, Switzerland.

Ducharme, S., B.S. Price, M. Larvie, et al. 2015. Clinical Approach to the Differential Diagnosis between Behavioral Variant Frontotemporal Dementia and Primary Psychiatric Disorders. *American Journal of Psychiatry* **172**(9):827–837.

Elbirt, D., K. Mahlab-Guri, S. Bezalel-Rosenberg, et al. 2015. HIV-Associated Neurocognitive Disorders (HAND). *Israel Medical Association Journal* **17**(1):54–59.

Elliot, R. 2003. Executive Functions and their Disorders. *British Medical Bulletin* **65**:49–59.

Erol, R., D. Brooker, and E. Peel. 2015. Women And Dementia: A Global Research Review. London: Alzheimer's Disease International www.alz.co.uk/sites/default/files/pdfs/Women-and-Dementia.pdf, accessed 28 January 2016.

Finger, E.C. 2016. Frontotemporal Dementias. *Continuum* **22**(2):464–469.

Folstein, M.F., S.E. Folstein, P.R. McHugh. 1975. "Mini-mental State": A Practical Method for Grading the Cognitive State of Patients for the Clinician. *Journal of Psychiatric Research* **12**:189–198.

Galik, E. 2016. Treatment of Dementia: Non-Pharmacological Approaches. M. Boltz, J.E. Galvin (eds.), *Dementia Care.* Springer International Publishing, Switzerland. pp. 97–112.

Galvin, J.E. 2016. Detection of Dementia. In M. Boltz and J.E. Galvin (eds.), *Dementia Care*, pp. 33–44. Switzerland: Springer International Publishing.

Geda, Y.E., L.S. Schneider, L.N. Gitlin, et al. 2013. Neuropsychiatric Symptoms in Alzheimer's Disease: Past Progress and Anticipation of the Future. *Alzheimer's & Dementia* **9**:602–608.

Geschwind, M.D. 2016. Rapidly Progressive Dementias. *Continuum* **22**(2):510–537.

Gitlin, L.K., K.A. Marx, I.H. Stanley, et al. 2014. Assessing Neuropsychiatric Symptoms in People with Dementia: A Systematic Review of Measures. *International Psychogeriatrics* **26**(11):1805–1848.

Gomperts, S. 2016. Lewy Body Dementias: Dementia with Lewy Bodies and Parkinson's Disease Dementia. *Continuum* **22**(2):435–463.

Grossberg, G.T., and A.K. Desai. 2006. Cognition in Alzheimer's Disease and Related Disorders. In C.G. Kruse, H.Y. Meltzer, C. Sennef, S.V. van de Witte (eds.), *Thinking about Cognition: Concepts, Targets and Therapeutics*, pp. 19–38. Washington, DC: IOS Press.

Haynes, N., A. Seifan, and R.S. Isaacson. 2016. Prevention of Dementia. In M. Boltz and J.E. Galvin (eds.), *Dementia Care*, pp. 9–32. Switzerland: Springer International Publishing.

Hallenbeck, J. 2015. Pain Management in American Nursing Homes – A Long Way to Go. *Journal of the American Geriatrics Society* **63**:642–643.

Herr K.A., Mobily, P.R., Kohout, F.J. et al. 1998. Evaluation of the Faces Pain Scale for Use with the Elderly. *Clinical Journal of Pain* **14**:29–38.

Inouye, S.K., van Dyck, C.H., Alessi, C.A., et al. 1990. Clarifying Confusion: The Confusion Assessment Method. A New Method for Detection of Delirium. *Annals of Internal Medicine* **113**:941–948.

Jacquin-Piques, A., G. Sacco, N. Tavassoli, et al. 2015. Psychotropic Drug Prescription in Patients with Dementia: Nursing Home Residents versus Patients Living at Home. *Journal of Alzheimer's Disease* **49**(3):671–680.

Jennings, L., and G.T. Grossberg. 2013. Antipsychotics Continue to Have a Place in the Management of Difficult Behavior Problems in Patients with Dementia. *Journal of the American Medical Directors Association* **14**:447–449.

Jeste, D.V., and J.E. Maglione. 2013. Treating Older Adults with Schizophrenia: Challenges and Opportunities. *Schizophrenia Bulletin* **39**(5):966–968.

Johnson, A.C., and J.S. Paulsen. 2014. *Understanding Behaviors in Huntington's Disease: A Guide for Professionals.* Huntington's Disease Society of America www.hdsa.org (accessed March 22, 2017).

Jost, B.C., and G.T. Grossberg. 1996. The Evolution of Psychiatric Symptoms in Alzheimer's Disease: A Natural History Study. *Journal of American Geriatric Society,* **44**(9):1078–1081.

Kales, H.C., L.N. Gitlin, and C.G. Lyketsos; Detroit Expert Panel on Assessment and Management of Neuropsychiatric Symptoms of Dementia. 2014. Management of Neuropsychiatric Symptoms of Dementia in Clinical Settings: Recommendations from a Multidisciplinary Expert Panel. *Journal of the American Geriatric Society* **62**:762–769.

Kimchi, E.Z., and C.G. Lyketsos. 2015. Dementia and Mild Neurocognitive Disorders. In D.C. Steffens, D.G. Blazer, M.E. Thakur (eds.), *The Textbook of Geriatric Psychiatry,* 5th ed., pp. 177–242. Arlington, VA: American Psychiatric Publishing.

Livingston, G., L, Kelly, E. Lewis-Holmes, et al. 2014. Non-Pharmacological Interventions for Agitation in Dementia: Systematic Review of Randomized Controlled Trials. *The British Journal of Psychiatry* **205**:436–442.

McGillick, J., and M. Murphy-White. 2016. Experiences and Perspectives of Family Caregivers of the Person with Dementia. In M. Boltz and J.E. Galvin (eds.), *Dementia Care,* pp. 189–214. Switzerland: Springer International Publishing.

Marano, C.M., P.B. Rosenberg, C.G. Lyketsos. 2013. Depression in Dementia. In H. Laveretsky, M. Sajatovic, C.F. Reynolds III (eds.), *Late-Life Mood Disorders,* pp. 177–205. Oxford: Oxford University Press.

Mitchell, S. 2015. Advanced Dementia. *New England Journal of Medicine* **272**:2533–2540.

Morley, J.E. 2012. Aging in Place. *Journal of the American Medical Directors Association* **13**(6):489–492.

Morley, J.E., and D.M. Cruz-Oliver. 2014. Cognitive Stimulation Therapy. *Journal of the American Medical Directors Association* **15**:689–691.

Nasreddine, Z.S., N.A. Phillips, V. Badirian et al. 2005. The Montreal Cognitive Assessment, MoCA: a Brief Screening Tool for Mild Cognitive Impairment. *Journal of the American Geriatrics Society* **53**:695–699.

National Institute of Health and Clinical Excellence 2012. Low Dose Antipsychotics in People with Dementia. https://www.nice.org.uk/media/default/About/what-we-do/Into-practice/education-learning-and-professional-development/academic-detailing-aids/low-dose-antipsychotics-in-people-with-dementia.pdf (last accessed on November 16, 2016).

Peisah, C., O.A. Sorinmade, L. Mitchell, and C. M. Hertogh. 2013. Decisional Capacity: Toward an Inclusionary Approach. *International Psychogeriatrics* **25**(10):1571–1579.

Petersen, R. 2016. Mild Cognitive Impairment. *Continuum* **22**(2):404–418.

Porteinsson, A.P., L.T. Drye, B.G. Pollock, et al. 2014. CITAD Research Group. Effect of Citalopram on Agitation in Alzheimer Disease: The CitAD Randomized Clinical Trial. *Journal of the American Medical Association* **311**(7):682–691.

Powers, R. and H.L. Herrington. 2016. Hospice Dementia Care. In M. Boltz and J.E. Galvin (eds.), *Dementia Care,* pp. 261–298. Switzerland: Springer International Publishing.

Rao, R., and B. Draper. 2015. Alcohol-Related Brain Damage. *Lancet Psychiatry* **2**:674–675.

Reisberg, B., J. Borenstein, S.P. Salob, et al. 1987. Behavioral Symptoms in Alzheimer's Disease: Phenomenology and Treatment. *Journal of Clinical Psychiatry* **48**(suppl 5):9–15.

Reisberg, B., S.H. Ferris, M.J. de Leon, and T. Cook. 1982. The Global Deterioration Scale for Assessment of Primary Degenerative Dementia. *American Journal of Psychiatry* **139**:1136–1139.

Ricker, J.H., and Axelrod, B.N. 1994. Analysis of an Oral Paradigm for the Trail Making Test. *Assessment* **1**(1), 47–51.

Rosen, J., L. Burgio, M. Kollar, et al. 1994. A User Friendly Instrument for rating Agitation in Dementia Patients. *American Journal of Geriatric Psychiatry* **2**(1):52–59.

Rowe, M.A., J. Farias, and M. Boltz. 2016. Interventions to Support Caregiver Well-Being. In M. Boltz and J.E. Galvin (eds.), *Dementia Care,* pp. 215–230. Switzerland: Springer International Publishing.

Saczynski, J.S. and S. Inouye. 2015. Delirium. In D.C. Steffens, D.G. Blazer, M.E. Thakur (eds.), *The Textbook of Geriatric Psychiatry,* 5th ed., pp. 155–176. Arlington, VA: American Psychiatric Publishing.

Saliba, D., J. Buchanan, M.O. Edelen, et al. 2012a. MDS 3.0: Brief Interview for Mental Status. *Journal of the American Medical Directors Association* **13**:611–617.

Saliba, D., S. DiFilippo, M.O. Edelen et al. 2012b. Testing the PHQ-9 Interview and Observational Versions (PHQ-OV) for MDS 3.0. *Journal of the American Medical Director's Association* **13**(7):618–625.

Sanders, A.E. 2016. Caregiver Stress and the Patient with Dementia. *Continuum* **22**(2):619–625.

Schmahmann, J. 2014. The Differential Diagnosis of Rapidly Progressive and Rare Dementia: A Clinical Approach. In B. Dickerson and A. Atri (eds.), *Dementia: Comprehensive Principles and Practice,* pp. 291–359. New York: Oxford University Press.

Scott, J.G., B. Ostermeyer, and A.A. Shah. 2016. Neuropsychological Assessment in Neurocognitive Disorders. *Psychiatric Annals* **46**(12):118–126.

Shapey, J., L.J. Glanez, and P.M. Brennan. 2016. Chronic Subdural Hematoma in the Elderly: Is It Time for a New Paradigm in Management? *Current Geriatrics Reports* **5**:71–77.

Shively, S., A.I. Scher, D.P. Pearl, and R. Diaz-Arrastia. 2012. Dementia Resulting from Traumatic Brain Injury: What Is the Pathology? *Archives of Neurology* **69**(10):1245–1251.

Small, G.W., and S. Greenfield. 2015. Current and Future Treatment of Alzheimer's Disease. *American Journal of Geriatric Psychiatry* **23**(11):1101–1105.

Spitzer, R, Kroenke, K., and Williams, J. 1999. Validation and Utility of a Self-Report Version of PRIME-MD: The PHQ Primary Care Study. *Journal of the American Medical Association* **282**: 1737–1744.

Stinton, C., I. McKeith, J. Taylor, et al. 2015. Pharmacologic Management of Lewy Body Dementia: A Systematic Review and Meta-Analysis. *American Journal of Psychiatry* **172**: 731–742.

Thakur, M.E. and L.P. Gwyther. 2015. Agitation in Older Adults. In D.C. Steffens, D.G. Blazer, and M.E. Thakur (eds.), *The Textbook of Geriatric Psychiatry*, 5th ed., pp. 507–526. Arlington, VA: American Psychiatric Publishing.

The Royal Australian and New Zealand College of Psychiatrists. 2016. *Antipsychotic Medication as a Treatment for Behavioral and Psychological Symptoms of Dementia. Professional Practice Guideline 10.* https://www.ranzcp.org/Files/Resources/College_Statements/Practice_Guidelines/pg10-pdf.aspx (last accessed November 16, 2016).

Trivedi, M.H., and T.L. Greer. 2014. Cognitive Dysfunction in Unipolar Major Depression: Implications for Treatment. *Journal of Affective Disorder* **152**:19–27.

van der Linde, R.M., T. Dening, C. Blossom, et al. 2016. Longitudinal Course of behavioral and Psychological Symptoms of Dementia: Systematic Review. *The British Journal of Psychiatry* **209**:266–377.

Vitalta-Franch, J., L. Calvo-Perxas, J. Garre-Olmo, et al. 2013. Apathy Syndrome in Alzheimer's Disease Epidemiology: Prevalence, Incidence, Persistence, and Risk and Mortality Factors. *Journal of Alzheimer's Disease* **33**:535–543.

Warden, V., A.C. Hurley, and L. Volicer. 2003. Development and Psychometric Evaluation of the Pain Assessment in Advanced Dementia. *Journal of the American Medical Directors Association* **4**:9–15.

Williams, M.A., and J. Malm. 2016. Diagnosis and Treatment of Idiopathic Normal Pressure Hydrocephalus. *Continuum* **22**(2):579–599.

Wood, S., J.L. Cummings, M. Hsu, et al. 2000. The Use of the Neuropsychiatric Inventory in Nursing Home Residents. *American Journal of Geriatric Psychiatry* **8**:75–83.

Yesavage, J.A., T.L. Brink, T.L. Rose, et al. 1983. Development and Validation of a Geriatric Depression Scale: A Preliminary Report. *Journal of Psychiatric Research* **17**:37–49.

Chapter 4

Delirium

Delirium is a clinical syndrome characterized by an acute change in a person's awareness, attention, and other cognitive functions and a fluctuating course (Inouye, Westendrop, and Saczynski 2014). It is often called acute confusional state or acute brain failure. Delirium is one of the most serious mental disorders in long-term care (LTC) populations and may be the only sign of a life-threatening medical condition. Even with appropriate treatment, mortality and morbidity due to delirium in LTC populations are high. Without treatment, it is often fatal. Delirium causes severe emotional distress and is accompanied by severe impairment of function. Hence, accurate early diagnosis and prompt treatment of the cause(s) and appropriate management are crucial for maintaining the person's quality of life and preventing premature mortality (Saczynski and Inouye 2015). Delirium is prevalent among LTC residents and often is poorly managed. Misdiagnosis of delirium as major neurocognitive disorder (MNCD), major depressive disorder (MDD), or a psychotic disorder is common in LTC populations, and early clinical manifestations of delirium are often missed.

The diagnosis of delirium can be made easily and reliably by using criteria established by the *Diagnostic and Statistical Manual of Mental Disorders*, fifth edition (*DSM-5*) (American Psychiatric Association 2013). Delirium is determined when a person has all four of the following characteristics:

- Acute onset (over hours to few days) and fluctuating course (severity of symptoms vary dramatically during the course of a day)
- Problems with attention (focus, maintain, and shift attention) and impairment in awareness (drowsiness or hyperalert state)
- Additional impairment in cognition (e.g. disorientation, memory impairment)
- There is evidence that the disturbance is a direct physiological consequence of one or more medical conditions (including substance intoxication or withdrawal).

Disturbed sleep-wake cycle, disturbed perception (illusions, hallucinations), change in mood (e.g. depression, elated mood), anxiety (e.g. frequent calls for assistance), disturbed behavior (e.g. agitation, disinhibition, bizarre behavior), and disturbed thinking (delusion, disorganization in thinking, incoherent thought process) typically accompany delirium (Meagher, Norton, and Trzepacz 2011). Subsyndromal delirium has been defined as one or more core symptoms of delirium that do not meet the diagnostic threshold for delirium. Delirium is often preceded by subsyndromal symptoms (also called prodromal symptoms) for hours to days.

Although the onset of symptoms is typically described as acute (often within hours to one or two days), subacute onset of delirium over days to weeks is not uncommon in LTC populations. Psychosis (especially visual hallucinations) and agitation can accompany delirium irrespective of cause. At the cellular level, delirium is considered to be a reversible dysregulation of neuronal membrane function. This involves a selective vulnerability of certain populations of neurons (such as the reticular activating system) and neurotransmitter dysfunction (such as acetylcholine, melatonin, and gamma amino butyric acid [GABA]). The health care provider (HCP) should always assume delirium to be reversible until proven otherwise. By identifying and removing the cause, the HCP can expect the person to return to the predelirium cognitive and functional baseline.

The prevalence of delirium is between 10 and 20 percent, and the annual incidence of delirium is between 20 and 25 percent in LTC populations. Up to 20 percent of residents admitted to a postacute facility have delirium at screening. Among LTC residents older than 85, up to 60 percent may have delirium at some point during their stay. Subsyndromal delirium is even more prevalent than delirium. The prevalence of delirium in LTC settings may be increasing as a result of the pressure to reduce the length of stay in a hospital.

Subtypes of Delirium

There are four subtypes of delirium.

Agitated (Hyperactive) Delirium

Agitated delirium is characterized by heightened arousal, hyperalertness/vigilance, psychomotor overactivity/agitation, aggression, and vivid hallucinations. It accounts for 25–30 percent of cases of delirium in LTC. Agitated delirium is often misdiagnosed as an acute psychotic disorder or mania.

Quiet (Hypoactive) Delirium

Quiet delirium is characterized by somnolence (the resident tends to sleep all the time), apathy, sluggishness, lethargy, and withdrawn behavior. It accounts for 50–55 percent of cases of delirium in LTC. Quiet delirium is more likely to be overlooked and hence carries a higher risk of mortality than agitated or mixed delirium. Often, quiet delirium goes unrecognized until the resident becomes stuporous (difficult to arouse) or comatose (unarousable). Quiet delirium is often misdiagnosed as MDD.

Delirium with Normal Psychomotor Activity

Delirium with normal psychomotor activity carries the lowest risk of mortality of all types of delirium. It is the least common, accounting for 5–10 percent of cases of delirium in LTC. Delirium with normal psychomotor activity is often misdiagnosed as MNCD.

Mixed Delirium

Mixed delirium is characterized by a pattern of fluctuating symptoms, including periods of agitation and periods of quiet confusion. Mixed delirium accounts for 15–20 percent of cases of delirium in LTC and often is misdiagnosed as MDD with significant anxiety, acute psychotic disorder, or mania with mixed symptoms.

BOX 4.1 **Risk Factors (Predisposing Factors) for Delirium in Long-Term Care Populations**

- Recent transfer from hospital for postacute stay in a LTC facility
- Recent surgery
- Pre-existing major neurocognitive disorder (MNCD)/dementia (especially advanced MNCD)
- Pre-existing mild cognitive impairment
- Advanced age (more than 85 years)
- Past history of delirium
- Moderate to severe cerebrovascular disease (large or small strategic stroke, lacunar infarct), history of stroke, history of TIA
- Vision and/or hearing impairment – especially abrupt
- Frailty
- Poor nutritional status (such as protein energy malnutrition, low serum albumin, low body mass index, morbid obesity)
- Alcohol use disorder
- Major depressive disorder
- Presence of polypharmacy (five or more medications), high anticholinergic burden (score of 6 or more on anticholinergic burden scale [scale available at www.agingbraincare.org]), psychoactive medication (see Box 4.2)
- Comorbid advanced physical condition (e.g. chronic heart failure, advanced COPD, end-stage renal disease)
- Hypertension
- Inadequate pain relief and severe pain
- Physical restraint
- Indwelling urinary catheter
- Certain medications (drug with high anticholinergic activity, benzodiazepine, opiate)
- Chronic end-organ failure (end-stage COPD, end-stage renal disease, end-stage liver disease)
- Metastatic cancer
- Prolonged sleep deprivation
- Social isolation
- Bedfast status

Risk Factors and Etiological Factors

The development of delirium is due to a complex interaction between the person's baseline vulnerability (diminished cognitive reserve) and acute neurotoxic insults. The higher the vulnerability, the less severe the neurotoxic insult required to cause delirium. LTC populations have multiple risk factors (predisposing factors) for delirium. (See Boxes 4.1 and 4.2.) Although all LTC residents have at least one risk factor for delirium, many have several, and these residents are at highest risk for delirium. In the majority of cases, delirium is due to one or more reversible (partially or completely) causes. (See Box 4.3.) Key irreversible causes of delirium in LTC populations include acute coronary event, stroke, brain metastasis, and traumatic brain injury. For

BOX 4.2 Psychoactive Medications with High Potential to Cause Delirium

Class of Medication	Common Examples in Long-Term Care Populations
Anticholinergic	Benztropine, belladonna, scopolamine, oxybutynin, hyocyamine
Antihistamine*	Diphenhydramine, hydroxyzine
Benzodiazepine	Lorazepam, alprazolam, diazepam, temazepam
Opioid	Hydrocodone, oxycodone, meperidine, codeine*
Non-opioid analgesic	Tramadol
Steroid	Prednisone
Muscle relaxant	Cyclobenzapine*, baclofen
Antidizziness medication	Meclizine*
Antipsychotic	Thioridazine*, chlorpromazine*, olanzapine*, quetiapine*
Hypnotic	Zolpidem
Anticonvulsant	Phenobarbital, phenytoin, carbamazepine*
Antidepressant	Amitriptyline, imipramine, doxepin, paroxetine
Cardiac medication	Digoxin, amiodarone
Anticoagulant	Warfarin

* Also has strong anticholinergic effect

BOX 4.3 DELIRIUM Mnemonic for Common Reversible Causes (Precipitating Factors) of Delirium in Long-Term Care Residents

D: Dehydration, deficient nutrition (such as Wernicke's encephalopathy due to thiamine deficiency in a person who has alcohol use disorder and or malnutrition)

E: Electrolyte imbalance (such as hyponatremia, hypercalcemia), Endocrine disorder (such as diabetes-related [insulin-induced hypoglycemia, hyperglycemia], thyroid disorder), end-organ failure (kidney, liver, lungs, heart), electrical disturbance in brain (seizures), ETOH (alcohol) induced (intoxication, withdrawal)

L: Lack of oxygen to the brain (hypoxia/hypoxemia) and hypercarbia (e.g. due to heart failure, myocardial infarction, acute blood loss, pulmonary embolism, COPD exacerbation, occult respiratory failure)

I: Injury (hip fracture, head injury after a fall or due to physical abuse [resulting in subdural hematoma]), intestinal obstruction and impaction (fecal)

R: Rule out psychiatric disorder (mania, depression, psychosis, acute stress disorder, PTSD)

I: Infection (such as urinary tract infection, pneumonia, cellulitis)

U: Urinary retention, unfamiliar environment

M: Medication (see Box 4.3; such as steroid, drug with high anticholinergic activity, benzodiazepine [intoxication, withdrawal], opiate), malignancy (includes paraneoplastic syndrome)

residents older than 85, an acute physical health condition (e.g. acute myocardial infarction) may present more often as delirium than as classic presentation (chest discomfort, shortness of breath due to acute myocardial infarction). In LTC populations, dehydration and infection are the two most common causes of delirium. Acute partial or complete bowel obstruction and drug-induced delirium are also common. In high-risk residents (e.g. residents who have advanced MNCD), a relatively benign insult, such as addition of a psychotropic medication (e.g. lorazepam for anxiety management), may be sufficient to precipitate delirium. Even after identifying one cause of delirium, the HCP should pursue a thorough evaluation to identify all causes and reversible predisposing factors.

Assessment and Management

The assessment and management of delirium involve confirming the diagnosis, identifying and treating the causes, managing and relieving symptoms, and preventing complications. Residents who have delirium are at high risk of recurrence. Therefore, instituting interventions to prevent delirium in the future is a crucial aspect of management.

Diagnosis and Work-Up to Identify Causes

Delirium is a clinical diagnosis; there is no laboratory test to diagnose it. Delirium is diagnosed via a thorough history, comprehensive mental status examination, and formal cognitive testing using standardized assessment tools for attention and other cognitive functions. Table 4.1 lists recommended bedside standardized cognitive assessment tools (Folstein, Folstein, and McHugh 1975; Inouye et al. 1990; Warden, Hurley, and Volicer 2003; Nasreddine et al. 2005; Saliba et al. 2012; Cummings-Vaughn et al. 2014). Because impaired attention is a core feature of the diagnosis of delirium, the HCP can use simple bedside tests for attention (months of the year or days of the week backward, serial sevens [serially subtracting 7 from 100 to reach 72 is normal], digit span backward [4 or more digits backward is normal]) to identify impaired attention. Less than perfect scores indicate attention deficits. The setting (such as post-acute stay) and the presence of several risk factors for delirium add to the diagnostic acumen.

Residents who have delirium usually cannot give an accurate history because of diminished awareness and impaired attention. Therefore, to establish an early accurate diagnosis, it is critical that the HCP obtain input from various staff members who know the resident well (e.g. certified nursing assistant [CNA], geriatric nursing assistant [GNA], licensed practical nurse [LPN], registered nurse [RN], dietary staff, housekeeping) and the resident's family regarding the onset and nature of change in mental status. Acute onset of impaired attention and dramatic fluctuation of symptoms within a day (usually some improvement in the day time and maximum impairment in the evening or at night) can be discerned from input from the staff familiar with the resident, the resident's family, and review of nursing notes. Comprehensive physical/neurological exam, review of medications, measurement of vital signs, pulse oximetry (to detect hypoxia), and finger stick for blood glucose are essential components of a thorough assessment and often give clues to the cause(s) of the delirium. Review of medication involves a thorough review of not only prescribed medications the resident is taking at the time of the assessment but also over-the-counter herbal remedies and supplements, any possibility of the resident's consuming (or being given) a family member's medication (e.g. spouse using sleep aids), and any recent change in medication.

Delirium is often missed, and diagnosis can be improved by looking for one or more of the following:

- Acute change in mental status (especially drowsiness, difficulty maintaining or shifting attention, CNA or housekeeping staff report the resident's "not acting like herself")
- Acute onset of disorientation (e.g. a resident who is generally oriented to place [aware that he or she is in a LTC facility] is now disoriented to place [thinks he or she is somewhere else])
- Acute onset of disorganization in thinking and/or speech
- Acute onset of "depression" (e.g. resident is withdrawn, not interested in activities, apathetic)
- Acute onset of illusion, delusion (e.g. persecutory delusion, grandiose delusion, bizarre delusion), and/or hallucination (especially visual and/or tactile hallucination)
- Acute onset of agitation and aggressive behavior with no obvious environmental precipitant
- Acute onset of sleep-wake reversal in a resident who has a normal sleep-wake cycle
- Acute decline in activities of daily living (e.g. unable to dress or toilet self, in contrast to baseline ability)
- Acute onset of suicidal and/or homicidal ideas

Residents who have MNCD (especially in advanced stages) are at very high risk of delirium, which often manifests as acute onset of psychotic symptoms and/or acute onset of agitation/aggression.

Tools for Screening and Diagnosis

The Confusion Assessment Method (CAM) is the gold standard tool for assessing delirium. It focuses on four core features of delirium: acute onset and fluctuating course, inattention, disorganized thinking, and altered level of consciousness. Diagnosis of delirium is made if the first and second features are present with either the third or the fourth feature. The CAM is available as a short version, long version, and three-minute version (www.hospitalelderlife.org). The Family Confusion Assessment Method (FAM-CAM) is another standardized tool that obtains input from family and caregivers, who are typically the first to detect acute change in a resident's mental status. The Three-Minute Confusion Assessment Method (3 M-CAM) and 4AT are two

Table 4.1 Standardized Bedside Assessment Tools for Evaluation and Management of Delirium in Long-Term Care Populations

Standardized Assessment Tool	Key Benefits	Key Limitations
Mini-Mental State Exam (MMSE)	Excellent tool to assess global cognitive function Excellent tool for diagnosis of delirium if baseline measurement available A significant drop in the scores within a few days is a good screening test for delirium	Copyright issues claimed by Psychology Assessment Recourses Inc. limit its routine use Requires staff training for its reliable use
Montreal Cognitive Assessment (MOCA)	Excellent tool to assess global cognitive function No cost for its use It is translated into 35 languages Excellent tool for diagnosis of delirium if baseline measurement available A significant drop in the baseline scores within a few days is a good screening test for delirium	Requires staff training for its reliable use
Saint Louis University Mental State (SLUMS)	Excellent tool to assess global cognitive function No cost for its use Excellent tool for diagnosis of delirium if baseline measurement available A significant drop in the baseline scores within a few days is a good screening test for delirium	Requires staff training for its reliable use Not as well validated as MMSE and MOCA
Brief Interview of Mental Status (BIMS)	Easy to use tool to assess global cognitive function that is a part of the Minimum Data Set 3.0 used in nursing homes in the United States Excellent tool for diagnosis of delirium if baseline measurement available A significant drop in the baseline scores within a few days is a good screening test for delirium	Not as well validated as MMSE, MOCA and SLUMS
Confusion Assessment Method (CAM) (Short version, Long version)	Gold standard screening tool for diagnosis of delirium No costs for its use	Primarily studied in hospitalized population and not as well studied in LTC population Requires staff training for its reliable use
Family Confusion Assessment Method (FAM-CAM)	Good screening tool for delirium using family input No cost for its use	Requires staff and family to be familiar with resident's baseline cognitive state
Three-Minute Confusion Assessment Method (3 M-CAM)	Excellent tool for diagnosis of delirium No cost for its use	Primarily studied in hospitalized population and not as well studied in LTC population Requires staff training for its reliable use
4AT	Good screening tool for delirium No cost for its use	Primarily studied in hospitalized population and not as well studied in LTC population Requires staff training for its reliable use

Table 4.1 (cont.)

Standardized Assessment Tool	Key Benefits	Key Limitations
Numerical Rating Scale (Likert scale)	Excellent tool to assess severity of pain in people who have mild to moderately severe delirium and monitor response to treatment Easy to use No cost for its use	Not reliable with people who have severe delirium and people who have significantly impaired receptive language
Pain in Alzheimer's Disease (PAIN-AD)	Excellent tool to assess severity of pain and monitor response to treatment in residents with severe MNCD and delirium No cost for its use	Requires staff training for its reliable use

other standardized assessment tools to screen for and diagnose delirium.

Delirium often is noticed in an agitated or noisy resident, but is easily missed in a quietly confused, apathetic resident and a resident who has psychomotor retardation and is staying in her room. Underlying MNCD, impaired vision, and being older than 80 years have also been associated with underdiagnosis of delirium. For many residents, delirium may be the only manifestation of a serious medical problem (for example, sudden onset of change in mental status without typical symptoms such as speech disturbance, focal neurological deficit [in case of stroke], or dyspnea, tachypnea [in case of respiratory failure], chest discomfort/pain [in case of myocardial infarction], shortness of breath [in case of heart failure], or fever, leukocytosis / leukopenia [in case of infection]). Asterixis (tremor of the hand when wrist is extended [flapping tremor]) may be seen in residents who have acute liver failure (hepatic encephalopathy) or acute renal failure (uremia). The HCP should have a high index of suspicion for occult infection in LTC residents who have acute change in mental status.

The HCP needs to consider new-onset falls in LTC residents an equivalent of delirium. The HCP should take subsyndromal delirium as seriously as delirium. In cases involving an uncooperative resident, it may not be possible to establish the diagnosis with certainty; it is reasonable to make a tentative diagnosis of delirium and search for reversible causes until further confirmation can be obtained.

Following the diagnosis of delirium, even if the cause of delirium is identified from physical exam, vital signs, pulse oximetry, or finger stick glucose test, the HCP should consider additional work-up to identify other common causes of delirium. Work-up usually involves tests (such as blood, urine) guided by history and physical exam. A comprehensive metabolic panel and complete blood count are typically done in the initial work-up. If the HCP suspects a urinary tract infection (UTI), a clean-catch urine specimen needs to be sent for culture and sensitivity. The need for further diagnostic testing (such as stool exam, electrocardiogram [EKG], thyroid function test, B_{12} or cortisol level test, drug levels or toxicology screen, ammonia level, chest radiograph, arterial blood gases) will be determined according to the individual resident's clinical picture. The goal of such a work-up is to identify all potential predisposing, precipitating, and aggravating factors. The HCP may consider neuroimaging in some cases (such as falls and head injury). A CT scan may be preferred to MRI to detect intracerebral or extracerebral bleed or for some residents who have advanced MNCD because of increased stress and anxiety associated with the need to be still for a longer time to obtain a high-quality MRI of the brain compared to a CT scan. If the HCP suspects meningitis (due to fever, neck rigidity) or encephalitis (fever, seizures) as the cause of delirium, examination of cerebrospinal fluid (CSF) is indicated. The HCP may also consider CSF examination if he or she suspects subarachnoid hemorrhage and for persistent or worsening delirium in which a thorough work-up has not identified a cause.

The HCP may consider prescribing electroencephalography (EEG) if he or she suspects occult seizure (e.g. nonconvulsive status epilepticus, atypical complex partial seizure) as the cause of delirium. In delirium due to other causes, the EEG shows diffuse slowing (increased

Table 4.2 Differentiating Delirium from Major Depressive Disorder and Major Neurocognitive Disorder due to Alzheimer's Disease

Feature	Delirium	Major Depressive Disorder (MDD)	Major Neurocognitive Disorder due to Alzheimer's Disease
Onset	Acute (over hours to few days)	Subacute (over weeks)	Insidious (over years)
Dramatic fluctuation of severity of symptoms within a day	Present (symptoms typically worse at night)	Occasionally present	Usually absent
Attentional impairment (e.g. difficulty following conversation)	Present and severity fluctuates	Usually absent	Absent (except in severe stages)
Altered level of consciousness (drowsiness or hyperalert state)	Usually present	Absent	Absent
Disorganization in thinking	Usually present	Absent	Absent (except in severe stages)
Reversal of sleep-wake cycle	Often present	Absent	Absent (except in severe stages)
Memory impairment	Present and is due to attentional impairment	Often present and is due to attentional and motivational impairment	Present and is due to impaired encoding
Depressed mood	Occasionally present	Present	Occasionally present
Feelings of hopelessness and helplessness	Usually absent	Frequently present	Usually absent (except when resident has insight into having AD)
Delusions	Often present (typically persecutory delusions)	Absent (except in MDD with psychotic symptoms)	Occasionally present (typically involving others stealing belongings)
Perceptual disturbances	Often present (typically visual hallucinations and illusions)	Absent (except in MDD with psychotic symptoms when auditory hallucinations may be present)	Absent in mild stages, may be present in advanced stages (typically visual hallucinations and illusions)
Course	Fluctuating, may progress to coma without treatment and is usually reversible with appropriate treatment	Slow worsening of symptoms without treatment and is usually reversible with appropriate treatment	Relentless and irreversible progression to more severe stages

theta and delta activity) and disorganization of background rhythm that correlates with the severity of the delirium. Thus, the EEG may also be useful with difficult-to-assess residents to differentiate delirium from other acute non-neurocognitive psychiatric disorder (e.g. mania, acute exacerbation of a chronic psychotic disorder) where the EEG does not show diffuse slowing.

Differential Diagnosis

Major Depressive Disorder. Delirium (especially quiet or hypoactive delirium) is often misdiagnosed as MDD. Signs and symptoms listed in Table 4.2 can help differentiate delirium from MDD. Residents who have depression demonstrate a normal level of alertness, intact thought processes, depressed affect, and poor motivation to participate. Onset is usually gradual over weeks to months. There is often a past history of a depressive episode.

MNCD with Delirium. At least two-thirds of cases of delirium occur when there is underlying MNCD. There is documented history of pre-existing MNCD or obvious history of cognitive decline before developing delirium. Cognitive symptoms (e.g. disorientation, memory impairment, inattention, thought organization) are worse in people who have delirium superimposed on MNCD than in people who have delirium alone. Residents who have MNCD with delirium often display significantly more agitation than residents who have MNCD without delirium.

MNCD without Delirium. In LTC residents, cognitive impairment due to delirium may be confused with a MNCD, especially if the staff are not familiar with the resident's baseline functioning. Signs and symptoms listed in Table 4.2 can help the HCP accurately differentiate delirium from MNCD. Residents who have MNCD, such as MNCD due to Alzheimer's disease (AD), have insidious onset of cognitive decline, progression is over months to years, and they demonstrate a normal level of alertness. MNCD due to Lewy Bodies (dementia with Lewy bodies [DLB]) shares some clinical features with delirium (e.g. visual hallucination, fluctuating symptoms), but the resident who has DLB also has signs of Parkinsonism and the progression of symptoms is over months to years. Major vascular neurocognitive disorder (vascular dementia [VaD]) may present with acute onset of cognitive impairment, but the characteristic features of delirium (e.g. fluctuating sensorium and inattention) are usually not seen. With advanced MNCD, residents may have inattention and speech may be aphasic, making differentiation from delirium challenging. The level of alertness is not impaired and the inattention and speech impairment have been progressing over several months. Disorientation and memory impairment do not help differentiate MNCD from delirium, as they may be seen in both. A good knowledge of resident's baseline functioning is critical to differentiating advanced stages of MNCD from delirium superimposed on MNCD.

Bipolar Disorder, Manic Episode. Residents who have bipolar disorder typically have a long history of psychiatric illness, have clinical symptoms of elated or irritable mood, excessive talking, flight of ideas, racing thoughts, decreased need for sleep, and grandiosity with a normal level of alertness. Steroid-induced delirium may have symptoms of mania (e.g. grandiosity, excessive talking) but usually have altered alertness and a fluctuating course.

Acute Exacerbation of a Chronic Psychotic Disorder. Exacerbation of pre-existing chronic psychotic disorder, such as schizophrenia or schizoaffective disorder, may present with acute onset agitation, hallucinations, and delusions, but dramatic fluctuation in orientation and attention are usually absent and there is a history of severe and persistent mental illness.

Acute Exacerbation of a Chronic Anxiety Disorder. Acute exacerbation of a chronic anxiety disorder, such as post-traumatic stress disorder (PTSD), may manifest as agitation, inattention, and hypervigilance, but there is no alteration in consciousness or disorganized thinking. Usually, the presence of other symptoms of PTSD (e.g. nightmare, flashback, history of abuse or trauma) and a history of similar symptoms help clarify the diagnosis.

Delirium along with Acute Psychiatric Illness. Residents who have mania or acute psychotic symptoms or severe depression may develop delirium for a variety of reasons (such as noncompliance with medication [e.g. diabetes medication], development of pneumonia). High index of suspicion, a thorough history, and time course of symptoms usually help the HCP identify the nature of the dual diagnosis.

Clinical Case 1: "I want to go home"

Mr. A was an 80-year-old male who had hypertension, benign prostatic hypertrophy, hyperlipidemia, and arthritis. In the hospital after hip fracture surgery, Mr. A became disoriented, insisting that he needed to go to work, trying to climb out of bed, and becoming aggressive when the staff tried to redirect him. He was given haloperidol (2 mg twice daily) and was recommended to continue haloperidol when he was transferred to a nursing home (NH) for rehabilitation. Mr. A developed drooling, tremors, and daytime sedation and continued to have periods of agitation. Psychiatric consultation was requested. The psychiatrist asked Mrs. A about Mr. A's cognitive functioning before surgery. Mrs. A insisted that Mr. A's memory was "quite good" but added, "He is quite old, you know." Mr. A's daughter reported that for the last two years, her father had been increasingly forgetful, repeating himself often, growing irritable, and in the last six months, started making mistakes in bill paying, became lost while driving, started avoiding social gatherings, and refused to wear a hearing aid. During examination, the psychiatrist found Mr. A somewhat drowsy, with poor attention and concentration. Mr. A stated to the psychiatrist, “I want to go home.” He did not recall having been hospitalized and had slurred speech. The psychiatrist reviewed the results of tests done in the hospital. A CT scan of the brain showed diffuse moderate cerebral atrophy, urine analysis was negative for infection, and the results of blood tests, including chemistry panel, thyroid profile, and folate levels, were within normal limits. Vitamin B_{12} was at the lower limit of normal (level of 220). The psychiatrist made the diagnosis of MNCD due to probable Alzheimer’s type (AD) with postoperative delirium, discontinued haloperidol due to adverse effects caused by it, added vitamin B_{12} 1000 mcg daily, and started donepezil 5 mg daily in the morning to be taken after breakfast. The psychiatrist also met with the family and staff to discuss various psychosocial environmental interventions to be instituted (such as listening to favorite music, aromatherapy with lavender lotion, one-to-one supervision at times, minimizing night-time noise, and lowering expectations for the resident to remember and follow directions). The psychiatrist then had a lengthy family meeting at which he explained his diagnosis to the family, recommended a support group for the wife and daughter, and discussed the prognosis. Over the next several days, Mr. A gradually became less agitated and started taking part in physical therapy (although he required constant reassurance, redirection, and encouragement). The drooling markedly reduced, tremors and slurred speech decreased significantly, and daytime sleepiness resolved completely. After six weeks, Mr. A was found to smile and joke, although he still asked when he could go home.

Teaching Points

Mild AD often goes unrecognized and undiagnosed. It predisposes the person to develop postoperative delirium. Hence, for any resident who has postoperative delirium, it is crucial that the HCP inquire about cognitive functioning before surgery. Also, it is common for delirium to be treated with much larger doses of haloperidol in the hospital, and patients are often discharged on haloperidol or another antipsychotic medication. Haloperidol is associated with a high incidence of extrapyramidal adverse effects in older adults who have MNCD, especially at doses larger than 1–2 mg/day (although extrapyramidal symptoms [EPS] can be seen at doses as low as 0.5 mg/day). Hence, in the management of delirium, it is important that the HCP discontinue haloperidol or any other antipsychotic as soon as possible, especially if adverse effects arise. Finally, besides treatment of the cause, management of delirium primarily involves psychosocial interventions, although cholinesterase inhibitors may also help residents who have AD recover from delirium.

Clinical Case 2: “I don’t feel well”

Mrs. S was a 72-year-old woman who had multiple chronic medical problems (diabetes for 30 years, hypertension, osteoarthritis, chronic liver disease due to alcoholism, peripheral neuropathy) and recently had right-sided hemiplegia due to stroke. After some initial anxiety and depression upon moving into an assisted living home, she had been doing well for the last three months. Mrs. S was a frail, petite woman who had a body mass index of 17. She was taking 12 different medications for her many medical conditions, including 10 mg amitriptyline for peripheral neuropathy pain and insomnia. Over the last several weeks, Mrs. S had developed urinary frequency and incontinence. A week ago, Mrs. S was started on oxybutynin 5 mg daily for suspected overactive bladder (OAB). Her urine analysis was negative for infection. The staff noticed that for the last five days, the resident had become more confused and irritable, had two falls (no injuries), and was unable to sleep more than two or three hours at night. The HCP recommended discontinuing amitriptyline, but the resident and family refused because she had been taking it for more than 15 years and it had helped her peripheral neuropathy pain and insomnia. A psychiatric consult was obtained. Mrs. S told the psychiatrist, “I don’t feel well,” but could not clarify what was bothering her. After assessment, the psychiatrist recommended discontinuing oxybutynin and following a scheduled toileting program to treat OAB. Over the next 72 hours, Mrs. S’s delirium resolved and she was back to her level of functioning before starting oxybutynin. The psychiatrist then met with the resident and her family, explaining the risk of cognitive impairment with amitriptyline and potential benefits of alternatives, such as gabapentin or nortriptyline. The family agreed to try switching to gabapentin with the assurance that if it did not help, the resident could restart the amitriptyline. The psychiatrist checked the resident's renal function before she started taking the gabapentin. Her serum creatinine was 1.8, indicating mild chronic kidney disease. Amitriptyline was decreased to 5 mg daily at bedtime for two weeks and then discontinued. Gabapentin was added at 100 mg daily at bedtime and over two weeks increased to 300 mg at bedtime. The resident had mild insomnia for a few days but no increase in peripheral neuropathy pain. To improve sleep, the staff was recommended to encourage Mrs. S to increase physical activity, increase exposure to sunlight, and minimize daytime napping. After two weeks of taking gabapentin, discontinuing amitriptyline, and beginning a regimen of individualized psychosocial environmental approaches, Mrs. S felt she was doing "quite well." The staff noticed that her constipation was replaced with mild diarrhea, which resolved once the medications for constipation (docusate sodium and senna) were discontinued.

Teaching Points

Adding an anticholinergic medication such as oxybutynin for a frail resident who already is taking other medications with high anticholinergic activity (amitriptyline in this case) and compromised neurological status (cerebrovascular disease in this case) puts that resident at high risk of drug-induced delirium. Drugs for OAB such as tolterodine and oxybutynin and other anticholinergic drugs (diphenhydramine, hydroxyzine) may precipitate delirium and should be used with great caution in residents who are frail, have pre-existing MNCD, have a history of liver disease, or are taking multiple drugs metabolized through the Cytochrome PCY450 system (American Geriatrics Society 2015). We recommend instituting a rigorous trial of scheduled toileting before prescribing drugs for OAB. Each assessment for change in mental status is also an opportunity to review the resident's medications and reduce the anticholinergic load. Gabapentin has no anticholinergic activity and is a much better choice than amitriptyline for the treatment of peripheral neuropathy in LTC residents. Because gabapentin is primarily excreted by the kidneys, it is important to start with a low dose in residents who have chronic kidney disease, and a very low dose may be sufficient for a therapeutic response. Also, for a resident who has been taking psychiatric medication for a long time, discontinuing such medication is a major decision and may be associated with significant anxiety. Hence, it is important that the HCP discuss the risks of continuing current psychiatric medications and the benefits of safer alternatives before instituting any change. Finally, anticholinergic medications are constipating, and most residents need medication to treat constipation caused by anticholinergic drugs. By reducing the anticholinergic load, the HCP may help residents be able to decrease the need for medication to treat constipation, thus reducing polypharmacy and its harmful consequences.

Complications

Delirium in LTC populations is associated with high mortality, high rates of hospitalization, increased risk of falls, wandering, injury, pneumonia, pressure ulcers, increased caregiver burden, and accelerated pre-existing cognitive decline (Witlox et al 2010). Delirium at the time of admission of postacute care residents is associated with five times increased risk of mortality at six months. With hospitalized older adults, delirium results in increased length of stay in the hospital and is highly predictive of future cognitive and functional decline and subsequent institutionalization. Delirium during hospitalization is also a risk factor for subsequent hospitalization. Even subsyndromal delirium carries significant morbidity and mortality. Delirium markedly and independently affects resident outcomes such as functional decline and loss of independent living. Complications associated with delirium are more likely with residents who have pre-existing unstable medical conditions (such as brittle diabetes, protein energy malnutrition, advanced Parkinson's disease) and residents who have advanced MNCD. Even after successful treatment of delirium, residents are often left with significant new cognitive impairment or worsening of pre-existing cognitive impairment, fatigue, mood change (e.g. irritability, apathy, sadness), anxiety, sleep disturbance, and agitation due to delusions and hallucinations that can last for several weeks. Residents who survived a critical illness and had a subsequent stay in an intensive care unit may develop PTSD-like symptoms.

Treatment

The HCP should consider delirium a medical emergency. The first step is to decide if the resident needs

BOX 4.4 Management of Delirium

Specific Area	Common Examples
Treat reversible cause(s)	Urinary tract infection Dehydration Pneumonia Hyponatremia Discontinue offending medication
Address reversible risk factors	Remove bed alarm and physical restraint Discontinue psychoactive medication Discontinue medication on the Beers list Other rational deprescribing strategies (geriatric scalpel)
Maintenance of resident safety	Protection of airway, prevention of aspiration Maintenance of hydration and nutrition Provision of safe early mobilization while preventing falls Prevention of skin breakdown Family/companion to be with the resident Verbal and nonverbal de-escalation techniques
Management of symptoms	Multicomponent interventions* Melatonin Antipsychotics**
Address distress of family	Emotional support Education of family regarding all aspects of delirium Guiding family in helping with symptom management
Postdelirium management	Institute strategies to prevent future recurrence of delirium Address postdelirium fatigue with physical therapy Address postdelirium depression with counseling Discuss palliative care goals for frail residents

* Multicomponent interventions: Frequent reorientation, engagement in cognitively stimulating activity, promotion of sleep with sleep-inducing stimuli (e.g. relaxation tapes, warm milk) and a sleep-promoting environment (e.g. noise reduction), encouragement of physical activity, and use of visual and auditory aids.

** Use of antipsychotic should be limited to situations in which the resident poses an imminent danger to self and/or others due to severe agitation and/or severe distressing psychotic symptoms that interfere with delivery of essential medical care. Antipsychotics can prolong duration of delirium, worsen associated cognitive impairment, increase risk of falls, and worsen outcomes. Lowest effective doses of antipsychotics should be used for shortest duration.

to be transferred to a local emergency department for hospitalization (e.g. has unstable vital signs). Most of the time, delirium can be safely managed in the LTC facility. See Box 4.4 for key aspects of the management of delirium. The HCP should always assume delirium to be reversible until proven otherwise. The goal of treating delirium is not only to control agitation or hallucinations but also to reverse the delirium and thereby mitigate associated risks of morbidity and mortality. Delirium in LTC residents requires prompt comprehensive treatment because the experience is frightening to residents and family, with increased risk of wandering, falls, self-harm, and death. Treatment of delirium is much more than treatment of its cause (such as UTI). Treatment also should address any and all predisposing and precipitating factors for delirium, because delirium in LTC populations is typically multifactorial. The treatment of delirium begins with a thorough evaluation of the causes and risk factors unless the resident is in the end stages of life, in which case palliative and hospice care are more appropriate and work-up may not be necessary. If the offending agent is obvious (e.g. diphenhydramine), discontinuing it may be sufficient intervention without the need for any tests. Addressing safety (falls, injury due to removal of tubes, etc.), preventing complications (seizures, coma), removing restraints, and treating agitation are also needed at the same time as treating the cause. Prompt treatment of a UTI should result in clearing of delirium.

Avoidance of and discontinuation of drugs with high anticholinergic activity whenever possible is a cornerstone of the management of delirium. We recommend rational deprescribing (geriatric scalpel) for all residents who have delirium; this includes discontinuing all nonessential medications, all medications with questionable benefit, medications with high anticholinergic activity, and medications on the Beers list of drugs inappropriate for elderly people whenever possible and if necessary replacing them with safer alternatives. We strongly recommend consulting with a geriatrician, geriatric psychiatrist, geriatric nurse practitioner, or pharmacist for rational deprescribing in complex situations.

Even after a thorough assessment and after all diagnostic tests are completed, the HCP may still not know the cause of delirium. We recommend close observation of the resident to ensure safety, to see if an obscure confusion perhaps related to a medication may clear up, or new clues to an underlying medical condition may appear.

Multimodal psychosocial-environmental interventions are the primary mode of treatment of delirium, and the HCP should institute them for all residents who have delirium. We recommend the use of bright or blue light for circadian rhythm disturbances, massage, soothing music, aromatherapy, one-to-one monitoring (encouraging the presence of family members, staff, use of sitters), reorientation strategies (clock, calendar, resident's daily schedule) as appropriate, and minimizing the need for physical restraint by using intramuscular injection to administer antibiotic instead of intravenous antibiotic. Sensory deprivation can be minimized by encouraging the use of hearing aids and eyeglasses when appropriate. For hearing impairment, we recommend the use of hearing aids, amplifying devices, and earwax disimpaction. We recommend a quiet environment with appropriate lighting, and the staff should make every effort to allow an uninterrupted period for sleep at night. Sleep deprivation should be addressed with interventions such as warm bedtime drinks (e.g. warm milk, herbal tea), relaxation tapes, and back massage. Aggravating environmental and other factors such as sleep deprivation, immobilization, sensory overload, or deprivation can place excessive demands on the cognitively compromised resident and should be identified and addressed. Ensuring adequate nutrition and hydration is another key component of the management of delirium.

Pharmacological interventions should be reserved for residents whose severe agitation/aggression or severe psychotic symptoms may result in interruption of essential medical therapies (e.g. intravenous therapies) or who pose a danger to themselves (such as vivid hallucinations causing the resident to jump out of a window) or others (because of physical aggression). Although antipsychotics are the first-line agents in the pharmacological management of severe agitation, aggression, and distress due to psychotic symptoms for people experiencing delirium, these drugs do not carry an indication from the US Food and Drug Administration (FDA) for the management of delirium (Kishi et al. 2016). In addition, antipsychotics can prolong the duration of delirium, exacerbate associated cognitive impairment, increase the risk of falls, and worsen outcomes (Inouye, Westendrop, and Saczynski 2014). Haloperidol is usually recommended because of its wide therapeutic margin of safety, ease of administration by a variety of routes (oral [pill and liquid], intramuscular, and intravenous), and relative lack of cardiopulmonary and anticholinergic effects at low doses. Oral (liquid) or intramuscular haloperidol is usually recommended for LTC residents, and the intravenous form of haloperidol is usually reserved for the treatment of delirium in the hospital setting. The recommended doses of haloperidol to treat delirium in LTC populations are very low (0.25–0.5 mg repeated every 30 minutes to achieve sedation [up to 2 mg/day]). Younger residents and residents who have a high body mass index may need higher doses. The major problems with the use of haloperidol are drug-induced Parkinsonism (DIP) and akathisia. DIP may be associated with discomfort, swallowing difficulties/choking during meals, falls by ambulatory residents, and increased immobility of nonambulatory residents. The use of liquid risperidone (0.125–0.25 mg repeated every 30 minutes to achieve sedation [up to 2 mg/day]) or orally dissolvable risperidone in place of haloperidol may also be appropriate. Adverse effects of risperidone are similar to those of haloperidol. With agitated residents, especially those who have Parkinsonism, low-dose quetiapine (12.5–25 mg one to three times a day and may be increased if initial doses are tolerated to up to 200 mg/day]) may also be useful. The use of quetiapine and less commonly risperidone may be associated with orthostatic hypotension. Norquetiapine, the active metabolite of quetiapine, has anticholinergic properties, whereas risperidone has minimal anticholinergic properties. Once initial sedation is achieved, one-half of the loading dose of medication may be given in divided doses (one to three times a day) for one to two more days with tapering doses over the next few days. The HCP may consider prescribing intramuscular ziprasidone (10–20 mg one to three times a day) for agitated delirious residents for whom the use of haloperidol is relatively contraindicated (such as residents who have Parkinsonism or Parkinson's disease) and residents refusing oral atypical antipsychotics, such as quetiapine. Olanzapine also has anticholinergic properties and is usually recommended only as a third- or fourth-line agent (after haloperidol, risperidone, and quetiapine). Olanzapine is available as an orally dissolvable tablet or intramuscular injection. Haloperidol (especially intravenous), ziprasidone, and quetiapine may prolong QT interval and thus increase the risk of potentially fatal Torsades de pointes (ventricular arrhythmias). Hence, the HCP needs to review an electrocardiogram before prescribing these medications and should avoid prescribing them for residents who have pre-existing arrhythmia or advanced heart block.

Considering the potential antipsychotic agent-related adverse effects of DIP, Torsades de pointes, hypotension (especially with intravenous haloperidol, high-dose quetiapine), and neuroleptic malignant syndrome, the HCP must evaluate the safety of these agents in the context of potential benefits. Titrating medications to resident-specific, goal-directed target sedation levels (resident is awake and manageable), rather than to "unresponsive resident" status (resident lethargic), may be helpful in reducing iatrogenically induced morbidity and mortality. Antipsychotics should be used only for short-term treatment (few days), using the lowest effective dose appropriate for a particular resident. Lorazepam and oxazepam may be useful for residents who are experiencing withdrawal from alcohol or sedative-hypnotic agents or if the HCP suspects seizures are a cause of delirium; otherwise their use may be associated with worsening of delirium, falls, and agitation. To date, the FDA has not approved any agent for the treatment of behavioral sequelae of delirium. Also, people who have pre-existing MNCD are at increased risk of stroke and stroke-like events and increased mortality with the use of antipsychotics. The HCP should weigh these risks of antipsychotics against the risk of not treating severe agitation in residents who have delirium and MNCD before instituting treatment. The HCP may consider prescribing melatonin to manage the symptoms of insomnia and circadian rhythm disturbances due to delirium.

Family members often experience considerable stress while witnessing a loved one's distress during delirium. The management of delirium should include inquiring about their stress, educating them regarding manifestations of delirium, and a team effort to address the resident's distress and provide guidance regarding the important role family members can play in reducing the resident's distress and keeping the resident safe.

After successful treatment of delirium, the HCP needs to continue addressing sequelae of delirium (e.g. depression, fatigue). The HCP should consider physical therapy to address fatigue and individual counseling (for residents who have relatively preserved cognitive function) to address depression and PTSD-like symptoms. For residents who have limited life expectancy, successful treatment of delirium should be followed by discussion with the resident and the family of the goals of palliative care. Delirium is a marker of brain vulnerability with diminished cognitive reserve, and residents who have delirium are at high risk of a recurrence of delirium.

Recovery

The goal of treatment is complete resolution of delirium and return of the resident to his or her predelirium level of functioning and cognition. Residents whose delirium resolves quickly (within two weeks) without recurrence usually regain 100 percent of the predelirium functional level, while those who do not will regain less than 50 percent. A substantial number of residents do not return to the predelirium level of cognition and function. Delirium can be a persistent issue for a given resident, persisting for months or even years. Follow-up to confirm the resolution of delirium once the cause is found and treated is essential, as persistent delirium or delirium of unknown etiology carries a high risk of morbidity and mortality.

The speed of resolution of delirium in residents newly admitted to a skilled nursing facility for rehabilitation after hospitalization correlates with the ability of those residents to carry out ADLs and reach prehospital functionality. If a resident has not reached prehospital functionality by six months, the prognosis for significant further recovery is poor.

Outcome

Complete Resolution over Days to Weeks. Complete resolution is usually seen in residents who have good baseline cognitive function, absence of preclinical degenerative changes in the brain, minimal cerebrovascular disease, and good premorbid cognitive reserve.

Persistent Delirium. Symptoms may persist for months to years. Persistent delirium is much more common than previously believed. It is usually seen in residents who have significant cerebrovascular disease and/or other medical comorbidity (e.g. end organ failure of liver, kidney, heart, lung), poor cognitive reserve, and impaired predelirium cognition (e.g. presence of MNCD, amnestic disorder in residents who have alcohol use disorder).

Delirium followed by MNCD due to Alzheimer's Disease. For this outcome, the resident usually has pre-existing pre-MNCD stage of AD (usually mild neurocognitive disorder due to AD and occasionally subjective cognitive impairment stage of AD), but symptoms are subtle or mild and further brain damage due to factors causing delirium results in manifestation of obvious symptoms of MNCD and subsequent typical progression. In this context, delirium has the effect of moderate to severe traumatic brain injury, accelerating the neurodegenerative pathology. Anesthetic agents may also have a role in accelerating neurodegenerative processes.

Delirium Causing MNCD. This outcome is controversial. There is growing evidence that delirium can be directly neurotoxic (similar to TBI) and a potential mechanism of permanent cognitive impairment (Inouye, Westendrop, and Saczynski 2014). Neuroimaging studies have documented regions of hypoperfusion in people who have delirium, suggesting that delirium may trigger a derangement in brain vascular function that may lead to MNCD in some cases.

Accelerated Cognitive Decline in People Who Have Pre-existing MNCD. This outcome is common in LTC populations. The resident may not recover to predelirium baseline but instead moves to the next stage of MNCD (e.g. from moderate stage of AD to severe stage of AD). Thus, because the resident developed delirium, cognitive decline was accelerated over days to weeks, which otherwise would have taken several months. The HCP should suspect the existence of delirium in a resident who has progressive MNCD such as AD and begins to show an abrupt downward course.

Prevention

Delirium is preventable in 30–40 percent of cases (Inouye, Westendrop, and Saczynski 2014). Evidence for successful prevention of delirium is strong and is targeted toward at-risk populations. All LTC populations should be considered at risk for delirium because of high medical comorbidity, limited cognitive reserve, and advanced age. Residents who have advanced MNCD, frail residents, and residents receiving palliative care are at highest risk for delirium and often develop delirium after minor stressors (e.g. hospitalization, addition of one medication with anticholinergic properties). See Box 4.5 for practical strategies to prevent delirium in LTC populations. For residents in severe or terminal stages of MNCD, aggressive work-up and treatment of cause (e.g. intravenous antibiotics to treat pneumonia) may pose substantial burden with questionable benefit. For these residents, palliative and hospice care is preferable if it is in keeping with the resident's values and wishes (as reflected in advance health care directives). The HCP should follow residents who have urinary incontinence due to OAB and have been prescribed antispasmodics for the development of drug-induced delirium. Trospium is eliminated as an unchanged drug and may be a safer treatment option for OAB than other medications (such as tolterodine or oxybutynin) in the context of polypharmacy or residents who have liver disease because of less risk of drug-drug interaction. Common precipitants of delirium in LTC populations include, but are not limited to, the presence of three or more medications, long-term use of broad-spectrum antibiotics, undernutrition, use of physical restraint, or use of a bladder catheter. By changing the processes of care, we can prevent delirium in many residents. Barriers to the early recognition of delirium (such as less time for staff to spend with the resident due to high workload, fragmentation of clinical care with lack of knowledge of the course of mental status changes, and lack of recognition of delirium as a medical emergency) need to be addressed at the administrative level to improve outcomes. Initial report suggests that ramelteon may help

BOX 4.5 Strategies to Reduce the Risk of Delirium in Long-Term Care Populations

- Screen cognition of all residents at the time of admission to obtain reliable baseline.
- Educate and train staff in early identification of delirium, appropriate use of bedside standardized cognitive assessment tools, and identifying common causes.
- Consult with geriatrician and/or geriatric psychiatrist and/or geriatric nurse practitioner proactively for recommendations to prevent delirium in high-risk residents (e.g. residents admitted from hospital for postacute care and rehabilitation, residents who have MNCD in severe or terminal stages, before and after planned surgery).
- Consult with a pharmacist proactively to identify inappropriate medication (based on Beers list of medications that are inappropriate for LTC populations) and medications with significant anticholinergic properties.
- Reduce and eliminate all psychoactive medication (especially anticholinergic medication, benzodiazepine, opioid) whenever possible and replace medication on Beers list with safer alternative.
- Minimize or eliminate use of physical restraint.
- Minimize or eliminate use of urinary catheter.
- Ensure early accurate diagnosis and treatment of MNCD with cholinesterase inhibitor and/or memantine as appropriate.
- Institute interventions to reduce risk of infection (pneumococcal and flu vaccine).
- Reduce inactivity and immobility, avoid bed rest, and maintain safe mobility and physical activity.
- Ensure optimal treatment of pain and depression.
- Institute sleep-enhancing strategies (to reduce chronic sleep deprivation).
- Ensure that residents who need them have glasses, hearing aids, and dentures.
- Improve nutritional status (to prevent dehydration, protein energy malnutrition, vitamin deficiencies).
- Institute fall precautions as appropriate.
- Ensure regular skin care and prevention of pressure ulcers as appropriate.
- Identify swallowing problems early to prevent aspiration pneumonia (e.g. coughing or choking during meals, food or medication "sticking" to the mouth).
- Ensure structure and keep to resident's normal routine.
- Ensure availability of robust therapeutic activities program/continuous activity programming (to prevent boredom, sensory deprivation).
- Reduce time resident spends in bed.
- Reduce ambient noise.
- Minimize and/or eliminate medical orders for bed rest.
- Encourage self-care.
- Increase exposure to outdoors, sunlight, and nature.
- Train staff to document accurate and specific findings (e.g. resident was inattentive and disoriented to place and this is not resident's baseline) in mental status rather than nonspecific words (e.g. the resident was confused).
- During rounds, health care professionals (HCPs) should routinely ask staff and family about any acute change in mental status. (Acute change in mental status in long-term care populations should be considered the sixth vital sign, after pulse, blood pressure, respiratory rate, temperature, and pain.)

reduce the risk of delirium for elderly people admitted to a hospital for acute care (Hatta et al. 2014). Its use for the prevention of delirium in LTC populations awaits further randomized controlled studies. We do not recommend the use of cholinesterase inhibitors or antipsychotics for the prevention of delirium (Barr et al. 2013). Box 4.6 lists web resources for improving the prevention, diagnosis, and management of delirium. Routine use of educational tools and implementation of care pathway resources listed in Box 4.6 along with strategies for the prevention of delirium listed in Box 4.5 can make successful prevention of delirium a reality for all residents.

Clinical Case 3: "My soul is in England"

Mrs. S was a 91-year-old retired schoolteacher, recovering from recent hospitalization for aspiration pneumonia. She had been lethargic for the first few days after

BOX 4.6 Internet Resources for Delirium

American Delirium Society (www.americandeliriumsociety.org) has a wealth of resources and tools (available at no cost) for HCPs to use in effort to improve delirium care. Key resources and tools include: anticholinergic burden scale, eCHAMP (Enhancing Care for Hospitalized Older Adults with Memory Problems) delirium protocol for physicians and nurses, delirium education cards, and educational videos.

European Delirium Association (www.europeandeliriumassociation.com) has a wealth of resources and tools (available at no cost) for HCPs to use in effort to improve delirium care. Key resources and tools include: care pathways for catheters, constipation, dehydration, pain, communication, environment, and medication.

Scottish Delirium Association (www.scottishdeliriumassociation.com) has a wealth of resources and tools (available at no cost) for patients experiencing delirium and their family.

Australasian Delirium Association (www.delirium.org.au) has an excellent list of links for HCPs regarding educational resources and research involving delirium. Newsletters available at this website also have a wealth of useful information for HCPs, including for pharmacists.

Hospital Elder Life Program (HELP) (www.hospitalelderlife.org) is a comprehensive, evidence-based patient care program that provides optimal care of older patients in the hospital. Dr. Sharon Inouye and colleagues at Yale University School of Medicine originally created HELP to prevent delirium in older hospitalized patients. The website has several validated delirium assessment tools (Confusion Assessment Method [short and long version], Family–Confusion Assessment Method, and Three-Minute Confusion Assessment Method) and corresponding training manuals that are available for free.

Mini-Mental State Exam: Available for purchase at www.parinc.com

Montreal Cognitive Assessment (MOCA): available at www.mocatest.org

Saint Louis University Mental State (SLUMS): available at http://aging.slu.edu/index.php?page=saint-louis-university-mental-status-slums-exam

Confusion Assessment Method (CAM), Family Confusion Assessment Method (FAM-CAM), and Three-Minute Confusion Assessment Method (3 M-CAM): all of these assessment tools available at www.hospitalelderlifeprogram.org/delirium-instruments/

4AT: available at www.the4at.com

Pain in Alzheimer's Disease (PAIN-AD): available at http://geriatrictoolkit.missouri.edu/cog/painad.pdf

American Medical Directors Association (AMDA) (www.paltc.org) has a wealth of resources for HCPs at its website, including 2013 Practice Guidelines for Management of Delirium and Acute Problematic Behavior in Long-Term Care Setting.

returning from the hospital and then started becoming more anxious, stating, "My soul is in England . . . I left it at the airport . . . When will it arrive back?" Psychiatric consultation was requested to start antipsychotics, as Mrs. S was severely distressed and agitated, yelled off and on for hours, had not slept for two consecutive days, could not be consoled or distracted, and hit staff during personal care. After comprehensive assessment, the psychiatrist diagnosed multifactorial delirium (due to pneumonia and high-dose prednisone [tapered off by the time of the assessment]), as work-up otherwise was negative. The psychiatrist educated the staff and Mrs. S's son that due to underlying moderate-stage VaD, advanced age, high medical comorbidity, and frailty, Mrs. S is at high risk of serious adverse effects from antipsychotics, has limited life expectancy, and is at high risk of recurrent delirium. This was Mrs. S's second aspiration pneumonia and second hospitalization in three months and, per her son, both hospitalizations were a "harrowing experience" for Mrs. S. The psychiatrist explained to Mrs. S's son and staff that pneumonia in this context can be seen as a friend rather than a foe and discussed the goals of palliative care, as the son shared that this would be in keeping with Mrs. S's values and wishes. The psychiatrist prescribed low-dose quetiapine (12.5 mg twice daily) after explaining serious risks, including risks of stroke, mortality, dysphagia, and ventricular arrhythmias (as Mrs. S had pre-existing prolonged QTc interval [512 msec] and quetiapine prolongs QTc interval). Her son wanted Mrs. S to be comfortable and not in so much distress. The psychiatrist chose quetiapine over haloperidol, risperidone, and olanzapine because Mrs. S had pre-existing mild Parkinsonism due to cerebrovascular disease. The psychiatrist also asked the facility chaplain to visit Mrs. S and recommended that the staff provide soothing hand massages with lavender lotion and make extra efforts to distract Mrs. S by showing her photos of her grandson and videos of the grandson's piano recital. Her son also started visiting more and giving the staff some breaks. Mrs. S's anxiety, agitation, and psychotic symptoms improved with these interventions and over the subsequent two weeks, quetiapine was decreased and discontinued. The son opted for Do Not Hospitalize intervention and comfort measures only if Mrs. S developed pneumonia again. The pharmacist and primary care team reviewed Mrs. S's medications and discontinued statins, vitamins, aspirin, clopidrogel, and calcium. Staff was educated about the importance of ensuring that Mrs. S regularly wears her glasses and uses her dentures to address visual deficits and prevent malnutrition, as both are reversible risk factors for delirium.

Teaching Points

The psychiatrist is often the first clinician to recognize the high burden of life-prolonging treatment for a resident who has limited life expectancy and high medical and neurocognitive comorbidity. It is important to explain to residents, their family, and staff about the significant burdens imposed by hospitalization, steroids, and antibiotics on residents who have advanced MNCD and the value of palliative care goals in ensuring that the last weeks and months of life are peaceful and dignified. The management of delirium also offers an opportunity for the psychiatrist to provide case-based education that is tailored to the staff's educational needs (in this case, poor recognition of the resident's limited life expectancy, limited understanding of the high burdens of life-prolonging care on many residents, and lack of recognition of the importance of inquiring into Mrs. S's values and wishes regarding palliative care).

Delirium in Palliative Care Settings and End-of-Life Delirium

Delirium is the most common mental disorder in palliative care settings, especially among LTC residents receiving end-of-life care. Delirium is one of the natural manifestations of the dying process. Among dying residents, delirium progresses to coma, preceding death. Dehydration and drug-induced delirium (particularly opiate-induced delirium) are among the most treatable causes of delirium at the end of life. Atypical antipsychotics or low-dose haloperidol may be considered for pharmacologic treatment of severe agitation associated with delirium. Benzodiazepines may worsen confusion, but may be needed in the final hours to days of life to facilitate calm and reduce the risk of seizure with the use of antipsychotics. Morphine along with lorazepam may be considered to relieve distress related to shortness of breath. It is not uncommon for some family members to request euthanasia or assisted dying when they witness a loved one in extreme distress in the context of end-of-life delirium. In such situations, we recommend palliative sedation. The HCP should counsel the family and staff that the goals of palliative sedation are relief of distress, not hastening of death. Palliative sedation (e.g. with combination of antipsychotics, benzodiazepines, and opioids) is ethical and appropriate if the resident is in severe emotional distress in the context of end-of-life delirium and all efforts to reduce distress have failed. Family of residents who have end-of-life delirium can experience significant distress and feelings of helplessness in their efforts to relieve the resident's suffering. Addressing the distress of family members and guiding them regarding ways they can help their loved one and at the same time address their own emotional needs is a key component of the management of end-of-life delirium.

Summary

Delirium is prevalent in long-term care populations and is associated with high morbidity and mortality. Some 30–40 percent of cases of delirium are preventable. Efforts to reduce and eliminate all psychoactive medications (especially anticholinergic medications, benzodiazepines, opioids) whenever possible and replacing medications on the Beers list with safer alternatives has the highest yield among strategies to prevent delirium. A high index of suspicion, prompt recognition, a thorough diagnostic assessment, appropriate work-up, and evidence-based treatment of delirium are essential to reduce morbidity and mortality. Treatment includes treatment of the cause, treatment of reversible risk factors, maintenance of resident safety, management of symptoms with multicomponent interventions, and institution of strategies to prevent delirium in the future. The use of antipsychotics to manage symptoms should be limited to situations of severe agitation and/or severe psychotic symptoms in which the resident poses an imminent danger to self and/or others or agitation is interfering with the delivery of essential treatment.

Antipsychotics can prolong the duration of delirium, exacerbate associated cognitive impairment, increase the risk of falls, and worsen outcomes.

Key Clinical Points

1. Long-term care staff should ensure good understanding of baseline cognitive function of all residents under their care and conduct prompt assessment for delirium for any resident who has an acute change in mental status, new onset of agitation, and/or a new onset of falls.
2. Periodically educating and training all staff (especially recently graduated) in the use of bedside standardized cognitive tools, including Confusion Assessment Method, the importance of early diagnosis of delirium, and simple strategies to reduce the risk of delirium is key to reducing the suffering, morbidity, and mortality associated with delirium in long-term care populations.
3. To reduce the risk of delirium for all residents, the health care provider should routinely reduce and eliminate all psychoactive medication (especially anticholinergic medication, benzodiazepine, opioid) whenever possible and replace any medication on the Beers list with a safer alternative.
4. Treatment of delirium includes treatment of the cause and reversible risk factors, maintenance of resident safety, management of symptoms with multicomponent interventions, and institution of strategies to prevent delirium in the future.
5. The use of antipsychotics to manage symptoms should be restricted to situations of severe agitation and/or severe psychotic symptoms in which the resident poses an imminent danger to self and/or others or when agitation is interfering with the delivery of essential treatment.

References

American Geriatrics Society. 2015. 2015 Updated Beers Criteria for Potentially Inappropriate Medication Use in Older Adults. American Geriatrics Society Beers Criteria Update Expert Panel. *Journal of the American Geriatrics Society* **63**:2227–2246.

American Psychiatric Association. 2013. Neurocognitive Disorders. *Diagnostic and Statistical Manual of Mental Disorders*, 5th edition, pp. 591–643. Arlington, VA: American Psychiatric Association Press.

Barr, J., G.L. Fraser, K. Puntillo, et al. 2013. Clinical Practice Guidelines for the Management of Pain, Agitation, and Delirium in Adult Patients in an Intensive Care Unit. *Critical Care Medicine* **41**(1):263–306.

Cummings-Vaughn, L.A., N. Chavakula, T.K. Malmstrom, et al. 2014. Veterans Affairs Saint Louis University Mental Status Examination Compared with the Montreal Cognitive Assessment and the Short Test of Mental Status. *Journal of the American Geriatrics Society* **62**:1341–1346.

Folstein, M.F., S.E. Folstein, and P.R. McHugh. 1975. "Mini-mental state": A Practical Method for Grading the Cognitive State of Patients for the Clinician. *Journal of Psychiatric Research* **12**:189–198.

Inouye, S.K., R.G.J. Westendrop, and J.S. Saczynski. 2014. Delirium in Elderly People. *Lancet* **383**:911–922.

Inouye, S.K., C.H. van Dyck, C.A. Alessi, et al. 1990. Clarifying Confusion: The Confusion Assessment Method. A New Method for Detection of Delirium. *Annals of Internal Medicine* **113**:941–948.

Kishi, T., T. Hirota, S. Matsunaga, and N. Iwata. 2016. Antipsychotic Medications for the Treatment of Delirium: A Systematic Review and Meta-Analysis of Randomized Controlled Trials. *Journal of Neurology Neurosurgery and Psychiatry* **87**(7):767–774.

Hatta, K, Y. Kishi, K. Wada, et al. 2014. Preventing Effects of Ramelteon on Delirium: A Randomized Controlled Trial. *Journal of the American Medical Association Psychiatry* **71** (4):397–403.

Nasreddine, Z.S., N.A. Phillips, V. Badirian et al. 2005. The Montreal Cognitive Assessment, MoCA: A Brief Screening Tool for Mild Cognitive Impairment. *Journal of the American Geriatrics Society* **53**: 695–699.

Meagher, D.J., J.W. Norton, and P.T. Trzepacz. 2011. Delirium in the Elderly. In M.E. Agronin and G.J. Maletta (eds.), *Principles and Practice of Geriatric Psychiatry*, 2nd ed., pp. 383–404. Philadelphia: Lippincott, Williams & Wilkins

Saczynski, J.S. and S. Inouye. 2015. Delirium. In D.C. Steffens, D.G. Blazer, and M.E. Thakur (eds.), *The Textbook of Geriatric Psychiatry*, 5th ed., pp. 155–176. Arlington, VA: American Psychiatric Publishing.

Saliba, D., J. Buchanan, M.O. Edelen, et al. 2012. MDS 3.0: Brief Interview for Mental Status. *Journal of the American Medical Directors Association* **13**:611–617.

Warden, V., A.C. Hurley and L. Volicer. 2003. Development and Psychometric Evaluation of the Pain Assessment in Advanced Dementia. *Journal of the American Medical Directors Association* **4**:9–15.

Witlox, J., L.S. Eurelings, J.F. de Jonghe, et al. 2010. Delirium in Elderly Patients and the Risk of Post-Discharge Mortality, Institutionalization, and Dementia: A Meta-Analysis. *Journal of the American Medical Association* **304**:443–451.

Chapter 5

Major Depressive Disorder, Other Mood Disorders, and Suicide

After major neurocognitive disorders (MNCDs), mood disorders (especially depressive disorders) are the most common mental disorders among residents in long-term care (LTC) facilities, with point prevalence ranging from 10 to 30 percent (Hui and Sultzer 2013; Beyer 2015). See Boxes 5.1, 5.2, and 5.3 for mood disorders prevalent in LTC populations and their common causes. In contrast to MNCDs, which are irreversible, comprehensive evidence-based treatment has been shown to be effective at alleviating symptoms for at least two-thirds of residents who have mood disorders and are receiving treatment. Response to treatment takes longer in LTC populations than in the age-matched community-dwelling population. Despite the availability of safe and effective treatment, mood disorders are often overlooked and undertreated in LTC populations. Box 5.4 lists consequences and complications, often fatal, of untreated or inadequately treated mood disorder. Thus, all efforts to prevent mood disorder and early

BOX 5.1 Common Mood Disorders in Long-Term Care Populations

Depression syndromes	Major depressive disorder (MDD) (single episode, recurrent)
	Adjustment disorder with depressed mood
	Adjustment disorder with mixed depression and anxiety
	Persistent depressive disorder
	Bereavement-related depression (includes complicated grief)
	Major depressive disorder due to general medical condition*
	Depressive symptoms during delirium
	Depression due to prescription medication
	Depression due to alcohol use disorder
	Demoralization syndrome
Hypomania/mania	Bipolar disorder (type 1, type 2)
	Cyclothymia
	Hypomania/mania due to general medical condition*
	Hypomanic/manic symptoms during delirium
	Hypomania/mania due to prescription medications
	Hypomania/mania due to stimulant use disorder
Apathy syndrome	See Box 5.8
Schizophrenia spectrum	Schizoaffective disorder (depressed type, bipolar type)
	Schizophrenia with symptoms of major depressive disorder
	Schizoaffective disorder with apathy
	Schizophrenia with apathy
Pseudobulbar affect	Pseudobulbar affect due to major neurocognitive disorder
	Pseudobulbar affect due to stroke
	Pseudobulbar affect due to traumatic brain injury
	Pseudobulbar affect due to amyotrophic lateral sclerosis
	Pseudobulbar affect due to multiple sclerosis

* General medical condition includes neurological condition and adverse effect of prescription medication.

BOX 5.2 Common Causes of Mood Disorder in Long-Term Care Populations

Cause	Common Examples
Primary psychiatric disorder	MDD (single episode, recurrent) Bipolar disorder (type I, type II) Cyclothymia Schizoaffective disorder (depressed, bipolar type) MDD in the context of schizophrenia
Mood disorder due to MNCD	MDD-like syndrome Apathy Hypomania/mania
Stroke/cerebrovascular disease	MDD-like syndrome Apathy
Parkinson's disease	MDD-like syndrome Apathy
Huntington's disease	MDD-like syndrome Hypomania/mania
Multiple sclerosis	MDD-life syndrome Hypomania/mania
Traumatic brain injury	MDD-like syndrome Hypomania/mania
Hypothyroid disorder	MDD-like syndrome
Hyperthyroid disorder	Hypomania/mania (primarily with irritability)
Cushing's disease	MDD-like syndrome Hypomania/mania
Addison's disease	MDD-like syndrome
Pancreatic cancer	MDD-like syndrome
Paraneoplastic syndrome	MDD-like syndrome
Chronic pain syndrome	MDD-like syndrome
Macular degeneration	MDD-like syndrome
Cerebral neoplasm	MDD-like syndrome Hypomania/mania Apathy syndrome
Systemic lupus erythematosus	MDD-like syndrome Hypomania/mania
Medication-induced mood disorder	See Box 5.3
Substance-induced mood disorder*	MDD-like syndrome Hypomania/mania

* Substance-induced mood disorder (especially alcohol but also cocaine, heroin, methamphetamine) can occur in the context of intoxication or withdrawal and is uncommon in LTC populations, but the prevalence is slowly increasing with the increase in the Baby Boomer generation entering LTC facilities.

diagnosis and comprehensive treatment of mood disorder are critical to improving the quality of life of LTC residents. Mood disorders include depression spectrum disorders, apathy syndrome, hypomania/mania, mood disorders in the context of schizophrenia spectrum disorders, and pseudobulbar affect. Self-injurious behavior and suicidality are two syndromes closely related to mood disorder.

Major Depressive Disorders

Major depressive disorders (MDDs) are not a natural consequence of aging or of living in a LTC facility (Blazer and Steffens 2015). Among depression spectrum disorders, MDDs (single episode, recurrent) are the most disabling. MDD in LTC populations is potentially lethal. MDD (either unipolar MDD or in

BOX 5.3 Common Medications Causing Mood Disorder in Long-Term Care Populations

Medication	Mood Disorder
Steroids	Hypomania/mania Depressive symptoms
Anticonvulsants*	Depressive symptoms
Opioids	Apathy
Benzodiazepines	Depressive symptoms
SSRIs	Apathy
Antipsychotics	Apathy
Interferon alpha	MDD-like syndrome
Propranolol	Depressive symptoms
Clonidine	Depressive symptoms
Tetrabenazine	MDD-like syndrome

Note: Some anticonvulsants, such as lamotrigine, may have antidepressant properties, and the FDA approved lamotrigine for the prevention of relapse of bipolar depression.

* Anticonvulsants: Barbiturates, vigabatrin, topiramate, levetiracetam, felbamate, zonisamide, tiagabine, clobazam

context of bipolar disorder) poses the greatest risk of suicide among all depressive spectrum disorders. Recognition and treatment of MDDs constitute a quality indicator in LTC facilities. Prevention and successful treatment of MDD are two key benefits of psychiatric consultation in LTC. Older adults have numerous risk factors for MDD (e.g. multiple losses, decline in physical health, cerebrovascular disease), yet the frequency of MDD for the first time among older adults living in the community is lower than that of younger adults. This may be because of the protective effects of wisdom, capacity to de-emphasize negative experiences, and ability to prioritize emotionally meaningful goals, all of which are thought to increase with aging. These protective factors also enable most residents to adjust to LTC without developing MDD.

Prevalence rates of MDD in LTC residents are three to five times those of older adults living in the community. Point prevalence of MDD in LTC populations ranges from 5 to 10 percent. Prevalence of MDD increases with increase in medical comorbidity (Taylor 2014).

BOX 5.4 Consequences and Complications of Untreated Mood Disorder

Depressive spectrum disorder and bipolar disorder	Suicide Nonsuicide mortality Reduced quality of life Impaired compliance with medical treatment Impaired compliance with rehabilitation therapy Increased risk of myocardial infarction Accelerated cognitive decline Worsening of diabetes Exacerbation of rheumatological conditions Lowered immune function, proneness to infections Undernutrition Increased rate of hospitalization Longer hospital stay Increased physical pain Decline in IADLs and ADLs Increased staff time to care Increased risk of institutionalization for resident who has MNCD
Apathy	Deconditioning Deep vein thrombosis Reduced quality of life Decline in IADLs and ADLs Increased staff time to care
Pseudobulbar affect	Social isolation Reduced quality of life

Screening for MDD in LTC populations is critical. Not only is the frequency of MDD high, but also suicidal ideation can be detected by screening. Standard use of screening tools such as the Patient Health Questionnaire–9 (PHQ-9), Geriatric Depression Scale (GDS), and Cornell Scale for Depression in Dementia (CSDD) may improve the recognition of depression in LTC populations. We recommend using them in conjunction with other standardized scales listed in Table 5.1 (Folstein et al. 1975; Yesavage et al. 1983; Reisberg et al. 1987; Inouye et al. 1990; Ricker and Axelrod 1994; Rosen et al. 1994; Cohen-Mansfield 1996; Alexopoulos et al. 1988; Spitzer et al. 1999; Woods et al. 2000; Elliot 2003; Warden et al. 2003; Nasreddine et al. 2005; Saliba et al. 2012a, 2012b; Cummings-Vaughn et al. 2014, Chakkamparambil et al. 2015). Standardized tests for cognition, pain, and behaviors can help clarify comorbidity and guide treatment decisions. Residents should be screened for MDD within one to two weeks after admission, every six months thereafter, and after any new onset of depressive symptoms.

Table 5.1 Standardized Bedside Assessment Tools for Evaluating and Managing Major Depressive Disorder, Neurocognitive Disorder, and Other Syndromes in Long-Term Care Populations

Standardized Assessment Tool	Key Benefits	Key Limitations
Mini-Mental State Exam (MMSE)	Excellent tool to assess global cognitive function Abnormal score after successful treatment of MDD may suggest need for evaluation of underlying MNCD	Copyright issues limit its routine use Often misses executive dysfunction, and executive dysfunction due to MDD is prevalent in LTC populations
Montreal Cognitive Assessment (MOCA)	Excellent tool to assess global cognitive function Is translated into 35 languages Reliably assesses executive function Abnormal score after successful treatment of MDD may suggest need for evaluation of underlying MNCD	Requires staff training for its reliable use
Saint Louis University Mental State (SLUMS)	Excellent tool to assess global cognitive function Reliably assesses executive function Abnormal score after successful treatment of MDD may suggest need for evaluation of underlying MNCD	Requires staff training for its reliable use
Brief Interview for Mental Status (BIMS)	Easy-to-use tool to assess global cognitive function that is part of Minimum Data Set 3.0 used in nursing homes in the United States	Often misses executive dysfunction, and executive dysfunction due to MDD is prevalent in LTC populations
Trail Making Test–Oral (TMT-Oral)	Easy-to-use tool to measure executive function quickly	Cannot be used as only test to assess executive function, as it can be normal in some individuals who have significant executive dysfunction
Controlled Oral Word Association Test (COWAT)	Easy-to-use tool to measure executive function quickly	Cannot be used as only test to assess executive function, as it can be normal in some individuals who have significant executive dysfunction

Table 5.1 (cont.)

Standardized Assessment Tool	Key Benefits	Key Limitations
Confusion Assessment Method (CAM)	Excellent screening tool for diagnosis of delirium, especially in resident who has MDD	Requires staff training for its reliable use
Functional Activities Questionnaire (FAQ)	Excellent tool to assess functioning in instrumental activities of daily living (IADLs) (e.g. keeping appointments, managing money), as executive impairment often impairs IADLs	With resident who has impaired insight (some residents who have MNCD), this tool requires a knowledgeable informant for accurate assessment
Patient Health Questionnaire–9 (PHQ-9)	Excellent tool to screen for MDD in LTC populations and monitor response to treatment Easy to use Well known in primary care	Not reliable for screening MDD in resident who has more advanced MNCD
Geriatric Depression Scale–15 (GDS)	Excellent tool to screen for MDD in LTC populations and monitor response to treatment Also available in 5-, 10-, and 30-item versions	Not reliable for screening MDD in resident who has more advanced MNCD Requires some staff training for its reliable use Not as easy to use as PHQ-9
Cornell Scale for Depression in Dementia (CSDD)	Excellent tool to screen for depression in LTC populations with moderate to severe MNCD and monitor response to treatment	Requires staff training for its reliable use
Saint Louis University AM SAD (SLU AM SAD)	Easy-to-use tool to screen for MDD in LTC populations and monitor response to treatment	Not as well studied as PHQ-9, GDS, and CSDD
Cohen-Mansfield Agitation Inventory (CMAI)	Excellent tool to measure severity of distress expressed as agitation in LTC populations with moderate to severe MNCD and monitor response to treatment (MDD may manifest as persistent agitation, tearfulness, irritability, anxiety, and insomnia.)	Requires staff training for its reliable use
Pittsburgh Agitation Scale (PAS)	Excellent tool to measure severity of distress expressed as agitation in LTC populations with moderate to severe MNCD and monitor response to treatment (MDD may manifest as persistent agitation, tearfulness, irritability, anxiety, and insomnia.)	Requires staff training for its reliable use
Neuropsychiatric Inventory–Nursing Home Version (NPI-NH)	Excellent tool to screen for behavioral and psychological symptoms in LTC populations with MNCD and monitor response to treatment (MDD may manifest as persistent agitation, tearfulness, irritability, anxiety, and insomnia.)	Requires staff training for its reliable use

Table 5.1 (cont.)

Standardized Assessment Tool	Key Benefits	Key Limitations
Behavioral Symptoms in Alzheimer's Disease (BEHAVE-AD)	Excellent tool to screen for behavioral and psychological symptoms in LTC populations with MNCD and monitor response to treatment (MDD may manifest as persistent agitation, tearfulness, irritability, anxiety, and insomnia.)	Requires staff training for its reliable use
Numerical Rating Scale (Likert scale)	Excellent tool to assess severity of pain in resident who has MDD and monitor response to treatment (Pain often accompanies MDD, and untreated pain is key factor in lack of improvement of MDD with treatment.) Easy to use	Not reliable with people who have severe MNCD and people who have significantly impaired receptive language
Pain in Alzheimer's Disease (PAIN-AD)	Excellent tool to assess severity of pain in resident who has severe AD and monitor response to treatment (Pain often accompanies MDD, and untreated pain is key factor in lack of improvement of MDD with treatment.)	Requires staff training for its reliable use

Many risk factors for MDD in LTC populations are different from those of age-matched populations living in the community and younger adults who have MDD. They are listed in Box 5.5. Various losses in old age may precipitate or exacerbate MDD. Physical illness (especially chronic pain) and disability are major factors that can contribute to the development and persistence of MDD in LTC populations. Recognition of risk factors such as recent loss is often a key to developing a plan for management.

Diagnosis

Accurate early diagnosis of MDD is key to successful outcome. There are currently no reliable biomarkers for MDD. Diagnosis of MDD is clinical and can be reliably differentiated from delirium and MNCD. See Table 5.2. The *Diagnostic and Statistical Manual of Mental Disorders*, fifth edition (*DSM-5*), defines MDD as the presence of five of the following symptoms nearly every day for most of the day for at least two weeks: depressed mood, lack of interest, appetite change or significant weight loss or gain, insomnia or hypersomnia, psychomotor agitation or retardation, loss of energy or fatigue, feelings of worthlessness or excessive guilt, difficulty with concentration or decision-making, and recurrent thoughts of death or suicide, plans or attempts (American Psychiatric Association 2013). The diagnosis of MDD also requires that at least one of the five symptoms be depressed mood or lack of interest. In addition, these symptoms should cause significant impairment in daily functioning. Subsyndromal MDD (often called minor depressive disorder/other specified depressive disorder) is clinically relevant, as it may impair function (albeit to a lesser extent than MDD) and diagnosis is made if the total number of symptoms is three or four rather than five. Box 5.6 lists common symptoms of MDD in LTC residents. These symptoms may be considered equivalent to typical symptoms of MDD in LTC populations. There are several subcategories of MDD. See Table 5.3.

The high prevalence of cognitive impairment, sensory impairment, apathy, and lack of adequate time and training of health care professionals (HCPs) in the recognition of MDD make accurate diagnosis in LTC populations challenging. Stigma and myths about aging also hinder early diagnosis and appropriate treatment. (See Box 5.7.) Furthermore, the symptom profile of MDD in older adults may not resemble

BOX 5.5 Key Risk Factors for Major Depressive Disorder in Long-Term Care Populations

Risk factors for MDD in older adults in general

- Stroke
- High medical comorbidity
- Chronic pain
- Severe functional disability (e.g. severe arthritis or end-organ failure of heart, lung, liver, kidney causing functional disability)
- Recent loss (e.g. loss of spouse, loss of driving ability, loss of one's own home)
- Persistent and disabling impairment in vision and/or hearing
- MNCD
- Parkinson's disease
- Past history of MDD
- Past history of suicide attempt
- Alcohol and/or drug use disorder
- Urinary incontinence
- Chronic insomnia
- Use of certain medications (e.g. interferon, benzodiazepine, opioid)
- Victim of abuse (verbal, physical, sexual, financial) and/or neglect
- Personality disorder

Risk factors for MDD related to institutionalization

- Admission to a LTC facility for the first time
- Admission to a LTC facility without adequate preparation for the move (emotional preparation of the resident and communication of resident's personal information [e.g. health, life history, preferences, dislikes] to the staff)
- Change from one LTC facility to another without adequate preparation for the move (emotional preparation of the resident and communication of resident's personal information [e.g. health, life history, preferences, dislikes] to the staff of the new facility)
- Change of room within the facility without adequate preparation for the move
- Change or loss of roommate or staff with whom the resident has developed a close positive relationship
- Loneliness, social isolation, boredom, and too much "down time" (time spent alone and without engagement in meaningful activities)
- Countertherapeutic staff approach and interaction (e.g. staff constantly correcting resident's recall of events, putting excessive burden on resident)
- Perceived inadequacy of care
- Inadequate exposure to sunlight, outdoors, and natural settings
- Excessive noise or interruption of sleep
- Meals or snacks not in keeping with resident's preference and/or ethnic and cultural background
- Cognitively less impaired resident being among those who are more impaired

Even when MDD is recognized, less than one-quarter of those diagnosed receive treatment, and when they are treated with medication, they often receive a suboptimal dose or inappropriate antidepressant polypharmacy (Hui and Sultzer 2013).

that in younger adults. LTC residents are less inclined to express feelings of low mood or sadness openly and are more apt to present with somatic complaint (e.g. weakness, fatigue, dizziness) or to display anxiety, irritability, ruminative thinking, loss of interest, anhedonia, loss of appetite, sleeplessness, or pessimism. Feelings of worthlessness, being a burden, loss of confidence, and decreased self-esteem commonly

Table 5.2 Differentiating Delirium from Major Depressive Disorder and Major Neurocognitive Disorder due to Alzheimer's Disease

Feature	Delirium	Major Depressive Disorder (MDD)	Major Neurocognitive Disorder due to Alzheimer's Disease
Onset	Acute (over hours to few days)	Subacute (over weeks)	Insidious (over years)
Dramatic fluctuation in severity of symptoms within a day	Present (symptoms typically worse at night)	Occasionally present	Usually absent
Impaired attention (e.g. difficulty following conversation)	Present and severity fluctuates	Usually absent	Absent (except in severe stages)
Altered level of consciousness (drowsiness or hyperalert state)	Usually present	Absent	Absent
Disorganization in thinking	Usually present	Absent	Absent (except in severe stages)
Reversal of sleep-wake cycle	Often present	Absent	Absent (except in severe stages)
Impaired memory	Present and is due to impaired attention	Often present and is due to impaired attention and motivation	Present and is due to impaired encoding
Depressed mood	Occasionally present	Present	Occasionally present
Feelings of hopelessness and helplessness	Usually absent	Often present	Usually absent (except when resident has insight into having AD)
Delusions	Often present (typically persecutory delusions)	Absent (except in MDD with psychotic symptoms)	Occasionally present (typically involving others stealing belongings)
Perceptual disturbances	Often present (typically visual hallucinations and illusions)	Absent (except in MDD with psychotic symptoms when auditory hallucinations may be present)	Absent in mild stages; may be present in advanced stages (typically visual hallucinations and illusions)
Course	Fluctuating, may progress to coma without treatment; usually reversible with appropriate treatment	Slow worsening of symptoms without treatment; usually reversible with appropriate treatment	Relentless and irreversible progression to more severe stages

accompany physical symptoms. Prominent agitation, aggressive behavior (verbal and/or physical), social withdrawal, and/or accelerated cognitive and functional decline may also be the predominant manifestation of MDD in LTC populations, especially among residents who have neurocognitive deficits. Clinical signs and symptoms of MDD may also be modified or masked by comorbidity or causative disease process, such as severe chronic pain or aphasia. Bradykinesia and flat affect of Parkinson's disease may be mistaken for depressive symptoms. Symptoms of poor appetite, fatigue, and sleep disturbance may overlap with

BOX 5.6 Main Features of Major Depressive Disorder in Long-Term Care Populations

Core symptoms

1. Lack of interest in daily activities
2. Depressed mood/affect

Additional symptoms

1. Lack of appetite or weight loss; increased appetite or weight gain
2. Insomnia or hypersomnia
3. Recurrent thoughts of suicide, wish to die, or suicide attempt
4. Decreased energy or fatigue
5. Hopelessness
6. Helplessness
7. Worthlessness
8. Inappropriate or excessive guilt
9. Loss of self-confidence
10. Staying in bed excessively
11. Multiple somatic complaints
12. Chronic pain not responding to pain medication
13. Hypochondriasis (excessive fear that one may have or will develop a serious illness)
14. Marked symptoms of anxiety
15. Agitation (especially by resident who has advanced MNCD)
16. Verbal aggression or verbally abusive behavior (especially by resident who has advanced MNCD)
17. Physical aggression (especially by resident who has advanced MNCD)
18. Decreased spontaneous speech
19. Psychomotor retardation or agitation
20. Refusing medication
21. Resisting care
22. Refusing to participate in therapy (physical, occupational, speech)
23. Sudden decline in cognition
24. Subjective memory complaint

symptoms of a wide variety of physical illnesses. There may be complaints of memory problems with MDD and lack of effort in answering memory questions, with "I don't know" answers being common. The HCP should suspect MDD if the resident has been staying in his or her room more, the resident "takes to bed" because of physical illness, or a therapist reports a failure of rehabilitation efforts during recovery from a stroke or hip fracture surgery. In the presence of coexisting depressive symptoms and physical illness, the HCP may incorrectly assume that the depressive symptoms are the result of a general medical condition. We recommend including all symptoms present (e.g. low appetite, low energy) as part of the depressive symptom cluster. If sufficient symptoms are present to meet the *DSM-5* criteria for MDD, then the HCP should diagnose MDD even if some symptoms may be partly due to comorbid physical health problems.

Although core depressive symptoms are similar across cultures, cultural factors may modify the presentation of MDD. For example, older depressed people from Southeast Asia often present with physical complaint (e.g. weakness, dizziness) without depressed mood. African Americans may present with irritability, hostility, or vague somatic complaint. Latinos may complain of having problems with "nerves" or having "heartache" (Lewis-Fernandez et al. 2005).

Table 5.3 Key Types of Major Depressive Disorders in LTC Populations

Type of MDD	Clinical Features	Implications for Treatment
Single episode	First episode of MDD	Treatment may be discontinued after 1 year of remission of symptoms unless depression has been life threatening.
Recurrent MDD	Two or more episodes of MDD	Treatment usually needs to be continued for at least 5 years after remission of symptoms and often lifelong. HCP should offer mindfulness-based CBT to prevent relapse in residents who have relatively intact cognitive functioning.
Mild, moderate, and severe MDD	Based on number of symptoms present and severity of functional impairment	Mild MDD may be treated without antidepressant. Resident who has severe MDD may need inpatient psychiatric treatment.
MDD with psychotic symptoms	Presence of delusions, hallucinations, and/or catatonic symptoms	ECT is the most effective treatment. Antipsychotics usually need to be added to antidepressant if ECT is not an option.
MDD with atypical features	Presence of mood reactivity (positive mood in response to positive events), reverse vegetative signs (increased appetite, weight gain, hypersomnia), leaden paralysis (feelings of heaviness in limbs), and lifelong pattern of sensitivity to interpersonal rejection	SSRIs and SNRIs may not be effective. MAOIs are preferred antidepressants.
MDD with melancholic features	Loss of pleasure in all activities, lack of positive response to positive events, despair, depressed mood worse in morning, awakening 2 hours before usual, marked agitation or psychomotor retardation, anorexia, weight loss, excessive feelings of guilt	Responds well to ECT and tricyclic antidepressant (e.g. nortriptyline)
MDD with significant anxiety symptoms	Anxiety symptoms, such as feeling tense, restless, excessive worries, fear that something terrible will happen, sense of loss of control of self	Short-term use of low dose of short-acting benzodiazepine (e.g. lorazepam) may be necessary along with antidepressant for treatment response.
MDD with mixed features	Presence of hypomanic symptoms, such as elated mood, grandiosity, talkativeness, racing thoughts, increased energy interspersed with typical depressive symptoms	May not respond to antidepressant and may need addition of atypical antipsychotic or mood stabilizer Significant risk factor for development of bipolar disorder

BOX 5.7 Myths about Depression and Suicide in Long-Term Care Populations

1. Trivialization (Wouldn't you be depressed too?)
2. Belittling of psychiatric treatment (therapeutic nihilism) (Does it really work for these people when it is too late, anyway?)
3. Older people do not want psychiatric treatment
4. Depression is a normal part of aging
5. Depression cannot be distinguished from normal aging
6. Depression is a normal part of adjusting to life in a LTC facility
7. Suicidal ideas are a normal part of aging or adjusting to life in a LTC facility

Major Depressive Disorder with Psychotic Symptoms

When residents who have MDD develop delusions, hallucinations, and/or catatonic symptoms, they are said to have MDD with psychotic symptoms (also called psychotic depression). These residents often have rigidity in thinking, have more severe depression, and exhibit delusions that are usually congruent to mood and can include delusions of guilt relative to past events, poverty, somatic illness (e.g. preoccupation with having a terminal illness, such as cancer), or paranoia. Hallucinations, which occur less commonly than delusions in these residents, are more likely to be auditory than visual or somatic. Residents who have psychotic depression are much more likely to have agitation – "the classic pacing and wringing of hands" – have greater cognitive disturbance, and are more likely to have a family history of MDD or bipolar disorder. A history of delusions in a depressive episode or profound anxiety in a depressed resident is a major clue to possible psychotic depression. Psychotic depression carries a high risk of suicide and does not respond to antidepressant alone; hence, it is important that the HCP diagnose this entity as early as possible. Additional antipsychotic is usually necessary along with antidepressant for treatment response. The HCP should consider hospitalization and electroconvulsive therapy (ECT) early in the course of treatment, and we strongly recommend them for life-threatening cases of psychotic depression. ECT can be used safely with this population and in severe cases of psychotic depression (e.g. with inanition or catatonia) may be lifesaving.

Late-Onset Major Depressive Disorder

Late age at onset or late-life MDD (Late-onset MDD) is defined as a first episode of depression occurring after age 60 years and is characterized by a greater degree of apathy, cognitive dysfunction, resistance to treatment, neuroimaging evidence of cerebrovascular disease (especially white matter hyperintensities), and age-related changes that are greater than normal, as compared to early age at onset late-life MDD (Grayson and Thomas 2013). Late-onset MDD may be a prodrome of Alzheimer's disease (AD), and MDD in midlife may be a risk factor for the development of AD. MDD in individuals who have mild neurocognitive disorder (mild cognitive impairment [MCI]) increases the likelihood of conversion of MNCD. Inflammation may be a common underlying neuropathophysiological mechanism for MDD and AD. Thus, the HCP should closely follow all residents who have late-onset MDD and no MNCD for signs of MCI and mild MNCD due to AD. A score of less than 24 on MOCA (or SLUMS or MMSE) or a decline of more than three points from a stable baseline is thought to be clinically significant and to warrant evaluation for MNCD.

Diagnostic Assessment and Work-Up

A variety of conditions can mimic MDD, cause MDD-like symptoms, or exacerbate MDD. We recommend a comprehensive diagnostic assessment and work-up when the HCP thinks that depressive symptoms are more than a normal reaction to a situational stressor and more disabling than an adjustment disorder. See Table 5.4 (Borson and Thompson 2011; Blazer and Steffens 2015; Nassan et al. 2016). The choice of tests and extent of work-up will depend on findings from a comprehensive assessment and examination of the resident. MDD may be the initial presentation of Parkinson's disease or Huntington's disease, as motor symptoms or involuntary movement may be subtle in early stages; hence the importance of neurological examination. MDD and undernutrition (dehydration, protein and/or energy malnutrition, severe weight loss, vitamin deficiencies) are a potentially fatal combination because immune functioning may be affected, and the HCP should consider this a psychiatric and medical emergency. The HCP needs to act quickly to provide nutritional supplementation and aggressive treatment of MDD to avert serious debility,

Table 5.4 Diagnostic Work-Up for Major Depressive Disorder in LTC Populations

Diagnostic Test	Key Examples	Key Implications for Treatment
Comprehensive assessment	Psychiatric history (including history of suicide attempt) Family history (including history of suicide) Review of medications Vital signs Physical examination (including height, weight, body mass index) Neurological examination Mental status examination Use of standardized assessment scales	Suicide risk assessment is primarily based on comprehensive assessment Findings from cognitive assessment are key to choosing treatment (e.g. psychotherapy for residents who have relatively preserved cognitive functioning)
Bedside test	Pulse oximetry	Hypoxia may contribute to depressive symptoms
Bedside test	Glucose fingerstick	Hypoglycemia and severe hyperglycemia may contribute to depressive symptoms
Laboratory test	Complete blood count	Identifying anemia, which may contribute to fatigue and resistance to treatment Leukocytosis or leukopenia may indicate coexisting infection
Laboratory test	Comprehensive metabolic panel	Identifying dehydration and electrolyte imbalance, which may contribute to depressive symptoms and resistance to treatment Identify decline in renal function, which may influence choice of medication to treat depression (e.g. avoiding lithium in resident who has renal insufficiency or closer monitoring of lithium levels) Low albumin is indicator of protein malnutrition
Laboratory test	Vitamin B_{12} and vitamin D levels	Vitamin B_{12} and vitamin D deficiency are common in residents who have MDD and contribute to resistance to treatment if not corrected
Laboratory test	Thyroid function tests (e.g. thyroid stimulating hormone level)	Undercorrection or overcorrection of hypothyroidism is prevalent in residents who have MDD and contributes to resistance to treatment if not corrected
Laboratory test	Lipid panel	Low cholesterol is indicator of malnutrition
Laboratory test	Serum drug levels	Serum levels of antidepressant (e.g. nortriptyline) may help adjust dose and avoid toxicity
Laboratory test	Erythrocyte sedimentation rate (ESR) and C-reactive protein (CRP)	Identify exacerbation of rheumatological conditions and occult cancers that may cause or contribute to depression

Table 5.4 (cont.)

Diagnostic Test	Key Examples	Key Implications for Treatment
Laboratory or bedside test	Electrocardiogram (EKG)	Avoid using antidepressants that have significant risk of QTc prolongation (e.g. citalopram, mirtazapine) with resident who has baseline prolonged QTc due to risk of Torsades de pointes
Neuroimaging	MRI of brain	Evidence of silent stroke (e.g. lacunar infarct in frontostriatal pathways) may indicate cerebrovascular factors causing or contributing to MDD and/or suggest vascular depression
Laboratory test	Psychotropic drug genetic testing using buccal swab	HCP should avoid prescribing antidepressants with significant metabolism by 2D6 (e.g. paroxetine, fluoxetine) or 2C19 (citalopram, escitalopram) system for resident who metabolizes 2D6 or 2C19 system poorly, respectively
Imaging	CT scan of abdomen and/or lung	MDD-like symptoms with severe weight loss may be initial manifestation of occult malignancy (e.g. pancreatic cancer, lung cancer)

hospitalization, and death. For residents who have life-threatening MDD (e.g. intense thoughts of suicide, suicide attempt, undernutrition, severe agitation due to psychotic symptoms), transfer to a local emergency department for acute inpatient psychiatric hospitalization, preferably in a geriatric psychiatry inpatient unit, may be a necessary first step before the HCP can complete a comprehensive work-up.

Prevention and Treatment

MDD in LTC populations is often preventable. See Table 5.5 (Beekman, Cuijpers, and Smit 2013). Most preventive approaches can be led by nurses. MDD in LTC populations is eminently treatable, and the goal of treatment can be achieved with a comprehensive holistic individualized treatment plan using a variety of evidence-based options (Taylor 2014). The goals of treatment should go beyond remission of symptoms and include prevention of relapse and promotion of wellness (happiness and meaningful engagement in life). We recommend implementing the Clinical Practice Guidelines for the Treatment of Depression in LTC residents, by the Society for Post-Acute and Long-Term Care Medicine (formerly called the American Medical Directors Association [AMDA] www.paltc.org). The choice of treatment options for MDD listed in Table 5.6 depends on the severity of depressive symptoms, past response to treatment, resident and family preference, and resident strengths (especially cognitive functioning) (Blazer and Steffens 2015; Smoski, Jenal, and Thompson 2015; Huang et al. 2015). We recommend a combination of antidepressant therapy and individualized strengths-based psychosocial environmental approaches for any resident who has MDD, especially if it is in keeping with the preferences of the resident and/or the family. If the resident and/or the family opposes the use of antidepressant (e.g. has a negative view of the use of psychotropic medication), a trial of individual psychotherapy, and in particular cognitive-behavioral therapy (CBT) and/or individualized pleasant activity schedule and other individualized psychosocial environmental approaches (e.g. bright light therapy), is appropriate for the mild first episode of MDD. For residents who have moderate to severe MDD, we strongly recommend treatment with antidepressant.

The choice of an antidepressant should be informed by individual medication and resident factors: the adverse effect profile of the medication, tolerability of treatment (including potential for interaction with other

Table 5.5 Prevention of Major Depressive Disorder in Long-Term Care Populations

Type of Prevention	Key Target Residents	Key Approaches
Indicated prevention (targets residents who have mild depressive symptoms that do not reach criteria for MDD; goal is to prevent MDD)	Resident who has adjustment disorder with depressed mood Resident who has persistent depressive disorder Resident who has demoralization syndrome Resident who has bereavement-related depression or complicated grief Resident who has Parkinson's disease and mild depressive symptoms	Staff education to improve detection of mild depressive symptoms and institution of prevention strategies Exercise and physical activity program Psychotherapy/counseling* (including self-help versions) for motivated resident who has relatively preserved cognitive functioning Antidepressant (e.g. for persistent depressive disorder and complicated grief) Individualized pleasant and meaningful activity schedule Bright light therapy for resident who has seasonal affective disorder and other residents open to this approach Stepped-care approach in which approaches start with exercise and self-help strategies and slowly step up to antidepressants and/or psychotherapy if symptoms continue Optimizing motor function in resident who has Parkinson's disease
Selective prevention (targets residents who have known risk factors for MDD; goal is to prevent MDD and relapse of MDD)	Resident who sustained new CVA/stroke All residents soon after admission (especially unplanned admission) Resident who has lost spouse Resident who has history of MDD Resident who has newly diagnosed serious or life-threatening illness (e.g. cancer, MNCD) Resident who has macular degeneration Resident taking interferon therapy Resident who has insomnia disorder Resident who has chronic pain Resident who has Parkinson's disease Resident who has MDD in remission	Staff education regarding risk factors for MDD and institution of prevention strategies in high-risk groups Exercise and physical activity program Psychotherapy/counseling* (including self-help versions) for motivated resident who has relatively good cognitive functioning to help cope with loss or living with serious illness or disability (e.g. problem-solving therapy for resident who has macular degeneration) Individualized pleasant and meaningful activity schedule Antidepressant (e.g. after CVA for resident who has history of MDD and is not taking antidepressant; for resident who has MDD and is in remission; SNRI for resident who has chronic pain that is not optimally controlled) Optimizing motor function in resident who has Parkinson's disease

Table 5.5 (cont.)

Type of Prevention	Key Target Residents	Key Approaches
Universal prevention (targets all LTC populations; goal is to prevent MDD and improve resilience)	All residents	Exercise and physical activity program Individualized pleasant and meaningful activity schedule Omega-3 fatty acids and vitamin D Optimal control of vascular risk factors (e.g. hypertension, diabetes) Optimal control of pain Periodic staff, resident, and family education and awareness campaign about signs and symptoms of MDD and prevention strategies

* Psychotherapy/counseling: Cognitive behavior therapy, interpersonal therapy, problem solving therapy, reminiscence therapy, life-review, music therapy, dignity therapy

Table 5.6 Evidence-Based Approaches to Treat Major Depressive Disorder in Long-Term Care Populations

Approach	Clinical Pearls	Key Concerns/Limitations
Antidepressant (e.g. SSRI, SNRI, bupropion, mirtazapine, TCA, MAOI)	SSRI and SNRI preferred over TCA and MAOI Bupropion may be preferred for resident who is obese due to its potential to promote weight loss Response may take several weeks after therapeutic dose is reached	Serotonin syndrome and seizure can occur with concomitant use of tramadol Use of SSRI and SNRI is associated with increased risk of bleeding with concomitant use of antiplatelets, anticoagulants, and omega-3 fatty acid
Behavioral Activation and Individualized Pleasant Activity Schedule (IPAS)	Residents are encouraged to get out of bed, become active physically, intellectually, and socially, and participate in activities that are pleasurable and tailored to their interests and values	Staff need education and training in implementation of IPAS Resident needs some motivation
Onsite individual counseling/ psychotherapy (cognitive behavioral therapy [CBT], mindfulness-based CBT, problem-solving therapy, interpersonal psychotherapy, supportive psychotherapy, meaning-centered psychotherapy)	Individual psychotherapy without concomitant use of antidepressant may be appropriate for mild MDD in motivated resident who has relatively preserved cognitive functioning Combination of antidepressant and psychotherapy is recommended for motivated resident who has relatively good cognitive functioning and is experiencing moderate to severe MDD and/or recurrent MDD	Lack of availability of counselors trained in providing psychotherapy to LTC populations Lack of availability of counselors visiting LTC facilities to provide psychotherapy Resident may need to leave LTC facility and visit local mental health clinic

Table 5.6 (cont.)

Approach	Clinical Pearls	Key Concerns/Limitations
Internet-based and telepsychiatry approaches	Cognitive restructuring (to address cognitive distortions), behavioral activation, and problem-solving strategies can be effectively administered via Internet and telepsychiatry by psychiatric nurse or other mental health professional Good option for motivated resident (especially resident comfortable using technology) who has relatively preserved cognitive function and lack of availability of on-site psychotherapy Preferably used with antidepressant	Resident needs to be motivated and have relatively good cognitive functioning Technophobia may be difficult barrier Needs involvement of mental health professional to monitor response to treatment
Psychoeducation and self-management	Providing pamphlets and other education materials on MDD and late-life depression can reduce stigma resident experiences	Cognitive deficit in resident may limit its benefit
Methylphenidate	Adding methylphenidate to SSRI may accelerate response to treatment and increase likelihood of remission	Use limited to resident at relatively low risk of serious adverse event related to use of methylphenidate
Antipsychotic (e.g. aripiprazole, quetiapine, olanzapine, cariprazine, brexpiprazole)	Recommended for treatment-resistant MDD and MDD with psychotic symptoms	Management by psychiatrist is recommended if there is need for antipsychotic due to high risk associated with use of antipsychotic medication
Neurostimulation therapy	Electroconvulsive therapy (ECT) for life-threatening MDD and treatment-resistant MDD Transcranial magnetic stimulation (TMS) may be useful for mild MDD and as adjuvant to antidepressant for treatment-resistant MDD Vagal nerve stimulation (VNS)	Lack of availability of professionals providing neurostimulation therapy in the community Lack of reimbursement from health insurance for neurostimulation therapy (especially TMS) VNS and ECT should be done in academic center
Omega-3 fatty acid supplementation	Eicosapentanoic acid (EPA) and ethyl-EPA dominant formulation recommended	Small risk of increased bleeding, especially with concomitant use of NSAID, anticoagulant, antiplatelet, SSRI, or SNRI
Vitamin D supplementation	Checking vitamin D levels is recommended, as vitamin D deficiency is prevalent in residents who have MDD and may require vitamin D replacement therapy	Hypervitaminosis D, although rare, can occur and manifest as headache and dizziness
Bright light therapy	May be used with antidepressant, especially if there is history of seasonal affective disorder (e.g. winter depression)	Staff education and training is required for appropriate use of bright light therapy box

Table 5.6 (cont.)

Approach	Clinical Pearls	Key Concerns/Limitations
Exercise/physical activity	Exercise and increasing physical activity can accelerate response to antidepressant and increase likelihood of remission	Lack of time available to staff to help resident increase physical activity is key barrier to its routine use
Rational deprescribing (geriatric scalpel) with input from pharmacist	Discontinuation of medication that may contribute to depression, discontinuation of unnecessary or inappropriate medication (based on Beers list), and reducing anticholinergic burden may improve cognitive and emotional functioning of resident and reduce adverse drug-drug interaction with antidepressant	None
Optimizing control of pain and other comorbid physical health problems (e.g. hypertension) and correction of reversible physical health problems (e.g. dehydration, constipation, vitamin B_{12} deficiency, vision and hearing impairment, thyroid disorder)	Recommended for all residents	None

current medication), response to prior treatment, and resident and family preference. (See Table 5.7.) For example, there is significant risk of bleeding with use of an SSRI if the resident is taking an anticoagulant (e.g. warfarin) and/or antiplatelet (e.g. aspirin). Bupropion carries significant risk of seizure in residents who have epilepsy. In addition, LTC populations often exhibit higher and more variable drug concentrations and a greater sensitivity to adverse drug effect. The earlier the antidepressant starts to work, the better the chance for a good outcome; research data support the correlation between earlier clinical improvement and more robust recovery. The key to successful pharmacotherapy for MDD is giving the resident an adequate dose of antidepressant for an adequate duration (at least six weeks).

Residents who have depression present three key challenges for treatment: comorbid medical condition that may complicate the treatment of depression, concomitant use of medication(s) that may contribute to depression or interact with antidepressant, and a slow metabolic rate. The presence of a neurovegetative symptom (e.g. severe appetite and weight loss), suicidal ideation, and psychotic symptoms may indicate a need for more vigorous and comprehensive therapy (e.g. higher medication dosage, multiple medication trials, or ECT). Referral to a mental health specialist with expertise in LTC psychiatry is appropriate when the diagnosis of depression is unclear, when the syndrome is severe, if a risk of suicide is present, when the resident does not respond to treatment, or when complicating factors that may affect the choice of treatment are present. The HCP may consider ECT and/or hospitalization to an inpatient psychiatric unit (preferably a geriatric psychiatry unit) for the treatment of life-threatening or refractory depression even for residents who have MNCD. To improve early recognition, accurate diagnosis, and prompt successful treatment of MDD in LTC populations, we suggest a collaborative care model for MDD (with modifications) that has transformed the care of adults who have MDD in outpatient primary care clinics. In this model for LTC, primary care clinicians work closely with a psychiatrist, either directly or through a mental health professional (typically a social worker or licensed counsellor). Psychiatrists in this model must be quickly available to primary care clinicians who are seeking guidance on a resident's treatment plan.

Table 5.7 Common Antidepressants Used to Treat Major Depressive Disorder in Long-Term Care Populations

Antidepressant (Therapeutic Dose Range)	Potential Mechanism of Action and Clinical Pearls	Key Concerns/Limitations
Citalopram (10–40 mg/day)	SSRI May be first-line antidepressant Among all antidepressants, citalopram has best evidence for efficacy in management of severe behavioral and psychological symptoms of MNCD	Potential to prolong QTc is a concern, especially at doses above 20 mg Baseline EKG recommended Risks similar to those of other SSRIs
Escitalopram (5–20 mg/day)	SSRI May be first-line antidepressant Potential to prolong QTc is lower than that of citalopram	Risks similar to those of other SSRIs
Fluoxetine (10–30 mg/day)	SSRI Considered second- or third-line antidepressant	Long half-life is a concern in LTC populations Risks similar to those of other SSRIs
Fluvoxamine (50–200 mg/day)	SSRI Considered third- or fourth-line antidepressant	Long half-life and high potential for drug–drug interaction limit its use in LTC populations Risks similar to those of other SSRIs
Paroxetine (10–30 mg/day) and Paroxetine controlled release (12.5–25 mg/day)	SSRI Considered second- or third-line antidepressant	Risk of anticholinergic adverse effect and risk of drug–drug interaction due to inhibitory effect on cytochrome P450 2D6 enzyme system limit its use Risks similar to those of other SSRIs
Sertraline (50–200 mg/day)	SSRI May be first-line antidepressant	Risks similar to those of other SSRIs
Trazodone (25–50 mg)	Increases serotonin neurotransmission Used primarily as adjuvant to SSRI or SNRI to improve sleep	Antidepressant dose (200–300 mg/day) is too sedating for LTC residents Potential for orthostatic hypotension
Venlafaxine extended release (75–225 mg/day)	Starts as SSRI and becomes SNRI at higher doses May be first-line antidepressant SNRI effect may also help with management of chronic pain	Risks similar to those of SSRIs and SNRIs
Duloxetine (30–90 mg/day)	SNRI May be first-line antidepressant Preferred over SSRIs for management of MDD for resident with management of co-occurring chronic musculoskeletal pain, diabetic neuropathy, and fibromyalgia	Higher cost may limit its use as first-line antidepressant Risks similar to those of SSRIs and other SNRIs
Mirtazapine (15–30 mg/day)	Increases serotonergic, noradrenergic, and histaminic neurotransmission May be first-line antidepressant Its potential to improve appetite and promote weight gain may make it preferable to other antidepressants for resident who has MDD associated with significant weight loss	Potential to prolong QTc interval Baseline EKG recommended Potential for daytime sleepiness

Table 5.7 (cont.)

Antidepressant (Therapeutic Dose Range)	Potential Mechanism of Action and Clinical Pearls	Key Concerns/Limitations
Bupropion sustained release (100–300 mg/day in two divided doses, last dose not after 4 p.m.) and Bupropion XL (150–300 mg/day)	NDRI (noradrenaline dopamine reuptake inhibitor) May be best choice for overweight resident who wants to lose weight Usually used as second-line antidepressant	Potential to increase risk of seizure
Methylphenidate (10–20 mg/day in two divided doses, last dose not after 4 p.m.)	Stimulant May be used as adjuvant to SSRI to accelerate response to treatment and improve chance of remission	Potential for adverse cardiovascular event, including sudden cardiac death Baseline EKG recommended
Nortriptyline (25–150 mg/day)	TCA Usually used as second- or third-line antidepressant Preferred over SSRI and SNRI for treatment of MDD in resident who has Parkinson's disease Therapeutic drug levels can help monitor risk for adverse event and therapeutic effect	Anticholinergic effect and risk of adverse cardiac event limit its routine use Nortriptyline has therapeutic window Baseline EKG recommended
Desvenlafaxine* (50 mg/day)	SNRI May be considered third- or fourth-line antidepressant	Minimal data on benefits and risks in LTC populations
Vilazodone* (10–40 mg/day)	SSRI plus 5HT1a agonist May be considered third- or fourth-line antidepressant	Minimal data on benefits and risks in LTC populations
Selegiline* patch (6–12 mg/day)	Increases dopaminergic neurotransmission May be considered third- or fourth-line antidepressant May be considered first-line antidepressant to treat MDD in resident who has Parkinson's disease	Minimal data on benefits and risks in LTC populations
Vortioxetine* (5–20 mg/day)	Increases release of several neurotransmitters (e.g. serotonin, noradrenaline, acetylcholine) May be considered third- or fourth-line antidepressant May have beneficial effect on cognitive function	Minimal data on benefits and risks in LTC populations
Levomilnacipran* (40–100 mg/day)	Strongest norepinephrine reuptake inhibition among SNRIs May be considered third- or fourth-line antidepressant	Minimal data on benefits and risks in LTC populations

* Therapeutic dose range is not clear due to limited research on its use in LTC populations.

Starting and Ending Antidepressants. Educating residents, family, and staff about what to expect in the course of antidepressant therapy is critical. Difficulties can develop at any time in the course of antidepressant therapy, but they seem to cluster at the beginning, during any increase in dosage, and during discontinuation of the drug. Although it usually takes weeks for a therapeutic response, most adverse effects (e.g. nausea, diarrhea, constipation, sedation, lethargy, headache, and agitation) appear shortly after the first dose and after any increase in dosage. Thus, it is vital that the HCP educate the resident and caregivers that adverse effects, when they occur, usually precede therapeutic effects. Usually, if the dose is started low and increased slowly, early adverse effects are mild, are self-limiting, and remit within a few days to two weeks. For residents who are particularly prone to developing adverse effects (especially anxiety and insomnia), the HCP can minimize the risk of adverse effect by reducing the antidepressant dose to an even smaller starting dose, increasing it even more slowly, and using a lower final dose.

With some of the commonly used antidepressants, if a resident abruptly discontinues taking it after taking it for several weeks or more, a discontinuation syndrome is common. The discontinuation syndrome involves manifestations of dizziness, paresthesia (typically electric shock-like sensations), muscle jerks and twitches, and agitation. Drugs such as paroxetine and venlafaxine carry the highest risk of discontinuation syndrome due to their short half-life. Discontinuation syndrome is milder with intermediate-acting antidepressant, such as citalopram, sertraline, and escitalopram. Typically, the discontinuation syndrome remits within one to two weeks. Treatment may involve reinstating the antidepressant and tapering it more slowly. “Serotonin syndrome” is a serious and potentially fatal condition that may develop with use of a high dose of SSRI or use of SSRI in combination with other medication that also increases serotonin neurotransmission (e.g. lithium, trazodone, tramadol). Clinical manifestation of “serotonin syndrome” includes hyperreflexia, agitation, insomnia, myoclonic jerks, autonomic instability, and delirium. Treatment involves discontinuing the offending drug, close monitoring of vital signs, and hospitalization for severe symptoms.

Treatment-resistant and Treatment-refractory MDD. Partial response to the first-line antidepressant monotherapy (adequate dose and duration) is common and may be seen in as many as 50 percent of cases (Unutzer and Park 2012). Further response often requires augmentation strategies, although increasing the dose of the antidepressant the resident is already taking may also be appropriate (Lenze et al. 2015). Residual symptoms are strong predictors of relapse that may place the resident at higher risk for suicide. Older adults who have limited mobility or who present with a history suggesting that MDD is superimposed on underlying persistent depressive disorder (double depression) may be most at risk for partial response. Addition of an adjuvant such as aripiprazole, quetiapine, brexpiprazole is considered the first-line treatment for treatment-resistant MDD, as the Food and Drug Administration (FDA) has approved these drugs for treatment-resistant MDD. The FDA has also approved a combination of fluoxetine and olanzapine for treatment-resistant MDD. Addition of methylphenidate to an SSRI can accelerate improvement and increase the likelihood of remission of MDD in older adults (Lavretsky et al. 2015). The HCP may consider prescribing a combination of an SSRI and methylphenidate for residents who have MDD and are at relatively low risk of serious adverse cardiovascular event due to use of methylphenidate. The HCP may also consider other strategies for augmentation, including another antidepressant (that targets neurotransmitter networks different from the first one), buspirone, or triiodothyronine, opioids, ECT, and psychotherapy (for residents who have relatively good cognitive function and initially declined psychotherapy). We do not recommend augmentation with lithium for most LTC residents because of the high risk of toxicity due to pre-existing medical and cognitive frailty. Augmenting one antidepressant by adding a second with a different mechanism of action (e.g. an SSRI with bupropion or mirtazapine) is a common practice in LTC but does not have good support from research and is associated with potentially serious risk (e.g. risk of delirium when bupropion is added to duloxetine because both are cytochrome P450 2D6 enzyme inhibitors that may result in a higher level of hydroxybupropion, which is implicated in delirium).

Up to 35 percent of patients may show partial or minimal improvement in depressive symptoms with treatment despite at least two adequate trials with antidepressants from two different classes. These patients are said to have treatment-refractory depression. True treatment refractoriness should be differentiated from pseudo-refractoriness. The HCP should consider nonadherence, although uncommon in LTC populations, as with community-dwelling older adults who have MDD, it is prevalent and the most common cause of nonresponse. Many patients do not get better because antidepressants are not given at an adequate dose for an adequate time to work and psychosocial approaches are not individualized and used vigorously. The HCP needs to educate family and professional caregivers that these medications take six to eight weeks to start to show noticeable results. The goal should be remission of symptoms. Unaddressed underlying triggers, such as pain, thyroid problem, anemia, or a malignancy, also might prevent an adequate response to antidepressant therapy. The presence of executive dysfunction, underlying MNCD, significant cerebrovascular burden (vascular depression), or frailty also increases the chance of inadequate response to treatment. Another prevalent factor in treatment resistance is an incorrect diagnosis (e.g. correct diagnosis is bipolar depression rather than unipolar MDD). If the first trial of an antidepressant at an adequate dose and duration fails, the HCP should initiate a second trial with another class of antidepressant. If the second trial also fails, then the HCP should try prescribing a secondary tricyclic antidepressant (TCA), such as nortriptyline, if there is no contraindication (e.g. severe heart disease). If symptoms continue to be disabling and are not responding to multiple trials of antidepressant (treatment-refractory MDD), the HCP should consider ECT. For residents who have a history of good response to ECT, the HCP should consider ECT early in the course of treatment. The HCP may also consider prescribing pramipexole and selegiline transdermal patch for refractory cases, especially for residents who have Parkinson's disease, as pramipexole and selegiline increase dopaminergic neurotransmission in the brain. The HCP may consider prescribing a trial of ketamine or buprenorphine in an academic setting to treat refractory severe MDD and for life-threatening MDD if ECT is not an option.

Nutraceuticals (supplements). The HCP should consider adjunctive use of omega-3 (primarily EPA or ethyl EPA [1–2 mg/day]), methylfolate (15–30 mg/day), S-adenosylmethionine (SAMe [800–1600 mg/day]), and vitamin D (1000–1500 IUs/day) with antidepressant for the treatment of MDD based on the preference of the resident and/or the family (Sarris et al. 2016; Merrill, Payne, Lavretsky 2013). We do not recommend prescribing St. John's wort for LTC populations because it has clinically significant drug-drug interaction with conventional antidepressants and other medication the resident may be taking. All supplements have some potential for adverse effect (typically constipation, diarrhea, stomach upset) and drug-supplement interaction (e.g. increased risk of bleeding with concomitant use of omega-3 and anticoagulants). Hence, the HCP should use them cautiously. Omega-3 and methylfolate should be used with caution for residents who have prostate cancer due to reports that their use may be associated with the risk for prostate cancer. The HCP should prescribe SAMe cautiously for residents who have bipolar disorder because of its potential to switch depression to hypomania/mania. Hypercalcemia and vascular calcification are risks associated with the use of high-dose vitamin D.

Neuromodulation Therapy/Brain Stimulation Therapy. Neuromodulation therapies include electroconvulsive therapy, transcranial magnetic stimulation, vagal nerve stimulation, electrical deep-brain stimulation, and deep transcranial magnetic stimulation. If the HCP is considering electroconvulsive therapy or vagal nerve stimulation as a treatment option for MDD in LTC populations, we recommend involving an academic center due to the high medical comorbidity and risk of cognitive adverse effect.

Electroconvulsive Therapy. Electroconvulsive therapy (ECT) is the most effective treatment for severe MDD and life-threatening MDD. ECT is a relatively safe treatment and is rapidly effective. Older adults seem to have greater responsiveness to ECT than their younger peers. For residents who have MDD complicated by suicidal ideas, undernutrition and cachexia, and/or catatonic symptoms, ECT can be lifesaving. Other indications for ECT include treatment-refractory MDD, MDD with psychotic symptoms, and any other situation in which rapid antidepressant effect is needed. Residents who have depression and MNCD can be given ECT with good effect, but post-ECT delirium is a greater risk.

Transcranial Magnetic Stimulation. Transcranial magnetic stimulation (TMS) is the safest neuromodulation therapy available. TMS is an excellent option for the treatment of mild MDD in residents due to its low risks, maybe even safer than antidepressant therapy. To date, the FDA has approved four TMS devices. TMS uses electromagnetic induction to create small currents to depolarize neurons in key mood-regulating areas of the prefrontal cortex (usually left dorsolateral prefrontal cortex). Typically, 30–40 sessions of high-frequency (10-Hz) TMS are needed for significant response. Benefits may sustain for up to a year. TMS is considered second-line treatment for mild MDD (antidepressant and/or psychosocial approach is first-line treatment) in LTC populations primarily because of challenges in getting the resident to comply with its requirements (e.g. sitting with eyes open for one hour during each session). For moderate to severe MDD, TMS is not recommended as the primary treatment but can be used as an adjuvant to antidepressant therapy, especially in treatment-resistant cases. Deep TMS involves the use of different coil configurations that allow for more direct stimulation of deeper structures (e.g. pathways associated with the reward system).

Vagal Nerve Stimulation. The FDA has approved vagal nerve stimulation (VNS) for the treatment of treatment-resistant MDD. VNS involves an outpatient surgical procedure to implant a vagal nerve stimulator. The stimulator delivers intermittent mild electrical pulses to the left vagal nerve, whose afferent fibers project to the nucleus of the solitary tract and in turn modulate activity of the locus coeruleus, raphe nucleus, and other neural circuits implicated in MDD. Significant response to VNS may take up to 10 months. VNS is expensive and poses more inherent risks for LTC populations. The device requires programming and adjustments by a clinician who has special training. VNS has not been studied in LTC populations but may be appropriate if the resident is experiencing severe distress due to MDD, the MDD is refractory to all treatments, and ECT is not an option. VNS is also approved for the treatment of epilepsy, so the HCP should consider VNS for residents who have refractory epilepsy and severe depression.

Deep-Brain Stimulation. Deep-brain stimulation (DBS) involves an invasive functional neurosurgical procedure using electrical current directly to modulate specific areas of the brain. Although DBS is not approved by the FDA for the treatment of MDD, the HCP may consider it for treatment-refractory severe MDD, especially for residents who have obsessive-compulsive disorder (OCD), dystonia, or Parkinson's disease, as the FDA approved DBS for the treatment of refractory OCD, dystonia, and Parkinson's disease.

Psychotherapy and Psychosocial Approaches. Psychosocial and environmental approaches are important for all types of depression and may prove more effective and safer than the use of antidepressant for milder disorders (Smoski and Arean 2015). Many residents feel that initiating action in an environment that cannot be changed is futile (learned helplessness). Many residents may have expectations that are not realistic, overgeneralize or overreact to adverse events, and personalize events (cognitive distortions). Perceived negative interpersonal events are also associated with depression, particularly in residents who demonstrate a high need for approval and reassurance in the context of interpersonal relationship. To achieve successful outcome, the HCP may need to address other psychosocial factors, such as mutual social and affective withdrawal between residents and their social environment (family, friends), inadequate compensation for lost interests, failure to optimize abilities, poor quality of social support (e.g. significant family conflicts). For ongoing loss-related depression, including sadness about loss of health, HCP can help the resident ventilate feelings and either reacquire what is lost (for example, reacquiring the ability to ambulate after stroke through physical therapy) or grieve and then adapt to the new situation. Some residents who have relatively good cognitive function may prefer psychotherapy instead of, or in addition to, medication. Moreover, psychotherapy may be the approach of choice for residents who have relatively intact cognitive function and are dealing with grief or other stressful situation or interpersonal problem. Social factors and perceptions of health and well-being may be important predictors of outcome in older adults who have MDD, and the HCP can address them during psychotherapy. Several types of psychotherapy have been found to reduce the symptoms of depression, including cognitive-behavioral therapy, interpersonal therapy, problem-solving therapy, family therapy, and brief psychodynamic therapy. The HCP may also consider life review/reminiscence psychotherapy, group therapy, music therapy, and meaning-centered therapy (logotherapy). Meaning-centered therapy is particularly helpful if the resident is experiencing demoralization or existential/spiritual distress. Psychosocial interventions, including psychoeducation, family counseling, and providing counseling to the spouse, may also be helpful.

Residents who have pre-existing personality disorder, a long-standing history of poor coping skills, and difficulty with interpersonal relationship may benefit from long-term psychotherapy in which the counsellor sees the resident every one to four weeks for months to years. Access to professionals able to provide psychotherapy to LTC populations is a significant barrier. In many instances, the resident may need to be sent to an outpatient clinic that provides such treatment. In an increasing number of LTC facilities, a social worker or psychologist with expertise in providing psychotherapy to LTC residents visits the home to provide psychotherapy to residents identified by the consulting psychiatrist as potentially benefitting from psychotherapy. Most of the social workers who work in LTC facilities do not have the time or training to provide formal psychotherapy to the residents.

Other Complementary and Alternative Treatment Options. Individualized daily pleasant activities schedules and increasing daily physical activity and regular exercise program are two approaches with the most research support for the treatment of MDD in LTC populations and thus we strongly recommend them. Physical activity and regular exercise can also have beneficial effect on cognitive deficit accompanying depression through neuroprotective effect possibly mediated by anti-inflammatory and neurotrophic effect and promotion of vascular health. The HCP should consider a trial of bright light therapy (adjunctive therapy) for all residents who have MDD, especially if they have a history of seasonal affective disorder (especially winter depression) and have minimal exposure to outdoors and sunlight. The HCP may also consider approaches such as Tai Chi, yoga, exposure to sunlight, music therapy, aromatherapy, engagement in spiritual-religious activities and rituals, encouraging engagement in creative activity (e.g. therapeutic coloring), mindfulness and breathing exercises, massage therapy, Reiki, gratitude journaling, pet therapy, and intergenerational activity for the treatment of depression in LTC populations in addition to conventional interventions (antidepressant, psychotherapy). The HCP should routinely ask about resident and family preferences for such approaches and match the approach with the resident's strengths. Family members of a resident may also express a wish to add these approaches to conventional treatment for depression. One advantage of including such approaches is that staff and family can be actively engaged in helping the resident recover from depression, thus indirectly addressing their stress and helping them feel useful.

Other Depressive Spectrum Disorders

Besides MDD, depressive symptoms are commonly seen in the context of a resident's normal reaction to loss, adjustment disorder, bereavement-related depression, persistent depressive disorder, demoralization syndrome, MNCD-related depression, poststroke and vascular depression, depression in residents who have Parkinson's disease, depression due to other general medical or neurological condition, and frailty and depression.

Depressive Symptoms as a Normal Reaction to Loss

Many residents experience sadness, lack of interest, sleep and appetite disturbance, anxiety, and irritability in response to loss (e.g. loss of independence) or to undertreated pain. These symptoms are often a normal reaction of stress, usually mild, transient, and highly responsive to supportive approaches, and the resident should not receive a diagnosis of a mental disorder such as MDD. Emotional support, treatment of pain, and time usually resolve these symptoms. Statements made by residents which may indicate MDD as opposed to normal sadness include but are not limited to "I don't care anymore," "I wish I were dead," and "Help me, help me."

Adjustment Disorder with Depressed Mood

People who have adjustment disorder have significant depressive symptoms in response to an identifiable stressor (other than bereavement), they have some functional impairment, and the symptoms do not meet the criteria for MDD. The HCP should take adjustment disorder seriously, as without treatment it may develop into MDD. After moving from their home to a LTC facility, new residents commonly experience adjustment disorder with depressed mood or with mixed anxiety and depressive symptoms. Other common situations in which residents may experience adjustment disorder include change in room or roommate, transfer to another LTC facility, sudden decrease in visits from close family/friends (due to hospitalization of spouse, for example), and change in staff that the resident has become attached to. Symptoms include tearfulness, insomnia, anxiety, restlessness, irritability, trying to leave, and sometimes aggression. Typically, these symptoms gradually decrease in intensity over one to two months. These symptoms are best managed by psychosocial environmental approaches, such as empathic support from family and staff, providing the resident an outlet to express distress (e.g. therapeutic listening), use of reminiscence, engagement in activities preferred by residents, and counseling family members regarding strategies to ease their loved one's transition to a LTC facility. On occasion, the HCP may consider short-term use of low-dose hypnotic (e.g. zolpidem) to treat severe insomnia or benzodiazepine (e.g. lorazepam or oxazepam) to treat severe symptoms of anxiety. In some residents, these symptoms may progress to MDD. In such situations, the HCP may need to add antidepressant to psychosocial environmental approaches.

Bereavement-Related Depression

Although bereavement is not a mental disorder and most people adjust without professional psychological intervention, it is associated with excess risk of mortality, particularly in the early weeks and months after loss (Smoski, Jenal, and Thompson 2015). Bereaved individuals report diverse psychological reactions, with feelings of emptiness and loss being most prevalent. The resident may express intense sadness, rumination about loss, difficulty sleeping, loss of appetite, and even weight loss in response to a recent loss (or losses) such as death of a spouse. After a lifetime together, often with increasing interdependence during retirement and dependence due to MNCD, the loss of a spouse may result in a chronic or inhibited bereaved state. A recent loss can also reactivate grief from a previous bereavement (especially if those feelings were not acknowledged and expressed). Differentiation of grief and bereavement from MDD can be difficult, especially in early stages of grief when symptoms are most severe. (See Table 5.8.) Diagnosis requires clinical judgment that takes into account the degree of functional impairment, the resident's history, and norms of expression of grief in the resident's culture. The duration of bereavement-related depression also varies. Usually,

Table 5.8 Differentiating Bereavement-Related Depression from Major Depressive Disorder

Feature	Bereavement-Related Depression	Major Depressive Disorder
Predominant emotions	Emptiness and loss	Pervasive sadness and inability to have pleasure in activities that were pleasurable
Fluctuation of symptoms	Typically, dramatic within a day and from day to day with pangs of grief interspersed with positive emotions and even laughter in response to specific memories and reminders	Pervasive sadness or dysphoria that does not fluctuate dramatically, not tied to specific thoughts or preoccupations, and typically, there is absence of positive emotions and laughter
Thought content	Preoccupation with memories and thoughts of the deceased and preserved self-esteem	Frequent presence of feelings of worthlessness, self-loathing, and preoccupation with self-critical and pessimistic thoughts about the future (hopelessness)
Course	Gradual decrease in intensity of negative emotions and thoughts over days to weeks	Persistence and even worsening of negative emotions and thoughts over days to weeks
Functional impairment	Typically, mild to moderate, worst initially but gradually improves over days to weeks	Significant and may worsen over days to weeks
Thoughts of suicide	Usually absent; when present, are transient and take the form of wish to be with the deceased	Often present and may be accompanied by intention to end one's life due to feelings of worthlessness and hopelessness and a suicide plan
Serious suicide attempt	Rare	Suicide is the most serious complication of MDD
Treatment	Supportive (in situations of complicated grief, psychotherapy to help adaptation to loss is recommended)	Comprehensive treatment plan with combination of a variety of evidence-based interventions (see Table 5.6) is indicated

Note: HCP should consider MDD in addition to normal reaction to loss.

symptoms of bereavement do not last beyond two years, although some widows and widowers experience symptoms of bereavement beyond two years. HCPs need to recognize that one does not get over the loss of a person who was deeply loved, and this sense of sadness is normal and expression of enduring love.

Symptoms that indicate complicated grief include difficulty accepting the death, inability to trust others since the death, excessive bitterness related to the death, feeling uneasy about moving on, detachment from formerly close others, feeling that life is meaningless without the deceased, feeling that the future holds no prospect for fulfilment without the deceased, and feeling agitated since the death. Psychotherapy that focuses on promoting adaptation to the loss and psychosocial approaches are primary approaches for the treatment of complicated grief in residents who have relatively good cognitive functioning. Residents who have significant cognitive impairment may need an antidepressant besides psychosocial approaches to reduce suffering associated with complicated grief. In residents who have cognitive impairment, distress associated with complicated grief may manifest as agitation, aggressive behavior, somatic symptoms, and accelerated cognitive and functional decline. It is also important to encourage bereaved residents to continue with spiritual observances that they have been engaging before bereavement-related depression.

Persistent Depressive Disorder

People with persistent depressive disorder (previously called dysthymic disorder) have depressive symptoms for two or more years, symptoms which do not meet the criteria for MDD. MDD may precede or occur during persistent depressive disorder (double depression). Some residents are admitted to the LTC facility having pre-existing persistent depressive disorder as a result of multiple losses related to aging (e.g. loss of health, independence, family) and decline in functional competence and other circumstance. Loss of personal autonomy related to life in a LTC facility often results in persistence and worsening of pre-existing depression. The clinical profile of late-life persistent depressive disorder may be different from that in younger adults. Late-life persistent depressive disorder is often associated with medical illness, institutionalization, progression to MDD, and inadequate response to antidepressant treatment. Early-onset persistent depressive disorder (onset in 20s and 30s) is often related to early loss of a parent in childhood, childhood abuse and neglect, substance use disorder, chronic disabling health problems that started in teens or 20s (e.g. insulin-dependent diabetes, multiple sclerosis, chronic migraine), and personality disorder. Many residents who have early-onset persistent depressive disorder have received antidepressant treatment and counseling services. All residents who have persistent depressive disorder are at risk of MDD due to adverse events after institutionalization (e.g. further decline in physical health) and are candidates for MDD-prevention strategies (see Table 5.5).

Demoralization Syndrome

Demoralization syndrome is characterized by feelings of being defeated by circumstances, loss of confidence to cope and maintain hope, sense of helplessness, hopelessness, and wanting to give up (Tecuta et al. 2015). There is usually an additional spiritual/existential dimension, such as a sense of meaninglessness and expression of being in a spiritual crisis. Depressed mood, anxiety, feelings of shame, feelings of being a burden, and anger often accompany this syndrome. It is often seen in residents who have incurable conditions (especially neurological conditions) and residents who have a life-threatening condition (e.g. cancer) and ongoing adversity (e.g. exhaustion of financial resources, persistent pain, persistent decline in health, lack of response to treatment, disabling adverse effects/complications of treatment, repeated need for hospitalization). The severity of symptoms may fluctuate in concert with the fluctuations in clinical situation. This is considered a normal response to persistent and/or overwhelming adversity but needs clinical attention due to its severe effect on motivation for further treatment and associated thoughts that life is not worth living and it is time to give up. Demoralization syndrome is best managed with emotional support, reassurance, and redoubling efforts to address the underlying adversity (e.g. inadequate pain control). If distress is persistent, we recommend individual psychotherapy (logotherapy [meaning-centered psychotherapy; if existential/spiritual issues predominant], cognitive behavioral therapy [if cognitive distortions about adversity prominent]), mobilizing increased involvement of the resident's support system, and spiritual support.

MNCD with Depression

MNCD with depression is probably the most common diagnosis in LTC residents who have depressive disorder. This is because of the high prevalence of MNCD in LTC populations and the high prevalence of depression in residents who have MNCD. The syndrome of MNCD with depression should be differentiated from normal sadness experienced by residents with MNCD in response to losses and environmental stressors. The presence of depression in residents who have MNCD is associated with accelerated cognitive and functional decline, higher rates of mortality, and impaired quality of life (Marano, Rosenberg, and Lyketsos 2013). In LTC populations, depressive symptoms have the strongest association with aggressive behavior, followed by delusions, hallucinations, and constipation. Depression occurs in approximately 20–40 percent of people who have AD, 30–40 percent of people who have Parkinson's disease depression, 35–50 percent of people who have vascular dementia, and 50–60 percent of people who have dementia with Lewy bodies at some point in the course of the MNCD. MDD can be reliably diagnosed in residents who have mild to moderate MNCD. Depressive symptoms in residents who have MNCD often fluctuate over time (crying spells in the evening but a bright affect in the morning), and they may have reduction in positive affect or pleasure (e.g. a resident who rarely or never smiles), irritability, verbal and physical aggression, social withdrawal, and isolation. The key sign of depression in people who have MNCD is "depressed affect." The resident who has depression and MNCD appears sad, is often tearful, has disturbed sleep and appetite, is easily discouraged, may withdraw socially, and may voice multiple vague somatic complaints (e.g. loss of energy, headache). Feelings or expressions of worthlessness ("I am stupid" or "I am useless"), hopelessness ("Why bother?" "Nothing is going to help me"), helplessness ("Help me, help me"), guilt ("I am a burden to my family"), wish to die ("I wish I was dead"), and having a plan for suicide may be present and indicate severe depression. The HCP should inquire into these symptoms even if the resident may not comprehend some of the questions. Diagnostic errors are common when attempting to distinguish between depression and MNCD. Marked forgetfulness often accompanies depression; as it worsens, memory loss may be misinterpreted as MNCD. Residents who have MNCD can appear apathetic and withdrawn. This can be especially true once executive function is impaired. Many residents who have MNCD say "No" when asked if they feel depressed, and usually say "Yes" to feeling lonely, bored, or useless. In advanced MNCD, depression may manifest as irritability, anger, verbal and physical aggression, lack of smile, agitation, persistent moaning, yelling, and wishes to go home. Comorbid delusions are often seen in residents who have MNCD and depression.

Mild levels of depression can produce significant functional impairment, and the severity of psychopathological and neurological impairments increases with increasing severity of depression. In a resident who has MNCD and has been stable, then either deteriorates rapidly or becomes acutely behaviorally disordered, in addition to the many causes of delirium, depression may also be the culprit. Differentiating MDD with cognitive impairment (and subjective memory complaints) from MCI plus depressive symptoms and mild AD with depressive symptoms is difficult. We recommend neuropsychological testing (preferably after treatment of depression) to clarify the presence of underlying neurocognitive disorder (MCI or MNCD). Gradual cognitive decline over several years with recent onset of depression, lack of insight about one's own obvious decline in a depressed resident, and continued cognitive decline despite improvement of depressive symptoms likely indicate a diagnosis of MCI or mild AD with depression. We recommend the SLU AM SAD, GDS, or PHQ-9 for assessing depression in cognitively impaired residents who have a MOCA score of 10 or higher, and we recommend CDDS if the score is less than 10.

Depression in residents who have MNCD is eminently treatable. The HCP should avoid prescribing antidepressant with significant anticholinergic properties, such as tricyclic antidepressant and paroxetine, because of the risk of direct cognitive toxicity and blunting the potential benefits of ChEIs. Treatment of depression in residents who have MNCD may also reduce other biopsychosocial-spiritual distress associated with depression, such as aggression, anxiety, agitation, insomnia, apathy, and even mild psychotic symptoms.

Clinical Case 1: "I feel terrible"

Mrs. U, a 90-year-old resident in a nursing home who had MNCD due to AD, had been experiencing severe depressive symptoms for the last four months. Symptoms included tearfulness, lack of interest in activities, severe anxiety, insomnia, lack of appetite, weight loss, and irritability. Referral to a psychiatrist was made, as Mrs. U was not responding to two trials of antidepressant. The psychiatrist found that patient had been tried on citalopram 20 mg daily for four weeks and then sertraline 50 mg for four weeks before the referral. The patient's primary care physician was reluctant to use higher doses of antidepressant because of the patient's advanced age and MNCD. In the week before evaluation by the psychiatrist, the resident had developed abdominal pain and was found to have a urinary tract infection and put on antibiotics. At the time of the interview, the psychiatrist found the resident to be severely depressed, tearful throughout the interview, expressing statements indicating hopelessness and a wish that she were dead. The resident was also distraught because she had developed mild antibiotic-induced diarrhea. Mrs. U told the psychiatrist, "I feel terrible." Her MOCA score was 13. The psychiatrist considered restarting one of the SSRIs but because of the risk of worsening antibiotic-induced diarrhea, decided to avoid SSRIs and start mirtazapine instead. The resident was put on 7.5 mg mirtazapine daily at bedtime and the dose was increased after seven days to 15 mg daily at bedtime. The resident started sleeping better after two weeks of treatment, the diarrhea resolved when the antibiotic course was over, the UTI resolved, and the abdominal pain improved. However, her tearfulness, daytime agitation, and hopelessness persisted. Hence, the dose of mirtazapine was further increased to 22.5 mg daily at bedtime for seven days. The resident was able to tolerate this dose without sedation or other adverse effect. An individualized pleasant activity schedule was created and initiated for Mrs. U, after consultation with the family and staff. The family and staff were counseled to try to walk with the resident daily, as Mrs. U had been active all her life. Bright light therapy was started (exposure to bright light for one hour every morning while Mrs. U was perusing her favorite magazines). Mrs. U enjoyed hugs from the staff, and staff who were comfortable hugging Mrs. U were encouraged to hug Mrs. U off and on throughout the day. Mrs. U enjoyed classical and instrumental music, and listening to this music was added to her daily schedule. The family hired a massage therapist to come twice a week. After eight weeks, her mood had improved significantly, her anxiety decreased, her appetite had returned to near normal, and her feelings of hopelessness had resolved.

Teaching Points

Even with the oldest old residents (residents above age 85), the HCP can cautiously increase the dose of antidepressant to final doses similar to those used with younger residents to treat severe depression. As long as the resident is being monitored closely for adverse effect, there is no reason not to try an adequate dose of antidepressant for an adequate time before abandoning the trial and trying another antidepressant. With this patient, it is possible that a higher dose of citalopram (up to 40 mg) or sertraline (up to 100 mg) may have improved the depression. Comprehensive individualized pleasant activity schedule and complementary and alternative treatment interventions (in this case, massage therapy) were also critical to the successful treatment outcome.

Clinical Case 2: "I don't care"

Mr. B was an 82-year-old retired accountant living in a NH. He had been experiencing lack of interest in activities, decreased appetite, decreased energy, and agitation during personal care, and was expressing statements such as "I don't care" for three months. The symptoms had started a few weeks after he was moved from an AL home to the NH due to advancing MNCD and recurrent falls. He also had a recent history of gastrointestinal bleeding due to peptic ulcer disease. Psychiatric consultation was requested. On clinical exam, the psychiatrist noted that Mr. B had depressed affect and poor eye contact. MNCD due to AD with MDD was diagnosed. The psychiatrist considered prescribing SSRIs but did not due to Mr. B's recent history of gastrointestinal bleeding and the potential for SSRI to increase the risk of bleeding. Mirtazapine was considered but not prescribed because of its propensity to cause weight gain and Mr. B had morbid obesity (body mass index [BMI] of 41)-related challenges (e.g. need for a Hoyer lift during care). Bupropion was started at 75 mg daily in the morning and after seven days increased to 75 mg in the morning and at 5 p.m. Individualized pleasant activity schedule was created for Mr. B after discussion with the resident, family, and staff. Family was encouraged to bring grandchildren to visit Mr. B, as they always cheered him up. Staff was recommended to bring Mr. B's former roommate to visit Mr. B, as they had become close friends over two years that they lived together in the AL home. Over the next four weeks, Mr. B gradually started talking more and eating more. The bupropion was changed to bupropion sustained-release preparation given as 150 mg once daily in the morning. After eight weeks Mr. B was attending activities and eating better and the agitation during personal care had reduced dramatically.

Teaching Points

The selection of antidepressants needs to take into account the patient's medical problems as well as what side effects of various antidepressants one wants or wants to avoid for a particular patient. There is no compelling evidence that one antidepressant works better than any other for the treatment of MDD in LTC populations. Antidepressants when used appropriately and in combination with an individualized psychosocial approach can dramatically improve depressive symptoms and the quality of life of residents who have MDD.

Poststroke Depression and Vascular Depression

The prevalence of MDD-like symptoms after stroke ranges from 30 to 60 percent and depends on the location and size of the stroke (stroke involving the left frontal lobe has the highest association with depression), physical disability after the stroke, presence of cognitive impairment with the stroke, whether the person had to move from home to a LTC facility after stroke (cerebrovascular accident [CVA]), and the extent of social support (Robinson and Jorge 2016). Onset of depression is usually acute, soon after stroke. A small group of patients have onset after weeks or months following a CVA. Association with left frontal lobe lesions is not seen in depressive syndromes that occur in the two to six months following stroke. The course of depression after stroke varies widely. For many people, the depression remits about one to two years after stroke. As many as 14 percent may have continued MDD symptoms and 18 percent may have persistent depressive disorder-like symptoms two years after stroke. Depression occurring within a few days after a stroke is more likely to be associated with spontaneous remission than is onset of depression several weeks after a stroke. The course of depression after stroke increases disability, adversely affects outcomes of rehabilitation, impairs recovery from illness, and contributes to an increased rate of mortality.

The term *vascular depression* is used to describe a subtype of late-onset depression associated with cerebrovascular risk factors (e.g. diabetes, hypertension, hyperlipidemia, obesity), accompanying executive dysfunction, evidence on brain imaging of significant cerebrovascular disease (especially periventricular white matter hyperintensities on MRI), and increased risk of being refractory to antidepressant medication monotherapy. Vascular depression may account for 5–20 percent of late-onset depression. Residents who have vascular depression usually have a later age of onset, may exhibit symptoms of motor retardation, slowness in thinking (bradyphrenia), apathy, poor insight, and impaired executive function. They may not score high on traditional scales to assess depression, such as the SLU AM SAD, GDS, and PHQ-9. Usually there is no family history of depression in older adults who have vascular depression.

Clinical Case 3: "I feel very lonely"

Mr. G, a 79-year-old resident who had sustained a stroke causing left hemiparesis four months ago, was referred for psychiatric consultation because of frequent episodes of irritation, hollering at staff, making sexually inappropriate comments, and attempts to touch them inappropriately during personal care. These symptoms were present for three months. Mr. G's wife (and legal surrogate decision maker) had refused antidepressant treatment for Mr. G from the primary care physician because Mr. G had become "wild" after initiation of an antidepressant (paroxetine) five years ago, after his first stroke. On mental status exam, Mr. G showed evidence of executive dysfunction and depressed mood. He enjoyed socialization and conversation with the psychiatrist and seemed to crave social interaction and personal attention. Mr. G told the psychiatrist, "Yes, I feel very lonely." A diagnosis of poststroke depression and impulse control disorder due to frontal lobe dysfunction was made. The psychiatrist reviewed previous records, which indicated that Mr. G was treated with 20 mg of paroxetine for depression five years ago. The psychiatrist reviewed with Mrs. G the possible adverse effects of antidepressants and potential benefits of a second trial with an antidepressant at a low dose. The psychiatrist assured Mrs. G that Mr. G would be closely monitored for any adverse effect and the antidepressant promptly discontinued if adverse effect was moderate to severe. Mrs. G agreed to this plan. A decision was made to start the resident on sertraline 12.5 mg daily each morning to be increased to 25 mg daily in the morning after seven days. Mr. G developed transient mild nausea and anxiety for three days, which resolved spontaneously. After treatment for four weeks, the staff noticed that Mr. G was less irritable but sexually inappropriate behaviors and occasional episodes of hollering (at least once a week) continued. After four weeks, his dose was increased to 37.5 mg daily for seven days and then 50 mg daily in the morning. The resident once again developed transient mild nausea and anxiety, which cleared up spontaneously over one week. After six more weeks of treatment, staff reported that sexually inappropriate behavior had decreased considerably and episodes of hollering now occurred only once a month.

Teaching Points

Some people may have an oversensitive subtype of serotonin receptor and/or poorly metabolize SSRI and may respond to small final doses of SSRI but may also be prone to develop adverse effects such as severe anxiety if the starting dose is not low. SSRIs (such as escitalopram, sertraline) are good first-choice antidepressants for people who have vascular disease (cardiovascular and cerebrovascular disease) because of negligible cardiac toxicity and anticholinergic properties. Paroxetine carries a small but significant anticholinergic effect and thus is not the SSRI of first choice for LTC residents. Fluoxetine and fluvoxamine are long-acting SSRIs with significant risk of drug-drug interaction and hence also not the first-line SSRI for LTC populations. SSRIs are also good first-choice antidepressants for people who have depression coexisting with sexually inappropriate behavior, as serotonin dysfunction has been found to be associated with impulse control disorders. Education of the family and staff in the management of adverse effects is also key to a successful outcome.

Depression in Residents Who Have Parkinson's Disease

Depression is common in people who have Parkinson's disease (PD). Symptoms of PD, such as flat affect and hypokinesia, may be mistaken for depression. Some people who have PD experience obvious worsening of depression during the motor "off" periods. Optimizing motor functioning often ameliorates depressive symptoms and hence is the first step in addressing depression for residents who have PD. The HCP should consider psychosocial approaches (e.g. counseling) and regular exercise (e.g. strength training using Pilates), especially for residents who have PD and relatively intact cognitive function. Pharmacotherapy for MDD-like symptoms in residents who have PD is complicated due to the high likelihood of adverse effect from antidepressant and frequent adverse drug–drug interactions between commonly used antidepressants and anti-PD medications. First-line antidepressants for residents who have PD include pramipexole, selegiline, or low-dose (5–25 mg) nortriptyline. Pramipexole and selegiline are approved by the FDA to treat motor symptoms of PD and may improve depression independent of their effect on motor symptoms. Besides improving depressive symptoms, mild anticholinergic activity of nortriptyline may also help reduce drooling, may inhibit overactive bladder, and its mild sedating effect may treat insomnia. For residents who have cognitive impairment, the HCP may need to avoid prescribing nortriptyline. SSRI, bupropion, venlafaxine, duloxetine, or mirtazapine may be appropriate as a second-line agent if a trial with a first-line agent has failed. SSRIs may worsen Parkinsonian symptoms, such as tremor, and may worsen REM sleep behavior disorder that some residents who have PD may have. Thus, use of SSRIs for residents who have PD requires close monitoring for these adverse effects. Because of its dopaminergic activity, bupropion may precipitate psychosis in residents who have PD, especially if they are taking dopaminergic drugs, such as carbidopa/levodopa. The anti-Parkinsonian medication selegiline is now also available in a patch form (besides a pill form) as an antidepressant, and the HCP may consider prescribing it for treatment of MDD-like symptoms in residents who have PD. Electroconvulsive therapy (ECT) is beneficial for residents who have PD whose MDD-like symptoms are severe and refractory to antidepressant trial and in situations in which depression is life threatening (e.g. the resident is suicidal, malnourished). ECT may also improve motor function (e.g. "on" and "off" phenomenon).

Depression due to General Medical or Neurological Condition

Box 5.2 lists general medical and neurological conditions that are often the cause of mood disorders in LTC populations. MNCDs, cerebrovascular disease, and pain are the three most common causes of depression in LTC populations. Treatment of the medical condition thought to cause depression often is not sufficient to resolve depressive symptoms. Antidepressants and a psychosocial approach are necessary to treat symptoms. Depression frequently results from and complicates the recovery of older patients who experience myocardial infarction and other heart conditions, diabetes, and hip fracture. Dispensing glasses to treat uncorrected refraction errors, other approaches to correct impaired vision and hearing, and aggressive treatment of pain can also lead to decreased symptoms of depression. Some 40 percent of individuals who have HD develop MDD-like syndrome, and tetrabenazine, the only FDA-approved treatment for HD frequently also causes MDD-like syndrome. Tetrabenazine-associated depression may improve with reducing its dose. Typically, LTC residents who have HD are in advanced stages and are taking tetrabenazine. The HCP should consider discontinuing tetrabenazine for residents who have HD and severe depression.

MDD and Frailty

MDD often contributes to the etiology of frailty. Residents who have MDD often lose weight, become less active, and can therefore lose muscle mass, strength, and exercise tolerance and may be more prone to acute illness. On the other hand, frailty may contribute to the etiology of MDD. Residents who are frail due to other factors, such as anemia, immune system dysfunction, undernutrition (such as being underweight, having sarcopenic obesity), advanced age, and high medical comorbidity may have loss of muscle mass, strength, and exercise tolerance, which can result in loss of pleasurable activities and subsequent depression. Strength training may increase muscle strength, break the cycle of frailty by stimulating increased activity, and thus prevent MDD in some residents.

Apathy Syndrome

Apathy as a symptom is common, occurring in up to 92 percent of residents who have MNCD at some point in the course. The Greek word *pathos* refers to passions. Apathy is characterized by lack of passion, indifference, often in situations that would normally arouse strong feelings or reactions (Orr 2011). Residents who have apathy lose initiative and drive for their usual activities. Residents often are unable to finish tasks. Family members and staff report that the resident is showing a lack of concern for daily events or even personal care and think the resident is depressed. Despite these issues, typically the resident appears emotionally absent or unconcerned. Apathy usually also includes lack of motivation, lack of interest and emotion, periods of sitting and staring blankly, and, in severe cases, self-neglect (not bathing or changing clothes for days or even weeks). It manifests in behaviors such as poor persistence, diminished initiation, low social interaction, indifference, and blunted emotional response. Apathy as a symptom can be seen in residents who have MDD. Apathy as a syndrome is distinct from MDD, although its symptoms are often mislabeled as MDD. Residents who have apathy lack dysphoria (tearfulness, expressions of sadness, irritability), suicidality, loss of appetite, agitation, anxiety, restlessness, insomnia, verbalization of hopelessness, worthlessness, and guilt seen in residents who have depression. Box 5.8 lists common causes of apathy syndrome in LTC populations. All the causes usually involve damage or impairment of the frontal lobe or connections to the frontal lobe. Most residents who have apathy also exhibit executive dysfunction. Apathy increases in severity as the MNCD progresses, in

BOX 5.8 Common Causes of Apathy in Long-Term Care Populations

Apathy syndrome secondary to physical illnesses/conditions

- Alzheimer's disease or other neurocognitive disorder
- Delirium
- End-organ failure of kidneys, liver, heart, lung
- Pain
- Medication (SSRI, antipsychotic, interferon)
- Stimulant withdrawal syndrome
- Infection (UTI, pneumonia, "flu")
- Brain tumor involving the frontal lobe or its connections
- Stroke involving the frontal lobe or its connections
- Head injury with damage to the frontal lobe or its connections
- Medical condition (dehydration, hyponatremia, hypothyroidism)
- Substance use disorder (especially stimulant use disorder)

Apathy accompanying primary psychiatric disorder

- Major depression or vascular depression
- Schizophrenia
- Schizoid personality disorder
- Schizotypal personality disorder

contrast to the decrease in prevalence of MDD with the progression of MNCD. Apathy is also commonly seen in residents who do not have MNCD, especially those who have delirium (especially quiet delirium) and after a stroke involving the frontal lobe or its connections. Apathy also often accompanies end organ failure of kidneys, liver, heart, or lungs. Apathy and depression in residents who have MNCD are often comorbid. Apathy should be differentiated from anhedonia. Anhedonia refers to diminished response to pleasurable activities. Differentiation is important, as apathy can occur in the absence of depression and anhedonia is typically a key symptom of depression.

By its nature, apathy prevents people from bringing up such issues with HCPs. Family or staff are the first to raise concerns. Treatment of apathy is treatment of its cause whenever possible (e.g. discontinuation of offending medication). For the majority of residents, apathy is due to MNCD or stroke, in which case treatment is primarily strength-based, personalized, psychosocial sensory spiritual environmental initiatives and creative engagement (SPPEICE). See Box 5.9 for approaches to treat apathy. Apathy is stressful for family and staff. Educating them about apathy, its neurobiological basis, its being different from depression is often useful in alleviating family and staff stress. Whenever possible, the HCP should discontinue medications that may cause or exacerbate apathy or lower the dosage. There are no FDA-approved medications to treat apathy syndrome. Occasionally, apathy in residents who have AD, DLB, or PDD improves to a modest extent with the use of ChEIs. In severe cases, the HCP may consider a judicious trial of dopaminergic agent such as stimulant (especially methylphenidate) or amantadine. Typically, apathy does not improve with antidepressant treatment. In fact, certain antidepressants, such as SSRIs, may exacerbate apathy. Apathy is often comorbid with depression, in which case the HCP may consider a trial of non-SSRI antidepressant (e.g. bupropion, duloxetine, or stimulants). For residents who have severe apathy and Parkinsonism, dopamine agonists may be preferred over stimulants. Apathy in the context of obstructive sleep apnea may respond to a trial of modafinil or armodafinil.

BOX 5.9 Approaches to Treat Apathy

Nonpharmacological approaches

- Education of family and staff regarding differences between clinical depression and apathy, neurological basis of apathy, and need to lower expectations for resident who has apathy
- Music (e.g. listening to preferred music, live music, singing group)
- Exercise
- Reminiscence
- Intergenerational approaches
- Animal-assisted therapy
- Nature (e.g. gardening, sunshine)
- Spirituality (e.g. going to church, listening to Bible, singing or listening to religious songs)

Medications to consider for the treatment of severe apathy*

- Stimulant (e.g. methylphenidate)
- Modafinil, Armodafinil
- Bupropion
- Dopamine agonist (e.g. selegiline, amantadine, pramipexole)
- Cholinesterase inhibitor (e.g. donepezil, galantamine, rivastigmine)
- Ginkgo biloba extract EGb 761

* The FDA has not approved any drug to treat apathy.

Clinical Case 4: "I am fine"

Mr. L, an 80-year-old married retired business entrepreneur, moved to an AL home after experiencing difficulty managing day-to-day activities and inability to take care of his home. He was also forgetting to take his medications. His wife of 48 years also moved with him, as Mr. L would not move otherwise and his wife was undergoing severe stress of caregiving and could not continue to care for Mr. L at home. Mrs. L had her own health problems, including severe rheumatoid arthritis. Over the last six months, Mrs. L had noticed that Mr. L had stopped initiating conversation, avoided going to social gatherings, and became irritated when his wife insisted that they attend at least some of the family functions that they had been attending for more than four decades. Mr. L would spend the major part of the day watching TV. Mrs. L also noticed that Mr. L would avoid changing clothes and would take baths only when Mrs. L became adamant that he do so. Mrs. L was concerned that her husband was depressed and requested a psychiatric consultation. Mrs. L told the psychiatrist that her husband had always enjoyed company, had many interests that he shared with friends and family (such as golf, hunting), and had always looked forward to family events. She related that Mr. L had bypass surgery one year ago and he had had a slow recovery. Some of the symptoms of lack of motivation may have started a month or two after the surgery, but Mrs. L noticed that in the last six months, Mr. L was "definitely not himself." Mr. L did not mind being interviewed by the psychiatrist, stated, "I am fine," and did not understand his wife's concerns. Mr. L had no history of depression and no family history of depression. Mr. L answered all of the psychiatrist's questions in short sentences and did not initiate any conversation. Mr. L denied feeling down, reported that he was content with his life, denied any problems with sleep or appetite, denied feeling pessimistic or hopeless, and did not feel he was a burden to others. He denied feeling that life is not worth living. He said that he had several interests but that he was "too old" for golf and hunting and enjoyed watching TV. His MOCA score was 21. A head CT showed lacunae in the right basal ganglia and pons. All other laboratory tests were normal. The psychiatrist diagnosed apathy in the context of mild major vascular neurocognitive disorder (vascular dementia [VaD]). Neuropsychological testing confirmed significant frontal lobe dysfunction (as indicated by severe executive dysfunction). Mr. L's wife was educated about apathy and how it was different from depression. The psychiatrist also explained various treatment options. Mrs. L preferred nondrug interventions as opposed to experimental medication trials. Mr. L had always loved music and agreed to see a music therapist once a week on an individual basis. He also agreed to help his great grandson with a life history project that would involve reminiscing about Mr. L's successful professional career. The psychiatrist counseled Mrs. L not to insist that Mr. L attend social and family events and to lower her expectations regarding daily bathing and be content with twice-weekly bathing. The psychiatrist also recommended that she see a social worker for individual counseling to address the stress of caregiving and the grief of losing parts of her husband's original personality. After 12 weeks, Mrs. L's depression had decreased significantly, and Mr. L showed mild interest in music therapy and in his life history project. He was agreeable to continuing these activities.

Teaching Points

Apathy can be reliably differentiated from depression by the absence of subjective depressed mood, lack of impairment in sleep and appetite, absence of psychomotor agitation or retardation, and lack of cognitive symptoms (hopelessness, guilt, worthlessness) or suicidal ideas. The occasional irritability in Mr. L could be considered mild depression, but because it was short lived and usually in the context of when his wife is trying to motivate him for social events, rather than a pervasive change in mood, it was more likely a part of apathy.

Mania

Mania involves a distinct period of abnormally and persistently elevated mood and/or irritable mood lasting at least one week along with other symptoms (excessive talking, pressure of speech [inability to interrupt speech], grandiosity, distractibility, increased goal-directed activity [or psychomotor agitation], lack of need for sleep) (American Psychiatric Association 2013). Classic mania is not hard to recognize. Mania in older adults often is characterized by mood incongruent persecutory delusion, irritability, dysphoria, hostility, resentment, and sexually inappropriate behaviors that are not characteristic of the individual and often surprise those closest to the patient. Euphoria, infectious elated mood, and flight of ideas are seen less often in older adults than in younger adults who have mania (Young and Mahgoub 2013). Symptoms of mania in older adults may also mimic delirium. Hypomania is a milder form of mania. Mania is uncommon in LTC but with the aging of population that has bipolar disorder, the prevalence is increasing. Manic and hypomanic symptoms due to MNCD and other general medical conditions are more prevalent than bipolar disorder in LTC populations. Grandiose delusions and irritability can also be seen in residents who have schizophrenia.

The differential diagnosis of mania includes:

- Primary mania or hypomania (e.g. bipolar I and bipolar II disorders, cyclothymia, schizoaffective disorder bipolar type)
- Secondary mania or hypomania (due to MNCD [e.g. FTD], medication, brain tumor, stroke, and in the context of delirium)
- Mixed (primary and secondary causes) (e.g. bipolar disorder and steroid-induced mania).

Bipolar Disorder

Bipolar disorder is a lifelong illness and confers susceptibility to recurrent depressive and manic (Bipolar I) or hypomanic (Bipolar II) episodes. Suicide risk and nonsuicide mortality are even higher in older adults who have bipolar disorder than in older adults who have MDD (Beyer 2015). As a result of the aging of the population, the number of older persons who have bipolar disorder will increase two- to threefold over the next several decades, with a corresponding increase in the prevalence of bipolar disorder in LTC facilities. Some 50 percent of residents in the Veterans Administration's bipolar disorder registry are over age 50, and the proportion of veterans who have bipolar disorder over age 65 increased fivefold since 1990. The majority of older adults who have bipolar disorder have age of onset before age 30 and have simply gotten older ("early-onset" bipolar disorder). About 10 to 15 percent of adults who have bipolar disorder experience onset of this illness after the age of 50 ("late-onset" bipolar disorder). Psychopathology of bipolar disorder among older adults can be severe, and both manic and depressive symptoms are more persistent in older adults who have bipolar disorder than in younger adults who have bipolar disorder. Morphologic abnormalities in the brain on neuroimaging (e.g. prominent deep frontal white matter, subcortical gray matter and periventricular signal hyperintensities, and/or silent infarcts on MRI of the brain indicating significant cerebrovascular disease and loss of tissue volume) appear to be more prevalent in late-onset cases, similar to what has been found in late-onset depression.

Medical comorbidity (especially diabetes, obesity, hyperlipidemia, heart disease, hypertension, metabolic syndrome, and COPD) is common in older adults who have bipolar disorder. Comorbid substance abuse is less common in older adults who have bipolar disorder than in younger adults who have bipolar disorder. However, the post–World War II Baby Boomer generation will have greater exposure to substances or street drugs, and thus the next wave of older adults who have bipolar disorder will be more likely than the current generation to have substance use disorder. Comorbid anxiety disorder (e.g. generalized anxiety disorder, panic disorder) is often seen in older adults who have bipolar disorder. A variety of cognitive deficits in people who have bipolar disorder persist between depressive and manic episodes. More than 40 percent of individuals older than age 60 who have bipolar disorder show cognitive impairment on cognitive screening tests. Older adults who have bipolar disorder have more rapid cognitive decline than age-matched peers, and diagnosis of MNCD at a later date increases in relation to greater number of prior exacerbations or episodes.

Older adults can and do experience the full range of manic and depressive symptomatology that characterizes bipolar disorder. Most people who have bipolar disorder spent a large part of their life experiencing depressive symptoms. Depression during bipolar disorder in older adults is often melancholic in nature and usually includes disturbances in sleep and appetite as well as cognitive impairment that can mimic MNCD. In people who have bipolar disorder, most episodes, and usually the first episode, are depressive. The first manic episode often occurs in the fifth or sixth decade and may result in psychiatric hospitalization for the first time. The interval between depression and mania can be more than a decade. The depressive episode meets the criteria for MDD. In individuals who have recurrent MDD, the HCP should always keep in mind the diagnosis of bipolar disorder, as the first manic or hypomanic episode may not occur for years to decades after the first episode of depression and may occur after many more episodes of depression. Differentiating bipolar depression from MDD is critical to successful treatment outcomes, as the treatment of the two disorders is different and antidepressants may worsen the symptoms and course of bipolar disorder. A history of hypomania or mania, a family history of bipolar disorder, early age of onset of MDD, a higher number of prior depressive episodes, and symptoms related to anxiety indicate bipolar depression rather than MDD. Work-up for bipolar disorder may include laboratory tests (e.g. CBC, CMP, vitamin B_{12} and vitamin D levels, TSH, EKG) as well as neuroimaging to clarify comorbidity and identify reversible factors that need to be treated to achieve successful remission of symptoms.

The goals of treatment of bipolar disorder are remission of symptoms, prevention of future mood episodes, and improvement in general function and well-being. Bipolar disorders are eminently treatable (Forester, Antognini, and Kim 2011). (See Table 5.9.) The incidence and severity of adverse effects due to psychotropic medication used to treat bipolar disorder are greater in LTC populations. In addition, LTC residents are more likely to be taking medications that may interact with medication used for bipolar disorder (e.g. diuretics and lithium) and are more likely to have comorbid physical and neurological conditions complicating psychotropic medication therapy (e.g. renal insufficiency increasing the risk of lithium toxicity). In older adults who have bipolar disorder, treatment resistance is common, recurrences are frequent,

Table 5.9 Evidence-Based Approaches to Treat Bipolar Disorder in Long-Term Care Populations

Approach	Clinical Pearls	Key Concerns/Limitations
Mood stabilizer (e.g. divalproate sodium, lamotrigine, lithium, carbamazepine, oxcarbazepine)	Divalproate, lamotrigine, and oxcarbazepine preferred over lithium and carbamazepine Response may take several weeks after therapeutic dose is reached	Use associated with significant risk of falls and delirium Use of divalproate is associated with increased risk of bleeding with concomitant use of antiplatelet, anticoagulant, or omega-3 fatty acid
Antipsychotic (especially second- generation antipsychotics)	Second-generation antipsychotic preferred over first-generation antipsychotic* Response may take several weeks after therapeutic dose is reached	Management by psychiatrist is recommended if there is need for antipsychotic due to high risk associated with use of antipsychotic medication
Antidepressant	May be considered adjuvant to mood stabilizer and/or antipsychotic for treatment of bipolar II depressive symptoms	May destabilize bipolar disorder (especially if used as monotherapy), cause rapid cycling, and switch depression to mania
Onsite individual counseling/ psychotherapy (e.g. cognitive behavioral therapy [CBT], mindfulness-based CBT, interpersonal and social rhythm therapy [IPSRT])	Psychotherapy is useful for relapse prevention and management of comorbid conditions (e.g. anxiety disorder, insomnia disorder)	Lack of availability of counselors trained in providing psychotherapy to LTC populations Lack of availability of counselors visiting LTC facilities to provide psychotherapy Resident may need to leave LTC facility and visit local mental health clinic
Internet-based and telepsychiatry approaches	Cognitive restructuring (to address cognitive distortions), behavioral activation and problem-solving strategies can be effectively administered via Internet and telepsychiatry by psychiatric nurse or other mental health professional for treatment of bipolar depression	Resident needs to be motivated and have relatively intact cognitive functioning Technophobia may be a difficult barrier Should be restricted to mild cases and in conjunction with antidepressants; close supervision is needed to monitor worsening of depression
Psychoeducation and self-management	Providing pamphlets and other education materials on bipolar disorder and late-life bipolar disorder can reduce stigma resident experiences	Cognitive deficit in resident may limit its benefit
Neurostimulation therapy	Electroconvulsive therapy (ECT) for life-threatening bipolar disorder and treatment resistant bipolar disorder Transcranial magnetic stimulation (TMS) as adjuvant to psychotropic medications for treatment of bipolar depression	Lack of availability of professionals providing neurostimulation therapy in the community Lack of reimbursement from health insurance for neurostimulation therapy (especially TMS)
Omega-3 fatty acid supplementation	Eicosapentanoic acid (EPA) and ethyl-EPA dominant formulation recommended	Small risk of increased bleeding, especially with concomitant use of NSAID, anticoagulant, antiplatelet, SSRI, or SNRI
Vitamin D supplementation	Checking vitamin D levels is recommended, as vitamin D deficiency is prevalent in residents who have bipolar disorder and may require vitamin D replacement therapy	Hypervitaminosis D, although rare, can occur and manifest as headache and dizziness

Table 5.9 (cont.)

Approach	Clinical Pearls	Key Concerns/Limitations
Bright light therapy	May be used with psychotropic medication to treat bipolar depression, especially if there is history of seasonal affective disorder (e.g. winter depression)	Staff education and training is required for appropriate use of bright light therapy box
Exercise/Physical activity	Exercise and increasing physical activity can accelerate response to psychotropic medication and increase likelihood of remission	Lack of time available to staff to help resident increase physical activity is key barrier to its routine use
Rational deprescribing (geriatric scalpel) with input from pharmacist	Discontinuation of medication that may contribute to bipolar symptom, discontinuation of unnecessary or inappropriate medication (based on Beers list), and reducing anticholinergic burden may improve cognitive and emotional functioning of resident and reduce adverse drug-drug interactions with medication used to treat bipolar disorder	None
Optimizing control of pain and other comorbid physical health problems (e.g. diabetes) and correction of reversible physical health problems (e.g. dehydration, constipation, vision and hearing impairment, thyroid disorder)	Recommended for all residents	None

* Second-generation antipsychotics: aripiprazole, quetiapine, olanzapine, risperidone, lurasidone, ziprasidone, paliperidone, iloperidone, cariprazine, brexpiprazole, asenapine

First-generation antipsychotics: haloperidol, fluphenazine, thioridazine, perphenazine, chlorpromazine, thiothixine

and there is a high incidence of mortality. Hence, bipolar disorder in LTC populations is best managed by a psychiatrist with expertise in LTC psychiatry.

Treatment strategies for controlling bipolar disorder consist of pharmacotherapy and psychosocial approaches. Pharmacotherapy involves mood stabilizer (e.g. valproate, carbamazepine, lamotrigine, oxcarbazepine) and atypical antipsychotic (e.g. risperidone, quetiapine, olanzapine, aripiprazole, paliperidone, iloperidone, lurasidone, ziprasidone, cariprazine, asenapine, brexpiprazole). The use of antidepressant by residents who have bipolar disorder type I is controversial because of the potential for antidepressant to worsen the course of bipolar disorder (e.g. switch to rapid cycling) and the potential for switching a resident who has depression to mania. This risk is especially higher with antidepressant that has serotonin and norepinephrine reuptake inhibition properties (e.g. tricyclic antidepressant, venlafaxine, duloxetine, desvenlafaxine). If an antidepressant is used, one of the SSRIs (e.g. sertraline, escitalopram, citalopram) or bupropion is preferred, added to a mood stabilizer and/or an atypical antipsychotic medication, and the resident closely monitored for switch to mania and rapid cycling. Antidepressants should not be used as monotherapy for bipolar depression. In type II bipolar disorder, use of antidepressant may carry less risk than bipolar disorder type I. Rapid cycling (four or more episodes of mania or hypomania or MDD in one year) is associated with a higher prevalence of hypothyroidism. Hence, all residents who have rapid cycling should have their thyroid-stimulating hormone (TSH) level checked. Even for residents who have rapid cycling and normal TSH, tri-iodothyronine (T3) augmentation may help control bipolar symptoms (especially depression). Although lithium is the gold standard of treatment for people who have bipolar disorder (especially those who have classic euphoric mania), LTC residents often develop toxicity with lithium even at very low doses in part due to lower renal clearance and to interactions with other medication (especially diuretics). Most common symptoms of toxicity with lithium in this population include neurocognitive adverse effect (e.g. disorientation, memory impairment), diarrhea, and tremor. LTC residents are also at higher risk of serious lithium toxicity involving delirium, myoclonic jerks, severe diarrhea, coma, cardiovascular collapse, and seizures compared to older adults in the community, who are at higher risk compared to middle-age and younger adults. Hence, we recommend that the HCP avoid prescribing lithium for LTC residents who have bipolar disorder unless they are already taking lithium, are tolerating it well, and have benefited from it. Also, for residents who have mixed symptoms (manic and depressive symptoms) and residents who have rapid cycling, lithium is not as effective as valproate, carbamazepine, or atypical antipsychotics. LTC residents tolerate valproate much better than lithium, and it may be considered one of the first-line agents for the treatment of bipolar mania, hypomania, and mixed episodes. Other first-line agents for the treatment of bipolar mania, hypomania, and mixed episodes include one of several atypical antipsychotics. Carbamazepine is considered a third-line agent because of a substantial risk of drug–drug interactions, hyponatremia, and other adverse effects. Atypical antipsychotics are preferred over mood stabilizers for bipolar symptoms associated with psychotic symptoms. Although olanzapine has lost its place as a drug of first choice for young adults who have bipolar disorder primarily due to its metabolic complication risks (weight gain, diabetes, hyperlipidemia, metabolic syndrome), in older adults who have bipolar disorder, it remains one of the first-line agents because the risk of metabolic complication is probably lower in older adults and weight gain may be beneficial for residents who have bipolar disorder and are underweight. The HCP should avoid initiating treatment with typical antipsychotic such as haloperidol, fluphenazine, chlorpromazine, or thioridazine for LTC residents who have bipolar disorder due to the much higher risk of adverse effects (e.g. Parkinsonism, falls, cognitive dysfunction, tardive dyskinesias) compared to atypical antipsychotics. For residents who are already taking one of the typical antipsychotics, are tolerating it well, and have benefited from it, continuing is appropriate, albeit with close monitoring for emergent adverse effects as the health of the resident declines. Lamotrigine is recommended for the treatment of bipolar depression to prevent future episodes. Quetiapine or lurasidone monotherapy or a combination of an SSRI (e.g. citalopram, sertraline, escitalopram) with olanzapine is recommended for the treatment of depressive episode of bipolar disorder. The HCP may consider prescribing cariprazine for treatment-resistant bipolar depression. In residents who have bipolar disorder and are stable taking psychotropic medications, adverse effects may develop with decline in physical and/or neurocognitive health. Small dose reductions in such situations may adequately address adverse effects without exacerbating bipolar symptoms. Many residents who have bipolar disorder may need complex medication regimens, including more than one mood stabilizer and an antipsychotic. Bipolar disorder is often comorbid with other psychiatric disorder, such as anxiety disorder (generalized anxiety disorder, panic disorder) and substance use disorder (especially smoking tobacco). The HCP should inquire into the presence of these comorbid disorders and, if present, appropriately treat them. The HCP may consider prescribing judicious short-term use of a low dose of a benzodiazepine (such as clonazepam or lorazepam) to control symptoms of severe agitation and/or severe anxiety. Residents who have bipolar disorder have a high risk of suicide, and hence the resident, staff, and family need to be educated regarding this risk. Also, we recommend close monitoring for suicidality during an acute episode of depression but also of mania. All statements of suicide, hopelessness, and wish to die should be taken seriously. The HCP should consider hospitalizing in a psychiatric unit (preferably a geriatric psychiatry unit) any resident who has suicidal ideas, suicide attempt, severe symptoms, psychotic symptoms, or symptoms not responding to treatment. The HCP should also consider ECT as one of the first-line treatment options for rapid control of manic, mixed, and depressive symptoms.

Psychosocial approaches primarily involve psychoeducational approaches for the resident, family, and staff. Residents, family members, and staff can be trained to recognize early signs of symptom exacerbation and adverse events. For residents who have relatively intact cognitive functioning, the HCP should consider individual psychotherapy (interpersonal and social rhythm therapy [IPSRT] and cognitive behavioral therapy [CBT]), as it may provide additional benefits of improved psychosocial well-being and reduced risk of future relapse of manic or depressive episode. Families of residents who have bipolar disorder may have been under considerable strain for decades before the resident entered the LTC facility. Thus, the HCP also needs to address their well-being.

Clinical Case 5: "I don't feel right"

Mrs. F, an 85-year-old resident, was recently admitted to the nursing home for rehabilitation after hip fracture surgery. She had a long history of bipolar disorder type I with multiple suicide attempts and hospitalizations but was stable for last 10 years taking olanzapine 5 mg at bedtime, lamotrigine 100 mg daily in the morning, and valproate extended release 500 mg at bedtime daily. The olanzapine was discontinued due to her experiencing "lethargy" and not participating in physical therapy. The daughter strongly opposed this intervention, and after Mrs. F started showing a recurrence of bipolar depression symptoms (frequent tearfulness, loss of appetite), the daughter insisted that olanzapine be restarted. The staff decided to seek input from the consulting psychiatrist. The psychiatrist obtained input from Mrs. F's daughter, who was her primary caregiver and had helped her through previous bouts of exacerbation of bipolar illness. The psychiatrist felt the daughter was knowledgeable about bipolar disorder and her mother's treatment history. The daughter was concerned about discontinuation of olanzapine due to the history of severe depression and serious suicide attempts. Mrs. F's valproate levels were 45. During the interview, Mrs. F told the psychiatrist, "I don't feel right." Upon reviewing Mrs. F's medications, the psychiatrist noted that she was prescribed hydrocodone (5 mg) as needed for pain that was being used three to four times daily. Laboratory tests indicated mild dehydration (BUN/creatinine 30 [20 and above indicates dehydration]). The psychiatrist recommended trying up to 3 grams/day of scheduled acetaminophen, encouraging intake of at least 1000 cc fluids daily, restarting olanzapine 5 mg at bedtime, and using low-dose (2.5 mg) hydrocodone (without acetaminophen) as needed for breakthrough pain. Over the next four weeks, as the use of hydrocodone decreased to once a day and dehydration resolved, the patient's "lethargy" cleared up, depressed mood lifted, appetite and sleep improved, and she started actively taking part in physical therapy.

Teaching Points

People whose bipolar disorder is well controlled by psychotropic medication should keep taking the same drugs as much as is possible, because bipolar disorder symptoms (especially depression) are usually difficult to treat. The management of bipolar disorder is complex, and the HCP should consult a psychiatrist before making any change in psychotropic medication. The HCP should look for other causes of lethargy (in this case, lethargy due to hydrocodone initiation and dehydration) before implicating psychotropic medication if the patient has been stable taking it for some time.

Secondary Mania

Secondary mania is mania due to general medical condition or medication. Manic symptoms can be due to a variety of general medical conditions, such as neurological conditions affecting the inferomedial frontal lobes (e.g. infarct, FTD, brain tumor, head injury), epilepsy (postictal mania), Huntington's Disease, multiple sclerosis, Cushing's syndrome, neurosyphilis, and medication induced (e.g. due to corticosteroids, stimulants). Right hemispheric lesions have been associated with mania, and euphoric mood is a common sequela of right hemispherectomy. Disinhibition syndromes that share some manic features have been linked to lesions in the medial orbitofrontal-subcortical circuits, including the thalamus and caudate nucleus. Residents who have MNCD may also develop hypomanic/manic symptoms. Older patients who have new-onset mania are more than twice as likely to have a comorbid neurological disorder, including silent cerebral infarct (65 percent in new-onset versus 25 percent in chronic illness). The HCP should consider all residents who have a first episode of mania to have secondary mania until proven otherwise. Treatment of secondary mania involves treatment of its cause (e.g. antibiotic for neurosyphilis). Most residents who have secondary mania also need medication (e.g. atypical antipsychotic, valproate) to treat the symptoms of mania. For residents who have moderate to severe symptoms, we recommend admission to an inpatient psychiatric unit (preferably a geriatric psychiatry unit) due to the high associated risk of morbidity and mortality (e.g. refusal of essential medication, physically aggressive behavior).

Clinical Case 6: "I am feeling great"

Mr. L, a 62-year-old realtor, was transferred to a nursing home after being treated for severe pneumonia in the hospital. He was diagnosed with bipolar disorder in the hospital and treated with haloperidol and lorazepam for aggressive behavior in the hospital. Mr. L was having falls and being belligerent with staff at the nursing home. Hence, he was referred to the consulting psychiatrist for "urgent" psychiatric evaluation. Mr. L had been having "mood swings" and aggressive verbal and physical behaviors that had progressively worsened over one and a half to two years before hospitalization for pneumonia. Mr. L had also been irritable and engaged in several failed schemes to make money by buying and selling real estate in impoverished areas over the last year. Mr. L had assaulted his friend at the friend's house and then decided to walk two miles in bitter cold to go home. As a result, he had developed pneumonia, refused antibiotics, and had to be hospitalized after developing high-grade fever, severe cough, and fatigue. Mr. L also had a history of making lewd comments during social situations and becoming verbally abusive toward the people he was working with. Mr. L had been a congenial and easygoing person all his life. Mr. L had no history of psychiatric problems. Mr. L had a brother who was diagnosed at age 59 with FTD. On mental status exam, Mr. L reported, "I am feeling great"; he felt that his friend "deserved" to be hit because the friend had declined Mr. L's offer to "make money" by buying some real estate for his friend. Mr. L's MOCA score was 25. On neurological exam, Mr. L had mild extrapyramidal symptoms (EPS) (tremor, stiffness, and hypokinesia).

After thorough assessment, including neuropsychological testing that showed significant executive dysfunction, MRI of the brain showing moderate to severe asymmetric atrophy of both the frontal lobes and insula, the HCP diagnosed FTD with secondary mania. Mr. L was started on valproate and quetiapine, haloperidol was discontinued, and lorazepam was switched from scheduled dosing to as-needed dosing. Over the next four weeks, Mr. L became much less aggressive and his behavior was more manageable by the staff. Haloperidol-induced EPS resolved completely.

Teaching Points

The HCP should consider a change in personality in a middle-aged person who has "mood symptoms" secondary mood disorder until proven otherwise. Long duration of "manic" symptoms and a family history of FTD in this resident's brother strongly suggested secondary mania rather than bipolar disorder. The HCP should avoid prescribing haloperidol to treat manic symptoms for patients who have secondary mania (as for all older adults) due to the higher risk of EPS (which led to falls in Mr. L). Lithium also should be avoided with people who have secondary mania due to the higher risk of lithium-induced adverse effect (especially delirium). Valproate and/or atypical antipsychotic with low risk of EPS, such as quetiapine, are usually drugs of choice for the treatment of manic symptoms in residents who have secondary mania.

Pseudobulbar Affect

Pseudobulbar affect (PBA) is a dramatic disorder of emotional expression and regulation characterized by a syndrome of uncontrollable laughter or crying that is unrelated or out of proportion to the eliciting stimulus (Frock, Williams, and Kaplan 2016). Residents who have PBA often feel embarrassed and, in severe cases, not only cause severe subjective emotional distress but also can be disruptive to the milieu. PBA can also lead to social isolation, obstruction of normal relationships with family and friends, and, rarely, choking if it occurs when the resident is eating or drinking. PBA is also known as involuntary emotional expression disorder (IEED), pathological laughing or crying, and emotional incontinence. PBA may relate to release of brainstem emotional control centers from regulation by the frontal lobes. Residents who have PBA tend to become emotional over trivial matters and typically cannot understand or explain these episodes. PBA is not associated with underlying depressed or happy mood and is not amenable to voluntary control. PBA is classically seen in individuals who have amyotrophic lateral sclerosis. PBA is uncommon in LTC populations, and AD is the most common cause of PBA in LTC residents. Other common causes of PBA in LTC populations include stroke, Parkinson's disease, traumatic brain injury, and multiple sclerosis. In most cases, education of resident, family, and staff caring for the resident and SPPEICE (distraction, reassurance, meaningful and stimulating activities) are recommended as first-line treatments. The FDA approved a combination of dextromethorphan and quinidine for the treatment of PBA. It should be used in moderate to severe cases. The most common side effects with dextromethorphan-quinidine include dizziness, diarrhea, and nausea, and potential drug interactions of other medication with dextromethorphan (especially with memantine, as both dextromethorphan and memantine are NMDA receptor antagonists) are also a concern. In addition, dextromethorphan can prolong QTc interval and pose a risk of ventricular arrhythmia, especially in residents who have prolonged QTc interval and/or concomitant use of other medication that prolongs QTc interval (e.g. citalopram). Second-line agents for the treatment of PBA include SSRIs and TCAs, although they are not approved by the FDA.

Suicide

Suicidality is one of the most serious complications of mood disorder (Turecki and Brent 2016). Manifestations of suicidality in residents range from passive suicidal ideation (e.g. life not worth living) to completed suicide. Completed suicide is a self-inflicted act with the intention to end one's life that results in death. Although completed suicide is rare in LTC populations, other manifestations of suicidality are prevalent, under-recognized, and undertreated. Much of the research findings about suicidality in older adults apply to LTC populations. Older adults are at a higher risk for suicide than any other age group. Suicidality in older adults is a complex phenomenon with multiple risk correlates interacting with protective factors. (See Tables 5.10 and 5.11.) Among all adults, older adults are most likely to die as a result of an attempt, with the ratio of completed to attempted suicides increasing

Table 5.10 Risk Factors for Suicide in Long-Term Care Populations

Risk Factor	Implication for Risk	Prevention/Therapeutic Implication
Age	Risk increases with age for men Risk increases with age for women until midlife and then levels off or drops	Staff education about myths of suicide in older adults (e.g. suicidal ideas are normal part of aging and/or normal part of living in LTC facility) is key prevention strategy
Race	Rates of suicide across the life cycle are higher among whites than non-whites Rates of suicide are lowest in African American women	Staff education about risk factors for suicide should include understanding of racial factors
Gender	Risk is higher in males than in females	Older white males are at highest risk among all demographic groups, and presence of suicidal idea and/or recent suicide attempt puts them at high risk
Suicide plan	Risk is higher if there is a resolved plan for suicide	Assessment of suicide risk should inquire about various ways the resident may have imagined attempting suicide and details of the plan
Attitude toward suicide	Risk is higher in residents who view suicide as reasonable strategy to cope with severe stress, express sense of competence about suicide, and even find suicide an act of courage	Assessment of suicide risk should inquire about resident's attitude toward suicide
Means to commit suicide	Risk is higher if resident has means to commit suicide (access to gun, cognitive capacity to hoard medication, and awareness of dangerousness of the medication)	Assessment of suicide risk should routinely inquire about resident's access to means to commit suicide, and suicide prevention plan should include strategies to limit access to lethal means

Table 5.10 (cont.)

Risk Factor	Implication for Risk	Prevention/Therapeutic Implication
Hopelessness	Presence of hopelessness increases risk	Resident who has hopelessness, even in absence of suicidal idea, should be considered at moderate to high risk
Feeling demoralized (wanting to give up and stop trying to overcome stress)	Presence of demoralization increases risk	Resident who has demoralization, even in absence of suicidal idea, should be considered at moderate to high risk
Burdensomeness	Perceived burdensomeness increases risk	Assessment of suicide risk should routinely evaluate presence of perceived burdensomeness
Autonomy and personal control	Any event or situation that poses direct threat to autonomy and personal control increases risk	Assessment of suicide risk should routinely evaluate presence of any threat to autonomy and personal control
Personality and coping style	Rigid independent personality increases risk Presence of obsessive traits increases risk Impulsive or careless problem-solving style increases risk	Assessment of suicide risk should routinely inquire about presence of these personality and coping styles
Major mental disorder	Presence of major mental disorder (e.g. MDD, bipolar disorder, schizophrenia) increases risk	HCP should consider all residents who have major mental disorder and express even transient suicidal ideas and/or hopelessness and/or demoralization at high risk
Medical comorbidity	Presence of seven or more illnesses increases risk ninefold	Assessment of suicide risk should routinely involve assessment of burden of medical comorbidity
Lack of social support	Absence of social support or recent significant decline in social network increases risk	Efforts to shore up social support is key component of reducing suicide risk in resident at risk of suicide who lacks social support or has recent decline in social network due to medical/neurological/mental illness
MNCD	Recent diagnosis of irreversible MNCD (e.g. Alzheimer's disease) increases risk	HCP should assess all residents for suicide risk after diagnosis of MNCD
Severe persistent pain	Increases risk	HCP should consider comprehensive pain strategies, referral to pain management specialist, and palliative care for resident who has severe persistent pain
History of suicide attempt	Increases risk	HCP should screen all residents who have history of suicide attempt for major mental disorder and assess suicide risk at time of admission
Family history of suicide	Increases risk	HCP should screen all residents who have family history of suicide for mood disorder (e.g. MDD, bipolar disorder) and assess suicide risk at time of admission

Table 5.11 Protective Factors for Suicide in Long-Term Care Populations

Protective Factor	Implication for Suicide Risk Assessment	Prevention/Therapeutic Implication for Residents at Risk of Suicide
Demographics	Older African American women have lowest risk of suicide among all demographic groups	Staff education about demographic factors that are protective
Family connections (includes connections with friends)	Strong family connections protect against suicide	Bolstering family connections (e.g. increased visits by children and grandchildren) and contact
Religious beliefs	Strong religious beliefs protect against suicide	Fortifying religious beliefs that help resident cope with life situation, preferably with help of preferred member of clergy
Social activities	Residents who are active in facility/community activities and organizations and have a hobby are at lower risk of suicide	Redoubling efforts to foster engagement in social activities and hobbies

from 1:200 in young adult women to 1:4 in older men. These statistics are primarily for community-dwelling older adults. Suicidality has not been rigorously studied in LTC residents, but preliminary studies indicate that suicidal ideas may be twice as common in LTC populations as in age-matched peers in the community. The prevalence of suicide, suicidal ideas, and suicide attempts in LTC is expected to increase over the next two decades with the increase in the population of baby boomers in LTC, a cohort that has carried relatively high suicide rates at each stage of life course development.

Self-harmful behaviors among LTC residents are strongly associated not only with mood disorder (especially MDD) but also with MNCD and may not necessarily reflect a wish to die. Self-harming behaviors associated with depression may take the form of refusal to eat, take medication, or undergo life-extending/life-saving interventions (e.g. dialysis). Most studies have not associated MNCD with suicidality, although for some individuals, diagnosis at early stages of AD when insight is preserved, there is lack of social support and/or strong aversion to loss of autonomy and becoming dependent on others, the risk of suicide can be considerable.

We recommend assessing for the risk of suicide all new residents and residents who have new onset of mood symptoms (depression as well as other mood symptoms, such as hypomanic/manic symptoms) or exacerbation of pre-existing mood disorder. Many at-risk residents may vehemently deny that they are depressed, may not report any dysphoria, but may acknowledge some feelings of disgust or discouragement. Hence, the HCP needs to inquire into the presence of a variety of negative emotional states as well as the absence of positive emotional states (e.g. happiness, contentment). Residents suspected to be suicidal may need their belongings searched for drugs on which they could overdose. It is also important to check for residents hoarding medications. The most common means of committing suicide in the community-dwelling older adult population is the use of a firearm. Residents who are suicidal and are requesting to visit their home should be screened for the presence of a firearm at home and interventions necessary to limit access to firearms should be implemented. Some residents (e.g. veterans, members of the military, residents who have a history of hobby of gun collection) can be resourceful in gaining access to a gun (e.g. borrowing a gun from a friend who is not aware of the resident's plan for suicide). Residents who have severe and persistent mental illness may attempt suicide by overdosing on medication they have hoarded, by hanging, or by throwing themselves out of a window. It is critical that the HCP involve family and friends (with the consent of the resident whenever possible) to help reduce the risk of suicide.

About 10 to 15 percent of individuals who have bipolar disorder commit suicide, and 25 percent attempt suicide. Among older adults who attempt suicide, the presence of bipolar disorder may be associated with a higher risk of suicide than any other psychiatric or medical disorder. The presence of other severe and persistent mental illness, such as schizophrenia or schizoaffective disorder, is also associated with a high risk of

BOX 5.10 Situations in which Residents Are Considered at Moderate to High Risk for Suicide

- Resident made a past attempt at suicide
- Resident expresses suicidal ideas with a plan for suicide
- Resident expresses suicidal ideas but does not have a plan for suicide
- Resident expresses a wish to die
- Resident expresses hopelessness
- Resident expresses a wish to give up (demoralization)
- Resident attempted suicide in the recent past (3–6 months)
- Resident has depression and family history of suicide

suicide. Although frail or confused LTC residents may have greater difficulty physically carrying out suicidal acts, the HCP should take any suicidal ideation seriously. Because 2 to 6 percent of deaths in HD are by suicide, all residents who have HD should undergo suicide assessment even if they don't have MDD-like syndrome.

The goal of suicide assessment is not only to attempt to predict whether resident will commit suicide or not but also to understand the basis for suicidality and generate a more individualized and informed suicide prevention care plan (Chan et al. 2016). (See Box 5.10.) Residents at imminent risk (a serious suicide attempt [evidence of high lethality {violent, near-lethal, premeditated attempt, precautions to avoid rescue}], or voicing suicidal ideas with plan or intent, severe depression with suicidal ideas, psychotic depression with suicidal ideas, poor judgment, refusal of treatment, medical complications) should be transferred to the emergency room of a local hospital for immediate evaluation and hospitalization to a psychiatric inpatient unit (preferably a geriatric psychiatry inpatient unit). Residents at moderate to high risk for suicide may need to be closely monitored (e.g. one on one, line of sight, check every 15 minutes) in the facility while assessment and treatment are under way.

Suicide in all age groups, including LTC populations, is a preventable cause of death. Among older adults who commit suicide, 85 percent or more have a treatable mental disorder (Conwell and O'Reilly 2013). MDDs account for more than two-thirds of treatable mental disorders in this group. The first step in suicide prevention is to address barriers head on. Usually, both family and professional caregivers have a harder time detecting emotional distress of residents at risk of suicide and engaging them in treatment. Residents may not be aware of their emotional state due to a combination of personality factors, cultural factors, and neurological deficit and/or minimize the gravity of their emotional state. Residents (especially older residents) are less likely to share thoughts of suicide and feelings of hopelessness than younger populations. For many residents, the stigma of mental illness adds a barrier to their accepting the need for comprehensive treatment (e.g. antidepressants plus counselling). Ageist attitudes are prevalent not only among LTC staff but also even among physicians and other HCPs, and myths (e.g. it is "normal" for a resident to wish for death) are commonly accepted. Staff education and training is key to successful prevention of suicide in LTC.

Suicide prevention programs in LTC involve the following four principles:

1. Identify at-risk populations (e.g. residents who have MDD, residents in severe persistent pain).
2. Assess suicide risk (low, moderate, high, imminent) in at-risk residents and share the finding with staff caring for the resident.
3. Institute a suicide prevention plan (matching the suicide risk severity in at-risk residents to ensure safety while prevention plan is under way) with involvement of a mental health professional early in the management.
4. Periodically monitor suicide risk and response to intervention, and modify the suicide prevention plan as necessary.

Summary

Mood disorders, especially MDD and apathy, are prevalent in LTC populations and are responsible for substantial excess morbidity and increased mortality. Suicide is the most serious complication of mood disorder. We recommend periodic screening for MDD for all residents and in particular recently admitted residents to increase the identification of MDD in LTC populations. We also recommend screening all new residents for risk of suicide, as suicidal thoughts can occur in the absence of MDD-like symptoms (e.g. accompanying demoralization syndrome). Mania, although uncommon in LTC populations, is associated with high morbidity and mortality. Suicide and self-harmful behaviors are more prevalent in LTC populations than previously thought. Residents who have depression that is not responding to treatment and residents who have made a suicide attempt and/or have persistent suicidal ideation, psychotic depression, and mania are best managed by a mental health clinician (psychiatrist, psychiatric nurse practitioner, psychiatric physician assistant) who has expertise in LTC psychiatry. Comprehensive assessment, prevention, and treatment strategies for all mood disorders and suicidality can dramatically improve the quality of life of all residents who have mood disorder and may be lifesaving.

Key Clinical Points

1. MDDs are seen in approximately 10 percent of LTC populations and are the most common reversible causes of disability and increased mortality.
2. Regular screening, accurate diagnosis, and successful prevention and treatment of MDDs constitute quality indicators in LTC facilities.
3. Suicide is the most serious complication of MDD and bipolar disorder.
4. The HCP should consider individual psychotherapy, exercise, individualized pleasant and meaningful activity schedule, bright light therapy, improving nutrition, and/or other psychosocial environmental approaches for all residents who have MDD or other mood disorder.
5. Moderate to severe MDD and bipolar disorder require appropriate psychotropic medication therapy and close follow-up, as the risks of adverse effect are higher in LTC populations than in community-dwelling older adults.

Suggested Resources

Depression Bipolar Support Alliance: www.dbsalliance.org. DBSA is a nonprofit organization providing support groups for individuals who have MDD and bipolar disorder and for their family and friends. Residents who have relatively preserved cognitive function and their family members may find this resource useful.

Relaxation Response Technique: www.relaxationresponse.org. A useful website providing instructions for eliciting relaxation response that may be printed free of charge. Relaxation response is an excellent intervention to reduce anxiety symptoms that often occur in residents who have mood disorder and may help prevent use of benzodiazepines for the treatment of anxiety symptoms.

Mindfulness Meditation: www.marc.ucla.edu/body.cfm. The website of UCLA Mindfulness Awareness Research Center provides free short audio recordings to engage in guided meditation. Mindfulness meditation is an excellent approach to reduce anxiety and depressive symptoms and to prevent MDD in motivated residents who have relatively preserved cognitive functioning.

Suicide Safe: A free suicide prevention app available for health care professionals from the Substance Abuse and Mental Health Services Administration. The app helps HCPs integrate suicide-prevention strategies into their practice and address suicide risk among their patients.

Shock: The Healing Power of Electroconvulsive Therapy, a book written by Kitty Dukakis, is an excellent resource to help educate residents and their family regarding potential benefits and risks of ECT and allay concerns regarding ECT.

References

Alexopoulos, G.S., R.C. Abrams, R.C. Young, and C.A. Shamoian. 1988. Cornell Scale for Depression in Dementia. *Biological Psychiatry* **23**:271–284.

American Psychiatric Association. 2013. Depressive Disorders. *Diagnostic and Statistical Manual of Mental Disorders*, 5th ed., pp. 155–188. Arlington, VA: American Psychiatric Association Press.

Beekman, A.T.F., P. Cuijpers, and F. Smit. 2013. Prevention of Depression in Later Life. In H. Lavretsky, M. Sajatovic and C.F. Reynolds III (eds.), *Late Life Mood Disorders*, pp. 516–531. New York, NY: Oxford University Press.

Beyer, J.L. 2015. Bipolar and Related Disorders. In D.C. Steffens, D.G. Blazer, and M.E. Thakur (eds.), *The Textbook of Geriatric Psychiatry*, 5th ed., pp. 283–308. Arlington, VA: American Psychiatric Publishing.

Blazer, D.G. and D. Steffens. 2015. Depressive Disorders. In D.C. Steffens, D.G. Blazer, and M.E. Thakur (eds.), *The Textbook of Geriatric Psychiatry*, 5th ed., pp. 243–282. Arlington, VA: American Psychiatric Publishing.

Borson, S. and D. Thompson. 2011. Major Depression and Related Disorders. In M.E. Agronin and G. J. Maletta (eds.), *Principles and Practice of Geriatric Psychiatry*, 2nd ed., pp. 405–422. Philadelphia, PA: Lippincott Williams & Wilkins.

Chakkamparambil, B, J.T. Chibnall, E.A. Graypel, et al. 2015. Development of a Brief Validated Geriatric Depression Screening Tool: The SLU "AM SAD." *American Journal of Geriatric Psychiatry* **23**(8):780–783.

Chan, M.K.Y., H. Bhatti, N. Meader, et al. 2016. Predicting Suicide Following Self-Harm: Systematic Review of Risk Factors and Risk Scales. *The British Journal of Psychiatry* **209**:277–283.

Cohen-Mansfield, J. 1996. Conceptualization of Agitation: Results Based on the Cohen-Mansfield Agitation Inventory and the Agitation Behavior Mapping Instrument. *International Psychogeriatrics* **8** supplement: 3:309–315.

Conwell, Y. and A. O'Riley. 2013. The Challenges of Suicide Prevention in Older Adults. In H. Lavretsky, M. Sajatovic and C.F. Reynolds III (eds.), *Late-Life Mood Disorders*, pp. 206–219. New York, NY: Oxford University Press.

Cummings-Vaughn, L.A., N. Chavakula, T.K. Malmstrom, et al. 2014. Veterans Affairs Saint Louis University Mental Status Examination Compared with the Montreal Cognitive Assessment and the Short Test of Mental Status. *Journal of the American Geriatrics Society* **62**:1341–1346.

Elliot, R. 2003. Executive Functions and Their Disorders. *British Medical Bulletin* **65**:49–59.

Folstein, M.F., S.E. Folstein, and P.R. McHugh. 1975. "Mini-Mental state": A Practical Method for Grading the Cognitive State of Patients for the Clinician. *Journal of Psychiatric Research* **12**:189–198.

Forester, B., F.C. Antognini, and S. Kim. 2011. Geriatric Bipolar Disorder. In M.E. Agronin and G. J. Maletta (eds.), *Principles and Practice of Geriatric Psychiatry*, 2nd ed., pp. 423–450. Philadelphia, PA: Lippincott Williams & Wilkins.

Frock, B., A. Williams, and J.P. Caplan. 2016. Pseudobulbar Affect: When Patients Laugh or Cry, But Don't Know Why. *Current Psychiatry* **15**(9):56–60.

Grayson, L. and A.J. Thomas. 2013. A Systematic Review Comparing Clinical Features in Early Age at Onset and Late Age at Onset Late-Life Depression. *Journal of Affective Disorder* **150**:161–170.

Huang, A.X., K. Delucchi, L.B. Dum, and J. Craig Nelson. 2015. A Systematic Review and Meta-Analysis of Psychotherapy for Late-Life Depression. *American Journal of Geriatric Psychiatry* **23**:261–273.

Hui, C., and D.L. Sultzer. 2013. Depression in Long-Term Care. In H. Lavretsky, M. Sajatovic and C.F. Reynolds III (eds.), *Late-Life Mood Disorders*, pp. 477–499. New York, NY: Oxford University Press.

Inouye, S.K., C.H. van Dyck, C.A. Alessi, et al. 1990. Clarifying Confusion: The Confusion Assessment Method. A New Method for Detection of Delirium. *Annals of Internal Medicine* **113**:941–948.

Lavretsky, H., M. Reinlieb, N. St Cyr, et al. 2015. Citalopram, Methylphenidate, or Their Combination in Geriatric Depression: A Randomized, Double-Blind, Placebo-Controlled Trial. *American Journal of Psychiatry* **172**:561–569.

Lenze, E., B.H. Mulsant, D.M. Blumberger, et al. 2015. Efficacy, Safety, and Tolerability of Augmentation Pharmacotherapy with Aripiprazole for Treatment-Resistant Depression in Late Life: A Randomized, Double-Blind, Placebo-Controlled Trial. *Lancet* **386**(10011):2404–2412.

Lewis-Fernandez, R., A.K. Das, C. Alfonso, et al. 2005. Depression in US Hispanics: Diagnostic and Family Considerations in Family Practice. *Journal of the American Board of Family Medicine* **18**:282–296.

Marano, C.M., P.B. Rosenberg, and C.G. Lyketsos. 2013. Depression in Dementia. In H. Lavretsky, M. Sajatovic and C.F. Reynolds III (eds.), *Late-Life Mood Disorders*, pp. 177–205. New York, NY: Oxford University Press.

Merrill, D., M. Payne, and H. Lavretsky. 2013. Complementary and Alternative Medicine Approaches for Treatment and Prevention in Late-Life Mood Disorders. In H. Lavretsky, M. Sajatovic and C.F. Reynolds III (eds.), *Late-Life Mood Disorders*, pp. 432–447. New York, NY: Oxford University Press.

Nasreddine, Z.S., N.A. Phillips, V. Badirian, et al. 2005. The Montreal Cognitive Assessment, MoCA: A Brief Screening Tool for Mild Cognitive Impairment. *Journal of the American Geriatrics Society* **53**:695–699.

Nassan, M., W.T. Nicholson, M.A. Elliot, et al. 2016. Pharmacokinetic Pharmacogenetics Prescribing Guidelines for Antidepressants: A Template for Precision Medicine. *Mayo Clinic Proceedings*, 1–11.

Orr, W.B. 2011. Executive Dysfunction in the Elderly: From Apathy to Agitation. In M.E. Agronin and G. J. Maletta (eds.), *Principles and Practice of Geriatric Psychiatry*, 2nd ed., pp. 659–673. Philadelphia, PA: Lippincott Williams & Wilkins.

Reisberg, B., J. Borenstein, S.P. Salob, et al. 1987. Behavioral Symptoms in Alzheimer's Disease: Phenomenology and Treatment. *Journal of Clinical Psychiatry* **48** (suppl 5):9–15.

Ricker, J.H., and B.N. Axelrod, 1994. Analysis of an Oral Paradigm for the Trail Making Test. *Assessment* **1**(1): 47–51.

Robinson, R.G., and R.E. Jorge. (2016). Post-Stroke Depression: A Review. *American Journal of Psychiatry* **173**:221–231.

Rosen, J. L. Burgio, M. Kollar, et al. 1994. A User Friendly Instrument for Rating Agitation in Dementia Patients. *American Journal of Geriatric Psychiatry* **2**(1):52–59.

Saliba, D., J. Buchanan, M.O. Edelen, et al. 2012a. MDS 3.0: Brief Interview for Mental Status. *Journal of the American Medical Directors Association* **13**:611–617.

Saliba, D., S. DiFilippo, M.O. Edelen et al. 2012b. Testing the PHQ-9 Interview and Observational Versions (PHQ-OV) for MDS 3.0. *Journal of the American Medical Director's Association* **13**(7):618–625.

Sarris, J., J. Murphy, D. Mischoulon, et al. 2016. Adjunctive Nutraceuticals for Depression: A Systematic Review and Meta-Analyses. *American Journal of Psychiatry* **173**:575–587.

Smoski, M.J. and P.A. Arean. 2015. Individual and Group Psychotherapy. In D.C. Steffens, D.G. Blazer, and M.E. Thakur (eds.), *The Textbook of Geriatric Psychiatry*, 5th ed., pp. 649–668. Arlington, VA: American Psychiatric Publishing.

Smoski, M.J., S.T. Jenal, and L.W. Thompson. 2015. Bereavement. In D.C. Steffens, D.G. Blazer, and M.E. Thakur (eds.), *The Textbook of Geriatric Psychiatry*, 5th ed., pp. 415–434. Arlington, VA: American Psychiatric Publishing.

Spitzer, R, Kroenke, K., and Williams, J. 1999. Validation and Utility of a Self-Report Version of PRIME-MD: The PHQ Primary Care Study. *Journal of the American Medical Association* **282**: 1737–1744.

Taylor, W.D. 2014. Depression in the Elderly. *New England Journal of Medicine* **371**:1228–1236.

Tecuta, L., E. Tomba, S. Grandi, and G.A. Fava. 2015. Demoralization: A Systematic Review on its Clinical Characterization. *Psychological Medicine*. **47**:673–691.

Turecki, G. and D.A. Brent. 2016. Suicide and Suicidal Behavior. *Lancet*. **387**:1227–1239.

Unutzer, J. and M. Park. 2012. Older Adults with Severe Treatment-Resistant Depression: "I Got My Mother Back." *Journal of the American Medical Association* **308**(9):909–918.

Warden, V., Hurley, A.C. and Volicer, L. 2003. Development and Psychometric Evaluation of the Pain Assessment in Advanced Dementia. *Journal of the American Medical Directors Association* **4**:9–15.

Wood, S., J.L. Cummings, M. Hsu, et al. 2000. The Use of the Neuropsychiatric Inventory in Nursing Home Residents. *American Journal of Geriatric Psychiatry* **8**:75–83.

Yesavage, J.A., T.L. Brink, T.L. Rose, et al. 1983. Development and Validation of a Geriatric Depression Scale: A Preliminary Report. *Journal of Psychiatric Research* **17**:37–49.

Young, R.C. and N.A. Mahgoub. 2013. Bipolar Disorder. In H. Lavretsky, M. Sajatovic, and C.F. Reynolds III (eds.), *Late-Life Mood Disorders*, pp. 104–128. New York, NY: Oxford University Press.

Chapter 6 Psychotic Disorders and Violence

Psychotic disorders are the third most common reversible cause of disability and increased mortality (after major depressive disorders [MDDs] and delirium) in LTC populations. Delusions and hallucinations are the hallmarks of psychotic disorders, although catatonic behavior, disorganized thinking (speech), and grossly disorganized behavior may also be evidence of impaired reality testing (American Psychiatric Association 2013). (See Table 6.1.) Delusions are false unshakeable beliefs (not amenable to change despite conflicting evidence) that are not in keeping with the individual's cultural beliefs. Persecutory delusions (belief that one is going to be harmed) are the most common type of delusion in LTC populations. Bizarre delusions are delusions that are clearly implausible (e.g. an entity is removing one's thoughts [thought withdrawal] and inserting dangerous thoughts [thought insertion], and controlling one's behavior [delusions of control]) and are hallmarks of schizophrenia, although they may be seen in other psychotic disorders. Hallucinations are perceptions (in any sensory modality) in the absence of appropriate external stimuli. In LTC populations, visual hallucinations are the most common hallucination, followed by auditory hallucinations, followed by other hallucinations (gustatory, tactile, or olfactory). In general, lack of insight, emotional distress, and impairment in daily functioning are required for symptoms such as hallucination and delusion to be considered part of a clinically significant psychotic disorder. Emotional distress due to psychotic symptoms may be experienced as fear, irritability, sadness, anger, and even panic. Not all residents who have delusion and/or hallucination experience emotional distress. Some delusions (e.g. false belief that family members are present in the facility, giving a sense of security to the resident) and hallucinations (e.g. feeling amused by seeing small children) may even be accompanied by positive emotion. Hallucinations that occur while falling asleep are called hypnagogic hallucinations, and hallucinations that occur while waking up are called hypnopompic hallucinations. Residents may have hypnagogic and hypnopompic hallucinations as part of normal experiences but need to be assessed, as these may herald an underlying psychotic and/or neurologic disorder (narcolepsy).

The point prevalence of psychotic disorder in LTC populations is 5–10 percent. Mild psychotic symptoms (e.g. transient delusions and/or hallucinations) are even more prevalent. (See Boxes 6.1 and 6.2.) Box 6.1 lists common psychotic disorders seen in LTC populations. Box 6.2 lists common medications that may cause or exacerbate psychotic symptoms. The majority of psychotic symptoms in LTC populations are in the context of delirium, major neurocognitive disorder (MNCD), Parkinson's disease (PD), and cerebrovascular disease. The prevalence of psychotic symptoms in people who have MNCD ranges from 50 percent in AD to more than 80 percent in MNCD due to Lewy bodies (dementia with Lewy bodies [DLB]) (Apostolova 2016; Gomperts 2016). The prevalence of schizophrenia and schizoaffective disorders in LTC populations is currently low (0.2–1 percent) but increasing primarily due to the aging of adults who have schizophrenia or schizoaffective disorder. LTC populations typically have multiple risk factors for the development of psychotic disorder. (See Box 6.3.)

Psychotic symptoms are a common cause of violence and aggressive behavior in LTC populations and one of the most common reasons for psychiatric consultation. (See Box 6.4.) Box 6.4 lists consequences and complications of untreated psychotic disorder in LTC populations. Comprehensive assessment, prevention, and treatment strategies for all psychotic disorders and aggression can dramatically improve the quality of life of all residents who have psychotic disorder and may be life saving (Desai and Grossberg 2017).

Table 6.1 Types of Psychotic Symptoms Commonly Seen in Long-Term Care Populations

Psychotic Symptom	Real-Life Examples	Clinical Implication/Complications
Persecutory delusion	Resident has delusional belief that nurse killed nurse's husband and is plotting to kill resident's husband Resident has delusional belief that there is a plot to kill him or her	Persecutory delusion is most common type of delusion and is seen in delirium, schizophrenia, and with MNCD
Delusion of reference (referential delusion)	Resident refuses to come out of room because of delusional belief that other residents and/or staff are constantly talking about him or her (in a negative manner)	Social isolation
Delusion of grandiosity (grandiose delusion)	Resident has delusional belief that he or she has multiple patents that are going to earn millions of dollars when sold	Financial ruin because resident may spend all financial assets
Delusion of jealousy (delusion of infidelity)	Resident is convinced that spouse/partner is having an affair with another resident	Violence toward spouse/partner and/or other resident believed to be involved More common in males than females
Erotomanic delusion (erotomania)	Resident is convinced that a celebrity is in love with him or her	Legal problems because of attempts to stalk the celebrity
Nihilistic delusion	Resident is convinced that there are no organs inside his or her body	High risk of suicide
Delusion of poverty	Resident is convinced that he or she has no money and cannot pay for any services	Risk of leaving the facility or refusing medical care
Somatic delusion	Resident is convinced that he or she has an untreated malignancy or contagious disease (e.g. HIV/AIDS)	High risk of suicide
Delusion of infestation	Resident has delusional belief that there are bugs on or under his or her skin even if no one can see them	Skin breakdown and even extensive excoriation due to attempts to remove bugs
Bizarre delusion	Resident has delusional belief that someone is controlling his or her thoughts and behavior	Classic symptom of schizophrenia
Delusional misidentification	Resident has delusional belief that family members visiting are imposters (Capgras syndrome) Resident has delusional belief that strangers he or she has encountered are actually family members pretending to be strangers (Fregoli syndrome)	Increases risk of aggressive behavior
Auditory hallucination	Resident can hear staff and other residents continuously talking about him or her and commenting on his or her behaviors even when they are in a different section of the facility	Classic symptom of schizophrenia

Table 6.1 (cont.)

Psychotic Symptom	Real-Life Examples	Clinical Implication/Complications
Visual hallucination	Resident sees intruders coming to his or her room	High risk of violence
Tactile hallucination	Resident can feel bugs crawling on his or her skin	Skin breakdown and even extensive excoriation due to attempts to remove bugs
Olfactory hallucination	Resident can smell poison being injected into the room	Refusal to sleep or be in his or her room
Gustatory hallucination	Resident can taste poison in the food	Refusal to eat or drink and consequent risk of malnutrition
Disorganized speech (formal thought disorder)	Resident has prominent derailment, loosening of association, and incoherence	Needs to be differentiated from speech disturbance due to aphasia (especially receptive but also expressive)
Catatonic excitement	Resident is in continuous frenzied activity/psychomotor agitation for hours to days	Exhaustion and potential to be fatal
Catatonic stupor	Resident is not moving (eyes are usually open and resident does show subtle signs of awareness of the environment)	Should be considered behavioral emergency requiring hospitalization
Catatonic mutism	Resident is not communicating (e.g. talking, writing) (and no evidence of aphasia)	May be mistaken for functional neurological symptom of mutism (conversion disorder)
Catatonic posturing and rigidity (waxy flexibility)	Resident remains in abnormal position/postures for hours	Risk of rhabdomyolysis
Other catatonic features	Echopraxia (mimicking other's movements), echolalia (mimicking other's speech), palilalia (mimicking other's words, syllables), mannerisms (odd caricature of normal actions), stereotypy (repetitive non-goal-directed movements), and grimacing	May need to be differentiated from tics
Grossly disorganized behavior	Resident behaves in a childlike silly manner Resident has unpredictable agitation	Availability of as-needed psychotropic medication may be necessary if episodes of agitation are moderate to severe

Diagnosis

Accurate early diagnosis of psychotic disorder is key to a successful outcome. There are currently no reliable biomarkers for any psychotic disorder, including schizophrenia (Maglione, Vahia, and Jeste 2015). The diagnosis of all psychotic disorders is clinical. Eliciting core symptoms of schizophrenia listed in Box 6.5, inquiring into all possible psychotic symptoms listed in Table 6.1, and clarifying associated functional impairment is key to accurate diagnosis. Schizophrenia can be reliably differentiated from other psychotic disorders, especially delirium with psychotic symptoms and MNCD with psychotic symptoms. (See Table 6.2.) Standardized scales, such as Neuropsychiatric Inventory–Nursing Home version (NPI-NH), can help improve the accuracy of diagnosis and assess the severity and comorbidity of other psychiatric symptoms. We recommend that NPI-NH be used in conjunction with other standardized scales listed in Table 6.3 (Folstein, Folstein, and McHugh 1975; Yesavage

BOX 6.1 Common Psychotic Disorders in Long-Term Care Populations

Primary psychotic disorders
- Affective psychoses (major depressive disorder [MDD] with psychotic symptoms, mania with psychotic symptoms)
- Schizophrenia
- Schizoaffective disorder: unipolar type, bipolar type
- Brief psychotic disorder
- Delusional disorder
- Hallucination during bereavement

Secondary psychotic disorders
- Major neurocognitive disorder with psychotic symptoms
- Parkinson's disease psychosis
- Delirium with psychotic symptoms
- Psychotic disorder due to another medical condition
- Medication-induced psychotic disorder (see Box 6.2)
- Substance-induced psychotic disorder (e.g. cocaine, alcohol, methamphetamine)

Mixed psychotic disorders
- Major neurocognitive disorder with psychotic symptoms and delirium with psychotic symptoms
- Schizophrenia and medical condition causing psychotic symptoms
- Other combinations of primary psychotic disorders and secondary psychotic disorders or two secondary psychotic disorders

BOX 6.2 Medications That Are Commonly Implicated in Causing Psychotic Symptoms

Anticholinergic drugs and other drugs with high anticholinergic activity (common reason for use):
- Diphenhydramine (allergies, insomnia)
- Brompheniramine (allergies)
- Chlorpheniramine (allergies)
- Trihexyphenidyl (antipsychotic-induced Parkinsonism)
- Biperiden (antipsychotic-induced Parkinsonism)
- Benztropine (antipsychotic-induced Parkinsonism)
- Orphenadrine (antipsychotic-induced Parkinsonism)
- Scopolamine (dizziness)
- Meclizine (dizziness)
- Oxybutynin (overactive bladder/urinary incontinence)
- Dimenhydrinate (allergies)
- Atropine (hypersalivation)
- Hyocyamine (hypersalivation)
- Hydroxyzine (itching)
- Doxylamine (sleep aid)
- Meperidine (opioid analgesic)
- Methocarbamol (muscle spasticity/tightness)

BOX 6.2 (cont.)

- Doxepin (insomnia, itching)
- Imipramine (MDD)
- Amitriptyline (sleep aid, headaches)
- Clomipramine (obsessive compulsive disorder)
- Desipramine (MDD)
- Nortriptyline (MDD)
- Chlorpromazine (schizophrenia)
- Thioridazine (schizophrenia)
- Olanzapine (schizophrenia, bipolar disorder, MDD, other psychotic disorders)
- Quetiapine (schizophrenia, bipolar disorder, MDD, other psychotic disorder)
- Clozapine (schizophrenia)

Dopaminergic drugs

- Ropinirole (Parkinson's disease, restless legs syndrome)
- Pramipexole (Parkinson's disease, restless legs syndrome)
- Rotigotine (Parkinson's disease)
- Levodopa (L-dopa), carbidopa (Parkinson's disease)
- Bromocriptine (Parkinson's disease)
- Amantadine (Parkinson's disease)
- Selegiline (Parkinson's disease, MDD [selegiline patch])

Cardiovascular drugs

- Digoxin (heart failure)
- Antiarrhythmics (e.g. lidocaine, quinidine, procainamide, amiodarone) (arrhythmia)

Steroids

- Corticosteroids (e.g. prednisone, dexamethasone) (exacerbation of COPD, rheumatological disease)

Gastrointestinal drugs

- Cimetidine (dyspepsia)

Sedative-hypnotics (intoxication or withdrawal)

- Benzodiazepines (severe anxiety, insomnia)
- Barbiturates (primidone used for essential tremors)
- Chloral hydrate (insomnia)

Analgesics (pain management)

- Hydrocodone
- Oxycodone
- Morphine
- Fentanyl
- Tramadol

et al. 1983; Reisberg et al. 1987; Inouye et al. 1990; Ricker and Axelrod 1994; Rosen et al. 1994; Cohen-Mansfield 1996; Alexopoulos et al. 1988; Spitzer, Kroenke, and Williams 1999; Woods et al. 2000; Elliot 2003; Warden, Hurley, and Volicer 2003; Nasreddine et al. 2005; Saliba et al. 2012a, 2012b; Cummings-Vaughn et al. 2014; Chakkamparambil et al. 2015). Standardized tests for cognition, pain, depression, and behaviors can help clarify comorbidity and guide treatment decisions.

BOX 6.3 Key Risk Factors for Psychotic Disorder

Risk factors for psychotic disorder in older adults in general:

- Recent transfer from hospital for postacute stay in LTC facility
- Older age
- Major neurocognitive disorder
- Stroke
- Polypharmacy (five or more medications), high anticholinergic burden (score of 6 or more on anticholinergic burden scale), psychoactive medication (see Box 6.2)
- Sudden vision loss
- Sudden hearing loss
- High medical comorbidity
- Bereavement
- Parkinson's disease
- History of psychotic disorder
- Family history of psychotic disorder
- Substance use disorder
- Chronic insomnia
- Use of certain medications (see Box 6.2)
- Victim of abuse (verbal, physical, sexual, financial) and/or neglect
- Personality disorder/personality traits (especially schizotypal, borderline, paranoid)

Risk factors for psychotic disorder related to institutionalization:

- Admission of resident without adequate preparation for move (emotional preparation of resident and communication of resident's personal information [e.g. health, life history, preferences, dislikes] to staff of new facility)
- Change from one LTC facility to another without adequate preparation for move (emotional preparation of resident and communication of resident's personal information)
- Change of room within facility without adequate preparation for move
- Countertherapeutic staff approach and interaction (e.g. staff constantly correcting resident's recall of events, putting excessive burden on resident, disrespectful and impatient attitude)

The high prevalence of cognitive impairment, sensory impairment, and apathy and lack of adequate time and training of health care professionals (HCPs) in the recognition of psychotic disorder make accurate diagnosis in LTC populations challenging. Prominent agitation, aggressive behavior (verbal and/or physical), social withdrawal, and accelerated cognitive and functional decline may be the dominant manifestations of psychotic disorder, especially among residents who have MNCD. The presence of delusion and/or hallucination may not be obvious but usually can be elicited during comprehensive assessment. Residents usually do not spontaneously report their psychotic symptoms but do share their thoughts and experiences if asked, "Has your mind been playing tricks on you?" The HCP should inquire into the range of delusions, hallucinations (in all modalities), and illusions (distortions of external stimuli [e.g. rope seen as a snake, blobs on a wall as someone's face]) and their frequency and severity in a gentle, nonjudgmental, and nonthreatening manner. This is important, as stigma against mental illness is prevalent in LTC populations. Some education of the resident at the time of the interview that the HCP is investigating potential adverse effect of medication or manifestation of a neurological problem (e.g. Parkinson's disease [PD], stroke) may make a resident more comfortable in sharing strange thoughts and frightening experiences. Residents who have relatively preserved cognitive function often appreciate learning about this.

For residents who have MNCD, staff and family input and review of staff notes may often shed

BOX 6.4 **Consequences and Complications of Untreated Psychotic Disorder**

Severe emotional distress
Suicide
Nonsuicide mortality
Homicide
Violence/physically aggressive behavior
Verbally aggressive behavior
Reduced quality of life
Impaired compliance with medical treatment
Impaired compliance with rehabilitation therapy
Accelerated cognitive decline
Malnutrition (weight loss [due to reduced food intake], obesity [due to excessive food intake])
Increased rate of hospitalization
Longer hospital stay
Decline in IADLs and ADLs
Increased staff time to care
Increased risk of institutionalization of individual who has MNCD or PD
Deconditioning (due to remaining in bed for prolonged periods)
Deep vein thrombosis (due to not moving, especially during catatonic symptoms)
Social isolation
Increased distress in family members and friends

light on the nature and severity of psychotic symptoms than information from the resident. Catatonic behavior and grossly disorganized behavior are under-recognized, and the HCP needs to routinely inquire into these during assessment of psychotic symptoms and/or violent behavior and look for them during interview (Tandon et al. 2013). Mental status exam may identify disorganized speech (formal thought disorder, such as frequent loosening of association, derailment, thought blocking, tangentiality, circumstantiality, incoherence [word salad]). History and mental status examination should also look for manifestation of negative symptoms in a resident who has psychotic symptoms. Two key negative symptoms are prominent decrease in emotional expression (flat affect or blunted affect on mental status examination) and dramatic decline in intentional purposeful activity (avolition). Other negative symptoms include apathy (decrease in drive/motivation), alogia (markedly diminished speech output), anhedonia (lack of positive emotions in response to positive events/pleasurable activities), and asociality (greatly diminished interest in social interactions). Flat affect and hypokinesia in a resident who has Parkinson's disease (PD) or

BOX 6.5 **Main Symptoms of Schizophrenia**

Core symptoms*

1. Delusion
2. Hallucination
3. Disorganized speech (prominent derailment, loosening of association, incoherence)
4. Grossly disorganized behavior and/or catatonic behavior
5. Negative symptoms (prominent avolition and diminished emotional expression)

Additional signs and symptoms

1. Lack of appetite or weight loss; increased appetite or weight gain
2. Insomnia or hypersomnia
3. Recurrent thoughts of suicide or wish to die or suicide attempt
4. Thoughts of wanting to harm others
5. Physically aggressive/violent behavior
6. Verbally aggressive behavior
7. Decreased energy or fatigue
8. Staying in bed excessively
9. Multiple somatic complaints (typically matching somatic delusions)
10. Chronic pain not responding to pain medication
11. Hypochondriasis
12. Marked symptoms of anxiety
13. Agitation (especially in resident who has comorbid MNCD)
14. Decreased spontaneous speech
15. Psychomotor retardation/agitation
16. Refusing medication
17. Resisting care
18. Refusing to participate in therapy (physical, occupational, speech)
19. Sudden decline in cognition
20. Subjective memory complaints

* For diagnosis of schizophrenia based on *DSM-5*, some symptoms need to be present for six months with at least one month of active phase symptoms (two of five core symptoms, with at least one being first three core symptoms)

Table 6.2 Differentiating Delirium with Psychotic Symptoms from Schizophrenia and Major Neurocognitive Disorder due to Alzheimer's Disease with Psychotic Symptoms

Feature	Delirium	Schizophrenia with Psychotic Symptoms	MNCD due to AD with Psychotic Symptoms
Onset of psychotic symptoms	Acute (over hours to few days)	Chronic with intermittent exacerbation or continuous symptoms (over months to years)	Subacute (over weeks)
Dramatic fluctuation of severity of symptoms within a day	Present (symptoms typically worse at night)	Usually absent	Occasionally present
Impaired attention (e.g. difficulty following conversation)	Present and severity fluctuates	Usually absent or mild	Absent (except in severe stages)
Altered level of consciousness (drowsiness or hyperalert state)	Usually present	Absent	Absent
Disorganized thinking	Usually present	Occasionally present	Absent (except in severe stages or presence of receptive aphasia)
Reversal of sleep-wake cycle	Often present	Absent	Absent (except in severe stages)
Impaired memory	Present and is due to impaired attention	Often present and is due to impaired attention and motivation	Present and is due to impaired encoding
Delusion	Often present (typically persecutory delusion)	Usually present, complex, and well formed (a variety of delusions including persecutory, reference, bizarre, grandiose)	Usually present but simple and not well formed (typically involving others stealing belongings)
Disturbed perception	Often present (typically visual hallucination and illusion)	Often present (typically auditory hallucination)	Absent in mild stages, may be present in advanced stages (typically visual hallucination and illusion)
Course	Fluctuating, may progress to coma without treatment, and is usually reversible with appropriate treatment	Chronic with periodic exacerbation	Relentless and irreversible progression to more severe stages

Parkinsonism due to other causes (e.g. antipsychotic, stroke, traumatic brain injury [TBI]) are often mistaken for negative symptoms of schizophrenia.

Symptoms of poor appetite, fatigue, and sleep disturbance accompanying psychotic disorder may overlap with a wide variety of physical illnesses. The HCP should assess a resident who has verbal or physical aggression for the presence of psychotic symptoms. In some cultures, visual or auditory hallucination with a religious content may be a normal part of religious experience (e.g. seeing the Virgin Mary, hearing God's voice) and should not be considered a manifestation of a psychotic disorder. In some religious ceremonies (e.g. Hindu religion), residents may report hearing voices from divine entities. Language barriers and cultural issues may pose barriers to accurate diagnosis

Table 6.3 Standardized Bedside Assessment Tools to Assist in the Evaluation and Management of Psychotic Disorders, Neurocognitive Disorders, and Other Syndromes

Standardized Assessment Tool	Key Benefits for Resident Who Has Psychotic Disorder	Key Limitations
Mini-Mental State Exam (MMSE)	Excellent tool to assess global cognitive function Abnormal score after successful treatment of psychotic disorder may suggest need for evaluation of underlying MNCD	Copyright issues and cost limit its routine use Often misses executive dysfunction, and executive dysfunction due to psychotic disorder is prevalent in LTC populations
Montreal Cognitive Assessment (MOCA)	Excellent tool to assess global cognitive function Available for use without cost Is translated into 35 languages Reliably assesses executive function Abnormal score after successful treatment of psychotic disorder may suggest need for evaluation of underlying MNCD	Requires staff training for its reliable use
Saint Louis University Mental State (SLUMS)	Excellent tool to assess global cognitive function Available for use without cost Reliably assesses executive function Abnormal score after successful treatment of psychotic disorder may suggest need for evaluation of underlying MNCD	Requires staff training for its reliable use Most as well researched as MOCA and MMSE
Brief Interview for Mental Status (BIMS)	Easy-to-use tool to assess global cognitive function that is a part of Minimum Data Set 3.0 used in nursing homes in the United States	Often misses executive dysfunction and executive dysfunction due to psychotic disorder
Trail Making Test–Oral (TMT-Oral)	Easy-to-use tool to measure executive function quickly	Cannot be used as only test to assess executive function, as it can be normal in some individuals who have significant executive dysfunction
Controlled Oral Word Association Test (COWAT)	Easy-to-use tool to measure executive function quickly	Cannot be used as only test to assess executive function, as it can be normal in some individuals who have significant executive dysfunction
Confusion Assessment Method (CAM)	Excellent screening tool for diagnosis of delirium, especially for resident who has MNCD	Requires staff training for its reliable use
Functional Activities Questionnaire (FAQ)	Excellent tool to assess functioning in IADLs (e.g. keeping appointments, managing money), as executive impairment often impairs IADLs	With resident who has impaired insight (some residents who have MNCD), this tool requires a knowledgeable informant for accurate assessment
Patient Health Questionnaire–9 (PHQ-9)	Excellent tool to screen for MDD (often comorbid with a psychotic disorder) and monitor response to treatment Easy to use Well known in primary care	Not reliable for screening MDD with resident who has more advanced MNCD

Table 6.3 (cont.)

Standardized Assessment Tool	Key Benefits for Resident Who Has Psychotic Disorder	Key Limitations
Geriatric Depression Scale–15 (GDS)	Excellent tool to screen for MDD and monitor response to treatment Also available in 5-, 10-, and 30-item versions	Not reliable for screening MDD with resident who has more advanced MNCD Requires some staff training for its reliable use Not as easy to use as PHQ-9
Cornell Scale for Depression in Dementia (CSDD)	Excellent tool to screen for MDD in resident who has moderate to severe MNCD and monitor response to treatment	Requires staff training for its reliable use
Saint Louis University AM SAD (SLU AM SAD)	Easy-to-use tool to screen for MDD and monitor response to treatment	Not as well studied as PHQ-9, GDS, and CSDD
Cohen-Mansfield Agitation Inventory (CMAI)	Excellent tool to measure severity of distress expressed as agitation in resident who has moderate to severe MNCD and monitor response to treatment (psychotic disorder may manifest as persistent agitation, tearfulness, irritability, anxiety, and insomnia)	Requires staff training for its reliable use
Pittsburgh Agitation Inventory (PAS)	Excellent tool to measure severity of distress expressed as agitation in resident who has moderate to severe MNCD and monitor response to treatment (psychotic disorder may manifest as persistent agitation, tearfulness, irritability, anxiety, and insomnia)	Requires staff training for its reliable use
Neuropsychiatric Inventory–Nursing Home Version (NPI-NH)	Excellent tool to screen for behavioral and psychological symptoms (including delusion and hallucination) in resident who has MNCD and monitor response to treatment	Requires staff training for its reliable use
Behavioral Symptoms in Alzheimer's Disease (BEHAVE-AD)	Excellent tool to screen for behavioral and psychological symptoms in resident who has MNCD and monitor response to treatment (psychotic disorder may manifest as persistent agitation, tearfulness, irritability, anxiety, and insomnia)	Requires staff training for its reliable use
Numerical Rating Scale (Likert scale)	Excellent tool to assess severity of pain in resident who has psychotic disorder and monitor response to treatment (pain often accompanies psychotic disorder, and untreated pain is a key factor in lack of improvement of psychotic disorder with treatment) Easy to use	Not reliable with people who have severe MNCD or significantly impaired receptive language
Pain in Alzheimer's Disease (PAIN-AD)	Excellent tool to assess severity of pain and monitor response to treatment in resident who has severe AD and psychotic symptoms (pain often accompanies psychotic disorder, and untreated pain is a key factor in lack of improvement of psychotic disorder with treatment)	Requires staff training for its reliable use

of psychotic symptoms, especially among residents who have MNCD. We recommend the use of an interpreter and input from family to distinguish cultural beliefs from delusional thinking. A resident who has confabulation (typically seen in people who have Korsakoff syndrome due to thiamine deficiency but also occasionally in people who have MNCD) or incoherent speech (e.g. residents who have Wernicke aphasia [receptive aphasia]) may be mistakenly diagnosed as having a psychotic disorder. Having a high index of suspicion and careful assessment of language and memory during the mental status exam will usually help the HCP differentiate psychotic symptoms (delusional thinking and formal thought disorder) from aphasia and confabulation.

We recommend a comprehensive diagnostic assessment and work-up of all distressing psychotic symptoms (Karim and Burns 2011). (See Table 6.4.) The goal of assessment is to clarify etiology and identify reversible comorbidity. The choice of tests and extent of work-up will depend on findings from the comprehensive assessment. Psychotic symptoms may be the initial presentation of delirium or MNCD (especially DLB), as cognitive symptoms may be subtle in early stages; hence the importance of detailed cognitive assessment. Psychotic symptoms and undernutrition (dehydration, protein and/or energy malnutrition, severe weight loss) are a potentially fatal combination because immune functioning may also be affected and should be considered a psychiatric and medical emergency. The HCP needs to act quickly to provide nutritional supplementation and aggressive treatment of psychotic disorder to avert serious debility, hospitalization, and death. For a resident who has life-threatening psychotic disorder (e.g. intense thoughts of suicide or violence, suicide attempt, severe aggressive behavior, undernutrition, severe agitation due to psychotic symptoms), transfer to a local emergency department (ED) for acute inpatient psychiatric hospitalization, preferably in a geriatric psychiatry inpatient unit, may be a necessary first step before the HCP can complete a comprehensive work-up.

Primary Psychotic Disorder

Primary psychotic disorders include affective psychoses (psychotic symptoms associated with MDD or mania), schizophrenia, schizoaffective disorder, delusional disorder, and brief reactive psychoses. These are serious disorders associated with high morbidity, risk for suicide, risk for violence and aggressive behavior, and increased mortality (with or without suicide).

Affective Psychosis

Residents who have affective psychosis typically experience psychotic symptoms along with significant mood symptoms (MDD or mania). Psychotic symptoms do not occur in the absence of mood symptoms, and family history is often positive for mood disorders. There may be a history of an affective episode (depression, mania) with or without psychotic symptoms.

Major Depressive Disorder with Psychotic Symptoms. When residents who have MDD develop delusions, hallucinations, and/or catatonic symptoms, they are said to have MDD with psychotic symptoms (also called psychotic depression). Psychotic symptoms are more common in depressed people whose first major depressive episode occurs later in life rather than in those who have early episodes. These people often have rigidity in thinking, have more severe depression, and exhibit delusions that are usually congruent to mood (e.g. delusions of guilt relative to past events, poverty, somatic illness), but occasionally exhibit delusions that are incongruent to mood (e.g. delusions of persecution). People who have psychotic depression often have more pronounced agitation or retardation. Examples include an individual who believes that he has an incurable illness or that he deserves punishment for "unforgivable sins" or that impending catastrophe affects a loved one. The presence of delusion appears to run true through repeated episodes. Hallucinations, which occur less commonly than delusions in these people, are more likely to be auditory than visual or somatic. People who have psychotic depression are much more likely to have agitation – "the classic pacing and wringing of hands" have greater cognitive disturbance, and are more likely to have a family history of MDD or bipolar disorder. A history of delusion in a depressive episode or profound anxiety in a depressed resident is a major clue to possible psychotic depression. Psychotic depression carries a high risk of suicide and does not respond to antidepressant alone. Hence, it is important that the HCP diagnose this entity as early as possible. Additional antipsychotic is usually necessary along with antidepressant for response to treatment. The HCP should consider hospitalization and ECT early in the course of treatment, and we strongly recommend them for

Table 6.4 Diagnostic Work-Up for Psychotic Disorder

Diagnostic Test	Key Examples	Key Implications for Treatment
Comprehensive assessment	Psychiatric history (including history of suicide attempt, violence, hospitalization) Family history (including history of suicide and treatment for major mental illness) Review of medication Vital signs Physical examination (including height, weight, body mass index) Neurological examination Mental status examination Use of standardized assessment scales Review of previous psychiatric records	Risk assessment for suicide and violence is primarily based on comprehensive assessment Findings from cognitive assessment are key to choosing treatment (e.g. avoiding antipsychotic with anticholinergic activity [e.g. olanzapine] for resident who has significant cognitive impairment; psychotherapy for resident who has relatively preserved cognitive function)
Bedside test	Pulse oximetry	Hypoxia may contribute to psychotic symptoms
Bedside test	Glucose fingerstick	Hypoglycemia and severe hyperglycemia may contribute to psychotic symptoms
Laboratory test	Complete blood count	Leukocytosis or leukopenia may indicate coexisting infection
Laboratory test	Comprehensive metabolic panel	Identifying dehydration and electrolyte imbalance that may contribute to psychotic symptoms and resistance to treatment Low albumin is indicator of protein malnutrition, often a complication of untreated psychotic disorder
Laboratory test	Vitamin B12, folate, and vitamin D levels	Vitamin B12 and vitamin D deficiencies are prevalent in residents who have psychotic disorder and contribute to functional impairment
Laboratory test	Thyroid function tests (e.g. thyroid stimulating hormone level)	Undercorrection or overcorrection of hypothyroidism is prevalent in residents who have psychotic disorder and contributes to resistance to treatment if not corrected
Laboratory test	Lipid panel	Low cholesterol is an indicator of malnutrition, often a complication of psychotic disorder Baseline lipid panel helps identify pre-existing dyslipidemia, which may influence choice of antipsychotic, as some antipsychotics can cause/worsen dyslipidemia (e.g. olanzapine)

Table 6.4 (cont.)

Diagnostic Test	Key Examples	Key Implications for Treatment
Laboratory test	Serum drug levels	Serum levels of antipsychotic (e.g. haloperidol, olanzapine) may help the HCP adjust the dosage and avoid toxicity Serum levels of digoxin may help clarify diagnosis of digoxin-induced psychotic disorder
Laboratory test	Erythrocyte sedimentation rate (ESR) and C-reactive protein (CRP)	Markedly increased levels may suggest exacerbation of rheumatological condition or occult cancer, which may cause or contribute to psychotic disorder
Laboratory or bedside test	Electrocardiogram (EKG)	HCP needs to avoid prescribing antipsychotic with significant risk of QTc prolongation (e.g. haloperidol, ziprasidone) for resident who has baseline prolonged QTc due to risk of Torsades de pointes
Neuroimaging	MRI of brain	Evidence of significant cerebrovascular disease on MRI (prevalent in residents who have psychotic disorder) may influence treatment, as cerebrovascular disease increases risk of antipsychotic-induced EPS
Laboratory test	Psychotropic drug genetic testing (pharmacogenomic testing) using a buccal swab Genetic testing for HLA-B 1502 allele for carbamazepine-induced Stevens-Johnson syndrome in residents with Asian descent	Activity of various liver enzymes in the cytochrome P450 system (poor metabolizers, ultrarapid metabolizers) may influence choice and dosage of antipsychotic (e.g. high dose of olanzapine may be used for resident who is ultrarapid metabolizer of 1A2 enzymes)
Imaging	CT scan of abdomen and/or lung	Psychotic symptoms with severe weight loss may be initial manifestation of occult malignancy (e.g. pancreatic cancer, lung cancer)
Laboratory test	Electroencephalography (EEG)	EEG may clarify diagnosis of psychotic disorder due to seizure (ictal, postictal, interictal psychotic symptoms)
Hearing and vision tests	Assessment for hearing and/or vision deficits	Hearing deficit often predisposes to paranoia; vision deficit may cause illusion and visual hallucination

life-threatening cases of psychotic depression. ECT can be used safely with this population and in severe cases of psychotic depression (e.g. with inanition or catatonia) may be life saving.

Clinical Case 1: "I am staying here illegally"

Mr. T, a 78-year-old divorced male, had been reporting fears of being put in jail because he had been living "illegally" in the nursing home. He was also having sleep impairment and lack of appetite with a 15-pound weight loss over the last three months (from 189 pounds to 174, height was 5' 8") and had been refusing to shave, change clothes, or bathe for the last three weeks. He was referred to the psychiatrist because in the past week, he had been saying that he would be better off dead. The psychiatrist noted that Mr. T had a history of "mini-stroke" six months ago and recently developed severe abdominal pain requiring gall bladder surgery. Mr. T was admitted to the nursing home (NH) for rehabilitation. After completing rehabilitation, he was transferred to the long-term care wing for continued stay, as there was no one to take care of him at home. He also had a history of recurrent falls, cognitive impairment, and refusal to take medication and required close monitoring of unstable diabetes. Family reported that Mr. T had been disappointed when he was told he could not return home, had since become withdrawn, stopped smiling, and even stopped watching sports on TV (one of his favorite activities in the past).

During the interview, Mr. T reported feeling nervous and explained that his reason for not shaving or bathing was fear that his skin would somehow "infect" his roommate. He felt that he could not ask for a room change because "I am staying here illegally." Mr. T further explained that he had no money to pay the high cost of the NH (Mr. T had apparently seen the monthly charge of his NH stay, which was approximately $6,000). Mr. T had a history of severe depression 15 years ago when he had retired but his daughters did not know the details and Mr. T could not give details except to confirm that he was given "nerve pills." There was no obvious history of previous manic or hypomanic episode. Mr. T had a family history of depression (sister) and suicide (brother). Medication review did not identify any medication that could cause or exacerbate psychiatric symptoms, and laboratory tests (including thyroid tests and vitamin levels) were unremarkable. On mental status exam, Mr. T exhibited a depressed mood and affect, delusions of persecution, and passive suicidal ideas (felt life was not worth living) but denied any specific suicidal intention or plan. His recall was 1 out of 3, MOCA score was 16, and GDS score was 20/30. Mr. T was diagnosed with recurrent major depressive disorder with psychotic features and probable vascular MNCD. The psychiatrist recommended hospitalization and ECT, but Mr. T declined both. There were insufficient grounds for involuntary commitment, as he agreed to treatment at the NH. Mr. T was started on sertraline 25 mg daily, and the dose was gradually increased every four days by 25 mg to 100 mg daily. He was also started on risperidone 0.25 mg at bedtime and it was increased to 0.5 mg at bedtime after one week. Behavioral activation with individualized pleasant activity schedule (IPAS) was initiated.

After four weeks, family and staff reported that Mr. T's appetite and sleep had improved but he was still refusing to shave and to come out of his room. His participation in exercise and IPAS was intermittent and brief. During interview, Mr. T continued to express delusional thinking and depressed affect. Over the next two weeks, risperidone was further increased to 0.25 mg daily in the morning and 0.5 mg at bedtime for seven days and then 0.5 mg daily in the morning and 0.5 mg daily at bedtime. After four more weeks, Mr. T for the first time reported he was feeling better and he started showing interest in watching sports on TV and allowed staff to shave him and help him bathe. His participation in exercise and IPAS also increased considerably. After four more weeks, he was shaving and bathing regularly and did not express any fears he had before. Mr. T still expressed sadness at not being able to go home and hoped the psychiatrist would help him return home. Mr. T's repeat GDS score was 8/30 and repeat MOCA score was 21.

Teaching Points

The first consideration in the management of any severe psychotic disorder is the safety of the patient and need for hospitalization to an inpatient psychiatric unit. ECT is the first-line treatment for psychotic depression. Psychotic depression may respond to a combination of antidepressant and atypical antipsychotic. Full therapeutic effects of medication may take 12 or more weeks. Although risperidone has been associated with a slightly increased risk of stroke and mortality ("black box warning") in people who have MNCD, the benefits of treating a potentially fatal illness such as psychotic depression outweigh this risk. Use of other SSRI, such as citalopram or escitalopram, in place of sertraline and other atypical antipsychotic, such as aripiprazole, quetiapine, or olanzapine, in place of risperidone may also have been appropriate. The improvement in the MOCA score underscores the fact that depression is often a reversible factor in the treatment of cognitive impairment in people who have MNCD.

Mania with Psychotic Symptoms. Psychotic symptoms are more common in older adults who have mania than in younger adults who have mania. Similar to middle-aged and younger adults, LTC residents who develop mania may have delusions of possessing great wealth, exceptional talents, and supernatural powers. The delusions accompanying mania often include themes of persecution. People who have mania and psychotic symptoms often have more pronounced agitation than people who have mania and no psychotic symptoms. Hallucinations, which occur less commonly than delusions in these patients, are more likely to be auditory than visual or somatic. Mania with psychotic symptoms may be misdiagnosed as delirium due to acute onset, severe inattention, and psychomotor agitation. Usually atypical antipsychotic with or without mood stabilizer is needed to achieve remission of symptoms. The HCP should consider hospitalization and ECT early in the course of treatment.

Schizophrenia

Approximately 13 percent of older persons who have schizophrenia live in NHs. In general, residents who have a diagnosis of schizophrenia are more likely to be younger and nonwhite (especially African American) than other residents. In addition, they have resided in NHs for longer periods (often longer than five years and some 10 years or more). More than half of residents who have schizophrenia receive inadequate mental health services. As the size of the population 65 years or older increases in the coming decades, it is likely that meeting the needs of LTC residents who have schizophrenia will be even more difficult. The diagnosis of schizophrenia is made using *DSM-5* diagnostic criteria (American Psychiatric Association 2013). (See Box 6.5.)

Schizophrenia has not been well studied in LTC populations, but much of the research involving older adults in the community applies to residents who have schizophrenia. There are reasons to be optimistic. In general, with aging, positive symptoms become less severe, comorbid substance use disorder is less common, and mental function improves. Aging is associated with complete remission in social deficit in more than 25 percent of those who have early-onset schizophrenia (onset before age 40 years), while another 40 percent show marked improvement in symptoms, especially positive symptoms. For some people who have schizophrenia, negative symptoms may increase with aging. A small but significant minority may even have remission of positive symptoms and may need only psychosocial therapy (cognitive behavioral therapy with social skills training) (Jeste and Maglione 2013). Hospitalization is usually due to acute physical health problems rather than psychiatric exacerbation.

Schizophrenia usually emerges between the late teens and mid-20s, although approximately 15 percent of individuals who have schizophrenia have onset after age 40 (termed late-onset schizophrenia for onset between 40 and 60 years and very-late-onset schizophrenia for onset after age 60 years). Among people who have late-onset or very-late-onset schizophrenia, there is a higher prevalence of the paranoid subtype; they have less severe negative symptoms; women are over-represented (versus a slight over-representation of men among those who have earlier-onset schizophrenia); and they require lower doses of antipsychotic medication than people who have earlier-onset schizophrenia.

LTC residents who have schizophrenia are usually two decades younger (chronologically) than their peers. Due to accelerated physiological aging and premature morbidity and mortality, residents who have schizophrenia in their 60s or 70s may be comparable medically with residents in their 80s or 90s. Many residents who have schizophrenia have been taking antipsychotic (often typical antipsychotic) for decades and have developed tardive dyskinesia (TD). Tobacco smoking is the most common substance use disorder.

There is remarkable heterogeneity among residents who have schizophrenia in symptom presentation, everyday functioning, response to treatment, and course of illness. Delusions and hallucinations are usually present along with negative symptoms. Some 30–40 percent of residents develop MDD at some point during the stay in LTC (usually in response to a stressor), which is associated with decline in function.

Neurocognitive deficit (especially attention, memory, executive function) is seen in the majority of people who have schizophrenia and typically is due to the neurobiology of schizophrenia and comorbid cerebrovascular disease. Neurocognitive deficit typically persists even when other symptoms are in remission and contributes to the disability of schizophrenia. Reversible etiologies (medication-induced, nutritional deficiency, poorly managed hypertension, diabetes, and dyslipidemia) of cognitive deficit are more common among people who have schizophrenia than among their peers who have cognitive deficit. Thus, identification and correction of reversible factors of cognitive deficit is one of the key approaches to improve the quality of life and functioning of residents who have schizophrenia. Some people who have schizophrenia may have comorbid MNCD (usually due to cerebrovascular disease but also to AD). Schizophreniform disorder is similar to schizophrenia in all features except the duration, which is more than one month but less than six months.

Compared to their peers, residents who have schizophrenia are at higher risk of suicide and violence during exacerbation of psychotic symptoms, but the risk is almost similar to that of their peers when the symptoms are mild and at baseline. If they have comorbid substance use disorder (e.g. cannabis, alcohol), then there is increased risk of suicide and violence during the drug intoxication phase. Comorbid MDD and hopelessness also increase the risk of suicide among residents who have schizophrenia. The risk of suicide is higher in the period after discharge from the hospital, after transfer from home to a facility (especially if unplanned), after transfer from one facility to another (especially if unplanned), and after a psychotic episode. Comprehensive assessment of the risks of suicide and violence and appropriate individualized preventive approaches should be a routine part of the treatment of all residents who have schizophrenia.

Treatment usually involves prescribing a low dose of antipsychotic and psychosocial approaches (e.g. supportive psychotherapy, CBT, social skills training, education of family and staff, SPPEICE [strength-based, personalized, psychosocial sensory spiritual environmental initiatives and creative engagement]). (See Tables 6.5, 6.6, and 6.7.) Atypical antipsychotic is preferred over typical/conventional antipsychotic primarily due to the relatively lower risk of adverse effect. Antipsychotic-related adverse effect (especially Parkinsonism/extrapyramidal syndrome [EPS]) is prevalent in residents who have schizophrenia, even at lower dosages. This is because EPS may occur with D2 receptor occupancies that are lower (35–75 percent) than those required in younger patients (80 percent). The HCP may consider short-term use of a low dose of short-acting benzodiazepine (e.g. lorazepam, oxazepam) for a resident who has schizophrenia and is experiencing severe anxiety, agitation, insomnia, or catatonic symptoms. Many residents who have schizophrenia have comorbid anxiety disorder (e.g. generalized anxiety disorder, panic disorder) and/or trauma-related disorder (e.g. post-traumatic stress disorder [PTSD]) and have been taking benzodiazepine for years before admission to a LTC facility. The HCP should consider gradual taper and discontinuation of benzodiazepine, as this may improve cognitive function and reduce the risk of falls. If anxiety symptoms are disabling and the resident is not motivated for CBT or not able to use CBT due to cognitive deficit, longer-term use of low-dose benzodiazepine to manage disabling anxiety symptoms may be necessary. Combination of antipsychotic and benzodiazepine is a high-risk approach (due to the increased risk of cognitive impairment, falls, and mortality) and hence we recommend involving a psychiatrist with LTC expertise. An antidepressant may need to be added to the antipsychotic to manage MDD and for comorbid anxiety disorder. ECT is a reasonable choice for catatonic symptoms and for severe depressive symptoms associated with suicidal behavior. Many residents who have schizophrenia may have been taking conventional antipsychotic at high dose for decades. These residents may benefit from a gradual (over months) reduction in antipsychotic with close monitoring for emergent tardive dyskinesia (TD). For a resident who has schizophrenia and has been taking conventional antipsychotic for most of his or her life, the HCP should consider switching to atypical antipsychotic if the resident is showing significant EPS (e.g. Parkinsonism, drooling, recurrent falls due to hypokinesia). A resident who is stable taking a low dose of conventional antipsychotic and tolerating the medication well should not be switched to atypical antipsychotic but closely monitored for emergent TD or worsening of pre-existing TD. Many residents who have schizophrenia have mild to moderate TD. The HCP should cautiously consider reducing the dosage of antipsychotic in this population due to the high risk of worsening TD, which in turn may adversely affect the resident's quality of life. A small but significant group of people who have schizophrenia show reduction or clearing of the delusion and hallucination in later life and may remain stable without antipsychotic medication.

Schizoaffective Disorder

In schizoaffective disorder, the criteria for MDD or a manic episode occur at the same time as symptoms

Table 6.5 Evidence-Based Approaches for the Treatment of Psychotic Disorder

Approach	Clinical Pearls	Key Concerns/Limitations
Antipsychotic (atypical antipsychotic and typical/ conventional antipsychotic)	Haloperidol may be first-line agent for behavioral emergency and for management of severe agitation in context of delirium Haloperidol is second-line agent for management of other psychotic disorder	Antipsychotics pose serious risks (see Box 6.6) and hence informed consent is crucial before starting antipsychotic (in behavioral emergency, antipsychotic may be given first and consent obtained once emergency is resolved)
Pimavanserin	Drug of choice for treatment of moderate to severe Parkinson's disease psychosis	Has not been well studied in LTC populations and hence should be used judiciously with close follow-up for adverse effect (e.g. pedal edema, confusion, hallucination, nausea)
Citalopram	Agitation due to psychotic symptoms in resident who has MNCD may decrease with citalopram Carries less risk than antipsychotic	Use is associated with prolonged QTc interval and FDA warning regarding this risk in adults age 60 or older for doses above 20 mg Increased risk of bleeding in resident taking anticoagulant and/or antiplatelet therapy Increased risk of hyponatremia in resident taking diuretic
Cholinesterase inhibitor (ChEI; donepezil, rivastigine, galantamine)	May have a modest effect in preventing emergence and worsening of psychotic symptoms in resident who has MNCD due to AD and Lewy bodies (DLB, PDD)	Not recommended for treatment of severe agitation due to psychotic symptoms in resident who has MNCD, as the role is more preventative
SPPEICE	First-line treatment for mild to moderate psychotic symptoms in context of MNCD	Staff are often not well trained in instituting SPPEICE and often do not have time or energy due to high workload and poor support from LTC facility leadership
Psychoeducation and self-management	Providing pamphlets and other educational material on schizophrenia and other psychotic disorder can reduce stigma the resident experiences	Cognitive deficit in resident may limit its benefit
Cognitive behavioral therapy (CBT) and cognitive training	CBT is useful with resident who has schizophrenia to reduce emotional distress due to psychotic symptoms and stigma Cognitive training is useful with resident who has schizophrenia to improve associated cognitive deficit and disability	Resident needs to be motivated and have relatively preserved cognitive function
Motivational interviewing (MI)	Is useful in motivating resident to engage in healthy lifestyle (e.g. nutrition, exercise, smoking cessation) to reduce metabolic and cardiovascular adverse effects of antipsychotic	Resident needs to be motivated and have relatively preserved cognitive function

Table 6.5 (cont.)

Approach	Clinical Pearls	Key Concerns/Limitations
Neuromodulatory therapy	Electroconvulsive therapy (ECT) for life-threatening psychotic symptoms, catatonic symptoms, and treatment-resistant psychotic symptoms	Lack of availability of professionals providing neurostimulation therapy in the community ECT should be done in an academic center because of potential for adverse event (e.g. post-ECT persistent delirium)
Omega-3 fatty acid supplementation (1000 mg/day)	Eicosapentanoic acid (EPA) and ethyl-EPA dominant formulation recommended	Small risk of increased bleeding, especially with concomitant use of NSAID, anticoagulant, antiplatelet, SSRI, and SNRI
N-acetyl cysteine (NAC) supplementation (500-600 mg twice daily)	May have small beneficial effect for resident who has schizophrenia	May increase pill burden and contribute to nonadherence
Vitamin D supplementation	Checking vitamin D levels is recommended, as vitamin D deficiency is prevalent in residents who have psychotic disorder and may require vitamin D replacement therapy	Hypervitaminosis D, although rare, can occur and manifest as headache and dizziness.
Bright light therapy	May be used with antipsychotic therapy to treat insomnia, agitation, and/or depressive symptoms that often accompany psychotic symptoms	Staff education and training is required for appropriate use of bright light therapy box
Physical activity/Exercise	Exercise and increasing physical activity can accelerate response to antipsychotic and increase likelihood of remission	Lack of time available to staff to help residents increase physical activity is key barrier to routine use
Rational deprescribing (geriatric scalpel) with input from pharmacist	Discontinuation of medication that may contribute to psychotic symptoms, discontinuation of unnecessary or inappropriate medication (based on Beers list), and reducing anticholinergic burden may improve cognitive and emotional function and reduce adverse drug–drug interaction with antipsychotic	None
Optimizing control of pain and other comorbid physical health problems (e.g. hypertension) and correction of reversible physical health problems (e.g. dehydration, constipation, vitamin B12 deficiency, vision and hearing impairment, thyroid disorder)	Recommended for all residents	None

Table 6.6 Evidence-Based Approaches for the Treatment of Schizophrenia and Schizoaffective Disorder

Approach	Clinical Pearls	Key Concerns/Limitations
Mood stabilizer (e.g. divalproex sodium, lamotrigine, lithium, carbamazepine, oxcarbazepine)	Divalproex, lamotrigine, and oxcarbazepine are better tolerated and hence preferred over lithium and carbamazepine Divalproex or oxcarbazepine may need to be added to antipsychotic medication to manage persistent aggressive behavior in resident who has schizophrenia and to manage manic/hypomanic symptoms in resident who has schizoaffective disorder Lamotrigine may need to be added to antipsychotic to manage recurrent MDD in resident who has schizoaffective disorder bipolar type	Use is associated with significant risk of falls and delirium Use of divalproex is associated with increased risk of bleeding with concomitant use of antiplatelet, anticoagulant, and omega-3 fatty acids
Antipsychotic (especially atypical/second-generation antipsychotic)	Atypical/second-generation antipsychotic preferred over typical/conventional/first-generation antipsychotic Response may take several weeks after therapeutic dose is reached	Management by a psychiatrist is recommended if there is need for antipsychotic due to high risk associated with use of antipsychotic medication
Antidepressant	May be considered adjuvant to mood stabilizer and/or antipsychotic for treatment of significant depressive symptoms	May destabilize schizoaffective disorder – bipolar type (especially if used as monotherapy), cause rapid cycling, and switch depression to mania
Onsite individual counseling/psychotherapy (cognitive behavioral therapy [CBT], cognitive behavioral social skills training, functional adaptation skills training)	Psychotherapy is useful to prevent relapse and manage comorbid conditions, such as an anxiety disorder and/or insomnia disorder	Lack of availability of counselors trained in providing psychotherapy to LTC populations Lack of availability of counselors visiting LTC facilities to provide psychotherapy services Resident may need to visit local mental health clinic for such services Resident needs to be motivated and have relatively preserved cognitive function
Internet-guided and telepsychiatry approaches	Cognitive restructuring (to address cognitive distortion), behavioral activation, and problem-solving strategies can be effectively administered via Internet and telepsychiatry by psychiatric nurse or other mental health professional for treatment of psychotic symptoms, depressive symptoms, and/or anxiety symptoms	Resident needs to be motivated and have relatively preserved cognitive function Technophobia (in residents as well as staff) may be a difficult barrier to overcome Should be restricted to mild to moderate cases and used in conjunction with antipsychotic; close supervision is needed to monitor worsening of psychotic symptoms

Table 6.6 (cont.)

Approach	Clinical Pearls	Key Concerns/Limitations
Psychoeducation and self-management	Providing pamphlets and other educational material on schizophrenia can reduce stigma the resident experiences	Cognitive deficit in resident may limit its benefit
Neurostimulation therapy	Electroconvulsive therapy (ECT) for life-threatening schizoaffective disorder and treatment-resistant schizoaffective disorder Transcranial magnetic stimulation (TMS) as adjuvant to psychotropic medication for treatment of treatment-resistant depression in resident who has schizophrenia or schizoaffective disorder	Lack of availability of professionals providing neurostimulation therapy in the community Lack of reimbursement from health insurance for neurostimulation therapy (especially TMS)
Omega-3 fatty acid supplementation	Eicosapentanoic acid (EPA) and ethyl-EPA dominant formulation recommended	Small risk of increased bleeding, especially with concomitant use of NSAID, anticoagulant, antiplatelet, SSRI, or SNRI
Vitamin D supplementation	Checking vitamin D levels is recommended, as vitamin D deficiency is prevalent in residents who have MDD and may require vitamin D replacement therapy	Hypervitaminosis D, although rare, can occur and manifest as headaches and dizziness
N-acetyl cysteine	May have small beneficial effect	May increase pill burden and contribute to nonadherence
Bright light therapy	May be used with psychotropic medication to treat depressive symptoms in resident who has psychotic disorder, especially if there is history of seasonal affective disorder (e.g. winter depression)	Staff education and training is required for appropriate use of bright light therapy box
Exercise	Exercise and increasing physical activity can accelerate response to psychotropic medication and increase likelihood of remission	Lack of time available to staff to help resident increase physical activity is key barrier to its routine use
Rational deprescribing (geriatric scalpel) with input from pharmacist	Discontinuation of medication that can cause/exacerbate psychotic symptoms, discontinuation of unnecessary or inappropriate medication (based on Beers list), and reducing anticholinergic burden may improve resident's cognitive and emotional function and reduce adverse drug–drug interaction with medication used to treat schizophrenia or schizoaffective disorder	None

Table 6.6 (cont.)

Approach	Clinical Pearls	Key Concerns/Limitations
Optimizing control of pain and other comorbid physical health problems (e.g. diabetes) and correction of reversible physical health problems (e.g. dehydration, constipation, vision and hearing impairment, thyroid disorder)	Recommended for all residents	None

Second-generation antipsychotics: aripiprazole, quetiapine, olanzapine, risperidone, lurasidone, ziprasidone, paliperidone, iloperidone, asenapine, cariprazine, brexpiprazole
First-generation antipsychotics: haloperidol, fluphenazine, thioridazine, perphenazine, chlorpromazine, thiothixine

Table 6.7 Common Antipsychotics Used to Treat Psychotic Disorder

Antipsychotic* (Therapeutic Dose Range)	Clinical Pearls	Key Concerns/Limitations**
Haloperidol (0.5-4 mg/day for resident who has MNCD; higher dosage for resident who has schizophrenia or schizoaffective disorder)	Availability of intramuscular and intravenous formulations makes it a drug of choice for management of behavioral emergency and for severe agitation in context of delirium Availability of long-acting depot preparation allows its use with resident who has schizophrenia and responded well to haloperidol but ongoing adherence to taking oral haloperidol is a concern	High risk of EPS and TD Potential to prolong QTc is a concern Baseline EKG recommended
Risperidone (0.25–2 mg/day for resident who has MNCD; higher dosage may be needed for resident who has schizophrenia or schizoaffective disorder)	First-line agent for treatment of severe agitation accompanying psychotic symptoms in resident who has MNCD	Higher risk of EPS and TD than other atypical antipsychotics
Olanzapine (2.5–10 mg/day for resident who has MNCD; higher dosage may be needed for resident who has schizophrenia or schizoaffective disorder)	Second-line agent (after risperidone) for treatment of severe agitation accompanying psychotic symptoms in resident who has MNCD	Higher risk of metabolic problems (e.g. weight gain, dyslipidemia, diabetes) than other atypical antipsychotics Has significant anticholinergic activity May rarely cause drug reaction eosinophilia and systemic symptoms (DRESS)
Quetiapine (12.5–200 mg/day for resident who has MNCD; higher dosage may be needed for resident who has schizophrenia or schizoaffective disorder)	Third-line agent (after risperidone, olanzapine, and aripiprazole) for treatment of severe agitation accompanying psychotic symptoms in resident who has MNCD due to AD Second-line agent (after pimavanserin) for treatment of PDP and first-line agent for treatment of DLB with psychotic symptoms	Metabolite Norquetiapine has significant anticholinergic activity Potential to prolong QTc is a concern. Hence, baseline EKG recommended

Table 6.7 (cont.)

Antipsychotic* (Therapeutic Dose Range)	Clinical Pearls	Key Concerns/Limitations**
Aripiprazole (2–10 mg/day for resident who has MNCD; higher dosage may be needed for resident who has schizophrenia or schizoaffective disorder)	Second-line agent (after risperidone) for treatment of severe agitation accompanying psychotic symptoms in resident who has MNCD Lower risk of metabolic adverse effect than risperidone, olanzapine, and quetiapine	May cause akathisia and insomnia May cause problem with impulse control (e.g. sexually inappropriate behavior, gambling behavior)
Ziprasidone (20–80 mg/day on full stomach for resident who has MNCD; up to 160 mg/day in two divided doses may be needed for resident who has schizophrenia or schizoaffective disorder)	Fourth-line agent for treatment of severe agitation accompanying psychotic symptoms in resident who has MNCD due to AD Second-line agent (after quetiapine) for treatment of DLB with psychotic symptoms and fourth-line agent (after pimavanserin, clozapine, and quetiapine) for PDP Lower risk of metabolic adverse effect than risperidone, olanzapine, and quetiapine	Not well studied in LTC populations and individuals who have MNCD Potential to prolong QTc is a concern. Hence, baseline EKG recommended May rarely cause DRESS
Clozapine (6.25–50 mg/day for resident who has PDP; higher dosage may be needed for resident who has schizophrenia or schizoaffective disorder)	Drug of third choice (after pimavanserin and quetiapine) for treatment of PDP First-line agent for treatment-refractory schizophrenia	Risk of leukopenia and burden of weekly blood draw on resident limit its use Has significant anticholinergic activity
Paliperidone (3–6 mg/day for resident who has MNCD; higher dosage may be needed for resident who has schizophrenia or schizoaffective disorder)	Long-acting once-a-month and once-every-3-month formulations are available for use with resident who has schizophrenia or schizoaffective disorder	Not well studied in LTC populations and individuals who have MNCD Risks similar to those of risperidone
Iloperidone (1–9 mg/day once a day or in two divided doses for resident who has MNCD; higher dosage may be needed for resident who has schizophrenia or schizoaffective disorder)	Potent alpha 1-blocking properties indicate potential use in treatment of nightmares for resident who has PTSD	Not well studied in LTC populations and individuals who have MNCD Risks similar to those of risperidone May cause leukopenia Should be avoided in resident who has significant cardiovascular illness due to risk of orthostasis (due to alpha 1-blocking effect)
Lurasidone (20-60 mg/day on full stomach for resident who has MNCD; higher dosage may be needed for resident who has schizophrenia or schizoaffective disorder)	First-line agent for psychotic symptoms in context of bipolar depression	Not well studied in LTC populations and individuals who have MNCD
Asenapine (2.5-5 mg/day for resident who has MNCD; higher dosage may be needed for resident who has schizophrenia or schizoaffective disorder)	Available only as orally dissolvable formulation	Not well studied in LTC populations and individuals who have MNCD

Table 6.7 (cont.)

Antipsychotic* (Therapeutic Dose Range)	Clinical Pearls	Key Concerns/Limitations**
Brexpiprazole (0.25–2 mg/day for resident who has MNCD; higher dosage may be needed for resident who has schizophrenia or schizoaffective disorder)	May be used as adjunct therapy for treatment-resistant depression	Not well studied in LTC populations and individuals who have MNCD
Cariprazine (1.5–3 mg/day for resident who has MNCD; higher dosage may be needed for resident who has schizophrenia or schizoaffective disorder)	Long half-life may make it preferable in resident taking medication erratically	Not well studied in LTC populations and individuals who have MNCD
Fluphenazine (2.5-5 mg/day for resident who has MNCD; higher dosage may be needed for resident who has schizophrenia or schizoaffective disorder)	Availability of long-acting depot preparation allows its use for resident who has schizophrenia and responded well to oral fluphenazine but ongoing adherence to taking oral fluphenazine is a concern	High risk of EPS and TD
Perphenazine (2–8 mg/day for resident who has MNCD; higher dosage may be needed for resident who has schizophrenia or schizoaffective disorder)	If resident who has schizophrenia or schizoaffective disorder is already taking this medicine, doing well, and tolerating it well, it may be continued with close monitoring for adverse effect	High risk of EPS and TD (lower than that of haloperidol)
Thiothixine (2–5 mg/day for resident who has MNCD; higher dosage may be needed for resident who has schizophrenia or schizoaffective disorder)	If resident who has schizophrenia or schizoaffective disorder is already taking this medicine, doing well, and tolerating it well, it may be continued with close monitoring for adverse effect	High risk of EPS and TD (lower than that of haloperidol)
Thioridazine (10–25 mg/day for resident who has MNCD; higher dosage is usually needed for resident who has schizophrenia or schizoaffective disorder)	If resident who has schizophrenia or schizoaffective disorder is already taking this medicine, doing well, and tolerating it well, it may be continued with close monitoring for adverse effect	High risk of adverse effect (orthostasis, daytime sedation, worsening cognition due to anticholinergic activity) severely limits its use
Chlorpromazine (10–25 mg/day for resident who has MNCD; higher dosage is usually needed for resident who has schizophrenia or schizoaffective disorder)	May be considered for refractory cases of schizophrenia and schizoaffective disorder Also used to treat refractory nausea and vomiting Intramuscular formulation available for management of behavioral emergency	High risk of adverse effect (orthostasis, daytime sedation, worsening cognition due to anticholinergic activity) severely limits its use

* Atypical antipsychotics usually preferred over typical/conventional antipsychotics because of better risk/benefit ratio

Atypical antipsychotics: risperidone, olanzapine, quetiapine, aripiprazole, ziprasidone, paliperidone, iloperidone, asenapine, lurasidone, brexpiprazole, cariprazine

Conventional/typical antipsychotics: haloperidol, fluphenazine, perphenazine, thiothixine, thioridazine, chlorpromazine

** All antipsychotics carry risks listed in Box 6.6.

that meet the diagnosis of an active phase of schizophrenia. In addition, psychotic symptoms must be present for at least two weeks in the absence of prominent mood symptoms. Treatment is similar to that of schizophrenia, although people who have significant manic symptoms may need a combination of antipsychotic and valproate. Symptoms of MDD may need antidepressant and/or lamotrigine added to antipsychotic. (See Tables 6.6. and 6.7.)

Clinical Case 2: "I am a worrier"

Ms. S was a 69-year-old, single woman living in a NH for the past two years due to sequelae of severe arthritis, obesity, congestive heart failure, chronic kidney disease, chronic pain, diabetes requiring insulin, poor mobility, and osteoporosis. She had a long history of schizoaffective disorder with multiple hospitalizations for serious suicide attempts, severe psychotic symptoms (paranoid delusions and auditory hallucinations), and severe depressive symptoms, but was stable for the last 7 years on a medication regimen that included olanzapine 10 mg at bedtime, mirtazapine 30 mg at bedtime, and lorazepam 0.25 mg four times daily. The psychiatrist was consulted for management of increased agitation (yelling out instead of using the call light, calling her roommate "the devil"), paranoia (accusing staff of stealing her clothes), and insomnia. Ms. S had relatively intact cognitive function (MOCA 28) and was able to give a detailed history of her psychiatric illness. She reported that the current medication regimen helped her more than all other medications she had tried since her 20s, and she had avoided hospitalization for the last seven years. Ms. S denied any history suggestive of hypomania or mania. She reported a lifelong history of excessive anxiety and added, "I am a worrier." The psychiatrist also noted that Ms. S had a history of recurrent UTI and was put on antibiotics two days before consultation for another UTI.

On mental status exam, Ms. S was found to be anxious and eager to please. She denied any suicidal or homicidal ideas or any current auditory or visual hallucination. She acknowledged that she had called her roommate "the devil" but reported that she was angry with the roommate because the roommate would keep her TV on until late in the night and Ms. S liked to go to sleep by 8 p.m. Staff acknowledged to the psychiatrist that this was an ongoing conflict between Ms. S and her roommate. Ms. S denied feeling that the staff were taking her belongings but felt that certain staff were "not nice" to her. The psychiatrist made a provisional diagnosis of schizoaffective disorder-depressed type and generalized anxiety disorder and felt that Ms. S's psychotic symptoms were controlled and hence did not recommend any change in antipsychotic dosage. The psychiatrist also recommended that the NH social worker address the conflicts between Ms. S and her roommate. The psychiatrist also requested records from previous psychiatrists. The psychiatrist recommended adding as-needed lorazepam 0.25 mg two times daily for anxiety in addition to scheduled lorazepam and to see if treatment of the UTI would also improve the agitation and paranoia. The social worker, over three meetings with Ms. S and her roommate, brokered an agreement that Ms. S's roommate could watch TV in their room until 9 p.m. and then go to a family room that had a TV if she wanted to continue watching TV.

After four weeks, staff reported that Ms. S's agitation was much better. She also reported feeling less anxious and irritable. Ms. S was given as-needed lorazepam once almost daily in addition to her scheduled dose for the first week but after that staff were able to manage Ms. S's anxiety without as-needed lorazepam. The psychiatrist considered switching olanzapine to another atypical antipsychotic with lower risk of metabolic complication (e.g. weight gain, hyperglycemia, risk of hyperlipidemia), such as aripiprazole or ziprasidone, and discussed this with Ms. S. Psychiatric records indicated that Ms. S had tried taking risperidone, quetiapine, haloperidol, thiothixene, sertraline, fluoxetine, and venlafaxine without adequate response. Records also confirmed the history obtained from Ms. S that she had several serious suicide attempts (primarily by overdose) in the past requiring repeated hospitalization and severe psychotic symptoms that had incapacitated her for several years. Ms. S was nervous about any change in medication and expressed awareness of metabolic risks with olanzapine and mirtazapine. The psychiatrist agreed with Ms. S that the risks of switching (destabilizing the psychiatric illness, relapse of severe depressive and psychotic symptoms, need for hospitalization, and suicide) outweighed the benefits (lower risk of weight gain, better control of diabetes and hyperlipidemia, improved mobility).

Teaching Points

Residents who have severe persistent mental illness, such as schizoaffective disorder, are as likely as those who do not have such illness to become agitated due to medical issues and/or environmental causes. The HCP should consider these factors before assuming that exacerbation of the underlying psychiatric illness is the cause of increased psychiatric symptoms. If a resident has been stable on a psychiatric drug regimen, it is advisable to avoid any major change in psychiatric drug regimen because obtaining a similar good therapeutic response from a different drug regimen is not predictable or assured. The HCP should decide to switch antipsychotic or antidepressant only after a thorough review of the patient's history and perspectives (and those of involved family) about changes and review of previous records. Although drugs like olanzapine and mirtazapine carry substantial metabolic risk (especially for people who are obese and have diabetes), for some people (such as Ms. S) the risk may not outweigh the benefit of stabilization of a serious psychiatric illness.

Delusional Disorder

Delusional disorder is characterized by the presence of nonbizarre and circumscribed delusions involving situations that could occur in real life (e.g. being monitored and targeted, being followed, being plotted against, having cancer, being poisoned or infected, spousal infidelity, being loved by another person [typically a prominent person]). The delusions are usually not associated with significant or prominent hallucination. Typically, there is lack of insight along with relatively good overall psychosocial functioning (as compared to schizophrenia). The duration of psychotic symptoms is typically months to years (even decades) but for diagnosis needs to be at least one month with some associated impairment in function. A resident who has delusional disorder may become aggressive toward the supposed persecutor; some residents may lock themselves in their rooms and live an isolated, reclusive life. The HCP may consider antipsychotic and supportive psychotherapy for a resident who has this disorder and develops significant agitation due to delusional thinking, although delusional disorder does not respond as well to antipsychotic as many other psychotic disorders. Also, individuals who have delusional disorder typically decline antipsychotic. Comorbid MDD is prevalent in this population, and the resident may be amenable to a trial of an antidepressant. Long-term individual supportive and problem-solving therapy has been found to be beneficial, and the HCP should offer it to a willing resident who has relatively preserved cognitive function.

Brief Psychotic Disorder

Brief psychotic disorder is characterized by a sudden onset of at least one of the following: delusion, hallucination, disorganized speech, grossly disorganized or catatonic behavior. It is usually (but not necessarily) in response to a stressor, lasts more than a day, and remits within a month. It is twice as common in females as in males. Treatment may involve short-term use of a low dose of atypical antipsychotic and/or a low dose of short-acting benzodiazepine to manage severe anxiety and insomnia and psychosocial approaches (e.g. supportive psychotherapy, family and staff education). Eventual full return to the premorbid social and interpersonal level of functioning occurs when the stressors subside and with the restoration of coping skills.

Hallucination during Bereavement

Hallucination during bereavement can occur in people who have intact cognition and typically is visual in nature; however, both auditory and tactile hallucinations have been described in people who recently lost a spouse. The grieving spouse/partner may report seeing, speaking to, or even touching the deceased spouse/partner. The majority of these experiences occur at night. The grieving individual usually acknowledges that the spouse looks different or "ghost like." Additionally, the individual does not believe the deceased spouse is truly present. In most cases, the individual describes the hallucinatory event as a positive experience. Treatment involves psychosocial approaches (e.g. emotional support, reassurance, and family and staff education).

Secondary Psychotic Disorder

Most residents who have psychotic symptoms have secondary psychotic disorder. Visual hallucinations in the absence of auditory hallucinations are usually suggestive of delirium and MNCD-related psychotic symptoms rather than schizophrenia. Psychotic symptoms due to an acute general medical or neurological condition typically occur in the context of delirium, although sometimes psychotic symptoms may be the only manifestation of a general medical condition. Failure to identify secondary psychotic disorder may result in inappropriate administration of antipsychotic, which may further obscure underlying medical conditions causing the psychotic symptom. Certain secondary psychotic disorders (e.g. delirium, psychosis due to a general medical condition), if not recognized and treated promptly, can be fatal.

Although the treatment of primary psychotic disorder usually requires atypical antipsychotic, secondary psychotic disorder can often be managed with psychosocial and environmental approaches and treatment of the underlying medical condition (e.g. UTI) or removal of offending medication. Use of atypical antipsychotic to manage psychotic symptoms due to secondary psychotic disorder is associated with even higher risk of adverse effect than for primary psychotic disorder, and thus the HCP should undertake it cautiously, preferably with input from a psychiatrist who has expertise in LTC psychiatry. Residents who have secondary psychotic disorder are at higher risk for serious adverse effect, such as EPS or TD, with conventional antipsychotic than those who have primary psychotic disorder. Many secondary psychotic disorders are iatrogenic (i.e. caused by a failure to make the correct diagnosis or by administration of inappropriate medication, such as anticholinergic, especially to a resident who has MNCD). Appropriate therapeutic choices may decrease the incidence of psychotic symptoms in LTC populations.

Major Neurocognitive Disorder with Psychotic Symptoms

Psychotic symptoms are among the most distressing and disabling complications of MNCD. The presence of visual hallucinations, more concrete or perseverative thought processes, gradual cognitive impairment before the onset of psychotic symptoms, and absence of long psychiatric history suggest psychotic disorder due to one of the MNCDs. Agitation and aggression (verbal and physical) frequently co-occur with psychotic symptoms in residents who have MNCD. Psychosis is often a trigger for agitation and aggressivity, which in turn may be in response to frightening visual hallucination. Depressive symptoms also frequently co-occur with delusion in residents who have MNCD. With increasing cognitive impairment, the complexity of delusion is reduced. Many people who have MNCD experience visual agnosia, in which they do not recognize a person or believe that they are someone else (e.g. spouse is identified as father, daughter is identified as sister).

Psychotic symptoms are common in residents who have AD, especially in moderate and severe stages. More than 50 percent of people who have AD have some form of psychosis at some point during the course of the illness. Delusions are much more common (20–30 percent-point prevalence) than hallucinations (5–7 percent point prevalence). The most common delusion in a resident who has AD is of people stealing, breaking in, or having intentions to persecute the resident or of food being poisoned. Often the delusional ideas in AD have an ad hoc quality: a purse is misplaced, and the delusion arises that someone is stealing personal items. Delusions, consisting largely of misconception or misidentification (e.g. of persons, objects, places, events), are common. Mistaken suspicion of marital infidelity, a belief that other residents or caregivers are trying to hurt the resident, and a belief that characters on television are real are also common delusions in residents who have AD. Anosognosia and depression often accompany delusions in AD. Elevated mood often accompanies grandiose delusions in AD.

Hallucinations are also found in residents who have AD. Visual hallucinations are the most common, followed by auditory hallucinations. Typical visual hallucinations include persons from the past (e.g. deceased parents), intruders, animals, complex scenes, or inanimate objects. Most auditory hallucinations tend to be benign (hearing a dead spouse or other relative) rather than persecutory, although the latter also occur. The resident who has advanced AD may not be able to verbalize the hallucination but may show hallucinatory behavior (reaching out to touch or grab imaginary people, objects, or bugs; carrying out conversations with imaginary people). Most residents who have hallucination associated with AD also have delusion.

Up to a third of residents in the advanced stages of AD have mild EPS (Parkinsonism, bradyphrenia). Residents who have AD and EPS have twice the frequency of psychosis of residents who have AD but not EPS. Residents who have AD and have a sibling who has AD and psychosis may be twice as likely to develop psychotic symptoms.

More than 50 percent of people who have DLB have delusions. The types of delusion are similar to those of residents who have AD. Delusions of misidentification (Capgras syndrome) may be seen in residents who have DLB. This syndrome is characterized by a belief that another person, usually closely related to the resident, has been replaced by an exact replica or double who impersonates the original person but is an imposter (e.g. a wife or husband would say, "He/she is not my spouse, although he/she looks like my spouse"). The presence of Capgras syndrome with visual hallucination may indicate DLB rather than AD. Vivid recurrent visual hallucinations are characteristic features of DLB and are seen in more than 80 percent of individuals who have DLB. Visual hallucinations occur early in the course of DLB, whereas they occur in moderate to severe stages of AD.

Vascular MNCD may be associated with paranoid psychotic features, with a prevalence ranging from 9 to 40 percent. Complex delusions are more likely in VaD than in AD. Psychotic symptoms are rare in FTD (Landquist et al. 2014). This may be due to limited temporal-limbic involvement in this disorder. When psychotic symptoms are present in FTD, they usually take the form of delusion. Paranoid, bizarre, and grandiose delusions may occur in people who have FTD. FTD with Parkinsonism linked to chromosome 17 (FTDP-17) is a rare familial form of FTD. Its presentation is much like other types of FTD but often includes psychiatric symptoms such as delusions and hallucinations.

Visual hallucinations in a resident who has MNCD may indicate a co-occurring delirium. Psychotic symptoms associated with MNCD wax and wane and are less persistent than those seen in residents who have schizophrenia. A significant number of residents who have MNCD develop transient psychotic symptoms that may remit spontaneously over time or with cholinesterase inhibitor (ChEI) therapy.

Treatment of psychotic symptoms in a resident who has MNCD includes a careful evaluation and treatment of general medical (e.g. UTI, an offending medication), environmental, or psychosocial problems that may be precipitating or causing psychotic symptoms. (See Tables 6.5 and 6.7.) If symptoms persist and are distressing, the HCP should institute strength-based SPPEICE (including removal of environmental triggers). If the resident poses an imminent danger to self or others, we recommend hospitalization to an acute inpatient psychiatric unit (preferably a geriatric psychiatry unit). ChEIs have been found to reduce the emergence of psychotic symptoms and may even reduce mild psychotic symptoms (especially hallucinations) in an individual who has AD, DLB, or MNCD due to Parkinson's disease (Parkinson's disease dementia [PDD]). The effect is modest and variable, and ChEIs do not help acute psychotic symptoms. They may be considered part of comprehensive prevention and treatment approaches for mild to moderate psychotic symptoms in a resident who has DLB, AD, or PDD. Antidepressants (e.g. citalopram) are also a good first-line psychotropic treatment option for reducing agitation and distress due to mild to moderate psychotic symptoms in a resident who has AD, even if depressive symptoms are absent (American Geriatrics Society 2011). For a resident who has MNCD, the HCP may consider judicious use of antipsychotic to treat psychotic symptoms that cause severe emotional distress and are not responding to psychosocial-environmental approaches, psychotic symptoms that cause severe agitation, and psychotic symptoms that pose a high safety risk for the resident and/or others (American Psychiatric Association 2016).

Deciding which antipsychotic to use is based on the relationship between the adverse effect profile of the various agents and the characteristics of the individual resident. Atypical antipsychotics are usually preferred over conventional antipsychotics for a resident who has MNCD because of the better overall adverse risk effect profile. Haloperidol, although usually a second-line agent, is an appropriate first choice for the management of behavioral emergency or severe agitation in the context of delirium. One of the suggestive features for a diagnosis of DLB is sensitivity to antipsychotic medications, both conventional and atypical. There have been case reports of a syndrome characterized by sedation, immobility, rigidity, postural instability, falls, and increased confusion due to antidopaminergic properties of antipsychotics. Hence, high-potency antipsychotics (haloperidol, risperidone, paliperidone) are relatively contraindicated for a resident who has DLB. If antipsychotic medication is needed for a resident who has DLB, quetiapine or aripiprazole is usually the drug of first choice. Any antipsychotic should be started at low dosage, preferably given at night, and the lowest possible effective dose should be used. The goal is not resolution of psychotic symptoms but reduction of the resident's distress and agitation and reduction in behavior that is dangerous to self and/or other. Family and staff often ask for an increase in the dosage of antipsychotic due to only modest improvement in agitation and aggressive

BOX 6.6 Potential Benefits and Risks of Antipsychotic Medication for the Treatment of Severe Psychotic Symptoms and/or Severe Agitation in Resident Who Has Major Neurocognitive Disorder

Potential benefits

- Prevent serious injury to self (e.g. fall and hip fracture due to severe agitation)
- Prevent serious injury to others (e.g. pushing another frail resident, who falls and sustains hip fracture or head injury)
- Prevent hospitalization
- Prevent suicide or mortality due to other self-harmful behavior (e.g. going out of facility in very cold weather in response to psychotic symptoms, refusal of life-sustaining medication, refusal to eat)
- Prevent fatal injury to others
- Decrease emotional distress and thus improve quality of life
- Staff better able to meet resident's basic needs (bathing, personal hygiene) after reduction in agitation and aggression caused by psychotic symptoms
- Decrease caregiver (family and professional) stress and burden

Potential risks

- Death due to heart-related events and infection, particularly pneumonia (2% increased risk versus placebo)
- Cerebrovascular adverse event (e.g. stroke) (2% increased risk versus placebo)
- Dysphagia
- Hospitalization
- Falls and serious injury (e.g. hip or vertebral fracture, skin tear, head injury)
- Neuroleptic malignant syndrome (rare)
- Tardive dyskinesia (especially with high-potency antipsychotic [e.g. haloperidol, fluphenazine, risperidone, paliperidone])
- Daytime sedation (and its risks, such as aspiration pneumonia)
- Accelerated cognitive and/or functional decline
- Akathisia
- Parkinsonian symptoms (e.g. tremors, muscle rigidity, hypokinesia, shuffling gait)
- Postural hypotension
- Prolonged QTc interval and ventricular arrhythmias
- Apathy

behavior. The HCP needs to educate family and staff that the benefits are modest and the risks dramatically increase at higher doses. It is better to be satisfied with modest benefit and redouble efforts to deliver SPPEICE for further reduction in agitation. It is essential that the HCP weigh the potential benefits and risks of antipsychotic with the resident and family. Risks for serious adverse effect due to antipsychotic are high in LTC populations in general and even higher in a resident who has MNCD. (See Box 6.6.) Treatment emergent sedation is associated with all antipsychotics. To minimize the risk of daytime sedation and falls, the HCP should discourage concomitant use of benzodiazepine with antipsychotic or limit it to short periods with careful observation. For a stable resident who has psychotic symptoms and MNCD, it is prudent to attempt to taper and discontinue the antipsychotic after 2-6 months of therapy. We urge the HCP to follow the American Psychiatric Association guidelines for the use of antipsychotics to manage agitation and psychotic symptoms in an individual who has MNCD (American Psychiatric Association 2016).

For a resident who has a problem with compliance or swallowing pills, the HCP may consider prescribing liquid preparations (e.g. liquid risperidone) or orally dissolvable preparations (available for risperidone, olanzapine, aripiprazole, asenapine) of atypical antipsychotic. Most atypical antipsychotics can be given as once-a-day dosing, preferably at night. The HCP may consider using behavioral observation scales, such as the Cohen-Mansfield Agitation Inventory (CMAI) or Neuro-Psychiatric Inventory–Nursing Home version (NPI-NH), to monitor response to treatment. We recommend periodic monitoring for the development of TD due to use of antipsychotic using the Abnormal Involuntary Movement Scale (AIMS).

Clinical Case 3: "Those children are cute"

Ms. L was an 84-year-old widowed woman who had MNCD due to probable AD and was admitted to an AL home because of increasing problems with agitation, incontinence, lack of self-care, and wandering. She had been in the AL home for more than six months. Family had noticed that even when Ms. L had been living in her home, she talked about children coming into her house and bringing cats and dogs. Over the last four months, Ms. L was having periods of agitation and anxiety over "little children" going through her belongings. She was also complaining of being upset with the AL staff because they would allow cats and dogs to roam freely into her room. Ms. L was referred to the psychiatrist for the management of hallucinations. On evaluation, she was not taking any medication that could have caused hallucination, nor was she having any physical aggression or depressive symptoms. Ms. L was taking memantine 10 mg twice daily and donepezil 10 mg daily besides medications for hypertension (hydrochlorothiazide and atenolol) and hyperlipidemia (simvastatin). She did not complain of any new physical health problems, and family and staff reported that the episodes of agitation and hallucination occurred once or twice a week. Staff reported that Ms. L participated in activities, slept well, and had a good appetite. When the psychiatrist inquired how staff and family dealt with Ms. L's complaints, they reported that they would try to convince Ms. L that she was imagining things and that there were no children or animals coming to her room. Staff and family said that often this would agitate Ms. L even more. The psychiatrist inquired about Ms. L's personality before the MNCD, and family reported that she had always been active and liked to be busy and "on the go." During the interview, Ms. L denied having any problems, denied being in physical pain, reported feeling "fine," said "yes" to feeling bored and lonely, but reported good sleep and appetite. She stated that "those children are cute" and did not seem bothered by their presence in her room. Her mental status exam showed significant short-term memory loss (recall was 0/3), and MOCA score was 12. The psychiatrist explained to the family and staff that visual hallucinations were a symptom of MNCD and that currently symptoms were best managed with SPPEICE and a small increase in donepezil to 15 mg daily. The psychiatrist recommended to family and staff not to correct or argue with Ms. L, but to try to reassure and then distract her. The psychiatrist together with family and staff devised a daily activity schedule that would involve more activities that staff and family could engage Ms. L in (e.g. reminiscing with old photos, listening to preferred music, reading the Bible to Ms. L) and a short nap in the afternoon. Ms. L continued to have transient visual hallucinations but her agitation during those periods gradually decreased and the staff became more adept at distracting Ms. L after reassuring her that they would "take care" of the problem promptly.

Teaching Points

Many residents who have MNCD (especially AD or DLB) often develop visual hallucination and agitation but can be safely and effectively managed by family and staff education, SPPEICE, and optimization of ChEI therapy. Antipsychotic may carry more risk than benefit in such situations because the severity of psychotic symptoms is not high and physical aggression is absent. Ms. L could be having psychotic symptoms due to AD or a combination of AD with some Lewy body pathology.

Clinical Case 4: "Those terrible men have left"

Mrs. S was a 78-year-old woman who had DLB and was living in an AL home. Over several months, she had been expressing concerns that men were in her "home" telling her to do inappropriate acts, like take down her pants. Mrs. S would start yelling at 3 p.m. that she can see "the man" on the trees looking into her room. She was not sleeping well and she used foul language toward staff during personal care. In the last four weeks Mrs. S had become physically aggressive toward staff (hitting, slapping, kicking, and biting them). SPPEICE had initially been successful but in the last four weeks her behavior was not manageable. She was referred to the consulting psychiatrist for management of aggression. On examination, the psychiatrist found that Mrs. S had mild muscle stiffness, restricted affect, and persecutory delusions. Medication review did not identify any medication as potential etiology. She was taking rivastigmine 3 mg twice daily with meals. She had a history of not tolerating a higher dose of rivastigmine and could not tolerate memantine. Laboratory tests were within normal limits and urine analysis was negative for infection. Staff and family were counseled regarding improving SPPEICE to reduce Mrs. S's agitation. For example, one staff member would engage Mrs. S from 2 p.m. onward in a coloring activity and another staff member would close her curtains so that when Mrs. S would go to her room, she would not be seeing trees outside her window. Also, only female staff were allowed to provide personal care. Family was explained the risk of stroke and premature death associated with the use of atypical antipsychotic but also the risk of not giving an antipsychotic (see Box 6.6). Family agreed to a trial of low-dose quetiapine. Mrs. S was started on quetiapine 12.5 mg in a.m. and at bedtime daily. She developed daytime sedation and hence her quetiapine was shifted to 25 mg daily at bedtime. After one week, her sleep had improved but the agitation and aggression persisted and hence the quetiapine was increased to 37.5 mg daily at bedtime and after four days to 50 mg daily at bedtime. She had mild daytime sedation, but it resolved over five days. Over the next two weeks, her agitation and aggression improved significantly, she allowed most ADL care, and stated, "I am so glad those terrible men have left" and felt relieved. She still expressed periodic concern that the men were coming and going through her suitcases and her drawers, but could be reassured and distracted most of the time. After three months, the quetiapine was tapered and then discontinued over four weeks. Mrs. S did not show any worsening of symptoms.

Teaching Points

For many residents who have MNCD with severe psychotic symptoms associated with physical aggression and/or severe agitation, SPPEICE may not adequately reduce emotional distress and an atypical antipsychotic may be necessary to substantially reduce agitation and aggression. Low doses for a short period (in this case, three months) often provide modest but clinically meaningful benefit. Close monitoring for adverse effect, such as daytime sedation or falls, is vital. The HCP should consider discontinuing the prescribed antipsychotic drug for the resident whose symptoms are stable.

Parkinson's Disease Psychosis

Parkinson's disease (PD) is a common neurodegenerative disease, affecting up to 1 percent of older adults. The population with PD in LTC is growing, primarily because individuals who have PD are living longer and due to aging of the population (Hoegh et al. 2013). The diagnosis of Parkinson's disease psychosis (PDP) is usually made when a resident who has PD has been experiencing psychotic symptoms continuously or recurrently for at least one month (Friedman 2013). PDP is primarily due to underlying pathophysiology of PD with overmedication or an idiosyncratic reaction to dopaminergic medication used to treat PD contributing to PDP. PDP is also directly associated with duration of PD, increasing severity of executive function impairment, global cognitive impairment, poor visual acuity, depression, anxiety, and older age. NMDA antagonists (e.g. memantine, dextromethorphan, methadone, ketamine) may also precipitate psychosis in a resident who has PD. PDP often precipitates or is the primary driver of institutionalization of individuals who have PD living at home. Evaluating for PDP should be a routine part of follow-up, as only 10–20 percent of individuals who have PDP spontaneously report psychotic symptoms. The HCP can use the section of hallucinations and psychosis in the Movement Disorder Society–Unified Parkinson's Disease Rating Scale (MDS-UPDRS) to document the presence and severity (absent, slight, mild, moderate, severe) of psychotic symptoms and track response to treatment (Goetz et al. 2008). Hallucinations are seen in up to 55 percent and delusions in 30 percent of residents who have PDD. The prevalence is much less in residents who do not have MNCD. Hallucinations are seen in only 18 percent of residents who have PD and no MNCD, followed by hallucinations plus delusions (4 percent), followed by delusions only (2 percent). The onset of psychotic symptoms in a resident who has PD often heralds the onset of MNCD or developing delirium. Persistent PDP is associated with greater functional impairment, caregiver burden, and death. Psychotic symptoms can be more disabling than motor symptoms.

Visual hallucinations are mostly complex (vivid scenes involving people and animals); preserved or disturbed insight relative to the nature of hallucinations is a major prognostic factor, although eventually all hallucinations will present with reduced insight. Initially, hallucinations are usually friendly (i.e.

"benign hallucinosis"). Residents often see vivid, colorful, and sometimes fragmented figures of beloved (deceased) persons and/or family animals. They talk to them and try to caress them or prepare drinks or food for them, only later displaying insight into their unreality. Visual hallucinations are often preceded by sleep disturbance, mild change in visual perception (e.g. sensation of a presence or a sideways passage of a person), or visual illusions. In time, however, reality testing further decreases and the content of the hallucinations may change. Frightening insects, rats, and serpents may predominate, accompanied by considerable anxiety and fear. Delusions of persecution and theft, television characters in the room, and spousal infidelity may accompany visual hallucinations. More than 50 percent of people who have PDP have comorbid significant depressive symptoms and/or restless legs syndrome. Rarely, PDP may present as part of a manic episode. Psychotic symptoms are rare in people who have untreated PD. Psychotic symptoms occurring early in the course of PD suggest a diagnosis of DLB or a coexisting primary psychotic disorder that, before the onset of PD, was not recognized and has been unmasked by dopaminergic therapy.

Treatment initially involves thorough evaluation and treatment of various potential etiological factors, such as general medical condition (e.g. dehydration, infection) and environmental and psychosocial problems. If psychotic symptoms are mild and not bothersome to the resident, reassurance and education of the resident and caregiver (family and professional) is sufficient. Severe symptoms and safety concerns (e.g. risk of suicide, violence, falls due to severe agitation, severe skin excoriation due to attempts to remove imaginary bugs from the skin) are best managed by transferring the resident to the local ER for evaluation and hospitalization. If psychotic symptoms are moderate to severe and accompanied by insomnia and agitation, pharmacologic therapy is necessary. Pharmacologic therapy involves reduction of anti-PD drugs and/or symptomatic treatment for PDP with psychotropic drugs. Involvement of a neurologist (preferably a movement disorder specialist) is crucial at this point, as a decrease in PD medication often worsens motor function. The goal of treatment of PDP is not resolution of symptoms but sufficient reduction in the severity of psychotic symptoms that the resident does not seem bothered (or only mild distress) and has begun to resume participation in daily activities and interests. If the resident is taking multiple dopaminergic drugs, the HCP should first discontinue the drug with the greatest psychosis-inducing potential and the least anti-Parkinsonian activity. Anti-PD drugs should be eliminated in the following order: first, adjunctive drugs (anticholinergics, amantadine, selegiline); second, dopamine agonists (pramipexole, ropinirole, rotigotine); and, finally, levodopa/carbidopa. Anti-PD drugs should be reduced to a point at which psychotic symptoms are reduced without a drastic worsening of motor symptoms. A reduction or discontinuation of medication taken in the evening and at bedtime may alleviate agitation in the evening, nocturnal hallucination, and insomnia. Dopamine agonists (e.g. ropinirole, pramipexole, rotigotine) have a much greater propensity to cause mental confusion, disorientation, and hallucination than does levodopa, especially for people who have MNCD. So in residents who have PD and have developed MNCD, to prevent the emergence of psychotic symptoms, the HCP should avoid using dopamine agonists as much as possible and use levodopa (with or without entacapone) and/or rasagiline to treat motor symptoms.

If moderate to severe psychotic symptoms do not improve with reduction in anti-PD drugs, or if such a reduction worsens motor symptoms significantly, symptomatic treatment with psychotropic medication is usually needed. Pimavanserin is the only FDA-approved medication for the treatment of PDP. Pimavanserin is not an antipsychotic, and it works on the serotonergic system, although the exact mechanism of action is unknown. The therapeutic dose is 34 mg daily (two 17-mg tablets). Although it can be started at this dose, we recommend starting at 17 mg once daily for seven days and, if the resident tolerates this dose well, increasing it to 34 mg daily. This is because pimavanserin has not been studied in LTC populations and LTC residents who have PD may be more prone to adverse effect due to higher frailty and comorbidity than community-dwelling individuals who have PD. If pimavanserin is not tolerated, not effective, or not available, the HCP should consider prescribing an antipsychotic with the least likelihood for exacerbating Parkinsonian symptoms, such as quetiapine, ziprasidone, or clozapine. Clozapine, quetiapine, and ziprasidone, at lower dosages, do not appear to worsen motor symptoms, although even at low dosages these agents may cause excessive daytime sedation and orthostatic hypotension. Conventional antipsychotics (e.g. haloperidol) and high-potency atypical antipsychotics (risperidone, paliperidone) are contraindicated due to the high risk of worsening Parkinsonian symptoms and increased mortality associated with their use by individuals who have PD. Olanzapine and aripiprazole have not been found to be beneficial. Newer antipsychotics, such as lurasidone, iloperidone, asenapine, brexpiprazole, and cariprazine, have not been studied well in individuals who have PD. After pimavanserin, clozapine has the best evidence for treatment of PDP. The weekly blood draw to monitor white blood cell count (because of the risk of agranulocytosis), which is needed for use of clozapine, is a significant burden for the resident who has PD. In addition, use of clozapine is associated with a risk of myocarditis, seizure, and orthostatic hypotension. Clozapine also has significant anticholinergic properties that may exacerbate cognitive impairment and precipitate delirium in residents who have PD and MNCD. Hence, quetiapine is the second-line agent (after pimavanserin) and ziprasidone the third-line agent. The HCP should consider prescribing clozapine for severe psychotic symptoms not responding to pimavanserin, quetiapine, or ziprasidone or if the resident cannot tolerate these drugs. The HCP should consider with great caution attempting to wean a stable resident who has PDP off pimavanserin or antipsychotic due to the high risk of recurrence of psychosis. Symptoms may be worse during recurrence than in the initial presentation and harder to control. If the resident who has PDP also has MNCD, cholinesterase inhibitor (especially rivastigmine, as it is the only ChEI approved by the FDA for the treatment of PDD) may help reduce psychotic symptoms (especially hallucination) or decrease the risk of worsening psychotic symptoms.

Delirium with Psychotic Symptoms

Psychotic symptoms are common in delirium and may be the predominant manifestation of delirium. Hallucinations are typically visual and often accompanied by illusion and paranoid delusion. Hallucinations are usually vivid, elaborate, and frightening. Delusions are transient and not well systematized. Treatment involves finding and treating the cause of delirium. The HCP may consider prescribing short-term use of a low-dose antipsychotic to treat severe agitation and aggression accompanying psychotic symptoms during delirium.

Psychotic Disorder Due to Another Medical Condition

Psychotic disorder due to another medical condition is more prevalent in LTC populations than in age-matched peers in the community. There may be a higher prevalence in females than males. On occasion, psychotic symptoms may be the only or initial manifestation of an underlying medical condition (e.g. UTI, thyroid dysfunction, electrolyte imbalance, epilepsy, dehydration, stroke, TBI, sleep apnea, brain tumor, SLE, encephalitis), especially among residents who have pre-existing MNCD. Olfactory hallucinations are typical in temporal lobe epilepsy. Visual hallucinations among residents who have retinal disease (e.g. macular degeneration) are common, underdiagnosed, and not associated with cognitive deficit, abnormal personality trait, or a family or personal history of psychiatric morbidity. Visual hallucination and illusion may also accompany other ocular pathology and decrease in visual acuity (e.g. cataract, glaucoma). In residents who have significant ocular pathology, hallucination may range from simple (e.g. dots, lines, shapes, patterns, flashes) to well formed and vivid (e.g. faces, people, landscapes, animals, objects) and can be miniaturized or distorted. In general, simple visual hallucinations are related to damage to the primary retinocortical visual system, and complex visual hallucinations are related to damage to higher cortical areas in occipital and parietal lobes. The occurrence of such persistent, complex visual hallucinations with preserved insight in people who have visual impairment and the absence of other etiologies (e.g. MNCD) is known as the Charles Bonnet syndrome. Among residents who have relatively good vision, hallucinations are associated with increased emotional distress and decreased quality of life. The HCP should consider the need for eyeglasses (or change in glasses), cataract surgery, and referral to an ophthalmologist for any resident who has visual hallucination. We recommend close monitoring for cognitive decline because the onset of complex visual hallucination in a resident who has intact vision may be an indication of early-stage MNCD (especially DLB). Psychotic symptoms due to deep brain lesion (e.g. basal ganglia) may resemble schizophrenia more closely than those seen with MNCD. Vivid, elaborate, and well-formed visual hallucination (so-called peduncular hallucinosis) may occur with disease (e.g. stroke) in the upper brain stem. Psychosis can be an uncommon but devastating consequence of traumatic brain injury. In residents who have neurological deficit (e.g. due to stroke, tumor), delusional thinking may be associated with denial of illness (anosognosia), denial of blindness (Anton syndrome), or reduplicative paramnesia (in which a person claims to be present simultaneously in two locations). Aging residents who have AIDS may develop central nervous system manifestations that often result in psychosis.

Careful consideration of various etiologies is critical to early and accurate diagnosis. Treatment involves identifying and treating the underlying medical condition. When psychosis develops in the context of epilepsy, the first step is to maximize anticonvulsant therapy in an effort to reduce the possible contribution of electrophysiologic disturbance. The HCP may consider prescribing benzodiazepine for ictal and postictal psychotic symptoms and agitation. Antipsychotics can lower the threshold for seizure and thus the HCP should use them cautiously to treat chronic psychotic symptoms (interictal) for a resident who has epilepsy. Symptomatic therapy with low-dose atypical antipsychotic may be necessary for a resident who has psychotic disorder due to a medical condition with severe agitation.

Medication-Induced Psychotic Disorder

Drugs used to treat Parkinson's disease (PD), anticholinergic drugs, benzodiazepines, and steroids often cause psychotic symptoms. Withdrawal from anxiolytics and sedative-hypnotics may also be associated with psychotic symptoms (especially visual hallucination along with illusion but occasionally tactile hallucination). (See Box 6.2.) The onset of psychotic symptoms usually correlates with the initiation or increase in the dosage of the offending medication. Serum drug levels (e.g. digoxin levels) may help clarify the diagnosis for some implicated medications. Psychotic symptoms may be seen even when digoxin levels are therapeutic. Treatment involves reducing and discontinuing the offending medication when feasible. The HCP should also discontinue other medication that is inappropriate for LTC populations based on the Beers list (American Geriatrics Society 2015). A low dose of atypical antipsychotic may be necessary if symptoms are severe and the offending medication (e.g. steroid) cannot be tapered and/or discontinued. Treatment of psychotic symptoms in the context of benzodiazepine intoxication involves gradual taper and discontinuation of benzodiazepine.

Psychotic Symptoms Associated with Alcohol Use Disorder

Psychotic symptoms typically occur during alcohol intoxication and withdrawal. Psychotic symptoms can also occur as a separate syndrome of alcohol-induced psychotic disorder with delusion (e.g. of infidelity) and/or hallucination (alcoholic hallucinosis). Diagnosis requires a high index of suspicion, as many residents continue to consume alcohol after admission to a LTC facility. Residents who have psychotic symptoms in the context of alcohol intoxication should be transferred to a local ER, where their behavior can be safely managed. The blood alcohol level may help clarify the diagnosis. In residents who have MNCD or frailty, even a small amount of alcohol may be sufficient to cause problems (intoxication or withdrawal). Treatment of alcohol withdrawal may require benzodiazepine, and if there is risk of withdrawal seizure (e.g. history of withdrawal seizure) and/or delirium (delirium tremens), the HCP needs to consider hospitalization.

Substance-Induced Psychotic Disorder

Although it is rare, some residents use cocaine, cannabis, synthetic cannabinoids, methamphetamine, phencyclidine, inhalants, LSD, or other street drugs after admission to a LTC facility (Taylor and Grossberg 2012). Psychotic symptoms are typically in the intoxication phase. Panic attacks, depersonalization symptoms, emotional lability, delusions of infestation, and tactile hallucinations (bugs or vermin crawling in or under the skin) often accompany persecutory delusions in residents experiencing substance-induced psychotic disorder. Residents usually have a history of drug abuse. Having a high index of suspicion is crucial for accurate diagnosis. Urine drug screen often helps clarify the diagnosis. Moderate to severe symptoms should be treated in a hospital due to the high risk of delirium, violence, and mortality.

Mixed Psychotic Disorder

Many residents may have two secondary psychotic disorders (e.g. MNCD with psychotic symptoms and superimposed delirium with psychotic symptoms) or a primary psychotic disorder (e.g. schizophrenia) comorbid with a secondary psychotic disorder (e.g.

delirium with psychotic symptoms). Inadequate psychiatric care in LTC facilities may result in the development of MNCD going unrecognized in a resident who has schizophrenia. Having a high index of suspicion and a comprehensive assessment are key to accurate identification of mixed psychotic disorders and appropriate treatment.

Violence and Aggression

Violent and aggressive behaviors are two of the most serious complications of psychotic disorder in LTC populations. Manifestations of violence and aggression in residents range from transient wishes to harm someone to impulsive aggressive behavior (e.g. hitting staff in response to stress) to preoccupation with plans to commit a violent act to completed homicide. Completed homicide is a self-inflicted act with intention to end someone's life that results in death of that person. Although homicide is rare in LTC populations, other manifestations of violence and aggression are prevalent, under-recognized, and undertreated. Homicide-suicide has been documented in the literature where a community-dwelling older adult (typically a white male) kills the spouse/partner (usually because the partner has advanced MNCD and the other adult cannot care for the spouse anymore) and then kills him- or herself. As more couples enter LTC, we urge the HCP to keep this potential risk in mind based on the individual risk factors of each resident. Aggressive behavior (e.g. hitting, scratching, biting) toward staff during personal care (e.g. bathing) is prevalent among residents who have advanced MNCD and is typically the resident's reaction to stress and perceived unwanted invasion of personal space rather than a manifestation of a psychotic disorder. Violence and aggression in LTC populations are a complex phenomenon with multiple risk correlates interacting with protective factors. (See Tables 6.8 and 6.9.)

We recommend violence risk assessment for any new resident (especially a resident who has new onset of psychotic symptoms, known history of violence, and/or pre-existing major mental illness [e.g. MDD, bipolar disorder, schizophrenia, schizoaffective disorder, other psychotic disorders, antisocial personality disorder, borderline personality disorder, intermittent explosive disorder, PTSD] or substance use disorder). Involving family and friends (with the consent of the resident whenever possible) to help reduce the risk of violence is critical. Although a frail or confused resident may have greater difficulty physically carrying out a violent act, the HCP should take seriously any expressed wish to harm others.

The goal of violence risk assessment is not only to predict whether a resident will commit an act of violence or not but also to understand the basis for a wish to harm others and generate a more individualized and informed violence prevention care plan. A resident at imminent risk (a serious attempt to harm others, or voicing homicidal idea with plan or intent, severe psychotic symptoms with aggressive behavior, poor judgment, refusal of treatment, medical complications) should be transferred to the ER of a local hospital for immediate evaluation and hospitalization in a psychiatric inpatient unit (preferably a geriatric psychiatry inpatient unit). A resident at moderate to high risk of harming others may need to be closely monitored (e.g. one on one, line of sight, check every 15 minutes) in the facility while assessment and treatment are under way. Involvement of law enforcement personnel and informing the person(s) who is the target of the resident's homicidal ideas may be necessary in certain situations.

Aggressive and violent behaviors in LTC populations are eminently preventable. (See Tables 6.8, 6.9, and 6.10.) Psychotic disorder, delirium, pain, and mood disorder are the most common treatable causes of violent and aggressive behavior in LTC populations. Staff education, rigorous training (especially in de-escalation techniques), and support are key to successful prevention of violence. We urge all LTC facilities to have an aggression/violence prevention team (preferably led by a psychiatrist with training in LTC psychiatry). A violence prevention program in LTC should involve the following steps:

Step 1: Identify at-risk populations (e.g. resident who has delirium, resident who has psychotic disorder).

Step 2: Assess violence risk (low, moderate, high, imminent) in at-risk resident and share the finding with staff caring for the resident.

Step 3: Institute a violence prevention plan (matching the severity of risk for danger to others in at-risk resident to ensure safety while the prevention plan is under way) with involvement of a mental health professional early in the management.

Step 4: Periodically monitor the risk for violence and response to treatment, and modify the violence prevention plan as necessary.

Table 6.8 Risk Factors for Violence and Aggressive Behavior in Resident Who Has Psychotic Disorder

Risk Factor	Risk Implication	Prevention/Therapeutic Implication
Age	Risk decreases with age	Staff education about risk factors is key prevention strategy
Gender	Risk is higher in males than in females	Staff education about risk factors is key prevention strategy
Plan for violence	Risk is higher if there is a resolved plan for violence	Violence assessment should inquire about various ways resident may have imagined attempting violence and details of plan
Attitude toward violence and aggressive behavior	Risk is higher in resident who views violence and aggressive behavior as a reasonable strategy to cope with perceived attack or injustice	Violence assessment should inquire about resident's attitude toward homicide
Thoughts of violence or wish to harm others	Risk is higher in resident who expresses having recurrent thoughts of wanting to harm others	Violence assessment should inquire about resident's preoccupation with thoughts of committing violent act/wish to harm others
Means to commit violence	Risk is higher if resident has access to means to commit violence (access to guns, cognitive capacity to use objects in the facility to harm others)	Violence risk assessment should routinely inquire about resident's access to means to commit violence, and violence prevention plan should include strategies to limit access to lethal means
Delusion	Presence of delusional belief (especially persecutory delusion and delusion of infidelity) increases risk	Resident who has delusional belief even in absence of wish to harm others should be considered at moderate to high risk of aggression
Auditory hallucination	Presence of command auditory hallucination telling resident to harm others increases risk	Resident who has command hallucination even in absence of wish to respond to the hallucination should be considered at moderate to high risk of aggression
Visual hallucination	Presence of visual hallucination involving intruder increases risk	Violence risk assessment should routinely evaluate presence of visual hallucination
Catatonic excitement	Presence of catatonic excitement increases risk	Catatonic excitement is behavioral emergency that should be rapidly controlled to reduce risk of imminent danger to others
Personality and coping style	Antisocial personality trait/disorder increases risk Short-tempered personality trait increases risk Impulsive or careless problem-solving style increases risk	Violence risk assessment should routinely inquire into presence of these personality and coping styles
Major mental disorder	Presence of major mental disorder (e. g. MDD, bipolar disorder, schizophrenia, schizoaffective	Any resident who has major mental disorder and expresses even transient wish to harm others

Table 6.8 (cont.)

Risk Factor	Risk Implication	Prevention/Therapeutic Implication
	disorder, intermittent explosive disorder) increases risk	should be considered at moderate to high risk of violence
Delirium	Presence of delirium increases risk	Violence risk assessment should routinely involve assessment for presence of delirium
MNCD	Presence of MNCD (especially with severely impaired executive function) increases risk	Violence risk assessment should be done for any resident after diagnosis of MNCD
Depression	Presence of depression is risk factor for verbally and physical aggressive behavior (e.g. yelling, use of foul language, hitting)	Violence risk assessment should routinely assess for presence of depression
Moderate to severe persistent pain	Presence of moderate to severe persistent pain increases risk	HCP should consider comprehensive pain strategy, referral to a pain management specialist, and palliative care for resident who has severe persistent pain
Substance use disorder	Intoxication and withdrawal phase (especially alcohol and stimulants) increase risk	High index of suspicion and good knowledge of resident's history of substance use disorder is important to reduce risk of violence
Prescription medication	Certain medications (e.g. benzodiazepine, drug that increases dopaminergic neurotransmission) increase risk (especially in resident who has damage to frontal lobe)	Violence risk assessment should routinely involve review of all medications the resident may be taking to identify medication-induced aggressive behavior
History of aggressive behavior and violence	History of aggressive/violent behavior increases risk	Any resident who has history of violence/aggressive behavior should be screened for major mental disorder and have violence risk assessment at time of admission
Exposure to violence	Current or past exposure to violence (especially in childhood) increases risk	Violence risk assessment should inquire into history of exposure to violence
Family history	Family history of violence may increase risk	Any resident who has family history of violence should be screened for mood disorder (e.g. MDD, bipolar disorder) and have violence risk assessment at time of admission
Staff approach and care practices	Countertherapeutic staff approach (e.g. arguing with a resident; disrespectful attitude, dismissing resident's experiences, ignoring resident's perspectives) and impatient care practices may increase risk	Staff education, training, and support are three of the most important aggression/violence prevention strategies

Table 6.9 Protective Factors for Violence and Aggressive Behavior in Resident Who Has Psychotic Disorder

Protective Factor	Implication for Violence Risk Assessment	Preventive Approach/Therapeutic Implication for Resident at Risk of Aggressive/Violent Behavior
Demographics	Older residents have relatively lower risk than younger residents Female residents have relatively lower risk than male residents	Staff education about demographic factors that are protective
Family connections (includes connections with friends) and support	Strong family connections and support may help resident cope with stress and thus reduce risk of aggressive/violent behavior	Bolstering family connections, support (e.g. increased visits by family and friends, family education) and contact (in person or via technology [FaceTime, Skype])
Religious/spiritual belief in nonviolence	Strong religious/spiritual belief in nonviolence may reduce risk of aggressive/violent behavior	Making robust efforts to support resident's engagement in religious/spiritual rituals and activities with like-minded individuals
Concrete support in times of need	Adequate services and support in time of crisis (e.g. access to community resources, peer support for resident who has addiction problem) reduce risk of aggressive/violent behavior	Staff education about in-house and community resources for various problems (e.g. financial, housing, addiction) that can quickly be accessed by resident, family, and staff
High-quality staff	Staff that receive regular education and rigorous training in prevention and management of aggressive/violent behavior and for simple strategies to bolster resilience of residents may dramatically reduce risk of aggressive/violent behavior	High-quality staff like working with LTC populations, are always respectful, and are well trained (especially in de-escalation techniques and in therapeutic and mindful care practices)
Adequate quantity of staff	Adequate staffing allows staff sufficient time to connect with resident and implement de-escalation strategies and reduce risk	Making adequate and high-quality staffing a reality depends on competency and resourcefulness of leadership team (especially administrators and directors of nursing) of LTC facilities
Adequate staff support	Staff that routinely have access to mentors and leadership team members and feel supported by them are able to engage with resident better, and this may help reduce risk	Leadership team should make themselves accessible to all staff, empower staff in day-to-day decision-making, support routine brief team meetings (huddles) to address challenging residents, and make other efforts so that all staff feel appreciated and valued and that their opinions and perspectives are respected
Social activities	Resident who is active in facility/community activities and organizations and has hobby is at lower risk of aggressive/violent behavior	Redoubling efforts to foster engagement in social activities and hobbies

Table 6.10 Prevention of Violence and Aggressive Behavior

Type of Prevention	Target Group of Residents	Examples of Preventive Approaches
Indicated prevention (targets resident who has mild agitation and/or aggressive or psychotic symptoms; goal is to prevent severe aggressive behavior and violence)	Resident who has moderate to severe psychotic symptoms Resident who has MNCD and mild agitation/aggression Resident who has schizophrenia or related disorder and is coping with acute stressor Resident who has PD and mild psychotic symptoms Resident who has delirium and subsyndromal delirium	Early diagnosis and prompt treatment of delirium Judicious use of antipsychotic for some residents who have moderate to severe psychotic symptoms Psychotherapy/counseling* (including self-help versions) for motivated resident who has relatively preserved cognitive function to help cope with frustration and stress of living in LTC facility (e.g. CBT for resident who has anger management problem) Antidepressant (e.g. citalopram for MNCD-related significant agitation) Optimizing anti-PD medication for resident who has PD Pimavanserin for moderate to severe Parkinson's disease psychosis (PDP) Optimizing psychotropic medication for resident taking psychotropic medication (especially helpful for resident who has serious mental disorder**) All interventions listed for universal prevention
Selective prevention (targets resident who has known risk factors for aggression/violence; goal is to prevent development of aggressive/violent behavior)	Resident who has history of aggressive/violent behavior Resident who has antisocial personality and/or borderline personality trait/disorder Resident who has MNCD and moderate to severe pain	Psychotherapy/counseling* (including self-help versions) for motivated resident who has relatively preserved cognitive function to help cope with frustration and stress of living in LTC facility (e.g. CBT for resident who has anger management problems) Optimizing psychotropic medication for resident taking psychotropic medication (especially helpful for resident who has serious mental disorder**) All interventions listed for universal prevention
Universal prevention (targets entire LTC population; goal is to prevent aggressive/violent behavior and improve resilience)	All residents	A robust exercise and physical activity program SPPEICE (especially helpful in prevention of aggression in resident who has MNCD) Geriatric Scalpel*** Optimal pain control Omega-3 fatty acids and vitamin D supplementation Optimal control of vascular risk factor (e.g. hypertension, diabetes) Periodic staff, resident, and family education and awareness campaign about risk and protective factors for aggressive/violent behavior and prevention strategies Education of all staff regarding person-centered bathing techniques (e.g. use of DVD titled *Bathing without a Battle*, created by University of North Carolina, Chapel Hill, to educate staff) Staff training in de-escalation techniques and mindful and therapeutic care practices

* Psychotherapy/counseling: cognitive behavioral therapy, interpersonal therapy, problem-solving therapy, reminiscence therapy, life-review, music therapy

** Serious mental disorders: schizophrenia, schizoaffective disorder, other psychotic disorders, bipolar disorder, major depressive disorder, post-traumatic stress disorder, intermittent explosive disorder

*** Geriatric scalpel: rational deprescribing (discontinuation of medication that is inappropriate for LTC populations based on Beers list and anticholinergic burden caused by medication with high anticholinergic activity)

Summary

Psychotic disorders (especially delirium with psychotic symptoms and MNCD with psychotic symptoms) are prevalent in LTC populations and are responsible for substantial excess morbidity and increased mortality. The prevalence of schizophrenia and schizoaffective disorder in LTC populations is low but increasing, due primarily to the aging of adults who have these disorders. Psychotic symptoms are a common cause of violence and aggressive behavior in LTC populations. Violence and aggressive behavior are more prevalent in LTC populations than usually recognized. We recommend violence risk assessment for all residents, and in particular recently admitted residents who have a history of violence, so that appropriate violence preventive approaches can be instituted. Residents who have psychotic symptoms that are not responding to treatment, residents who have aggressive behavior, and residents who have schizophrenia and schizoaffective disorder are best managed by a team led by a psychiatrist with expertise in LTC psychiatry. Comprehensive assessment, prevention, and treatment strategies for all psychotic disorders and aggression can dramatically improve the quality of life of all residents who have psychotic disorder and may be life saving.

Key Clinical Points

1. Psychotic disorders are seen in approximately 5–10 percent of LTC populations and are the third most common reversible cause of disability and increased mortality (after MDD and delirium).
2. Violence and serious harm to others are the most serious complications of untreated psychotic disorder in LTC populations.
3. Early accurate diagnosis and comprehensive treatment of psychotic disorder can prevent violence and dramatically improve the quality of life of residents who have psychotic disorder.
4. Therapeutic and mindful staff approach, SPPEICE, de-escalation strategies, individual psychotherapy (for residents who have relatively preserved cognitive function), and, if necessary, judicious short-term use of a low dose of atypical antipsychotic or other appropriate psychotropic medication can successfully treat psychotic disorder in LTC populations.
5. The use of antipsychotics in LTC populations carries a high risk because LTC residents are at higher risk for antipsychotic-induced adverse effect, such as Parkinsonism, tardive dyskinesia, falls, and daytime sedation.

References

Alexopoulos, G.S., R.C. Abrams, R.C. Young, and C.A. Shamoian. 1988. Cornell Scale for Depression in Dementia. *Biological Psychiatry* **23**:271–284.

American Psychiatric Association. 2013. Schizophrenia Spectrum and other Psychotic Disorders. In: *Diagnostic and Statistical Manual of Mental Disorders*, 5th ed., pp. 87–122. Arlington, VA: American Psychiatric Association Press.

American Psychiatric Association. 2016. The American Psychiatric Association Practice Guideline on the Use of Antipsychotics to Treat Agitation or Psychosis in Patients with Dementia. http://psychiatryonline.org/doi/pdf/10.1176/appi.books.9780890426807 (accessed May 5, 2016).

American Geriatrics Society. 2011. Guide to the Management of Psychotic Disorders and Neuropsychiatric Symptoms Associated with Dementia in Older Adults. http://dementia.americangeriatrics.org/GeriPsych_index.php (accessed December 29, 2014).

American Geriatrics Society. 2015. 2015 Updated Beers Criteria for Potentially Inappropriate Medication Use in Older Adults. American Geriatrics Society Beers Criteria Update Expert Panel. *Journal of the American Geriatrics Society* **63**:2227–2246.

Apostolova, L.G. 2016. Alzheimer's Disease. *Continuum* **22**(2):419–434.

Chakkamparambil, B, J.T. Chibnall, E.A. Graypel, J.N. Manepalli, A. Bhutto, G.T. Grossberg, et al. 2015. Development of a Brief Validated Geriatric Depression Screening Tool: The SLU "AM SAD." *American Journal of Geriatric Psychiatry* **23**(8):780–783.

Cohen-Mansfield, J. 1996. Conceptualization of Agitation: Results Based on the Cohen-Mansfield Agitation Inventory and the Agitation Behavior Mapping Instrument. *International Psychogeriatrics* **8** supplement: 3:309–315.

Cummings-Vaughn, L.A., N. Chavakula, T.K. Malmstrom, et al. 2014. Veterans Affairs Saint Louis University Mental Status Examination compared with the Montreal Cognitive Assessment and the Short Test of Mental Status. *Journal of the American Geriatrics Society* **62**:1341–1346.

Desai, A.K., and G.T. Grossberg. 2017. Psychiatric Aspects of Long-Term Care. In B.J. Saddock, V.A. Saddock, and P. Ruiz (eds.), *Comprehensive Textbook of Psychiatry*, 10th ed., pp. 4221–4232. Virginia: American Psychiatric Press Inc.

Elliot, R. 2003. Executive Functions and Their Disorders. *British Medical Bulletin* **65**:49–59.

Folstein, M.F., S.E. Folstein, and P.R. McHugh. 1975. "Mini-Mental state": A Practical Method for Grading the Cognitive State of Patients for the Clinician. *Journal of Psychiatric Research* **12**:189–198.

Friedman, J.H. 2013. Parkinson's Disease Psychosis: Update. *Behavioral Neurology* **27**(4):469–477.

Goetz, C.G., B.G. Tilley, S.R. Shaftman, et al. 2008. Movement Disorder Society-Sponsored Revision of the Unified Parkinson's Disease Rating Scale (MDS-UPDRS): Scale Presentation and Clinimetric Testing Results. *Movement Disorders* **23**(15):2129–2170.

Gomperts, S. 2016. Lewy Body Dementias: Dementia with Lewy Bodies and Parkinson's Disease Dementia. *Continuum* **22**(2):435–463.

Hoegh, M., A.K. Ibrahim, J. Chibnall, and G.T. Grossberg. 2013. Prevalence of Parkinson's Disease and Parkinson's Disease Dementia in Community Nursing Homes. *American Journal of Geriatric Psychiatry* **21**(6):529–535.

Inouye, S.K., C.H. van Dyck, C.A. Alessi, et al. 1990. Clarifying Confusion: The Confusion Assessment Method. A New Method for Detection of Delirium. *Annals of Internal Medicine* **113**:941–948.

Jeste, D. and J.E. Maglione. 2013. Treating Older Adults with Schizophrenia: Challenges and Opportunities. *Schizophrenia Bulletin* **39**(5):966–968.

Karim, S. and A. Burns. 2011. Psychotic Disorders in Late-Life. In M.E. Agronin and G. J. Maletta (eds.), *Principles and Practice of Geriatric Psychiatry*, 2nd ed., pp. 465–476. Philadelphia, PA: Lippincott Williams & Wilkins.

Landquist, W.M., L. Gustafson, U. Passant, and E. Englund. 2015. Psychotic Symptoms in Frontotemporal Dementia: A Diagnostic Dilemma? *International Psychogeriatrics* **27**(4):531–539.

Maglione, J.E., I.V. Vahia, and D.V. Jeste. 2015. Schizophrenia Spectrum and Other Psychotic Disorders. In D.C. Steffens, D.G. Blazer, and M.E. Thakur (eds.), *The Textbook of Geriatric Psychiatry*, 5th ed., pp. 309–332. Arlington, VA: American Psychiatric Publishing.

Nasreddine, Z.S., N.A. Phillips, V. Badirian, et al. 2005. The Montreal Cognitive Assessment, MoCA: A Brief Screening Tool for Mild Cognitive Impairment. *Journal of the American Geriatrics Society* **53**: 695–699.

Reisberg, B., J. Borenstein, S.P. Salob, et al. 1987. Behavioral Symptoms in Alzheimer's Disease: Phenomenology and Treatment. *Journal of Clinical Psychiatry* **48**\(suppl 5):9–15.

Ricker, J.H., and Axelrod, B.N. 1994. Analysis of an Oral Paradigm for the Trail Making Test. *Assessment* **1**(1):47–51.

Rosen, J., L. Burgio, M. Kollar, et al. 1994. A User Friendly Instrument for Rating Agitation in Dementia Patients. *American Journal of Geriatric Psychiatry* **2**(1):52–59.

Saliba, D., J. Buchanan, M.O. Edelen, et al. 2012a. MDS 3.0: Brief Interview for Mental Status. *Journal of the American Medical Directors Association* **13**:611–617.

Saliba, D., S. DiFilippo, M.O. Edelen et al. 2012b. Testing the PHQ-9 Interview and Observational Versions (PHQ-OV) for MDS 3.0. *Journal of the American Medical Director's Association* **13**(7):618–625.

Spitzer, R, K. Kroenke, and J. Williams. 1999. Validation and Utility of a Self-Report Version of PRIME-MD: The PHQ Primary Care Study. *Journal of the American Medical Association* **282**: 1737–1744.

Tandon, R., S. Heckers, J. Bustillo, et al. 2013. Catatonia in DSM V. *Schizophrenia Research* **150**:26–30.

Taylor, M.H. and G.T. Grossberg. 2012. The Growing Problem of Illicit Substance Abuse in the Elderly: A Review. *Primary Care Companion CNS Disorders* **14**(4): PCC.11r01320. doi:10.4088/PCC.11r01320

Warden, V., Hurley, A.C. and Volicer, L. 2003. Development and Psychometric Evaluation of the Pain Assessment in Advanced Dementia. *Journal of the American Medical Directors Association* **4**:9–15.

Wood, S., J.L. Cummings, M. Hsu, et al. 2000. The Use of the Neuropsychiatric Inventory in Nursing Home Residents. *American Journal of Geriatric Psychiatry* **8**:75–83.

Yesavage, J.A., T.L. Brink, T.L. Rose, et al. 1983. Development and Validation of a Geriatric Depression Scale: A Preliminary Report. *Journal of Psychiatric Research* **17**:37–49.

Chapter 7

Anxiety Disorders, Trauma- and Stress-Related Disorders, Obsessive-Compulsive and Related Disorders, and Sleep-Wake Disorders

Anxiety disorders, trauma- and stress-related disorders, obsessive-compulsive and related disorders, and sleep-wake disorders are prevalent in long-term care (LTC) populations (Streim 2015). They often co-occur with mood and psychotic disorders and are common causes of treatment resistance of mood and psychotic disorders. (See Boxes 7.1, 7.2, and 7.3.) Box 7.1 lists common anxiety disorders, trauma- and stress-related disorders, and obsessive-compulsive and related disorders, and Box 7.2 lists common sleep-wake disorders. Box 7.3 lists common consequences and complications if these disorders are not treated. Boxes 7.4 and 7.5 list common medications that may cause or exacerbate anxiety and sleep-wake disorders. These disorders are often misdiagnosed and inappropriately treated (e.g. with long-term use of benzodiazepine).

Anxiety Disorders

Anxiety is defined as a vague, uneasy feeling, the source of which often is nonspecific or unknown to the individual who is experiencing it. Fear is anxiety related to a specific object, event, or situation. Anxiety disorders are less prevalent in older adults than in young adults, but the rates of subsyndromal anxiety disorders are nearly as high in older adults as in their younger cohorts (Lenz, Mohlman, and Wetherell 2015). Point prevalence of anxiety disorders in LTC populations is 5–10 percent. Mild anxiety symptoms are even more prevalent. The majority of anxiety symptoms in LTC populations are in the context of acute stress, adverse effects of medication, delirium, major neurocognitive disorder (MNCD), Parkinson's disease (PD), and cerebrovascular disease. Anxiety symptoms are a common cause of agitation and verbal and physical aggression in LTC populations (Desai and Grossberg 2017). More than one-third of older adults who have major depressive disorder (MDD) also have a concurring comorbid anxiety disorder. Likewise, severe anxiety symptoms have been seen in as many as one-half of individuals who have late-life MDD. Comorbid anxiety disorder in late-life

BOX 7.1 Common Anxiety Disorders, Trauma- and Stress-Related Disorders, and Obsessive-Compulsive and Related Disorders in Long-Term Care Populations

- Anxiety disorders
  - Generalized anxiety disorder
  - Panic disorder with or without agoraphobia
  - Social anxiety disorder
  - Specific phobias (e.g. fear of falling, fear of injections, fear of hospitals, fear of blood, fear of medical procedures)
  - Major neurocognitive disorder with anxiety symptoms
  - Medication-induced anxiety disorder
  - Anxiety disorder due to Parkinson's disease
  - Anxiety disorder due to stroke or cerebrovascular disease
  - Medical condition-induced anxiety disorder
  - Substance-induced anxiety disorder (e.g. caffeine, alcohol, methamphetamine)
  - Anxiety symptoms due to delirium
- Trauma- and stress-related disorders
  - Post-traumatic stress disorder
  - Other specific trauma-related disorders (e.g. subsyndromal post-traumatic stress disorder)
  - Adjustment disorder with anxiety
- Obsessive-compulsive and related disorders
  - Obsessive-compulsive disorder
  - Hoarding disorder
  - Excoriation (skin picking) disorder

BOX 7.2 Common Sleep-Wake Disorders in Long-Term Care Populations

Insomnia disorder
Non-24-hour sleep-wake disorder
Nightmare disorder
REM sleep behavior disorder
Restless legs syndrome
Obstructive sleep apnea hypopnea syndrome
Major neurocognitive disorder with sleep-wake disturbance (e.g. insomnia, hypersomnia, REM sleep behavior disorder)
Medication-induced sleep-wake disorder
Medical condition-induced sleep-wake disorder

depression is also associated with future diagnosis of MNCD due to Alzheimer's disease (AD), indicating that anxiety and depression may be prodromal symptoms of future MNCD due to AD.

Diagnosis

Anxiety disorders can be accurately diagnosed in LTC populations using *DSM-5* diagnostic criteria. Accurate early diagnosis of anxiety disorder is key to successful treatment. There are currently no reliable biomarkers for any anxiety disorder. Diagnosis is clinical. Standardized scales can help improve the accuracy of diagnosis and assess the severity and comorbidity of other psychiatric symptoms. We recommend the health care provider (HCP) use the Geriatric Anxiety Inventory (www.gai.net.au) and the anxiety domain of the Neuropsychiatric Inventory–Nursing Home version (NPI-NH) to assess anxiety symptoms in conjunction with other standardized scales (Wood et al. 2000; Pachana et al. 2007). Standardized tests for cognition, pain, depression, and behavior can help clarify comorbidity and guide treatment decisions. The HCP should assess a resident who has verbal or physical aggression for the presence of anxiety disorder. (See Table 7.1.) Differential diagnosis of anxiety disorder includes adjustment disorder with anxiety and anxiety symptoms as part of another major mental disorder (e.g. MDD, bipolar disorder, schizophrenia, PTSD). We recommend a comprehensive diagnostic assessment and work-up of disabling anxiety disorder. (See Table 7.2.) The goal of assessment is to clarify the etiology and identify reversible comorbidity. The choice of tests and extent of work-up will depend on findings from the comprehensive assessment. Anxiety symptoms may be the initial presentation of delirium, as cognitive symptoms may be subtle in early stages, hence the importance of detailed cognitive assessment.

BOX 7.3 Consequences and Complications of Untreated Anxiety Disorder, Trauma- and Stress-Related Disorder, Obsessive-Compulsive and Related Disorders, and Sleep-Wake Disorder

Increased mortality
Increased risk of cerebrovascular disease
Increased risk of cardiovascular disease
Severe emotional distress (e.g. depression, anxiety, irritability)
Cognitive impairment (e.g. poor concentration and memory, slower reaction time)
Agitation (e.g. verbal aggression, physical aggression, increased psychomotor activity)
Increased risk of suicide
Reduced quality of life
Resistance to treatment when comorbid with a mood and/or psychotic disorder
Impaired adherence to treatment
Failure to progress with rehabilitation therapy
Decreased participation in activities
Decline in IADLs and ADLs
Hospitalization
Increased staff time to care
Increased risk of institutionalization (premature institutionalization) in an individual who has major neurocognitive disorder or Parkinson's disease
Social isolation
Increased distress in family members and friends

Treatment

Any resident who has anxiety disorder should receive comprehensive care with a variety of treatments tailored to the diagnosis, needs, and strengths. (See Table 7.3.) Although benzodiazepines are the most common treatment for anxiety disorder in LTC populations, their use should be minimized due to high risks. (See Box 7.6.) In general, an anxious resident may experience anticipatory dread about

BOX 7.4 Medications Linked to Anxiety Symptoms and/or Insomnia

- Sympathetomimetics
  - Phenylephrine
  - Phenylpropanolamine
  - Pseudoephedrine
- Medication used to treat COPD
  - Beta-adrenergic inhalers
  - Theophylline
- Thyroid medication
  - Levothyroxine (T4)
  - Tri-iodothyronine (T3)
- Stimulants
  - Methylphenidate
  - Dextroamphetamine
- Antidepressants
  - SSRI
  - Bupropion
  - Venlafaxine
  - Duloxetine
  - Desvenlafaxine
  - Vortioxetine
- Antipsychotics that may cause anxiety and/or insomnia
  - Aripiprazole
  - Brexpiprazole
  - Ziprasidone
  - Cholinesterase inhibitor (may cause insomnia)
  - Memantine (may cause excessive daytime sleepiness)
- Dopaminergic drugs
  - Ropinirole
  - Pramipexole
  - Rotigotine
  - Levodopa (L-dopa), carbidopa
  - Bromocriptine
  - Amantadine
  - Selegiline
- Other medications and substances that may cause anxiety and/or insomnia
  - Corticosteroid
  - Modafinil
  - Armodafinil
  - Nicotine (in patch form, nicotine gum)
  - Caffeine
  - Diuretic (may cause insomnia by causing nocturia and anxiety/insomnia by causing electrolyte imbalance)
- Withdrawal of sedating drugs and substances
  - Opioid
  - Benzodiazepine
  - Zolpidem
  - Barbiturate
  - Alcohol

the adverse effect of prescribed antianxiety medication, may be vigilant about potential adverse effect, and may have a tendency to catastrophize about it. Often, some caregivers (family and professional) share these fears. Thus, we recommend that the HCP educate residents, family, and staff in advance about potential adverse effect of medication and reassure them that the HCP will closely monitor the resident for adverse effect.

Generalized Anxiety Disorder

Generalized anxiety disorder (GAD) is characterized by at least six months of excessive uncontrollable worry accompanied by symptoms of motor tension and vigilance (American Psychiatric Association 2013a). GAD may manifest as agitation, pacing, restlessness, verbal and/or physical aggression, irritability, and insomnia. GAD has a high level of comorbidity with other psychiatric disorder (MDD and MNCD being most common). Most residents who have GAD usually have chronic symptoms that have been ongoing for years to decades without interruption but with some waxing and waning. Early-onset (before age 50) GAD constitutes a higher proportion (60 percent) of GAD in late life than late-onset (after 50) GAD (40 percent). Older adults who have early-onset GAD have a higher rate of psychiatric comorbidity, use of psychotropic medication (including use of benzodiazepine for years to decades), and more severe worry. Older adults who have late-onset GAD have more functional limitation due to physical problems. A variety of evidence-based approaches are available to treat GAD. (See Table 7.3.) Many residents who have GAD have been taking benzodiazepine for decades before entering the LTC facility. For these residents, the HCP should consider tapering benzodiazepine due to the risk of

BOX 7.5 Prescription and Over-the-Counter Medications Linked to Hypersomnia and Excessive Daytime Sleepiness

Antidepressants
- Mirtazapine
- Vilazodone
- Nefazodone
- Trazodone
- Tricyclic antidepressant
- Selegiline patch

Antipsychotics
- Quetiapine
- Olanzapine
- Clozapine
- Risperidone
- Paliperidone
- Iloperidone
- Lurasidone
- Cariprazine
- All conventional/typical antipsychotics (e.g. haloperidol, fluphenazine)

Medications used to treat major neurocognitive disorder
- Memantine

Sedative hypnotic drugs
- Benzodiazepines (e.g. lorazepam, diazepam, clonazepam)
- Nonbenzodiazepine hypnotics (e.g. zolpidem, eszopiclone)
- Barbiturates
- Chloral hydrate

Analgesics used to treat nociceptive and neuropathic pain
- Opiates
- Tramadol
- Gabapentin
- Pregabalin

Muscle relaxants
- Methocarbamol
- Carisoprodol
- Cyclobenzaprine

Anticholinergic drugs and other drugs with high anticholinergic activity
- Diphenhydramine
- Brompheniramine
- Chlorpheniramine
- Trihexyphenidyl
- Biperiden
- Benztropine
- Orphenadrine
- Scopolamine
- Meclizine
- Oxybutynin
- Dimenhydrinate
- Atropine
- Hyocyamine
- Hydroxyzine
- Doxylamine

Anticonvulsants
- Valproate
- Oxcarbazepine
- Clobazam
- Eslicarbazepine
- Lacosamide
- Carbamazepine
- Lamotrigine
- Topiramate
- Phenytoin

Dopaminergic drugs
- Ropinirole
- Pramipexole
- Rotigotine
- Levodopa (L-dopa), carbidopa
- Bromocriptine
- Amantadine
- Selegiline

Other drugs
- Digoxin
- Clonidine
- Primidone

cognitive impairment, falls, and fracture. The taper should be extremely slow (over several months). A small group of residents who have severe GAD may need low-dose benzodiazepine for the rest of their lives even in a LTC facility. For these residents, the HCP should prescribe the lowest possible dose of benzodiazepine and closely monitor them for adverse effect.

Table 7.1 Anxiety Disorders Commonly Seen in Long-Term Care Populations

Anxiety Disorder	Key Clinical Features	Therapeutic Pearls
Generalized anxiety disorder	Persistent worries in multiple areas (e.g. finances, health, family) for more than 6 months accompanied by significant anxiety symptoms and impaired function Resident may have been "lifelong worrier" and develops disabling anxiety after onset of MNCD	Avoid benzodiazepine, as it is a chronic disorder Routine engagement in relaxation strategies and activities SSRI or buspirone is first-line psychotropic option if symptoms are severe CBT for motivated resident who has relatively intact cognitive function
Panic disorder (with or without agoraphobia)	One or more episodes of panic attack (acute-onset severe anxiety symptoms reaching peak in 10 minutes and lasting 30 minutes to an hour)	HCP may prescribe low-dose short-acting benzodiazepine for acute panic attack if relaxation/distraction strategies do not help SSRI is first-line psychotropic option but should be started at low dose and slowly increased, as otherwise it may worsen anxiety initially Routine engagement in relaxation strategies and activities CBT for motivated resident who has relatively intact cognitive function
Specific phobia	Fall phobia is most disabling of all specific phobias in LTC populations Resident has fear of falls that prevents her from taking part in physical therapy and prefers to use wheelchair	Physical therapist and other team members need to have high index of suspicion for fall phobia to be identified as early as possible so that appropriate intervention can prevent complication (e.g. failure of rehabilitation) Treatment involves combination of relaxation strategies, graded exposure, and, if necessary, SSRI
Social anxiety disorder	Usually a life-long disorder that may be exacerbated by new challenge (e.g. memory deficit, expressive aphasia) Pseudobulbar affect can cause social anxiety disorder	SSRI may be appropriate to treat disabling social anxiety disorder CBT for motivated resident who has relatively intact cognitive function
Anxiety symptoms during grief	Anxiety symptoms during grief may take the form of panic attack, separation anxiety symptoms, or persistent worries	HCP should look for comorbid complicated grief and MDD, as it is often missed due to prominent anxiety symptoms
Major neurocognitive disorder with anxiety symptoms	Generalized anxiety symptoms and panic attack are common complications of MNCD	Benzodiazepines increase risk of falls and thus HCP should avoid prescribing them for resident with MNCD
Poststroke anxiety	Generalized anxiety symptoms and panic attack are common but under-recognized sequelae of stroke	Benzodiazepines increase risk of falls and thus HCP should avoid prescribing them for resident recovering from stroke

Table 7.1 (cont.)

Anxiety Disorder	Key Clinical Features	Therapeutic Pearls
Delirium-related anxiety	Acute onset of anxiety symptoms may be presenting feature of delirium even in absence of delirium-related psychotic symptoms Anxiety symptoms may dominate clinical picture in sedative-hypnotic and alcohol withdrawal delirium	Acute onset of disabling anxiety symptoms should prompt assessment and work-up similar to that for delirium Without prompt treatment with benzodiazepine, anxiety symptoms due to sedative-hypnotic and alcohol withdrawal may be followed by seizures and/or psychotic symptoms with severe agitation
Parkinson's disease with anxiety symptoms	Generalized anxiety symptoms and panic attack are prevalent in residents who have PD, especially after onset of PDD	Even low-dose benzodiazepine can precipitate delirium in resident who has PD, and hence should be avoided HCP may consider prescribing very low dose quetiapine (12.5 mg once or twice daily) for disabling and persistent anxiety symptoms in resident who has PD
Medication-induced anxiety disorder	Interdose withdrawal from inappropriately used benzodiazepine and beta-agonist inhaler (used to treat COPD) use are two most common causes of medication-induced anxiety disorder	High index of suspicion is key to early accurate diagnosis and treatment
Pain-induced anxiety symptoms	Pain may cause phobia for therapy and anxiety symptoms may cause pain to be treatment resistant	Comprehensive pain management can reduce anxiety, and comprehensive anxiety management can reduce pain and use of pain medication
Anxiety disorder induced by another medical condition	Overcorrection of thyroid disorder and hypoxia-hypercapnia in resident who has COPD are two most common other medical conditions that cause anxiety disorder	Optimization of treatment of underlying medical condition usually reduces anxiety symptoms
Substance use-related anxiety disorder	Prevalence of anxiety disorder related to alcohol use disorder is increasing in LTC populations	Education of resident and family is key to successful outcome, as resident may consider use of alcohol an important factor in quality of life and both residents and family may underestimate its risks
Mixed anxiety disorder	Most residents who have disabling anxiety have multiple factors contributing to anxiety symptoms (e.g. chaotic environment, lack of involvement of resident in decision-making, medication, electrolyte imbalance, pain, cognitive deficit)	Even when HCP identifies specific anxiety disorder and initiates treatment, comprehensive assessment to identify other causes of anxiety symptoms is key to successful outcome

Table 7.2 Diagnostic Work-Up for Anxiety Disorder

Diagnostic Test	Key Examples	Key Implications for Treatment
Comprehensive assessment	Psychiatric history (including history of use of benzodiazepines) Family history Review of medication Vital signs Physical examination (including height, weight, body mass index) Neurological examination Mental status examination Use of standardized assessment scales Review of previous psychiatric records	Most residents who have disabling anxiety have multiple factors contributing to anxiety symptoms (e.g. chaotic environment, lack of involvement in decision-making, medication, electrolyte imbalance, pain, cognitive deficit) in addition to one or more specific anxiety disorders Findings from cognitive assessment are key to choosing treatment (e.g. avoiding antipsychotic with anticholinergic activity [e.g. hydroxyzine] for resident who has significant cognitive impairment; psychotherapy for resident who has relatively intact cognitive function)
Bedside test	Pulse oximetry	Hypoxia may contribute to anxiety symptoms
Bedside test	Glucose fingerstick	Hypoglycemia may cause or contribute to anxiety symptoms (especially panic attack)
Laboratory test	Comprehensive metabolic panel	Identifying dehydration and electrolyte imbalance that may contribute to anxiety symptoms and resistance to treatment
Laboratory test	Thyroid function tests (e.g. thyroid stimulating hormone level)	Overcorrection of hypothyroidism contributes to or causes anxiety symptoms
Laboratory test	Serum drug levels	Serum levels of digoxin may help clarify diagnosis of digoxin-induced anxiety disorder
Laboratory or bedside test	Electrocardiogram	Arrhythmia may contribute to or cause anxiety symptoms (especially panic attack)
Laboratory test	Psychotropic drug genetic testing using buccal swab (pharmacogenomic testing)	HCP should avoid prescribing antidepressant (used to treat anxiety disorder) with significant metabolism by 2D6 (e.g. paroxetine, fluoxetine) or 2C19 (citalopram, escitalopram) system for resident who is poor metabolizer of 2D6 or 2C19 system, respectively
Laboratory test	Electroencephalography	EEG may clarify diagnosis of anxiety disorder due to seizure (ictal, postictal, interictal anxiety symptoms)

Clinical Case 1: "My vision has been worsening in the last two weeks"

Mrs. U was a 96-year-old widowed woman who was admitted to the nursing home (NH) because of frailty, blindness due to macular degeneration, and recurrent falls. She had a sister who was two years younger and in good health, one son, three grandchildren, eight great-grandchildren, and one great-great-grandchild. For 8–9 months, Mrs. U had been having increased anxiety and nervousness, used her call light excessively, shouting "Help, help" for long periods of time, grabbing passers by, and asking them to help her. Mrs. U had been in the NH for several years and had always been somewhat anxious, but these symptoms were much more severe and apparently triggered by a severe UTI nine months ago. The staff was able to initially manage her behavior with psychosocial approaches, such as taking her to church service twice a day (Mrs. U was a Methodist, religious but did not mind attending church services of different denominations), hand massage, and soothing music. But over the last five months, the symptoms became severe and difficult to manage. Mrs. U usually slept well and, although she was eating less in the last few weeks, had no weight loss. The family started decreasing their visits because they felt Mrs. U became

Table 7.3 Evidence-Based Approaches to Treat Anxiety Disorder

Approach	Clinical Pearls	Key Concerns/Limitations
Antidepressants	Reserved for treatment of persistent and disabling anxiety disorder Starting dose needs to be lower than that for MDD, but most effective dose may be as high as that for MDD Clinically obvious benefit may take 6 or more weeks at highest tolerated dose	There may be transient increase in anxiety symptoms during initiation of antidepressant and during increase in dosage
Buspirone	First-line treatment for moderate to severe GAD	Resident taking benzodiazepine may not obtain significant benefit from buspirone Takes 2–4 weeks to "kick in"
Benzodiazepines	Low-dose short-acting benzodiazepine (e.g. lorazepam) may be needed to treat panic attack and before situation (e.g. brain scan with MRI) that may trigger severe anxiety attack	Long-term (more than 3 months) use of benzodiazepine carries high risk of serious adverse event (e.g. falls and injury, accelerated cognitive and functional decline, delirium)
Onsite individual counseling/ psychotherapy (cognitive behavioral therapy [CBT], mindfulness-based CBT, supportive psychotherapy)	Psychotherapy is first-line treatment for motivated resident who has disabling GAD, panic disorder, specific phobia, or social anxiety disorder and relatively intact cognitive function	Lack of availability of counselors trained in providing psychotherapy to LTC populations Lack of availability of counselors visiting LTC facilities to provide psychotherapy services Resident may need to visit local mental health clinic for such services
Internet-guided or telepsychiatry treatment	Cognitive restructuring (to address cognitive distortion) and relaxation training can be effectively administered via Internet and telepsychiatry by psychiatric nurse or other mental health professional to treat anxiety symptoms	Resident needs to be motivated and have relatively intact cognitive function Technophobia (in resident as well as staff) may be a difficult barrier to overcome
Psychoeducation and self-management	Providing pamphlets and other educational materials on late-life anxiety disorder and relaxation strategies	Cognitive deficit in resident may limit its benefit
Exercise	Exercise and increasing physical activity can accelerate response to other approach and increase likelihood of remission	Lack of time available to staff to help resident increase physical activity is key barrier to routine use
Rational deprescribing (geriatric scalpel) with input from consultant pharmacist	Discontinuation of medication that can cause/exacerbate anxiety symptoms, discontinuation of unnecessary or inappropriate medication (based on Beers list), and reducing anticholinergic burden	None
Optimizing control of pain and other comorbid physical health problem (e.g. diabetes) and correction of reversible physical health problem (e.g. dehydration, constipation, vision or hearing impairment, thyroid disorder)	Recommended for all residents	None

BOX 7.6 Potential Benefits and Risks of Using Benzodiazepine to Treat Severe and Disabling Anxiety Symptoms

Potential benefits
- Rapid onset/relief of symptoms
- Decreased emotional distress and thus improved quality of life
- Improved sleep
- Improved participation in daily activities
- Reduced agitation and aggressive behavior
- Staff better able to meet resident's basic needs (e.g. bathing, personal hygiene) after reduction in agitation and aggression caused by anxiety symptoms
- Decreased caregiver (family and professional) stress and burden

Potential risks
- Death due to falls and fatal injury and/or delirium
- Delirium
- Dysphagia
- Falls and serious injury (e.g. hip or vertebral fracture, skin tear, head injury)
- Daytime sedation (and its risks, such as aspiration pneumonia)
- Accelerated cognitive and/or functional decline
- Paradoxical disinhibition and increased agitation/aggressive behavior

more agitated when they visited and asked her how she was feeling. The family felt helpless when they could not calm Mrs. U down and the staff told the family that Mrs. U was having "another bad day." The primary care physician (PCP) had tried citalopram and mirtazapine with her, but Mrs. U could not tolerate either of these medications. Hence, the PCP referred Mrs. U to the consulting psychiatrist. The psychiatrist found Mrs. U to be pleasant and talkative, and she anxiously stated, "My vision has been worsening in the last two weeks." She described herself as being a "worrier," and her son confirmed that she had always been extremely nervous and impatient, would be "easily stressed," and thought and feared the worst in any situation. Mrs. U denied any depressive symptoms, and her son confirmed that she had not had any significant depressive symptoms in the past. Mrs. U's PCP evaluated her for a UTI, constipation, pain, electrolyte imbalance, thyroid dysfunction, and vitamin deficiency and did not find any problems. Mrs. U's vision complaints were not new and were due to macular degeneration, which was being addressed by the ophthalmologist. The pharmacist reviewed Mrs. U's medications, recommended discontinuing cyclobenzaprine (which the PCP subsequently discontinued), but did not find any other medication that could cause anxiety. Mrs. U's Montreal Cognitive Assessment (MOCA) score was 24 (indicating relatively intact cognitive function, given her age and vision problems), and her Geriatric Depression Scale (GDS) score was 5 (suggesting minimal depression). The psychiatrist diagnosed Mrs. U as having GAD and mild cognitive impairment. The psychiatrist started Mrs. U on buspirone 5 mg twice daily and after one week increased it to 10 mg twice daily. After two weeks, the dosage was further increased to 15 mg twice daily. The psychiatrist also recommended that the family visit as often as possible, have an "active visit" rather than asking questions, and counseled the family regarding some of the activities they could do with Mrs. U. The family would sit with Mrs. U and encourage her to tell stories about her younger days on the farm. The family would also take Mrs. U for a 10-minute walk each time they visited, listen to Mrs. U's favorite music and reminisce, and watch baseball games on TV and keep Mrs. U informed about the game. The staff were encouraged to avoid telling the family that Mrs. U "was not doing well" but instead to reassure the family that with time, Mrs. U should start feeling better with the current care plan. After four more weeks, the family and staff noticed that Mrs. U was better and her anxiety was less. Over the next three months, Mrs. U continued to show further improvement, with only one to two episodes of anxiety and yelling per week.

Teaching Points

It is not uncommon for a resident to need to try multiple medications to manage anxiety disorder before finding a psychotropic that is tolerated and effective. Although antidepressant is usually the first-line agent for pharmacotherapy of GAD, the HCP should also consider prescribing buspirone as a first-line treatment option for a resident who has GAD. The full effects of medication for anxiety disorder may take a few months. Specific guidance and counseling of family and staff regarding psychosocial approaches has a much higher success rate than nonspecific recommendations.

Panic Disorder and Agoraphobia

Panic disorder involves recurrent panic attacks associated with persistent concern about having more attacks and/or about the implication of an attack (for more than a month) (American Psychiatric Association 2013a). A panic attack involves a discrete period of intense fear or discomfort developing abruptly and reaching a peak within 10–15 minutes. During this period, the person may experience pounding of the heart, sweating, trembling, sensations of shortness of breath, chest pain or discomfort, nausea or abdominal distress, feeling dizzy, unsteady, lightheaded, or faint, fear of losing control or going crazy, fear of dying, numbness or tingling sensations, chills or hot flashes, and/or feeling of choking. Residents who have panic disorder usually have a long-standing history of panic attacks and anticipatory anxiety that significantly impaired their daily functioning. Residents who have panic disorder typically have been treated for anxiety symptoms with medication (antidepressant and/or benzodiazepine) by their HCP. Panic disorder may be accompanied by agoraphobia. Panic disorder may have onset in late life, with typical presentation being an older woman who was recently widowed (in the last year) and is experiencing chest pain and no evidence of coronary artery disease is found. Agoraphobia involves disabling anxiety about being in places or situations from which escape might be difficult (or embarrassing) or in which help may not be available in the event of having an unexpected panic attack. Agoraphobia may also occur in the absence of panic disorder and may have onset in later life. Most individuals who have late-onset agoraphobia do not have a history of panic attack and the illness often starts after a traumatic event.

Panic attack occurring for the first time in a resident usually is due to a condition other than panic disorder. Bereavement, alcohol withdrawal, benzodiazepine withdrawal, caffeine intoxication, cardiac arrhythmia, and pheochromocytoma are some conditions that may cause panic attack.

See Table 7.3 for evidence-based options for the treatment of panic disorder. A resident who has panic disorder should start on a low dose of antidepressant medication to avoid initial exacerbation of anxiety (but then gradually increase the dosage to the therapeutic range). Given the delayed onset of action of antidepressant medication (8–12 weeks), short-term use of an adjunctive low-dose short-acting benzodiazepine, such as lorazepam, in the first few weeks of treatment may be appropriate for a resident who has disabling anxiety. The HCP should continue a resident who has long-standing panic disorder and is stable taking antidepressant at the same dose but periodically evaluate her to detect any adverse effect that may occur due to the change in pharmacodynamic and pharmacokinetic physiologic processes related to aging, advancing MNCD, or worsening medical comorbidity. A resident who has panic disorder and has been taking benzodiazepine for decades and is stable may need to continue taking the drug because of the high morbidity associated with poorly controlled panic disorder. We recommend close monitoring for potential adverse effect of benzodiazepine (e.g. falls, sedation, cognitive impairment) and a gradual reduction in dosage as the resident ages or develops frailty or reduced clearance due to progressive kidney and/or liver disease. We recommend psychotherapy (e.g. cognitive behavioral therapy) and relaxation exercise for the motivated resident who has relatively intact cognitive function.

Clinical Case 2: "I am not addicted to Valium"

Ms. F was a 70-year-old resident who had a long history of severe panic disorder with agoraphobia. She had been stable for decades taking 5 mg of diazepam twice daily for the last 30 years along with 0.25 mg of alprazolam as needed once a day and imipramine 25 mg daily at bedtime. She was admitted to the NH for rehabilitation after receiving a second kidney transplant. Her PCP, who had prescribed her psychiatric medications for decades, had recently passed away and a young family practitioner took over her care. He felt that Ms. F carried a high risk of fall and confusion due to diazepam, as-needed alprazolam, and imipramine. He also felt that Ms. F had become addicted to diazepam. He scheduled a withdrawal regimen. Within a few weeks, Ms. F was severely agitated and required hospitalization to a psychiatric unit. She clearly told the psychiatrist, "I am not addicted to Valium." The psychiatrist discussed treatment options with Ms. F, including switching to an SSRI or mirtazapine or nortriptyline versus reinstating her original medications. Ms. F chose restarting her original medications, as they had helped her for several years and she was willing to risk the potential adverse effects, including cardiac risks, falls, and cognitive impairment. The psychiatrist reinstated Ms. F's original medication regimen, and Ms. F was back to her baseline level of functioning within a couple of weeks.

The psychiatrist also collaborated with the new PCP, explained the severity of the panic disorder and the plan for frequent outpatient follow-up visits to closely monitor risks for falls and cognitive impairment. The PCP agreed as long as the psychiatrist would continue to manage Ms. F's panic disorder.

Teaching Points

Panic disorder can be disabling. For a resident who has severe symptoms, it may be more prudent to continue benzodiazepine and/or tricyclic antidepressant (TCA) if the resident is tolerating it relatively well and has been stable. This is because reducing the dosage can quickly decompensate panic disorder, and alternative options (e.g. SSRI) may not have as good a therapeutic effect as the medications that initially were therapeutic. Close monitoring and thorough discussion of risks and benefits of benzodiazepine and TCA, including risks of falls and fracture, delirium, and cardiac toxicity, are necessary. The HCP should also discuss alternative treatment options, such as SSRI, mirtazapine, and cognitive behavioral therapy (CBT).

Social Anxiety Disorder (Social Phobia)

A resident who has social anxiety disorder typically has a long history of marked and persistent fear of one or more social or performance situations in which he is exposed to unfamiliar people or to possible scrutiny by others. The resident fears that he will act in a way (or show anxiety symptoms) that will be humiliating or embarrassing. The resident who has this disorder may avoid participating in group activities in the LTC facility. Management involves one or two staff members (e.g. social worker) establishing a trusting relationship with the resident, providing reassurance, and instituting a graded and gradual exposure to other residents and group activity. For severe and disabling symptoms, trial of one of the SSRIs may be necessary.

Specific Phobias

A resident who has a specific phobia has a long history of marked and persistent fear that is excessive or unreasonable, cued by the presence or anticipation of a specific object or situation (e.g. animals, receiving an injection, seeing blood, hospitals, flying, heights, storms). The resident may refuse blood tests or injections or become agitated and anxious during such tests. Specific phobias are best managed by psychosocial environmental approaches, such as helping the resident avoid the trigger when possible. For phobia involving injection and blood draw, this could mean preparing the resident emotionally for a blood test or injection and holding the resident's hand and, with a soothing voice and gentle approach, constantly reassuring her during a test or before receiving an injection.

The fear of falling is a specific phobia that is particularly prevalent in LTC populations. Fall phobia has been recognized as an important consequence of having experienced a fall. Between 30 and 73 percent of older adults who have fallen acknowledge a persistent fear of falling. Fear of falling is more common in LTC residents than in community-dwelling peers. This fear frequently leads residents voluntarily to restrict ambulation (even take to using a wheelchair) and activities, limiting their independence and ability to engage in routines and participate in activity programs in the LTC facility. This fear is best managed with psychosocial environmental approaches, such as reassurance using a soothing voice and gentle approach, encouragement, and positive reinforcement of desired behavior (e.g. efforts to walk despite fear). Working actively with physical therapy may be useful. If the phobia is persistent and disabling, the HCP should consider CBT for a resident who has relatively good cognitive function and/or a trial of an SSRI.

Anxiety Disorder due to or in the Context of Major Neurocognitive Disorder

Individual symptoms of anxiety (e.g. tension, restlessness, irritability, fear of being left alone, anxious or worried expression, fidgeting, pacing, anger, agitation, apprehension) are common among people who have MNCD. Symptoms of GAD have been reported in 5–6 percent of individuals who have AD. People who are in mild to moderate stages of AD may experience a sense of fear about an upcoming event (Godot syndrome) and therefore may ask questions about it repeatedly (often emotionally exhausting the family), or they may experience excessive fear of being left alone and as a result shadow the caregiver. Expecting more than what a resident who has MNCD is capable of (overexpectation) and changing routines are two of the most common triggers for significant anxiety symptoms and catastrophic reactions (emotional outbursts with severe agitation in response to feelings of helplessness). In addition, anxiety in a resident who has MNCD may be a reflection of the caregiver's stress, because people who have MNCD tend to mirror the emotions of those around them. Anxiety symptoms correlate with the severity of cognitive impairment. Anxiety symptoms in a resident who has MNCD are often comorbid with depression, hallucination, delusion, aggressiveness, angry outbursts, and disturbed activity, such as wandering. Some individual symptoms of anxiety disorder can be easily confused with MNCD. These symptoms include impairment in memory, attention, and concentration. Many residents who have MNCD may have undiagnosed premorbid anxiety disorder (especially GAD) that may worsen after the resident develops AD. Reliable and valid diagnostic tools to diagnose and quantify anxiety symptoms in individuals who have MNCD are lacking. Hence, we recommend that clinicians have a high index of suspicion for premorbid anxiety disorder in a resident who has MNCD and disabling anxiety symptoms.

Treatment primarily involves psychosocial spiritual and environmental approaches (e.g. hand massage, soothing music, aromatherapy, meaningful activity, spending time in natural surroundings, spending time with pets, avoiding and removing environmental triggers [e.g. countertherapeutic approach, such as being impatient, poor lighting causing shadows]). As a result of short-term memory loss, every day is a new and potentially stressful experience for the person who has MNCD. However, procedural memory is retained longer than the ability to form new memories. Therefore, rituals, consistency in routine, and consistency in caregivers go a long way to prevent anxiety. A calm and patient approach, frequent reassurance, and avoiding arguments with residents are key staff-oriented approaches to reduce anxiety. Reducing stress by modifying the environment (e.g. reducing the noise level by moving a resident from an activity with lots of sounds [singing and playing live music] to an activity that is relatively quiet [water coloring]) and reducing unrealistic demands on the resident who has MNCD (expecting the resident not to become agitated in response to another resident who is yelling or expecting a resident who has receptive aphasia to understand simple spoken language) can also reduce anxiety. Bathing can be anxiety provoking for a resident who has MNCD and can be better managed with towel baths by two staff members (one gently cleaning and the other soothing and distracting the resident) rather than a shower assisted by one staff member. We strongly recommend staff education and training using the DVD *Bathing without a Battle* (created by University of North Carolina, Chapel Hill) to reduce the fear of bathing and associated physical aggression in residents who have MNCD.

A resident who has MNCD and is experiencing severe anxiety symptoms may benefit from a trial of antidepressant or buspirone. Use of benzodiazepine (short acting, such as lorazepam or oxazepam) for anxiety symptoms should be restricted to the management of acute anxiety attacks or for short-term use to give antidepressant or buspirone time to start helping. Extreme anxiety before a visit to a dental clinic (or similar situation) can be aborted with a one-time use of low-dose benzodiazepine, such as 0.5 mg of lorazepam one hour before the visit.

Clinical Case 3: "Of course, I worry about him"

Mrs. B was a 91-year-old woman admitted to an AL home six months ago because of increasing agitation and anxiety. Mr. B, who was 93 years old, could no longer take care of her. Mrs. B had been diagnosed with MNCD due to AD three years ago, could not tolerate cholinesterase inhibitors (ChEIs) due to nausea and diarrhea, and had been taking memantine 10 mg twice daily for the last two years. Over the last year, she would become increasingly anxious and agitated and start yelling for her husband if she was left alone for even a few minutes. Mrs. B would worry that something terrible happened to Mr. B. She would not allow her husband to go anywhere, even if one of their three daughters agreed to stay with her. Mrs. B would try to leave the house to look for Mr. B and would become aggressive if someone tried to stop her. She showed the same behavior in the AL home, and although lorazepam 0.5 mg three times a day prescribed by her PCP had helped, she became more anxious on taking 50 mg sertraline. The family was growing increasingly frustrated because they would spend several hours with Mrs. B without success. Mr. B would become irate with Mrs. B, and her daughters could not understand why Mrs. B was "so stubborn." The psychiatrist was consulted at this point. The psychiatrist found out from Mrs. B's sister that Mrs. B had lost her younger brother through accidental drowning when she was 10 years old. Mrs. B was the oldest of six children and did not have any role in the drowning. Mrs. B's mother was overwhelmed with working on the farm and raising 6 children and had put a lot of responsibility on Mrs. B for housework and looking after her younger siblings. Mrs. B had expressed guilt off and on to her sister for several years and had always been an anxious and shy person who liked to be in her home and take care of her husband and three daughters. There was no history of her anxiety and shyness having caused significant impairment in daily functioning. Mrs. B was otherwise in good health. She denied any depressive symptoms during the interview. She reported that she had a difficult life, that her worries about her husband were "normal," and added, "Of course, I worry about him." Mrs. B denied her husband's report that she would become "belligerent." Mrs. B could not give a detailed history because of her MNCD, her MOCA score was 16, and her Geriatric Depression Scale–15 (GDS-15) score was 7. The psychiatrist diagnosed severe anxiety disorder with MNCD (with separation anxiety disorder like symptoms) and started her on 12.5 mg of sertraline and increased it every two weeks to a total of 50 mg. The psychiatrist also informed the staff at the AL home about Mrs. B's childhood trauma. The staff and family were also counseled that MNCD makes her more susceptible to emotional disorders because of past trauma. The staff became more sympathetic and allowed the medication more time to work and tried harder to distract Mrs. B. The family and staff were educated that SSRI such as sertraline may cause an initial increase in anxiety, especially in a patient who is already anxious, before improving anxiety. After eight weeks, the staff and family reported mild improvement in Ms. B's agitation and anxiety, especially her episodes of yelling and disrupting the environment. The psychiatrist further increased sertraline to 62.5 mg daily for two weeks and then to 75 mg daily. After eight more weeks, the anxiety and agitation were substantially less and yelling episodes were occasional and easily managed. The lorazepam was gradually decreased and changed to as-needed. Mrs. B used it on average once or twice a week.

Teaching Points

The starting dose of antidepressants for a person who has severe anxiety needs to be much lower and increased more slowly than for someone who has depression, and the time for response may be much longer. Explaining the possible impact of earlier trauma on the resident's current problems may allow the staff and family to view the resident with more empathy and patience.

Medication-Induced Anxiety Disorder

Many commonly prescribed and over-the-counter medications (including herbs and supplements) can cause anxiety symptoms and can mimic an anxiety disorder (Kotlyar et al. 2011; American Geriatrics Society 2015). (See Box 7.4.) Treatment involves discontinuing the offending drug or lowering its dosage. If this cannot be done (e.g. steroids cannot be reduced or discontinued), treatment of anxiety symptoms with psychosocial approaches and, in severe cases, medication (e.g. low-dose benzodiazepine) may be necessary.

Anxiety Disorder due to or in the Context of Parkinson's Disease

Anxiety disorder is seen in up to 40 percent of people who have Parkinson's disease (PD) (Chen and Marsh 2014). The most common anxiety disorders in people who have PD are panic disorder, GAD, social anxiety disorder, and anxiety coexisting with MDD-like symptoms. Assessing the timing of anxiety symptoms in people who have PD is important. If anxiety symptoms occur during the "on-off" period of motor fluctuations, adjustment of anti-Parkinsonian medication may reduce or resolve the anxiety symptoms. Assessment and treatment options are similar to those of other anxiety disorders listed in Tables 7.2 and 7.3.

Anxiety Disorder due to Other Medical Conditions

Medical conditions causing anxiety disorders or anxiety symptoms include but are not limited to pain, hypoglycemia, hyperthyroidism, migraine, pheochromocytoma, hyperadrenalism (Cushing disease), cardiac arrhythmia, COPD, stroke, and brain tumor (Lenz, Mohlman, and Wetherell 2015; Campbell Burton et al. 2013). Residents who have anxiety symptoms or disorder due to medical conditions typically have other signs of these medical conditions and do not have a long history of anxiety disorder, and a thorough history and physical exam, laboratory tests, and/or neuroimaging usually pinpoint these medical conditions. An acute episode of anxiety attack for the first time in a resident who has no prior history of anxiety disorder should prompt a thorough investigation to evaluate for a medical cause of anxiety symptoms if review of medication does not identify any obvious etiology. Treatment involves treating the cause. For example, an acute attack of anxiety may be secondary to hypoglycemia due to an antidiabetic agent or an attack of asthma. For a resident who has severe anxiety symptoms due to a medical condition (e.g. hyperthyroidism), symptomatic treatment with a psychiatric drug such as benzodiazepine (lowest possible dose, shortest possible time to treat acute severe anxiety symptoms) and/or antidepressant (especially for chronic anxiety symptoms) may be warranted.

Substance-Induced Anxiety Disorder

Alcohol withdrawal, caffeine intoxication (or excessive use of caffeine), opiate withdrawal, stimulant (e.g. cocaine, amphetamine) use, and cannabis use can trigger anxiety or panic symptoms and mimic any of the anxiety disorders previously mentioned. Management involves having a high index of suspicion, urine drug screen or serum alcohol levels as indicated, and administration of benzodiazepine for a short period of time for severe symptoms.

Anxiety Symptoms Associated with Delirium

Anxiety symptoms are common among residents who have delirium and usually occur along with illusion, visual or other hallucination, and paranoia, although they can occur in the absence of these symptoms. Dramatic fluctuation in sensorium and acute onset usually help differentiate this condition from other anxiety disorders. The HCP should avoid prescribing benzodiazepine to treat anxiety and agitation associated with delirium because of the high risk of exacerbating cognitive impairment in a resident who has delirium. Benzodiazepine may be prescribed for an anxious and agitated resident who has delirium in the last hours or days of life. Benzodiazepine is the drug of choice to treat delirium associated with alcohol and sedative-hypnotic withdrawal.

Trauma- and Stress-Related Disorders

Post-traumatic stress disorder (PTSD) and subsyndromal PTSD are the most serious trauma-related disorders seen in LTC populations. War veterans in veterans' homes and other LTC facilities have a high prevalence of PTSD. Lifetime exposure to traumatic events in older adults is high (40–70 percent). With the aging of the population, the prevalence of PTSD and other trauma-related disorders is expected to increase in LTC populations. Adjustment disorders are the most prevalent stress-related disorders in LTC populations.

Post-Traumatic Stress Disorder

The resident who has post-traumatic stress disorder (PTSD) has a history of being exposed to a traumatic event(s) that involved actual or threatened death or serious injury or a threat to the physical integrity of self or others (American Psychiatric Association 2013b). Examples of such traumatic events include being in war (as a civilian [e.g. Holocaust survivor] or as a soldier [in active combat and/or prisoner of war]), physical abuse, sexual abuse or rape or other violent crime, domestic violence, terrorist attack, mass shooting, natural disaster, or motor vehicle accident. Aging combat veterans make up the majority of residents who have PTSD (Barak 2011). Symptoms of PTSD involve persistently re-experiencing the traumatic event through recollections of images, thoughts, or perceptions, distressing dreams of the event, or acting as if the traumatic event were recurring (sense of reliving the experience [e.g. resident who is a war veteran acts as if bombs are falling and people are dying]); persistent avoidance of stimuli associated with the trauma (e.g. avoiding conversation about the trauma, efforts to avoid places or people that arouse recollections of the trauma); and symptoms of severe anxiety (irritability, outbursts of anger, impaired sleep). PTSD is a debilitating disorder. (See Box 7.3.) PTSD is associated with accelerated aging process and increased risk of future MNCD.

Events of later life may awaken long-suppressed memories and feelings and yield emotional or behavioral problems that are evidence of an early traumatic experience. These residents may under-report PTSD symptoms or the symptoms may be masked by other diagnoses. PTSD is often associated with MDD, substance use disorder (especially alcohol and cigarette smoking), panic disorder, GAD, and social anxiety disorder. PTSD-like symptoms can develop for the first time after the onset of MNCD if the resident was exposed to a traumatic event. Alternatively, a resident may have a history of PTSD that was under fairly good control until the onset of MNCD. The neurodegeneration of memory pathways may disinhibit symptoms of PTSD. The discussion of acts of terrorism and war may be particularly disturbing for a resident who survived traumatic events in the past. Thus, any LTC resident who has a history of being in active combat should be screened for PTSD. Veterans who have PTSD have higher rates of MNCD (especially AD and MNCD due to cerebrovascular disease). Residents who have more severe trauma (prisoners of war) are at high risk of developing paranoia and even psychotic symptoms along with PTSD. A violent outburst related to PTSD symptoms in a resident who has MNCD may precipitate an emergency department visit or police involvement. Many residents who have been in an intensive care unit recently may have PTSD-like symptoms, especially if they were in physical restraint without sedation, were in deep sedation, or could recall delusional memories (e.g. interpreting a simple injection as an attempted homicide). A resident who has a history of psychological problems may be at increased risk of PTSD after a stay in the ICU. For a considerable number of older adults, losing a spouse in late life appears to be a traumatic experience. Some bereaved residents may experience subsyndromal PTSD-like symptoms.

A variety of evidence-based approaches are available to treat PTSD. (See Table 7.4.) Treatment of a

Table 7.4 Evidence-Based Approaches to Treat Post-Traumatic Stress Disorder

Approach	Clinical Pearls	Key Concerns/Limitations
SSRIs	First-line pharmacological treatment for disabling PTSD symptoms Clinically obvious benefit may take 12 or more weeks at highest tolerated dose	There may be transient increase in anxiety symptoms during initiation of SSRI and during increase in dosage
Prazosin (1–3 mg daily at bedtime)	First-line treatment for disabling nightmare in context of PTSD	Orthostatic hypotension and drug-drug interaction with antihypertensive, alpha-one antagonist, and other cardiovascular drugs is serious concern
Benzodiazepine	Short-acting benzodiazepine (e.g. lorazepam) may be used to treat acute anxiety attack related to PTSD	Falls risk and worsening of cognitive impairment are key concerns
Onsite individual counseling/ psychotherapy (trauma-focused cognitive behavioral therapy [TFCBT], prolonged exposure therapy [PE], cognitive reprocessing therapy, supportive psychotherapy, mindfulness-based therapy, eye movement desensitization and reprocessing [EMDR])	TFCBT, cognitive reprocessing therapy and PE are first-line treatment for motivated resident who has PTSD and relatively intact cognitive function HCP should also consider supportive psychotherapy, and EMDR for resident who has relatively intact cognitive function	Lack of availability of counselors trained in providing psychotherapy services for LTC populations Lack of availability of counselors visiting LTC facilities to provide psychotherapy services Resident may need to visit local mental health clinic for such services
Internet-guided or telepsychiatry treatment	Cognitive restructuring (to address cognitive distortion) and relaxation training can be effectively administered via Internet or telepsychiatry by psychiatric nurse or other mental health professional to treat many PTSD symptoms (e.g. anxiety, insomnia, avoiding social situations)	Resident needs to be motivated and have relatively intact cognitive function Technophobia (in resident as well as staff) may be a difficult barrier to overcome
Psychoeducation and self-management	Providing pamphlets and other educational material on PTSD and related disorders and relaxation strategies	Cognitive deficit in resident may limit its benefit
Support group	Adjuvant to other treatment for motivated resident who has relatively intact cognitive function VA home is ideal LTC facility for support group	Most LTC facilities may have difficulty identifying three or more residents who have PTSD and would be appropriate for support group

Table 7.4 (cont.)

Approach	Clinical Pearls	Key Concerns/Limitations
Omega-3 fatty acid supplementation	Eicosapentanoic acid (EPA) and ethyl-EPA dominant formulation recommended	Small risk of increased bleeding, especially with concomitant use of NSAID, anticoagulant, antiplatelet, SSRI, or SNRI
Rational deprescribing (geriatric scalpel) with input from consultant pharmacist	Discontinuation of unnecessary or inappropriate medication (based on Beers list) and reducing anticholinergic burden may improve resident's cognitive and emotional functioning and reduce adverse drug–drug interaction with medication used to treat PTSD	None
Optimizing control of pain and other comorbid physical health problem (e.g. diabetes) and correction of reversible physical health problem (e.g. dehydration, constipation, vision or hearing impairment, thyroid disorder)	Recommended for all residents	None

resident who has PTSD involves antidepressant. Benzodiazepine may be needed for short-term treatment of severe anxiety and antipsychotic if the resident develops severe psychotic symptoms with agitation. A resident who has PTSD and is motivated and has relatively preserved cognitive function may benefit from psychotherapy. The HCP should consider recommending that a resident who has a history of being in war or having witnessed a terrorist attack avoid news from TV, radio, or newspaper.

Clinical Case 4: "Bombs are falling! Run, run!"

Mr. M was a 92-year-old resident living in a NH. He had been experiencing nightmares, verbal and physical aggression, anxiety, and hypervigilance. He would also shout, "Bombs are falling! Run, run!," thereby agitating other residents. He was also isolating himself for several weeks. These symptoms started after Mr. M watched images of recent terrorist attacks on the TV. The staff at the NH felt that he should be hospitalized in a psychiatric unit, as he was "psychotic." The consulting psychiatrist was asked to help facilitate the hospitalization. The psychiatrist made an emergency psychiatric evaluation of Mr. M, and Mr. M's wife reported that he was an Army infantry man from 1942 to 1945. He had been in prolonged, intense combat in Sicily and Normandy. He had experienced mild PTSD symptoms and severe depression from 1946 to 1949. Symptoms gradually decreased after he started meeting regularly with a group of friends who were also in World War II. Married for 57 years, Mr. M had four children and 11 grandchildren; his wife reported that Mr. M was an easygoing person who seemed to enjoy life until he entered the NH due to multiple medical problems. He had a successful career as a banker and never abused drugs or alcohol. He developed severe peripheral vascular disease, resulting in bilateral above-knee amputation of his legs for the treatment of gangrene. He subsequently developed severe congestive heart failure and was admitted to the NH, as his wife could no longer take care of his increasing physical needs at home. The psychiatrist after evaluation counseled the family and staff that Mr. M's behaviors could be managed in the LTC facility if everyone collaborated in helping Mr. M and that hospitalization carried its own risks of increased confusion, delirium, functional decline, falls, and other iatrogenic problems. The psychiatrist recommended starting sertraline 12.5 mg daily and increased it every seven days to a total of 50 mg daily. The psychiatrist also started Mr. M on clonazepam 0.25 mg in the morning and at bedtime but due to daytime sedation, discontinued the morning dose. Family were encouraged and successful in finding a World War II veteran to visit Mr. M several times a week. Only comedy and game shows were kept on the TV in his room as well as at other places by astute staff. The psychiatrist also recommended to the family and staff to avoid discussion of the terrorist attacks with Mr. M and to have him avoid watching news on TV. A list of topics for conversation that did not involve war, politics, religion, or terrorist attacks was devised in consultation with the staff and family. After two weeks, Mr. M was less agitated but continued to have nightmares, aggression, and nighttime agitation. The psychiatrist discussed the use of prazosin for nightmares but because of significant risk of orthostatic hypotension, it was not started. The psychiatrist increased the dosage of clonazepam to 0.5 mg at bedtime, but Mr. M had two falls (no injuries) and the dose was decreased to 0.25 mg. The psychiatrist added mirtazapine 7.5 mg at bedtime and Mr. M started sleeping better over the next two weeks. Over the next three months, Mr. M gradually became significantly less anxious, started sleeping better regularly, and his verbal and physical aggression resolved.

Teaching Points

Treatment of disabling PTSD may involve multiple medications. A comprehensive plan, team approach, aggressive psychosocial approaches, close monitoring of adverse effect, and prompt change in medication that causes adverse effect often allow the disorder of the resident who has severe PTSD to be managed safely in the LTC facility and can avoid hospitalization.

Adjustment Disorder with Anxiety

Residents who have adjustment disorder with anxiety develop significant anxiety symptoms (worries, muscle tension, nervousness, agitation, jitteriness) in response to an identifiable stressor(s) (e.g. hospitalization of spouse). Anxiety symptoms usually occur within three months of the onset stressor(s). Treatment usually is reassurance, emotional support, and other psychosocial environmental approaches. In severe cases, low-dose benzodiazepine for a few days as needed may be warranted.

Obsessive-Compulsive Disorder

Obsessions involve recurrent and persistent thoughts, impulses, or images that are intrusive and unwanted and that cause marked anxiety. Compulsions are repetitive behaviors (e.g. hand washing, ordering, checking) or mental acts (e.g. praying, counting, repeating words silently) that the person feels driven to perform in response to an obsession or according to rules that must be applied rigidly. Obsessive-compulsive disorder (OCD) is diagnosed in a person who has obsessions and/or compulsions that last one or more hours per day and cause significant suffering and impairment in daily functioning (American Psychiatric Association 2013c). OCD usually starts in young adulthood and often persists into later life. Thus, residents who have OCD have a long-standing history. Up to 20 percent of individuals may experience remission of symptoms by middle and older age, and another 20 percent may have substantial reduction in symptoms in late life. Older individuals who have OCD have fewer concerns about symmetry, need to know, and counting rituals than do younger individuals who have OCD. Handwashing and fear of having sinned may be more common in older adults who have OCD than in younger people who have OCD. OCD symptoms for the first time in the older adults are rare and usually due to neurological disorder, such as a stroke in the basal ganglia. A variety of evidence-based approaches are available for the management of OCD (Grant 2014). (See Table 7.5.) Treatment of a resident who has OCD is primarily with one of the SSRIs. A motivated resident who has relatively intact cognitive function should be offered exposure and response prevention (ERP) therapy and CBT. Educating the staff about OCD and the need to accommodate the resident's compulsive behavior is the most important psychosocial approach.

Hoarding Disorder

Hoarding disorder is characterized by persistent difficulty parting with or getting rid of possessions (e.g. clothes, furniture, mail, bags, books) due to a strong need to save due to perceived utility or value or sentimental attachment. There is considerable distress associated with any effort to discard possessions. Excessive collecting of items that are not needed (e.g. leaflets, items discarded by others) often accompanies these symptoms. Over months to years, the house of a person who has hoarding disorder becomes severely cluttered and ability to live safely can be compromised (e.g. clutter increases fall risks and poses a fire hazard). Onset is before age 30, and late-onset hoarding disorder is typically due to stroke, TBI, or other lesion affecting basal ganglia and related networks. Hoarding disorder may be the most common obsessive-compulsive and related disorder in older

Table 7.5 Evidence-based Approaches to Treat Obsessive-Compulsive and Related Disorders

Approach	Clinical Pearls	Key Concerns/Limitations
SSRI	First-line treatment for OCD Starting dose needs to be lower than that for MDD, but most effective dose for OCD may be higher than that for MDD Clinically obvious benefit may take 12 or more weeks at highest tolerated dose	There may be transient increase in anxiety symptoms during initiation of SSRI and during increase in dosage
Clomipramine	Second-line treatment for OCD	Cognitive impairment due to its anticholinergic activity severely limits its use
Atypical antipsychotic	May be appropriate as augmentation therapy (e.g. augmenting SSRI or clomipramine) for incapacitating symptoms	High risks associated with use of atypical antipsychotic in LTC populations limit its use
Onsite individual counseling/ psychotherapy (cognitive behavioral therapy [CBT], exposure and response prevention [ERP], and supportive psychotherapy)	Psychotherapy is first-line treatment for motivated resident who has obsessive-compulsive or related disorder and relatively intact cognitive function	Lack of availability of counselors trained in providing psychotherapy to LTC populations Lack of availability of counselors visiting LTC facilities to provide psychotherapy services Resident may need to visit local mental health clinic for such services
Internet-guided or telepsychiatry treatment	Cognitive restructuring (to address cognitive distortion) and relaxation training can be effectively administered via Internet or telepsychiatry by psychiatric nurse or other mental health professional to treat anxiety symptoms	Resident needs to be motivated and have relatively intact cognitive function Technophobia (in resident as well as staff) may be a difficult barrier to overcome
Psychoeducation and self-management	Providing pamphlets and other educational material on obsessive-compulsive and related disorders and relaxation strategies	Cognitive deficit in resident may limit its benefit
Neuromodulation therapy	FDA approved deep brain stimulation for treatment-refractory and incapacitating OCD	Need for involvement of psychiatrist at academic center that specializes in this treatment option Higher risks in LTC populations limit its use
Neurosurgery	Ablation neurosurgery (cingulotomy, capsulotomy) for treatment-refractory and incapacitating OCD	Need for involvement of psychiatrist at academic center that specializes in this treatment option Higher risks in LTC populations limit its use
Omega-3 fatty acid supplementation	Eicosapentanoic acid (EPA) and ethyl-EPA dominant formulation recommended	Small risk of increased bleeding, especially with concomitant use of NSAID, anticoagulant, antiplatelet, SSRI, or SNRI

Table 7.5 (cont.)

Approach	Clinical Pearls	Key Concerns/Limitations
Rational deprescribing (geriatric scalpel) with input from consultant pharmacist	Discontinuation of unnecessary or inappropriate medication (based on Beers list) and reducing anticholinergic burden may improve resident's cognitive and emotional functioning and reduce adverse drug–drug interaction with medication used to treat obsessive-compulsive or related disorder	None
Optimizing control of pain and other comorbid physical health problem (e.g. diabetes) and correction of reversible physical health problem (e.g. dehydration, constipation, vision or hearing impairment, thyroid disorder)	Recommended for all residents	None

adults. Hoarding symptoms are three times more prevalent in older adults as in younger adults (American Psychiatric Association 2013c). Like OCD, it is a chronic disorder, but unlike OCD, in the majority of residents, it usually has not been formally diagnosed unless there have been severe complications. Typically, diagnosis is first made after the resident enters a LTC facility and characteristic manifestations begin to severely impair the resident's ability to adjust to living in a LTC facility. Treatment involves accommodating some of the resident's hoarding behaviors and emotional support. If symptoms are disabling, CBT for a motivated resident who has relatively intact cognitive function is the first-line treatment and/or a trial of an SSRI may be warranted.

Excoriation (Skin Picking) Disorder

Excoriation disorder is characterized by recurrent skin-picking behavior that results in multiple skin lesions. Skin picking is not in response to a specific dermatologic or other medical condition. Like other obsessive-compulsive and related disorders, it is a chronic disorder (with some waxing and waning of symptoms) with onset usually before age 30. A resident who has this disorder may have had remission of symptoms for years and may have a recurrence due to stress after entering a LTC facility. We strongly recommend seeking input of a dermatologist, as comorbid skin condition that causes itching (e.g. scabies, eczema, opioids) may be prevalent and needs to be diagnosed early so that comprehensive treatment of excoriation disorder as well as other dermatologic problem can be promptly instituted and serious complication (e.g. cellulitis) prevented.

Sleep-Wake Disorders

Several sleep-wake disorders are prevalent in LTC populations (Neikrug and Ancoli-Israel 2010). (See Box 7.2.) Point prevalence of sleep-wake disorders in LTC populations ranges from 10 to 20 percent. Sleep-wake disorders can be debilitating. (See Box 7.3.) The immense stress on family caregivers, who are repeatedly awakened by the affected loved one with nighttime awakening and behavioral disturbance night after night, often leads to admission to LTC of the person who has MNCD. Insomnia often plays a role in both the etiology and the presentation of delirium for a resident who has MNCD. The insomnia and resultant attempts at pharmacological treatment are equally implicated in the potential sequelae, ranging from excessive daytime somnolence to falls, accidents, and injury (e.g. hip fracture, subdural hematoma). Sleep disorders, in particular, nighttime behavioral disturbances, can also have a negative effect on the quality of life of other residents (especially roommates) and increase stress on staff. Hence, recognition and treatment of sleep-wake disorders is important in improving the quality of life of residents. We

Table 7.6 Diagnostic Work-Up for Sleep-Wake Disorder

Diagnostic Test	Key Examples	Key Implications for Treatment
Comprehensive assessment	Psychiatric history (including history of use of hypnotics, benzodiazepines) Daily sleep diary (2–4 weeks) Family history (including history RLS) Review of medication Vital signs Physical examination (including height, weight, body mass index) Neurological examination Mental status examination Use of standardized assessment scales Review of previous psychiatric records	Most residents who have disabling insomnia or excessive daytime sleepiness (EDS) have multiple factors contributing to symptoms (see Boxes 7.6 and 7.9) in addition to one or more specific primary sleep disorders Findings from cognitive assessment are key to choosing treatment (e.g. CBT-I for resident who has relatively intact cognitive function)
Bedside test	Pulse oximetry	Hypoxia may contribute to sleep-wake disturbance
Bedside test	Glucose fingerstick	Hypoglycemia may cause or contribute to sleep-wake disturbance
Laboratory test	Comprehensive metabolic panel	Dehydration and electrolyte imbalance may contribute to or cause sleep-wake disturbance and resistance to treatment of primary sleep-wake disorder
Laboratory test	Thyroid function tests (e.g. thyroid stimulating hormone level)	Thyroid dysfunction may contribute to or cause sleep-wake disturbance and resistance to treatment of primary sleep-wake disorder
Laboratory test	Serum drug levels	Serum levels of digoxin may help clarify diagnosis of digoxin-induced sleep-wake disturbance
Laboratory or bedside test	Electrocardiogram	Arrhythmia may contribute to or cause sleep-wake disturbance
Laboratory test	Electroencephalography	EEG may clarify diagnosis of sleep-wake disorder due to seizure in daytime (sleep-wake disturbance during ictal, postictal, interictal states) and nocturnal seizure (may mimic RBD)
Laboratory test	Polysomnography	Referral to a sleep disorder specialist for polysomnography is recommended if HCP suspects OSA, RLS, RBD, or PLMD or usual treatment approaches are not effective

recommend comprehensive assessment for any disabling sleep-wake disturbance (Krystal and Thakur 2015). (See Table 7.6.) Review of all current medications given by the LTC facility as well as medications (over-the-counter medications, herbal remedies, and supplements) taken by the resident (or given by family caregivers without the knowledge of or documentation by the staff) and timing of medications is crucial, as medication-induced sleep-wake problems are the most prevalent reversible factor. The HCP should also inquire into the resident's daily intake of caffeine, chocolate, fluids, alcohol, and smoking. Resident or caregiver reports or diary of sleep for the preceding two to four weeks can be useful in determining a pattern of sleep disruption that includes the onset, duration, total sleep time, frequency, and severity of sleep disturbances. The HCP should also evaluate the resident's lifestyle in relation to sleeping habits (e.g. diet, times of meals and snacks, regularity of sleep and awakening times, use of bed for activity other than sleep (e.g. watching TV, eating, reading) for a resident who has persistent sleep-wake disturbance. If the HCP suspects obstructive sleep apnea (OSA), restless legs syndrome (RLS), or RBD and in treatment-resistant cases, we recommend referral to a sleep disorder specialist (e.g. sleep disorders fellowship-trained psychiatrist, pulmonologist, neurologist, internist, family medicine physician).

Physiological changes associated with aging (fragmented nocturnal sleep, increased daytime napping, and decrease in slow-wave sleep), psychosocial-environmental factors, and medication are most commonly implicated in the etiology of sleep-wake disorders (Sorathia and Ghori 2016). (See Boxes 7.4, 7.5, and 7.7.) Other major causes of sleep disturbance in these populations include pathological involvement of suprachiasmatic nucleus (e.g. due to MNCD, stroke, TBI, PD) and the effects of co-occurring medical disorder (e.g. untreated pain, sleep apnea, RLS) and/or psychiatric disorders (e.g. MDD, GAD).

BOX 7.7 Common Environmental and Psychosocial Factors Causing or Contributing to Sleep-Wake Disorder

Environmental factors
- Inadequate exposure to light in daytime (low daytime indoor illumination, little time spent outdoors)
- Excessive exposure to light at night (light suppresses melatonin secretion)
- Excessive noise at night
- Uncomfortable bed
- Room is too hot or too cold
- Room is too dry or too humid
- Sleep interrupted by staff or other resident

Poor sleep hygiene/lifestyle factors
- Excessive daytime napping
- Spending too much time in bed
- Keeping irregular sleep-wake schedule
- Lying down in bed for activity other than sleep (e.g. watching television, eating, reading)
- Sedentary lifestyle/being physically inactive
- Inadequate social, intellectual, and physical stimulation
- Routine use of product that may interfere with sleep (e.g. caffeine, nicotine, alcohol)

Change in living situation
- Newly admitted resident
- Moving to a different LTC facility
- Change of room
- Change of roommate

Sleep-wake disorders should be differentiated from other psychiatric disorders associated with sleep-wake disturbance. Acute delirium due to any etiology can have insomnia or excessive daytime sleep (EDS) as a dominant feature of the initial presentation. A hallmark sign of untreated or undertreated (partially improved) MDD (especially in a resident who has MNCD) can be nighttime agitation or insomnia. Nightmares are one of the key symptoms of PTSD, and RBD may also occasionally be seen in a resident who has a history of PTSD.

Persistent distressing insomnia is neither a normal part of aging nor a typical consequence of living in a LTC facility. Self-reported difficulty with sleep is even more common and more severe among LTC residents than among older adults living in the community. Residents are commonly asleep intermittently at all hours of the day, even during mealtime periods. The sleep of LTC residents is distributed across the 24-hour day rather than being consolidated to the nighttime hours. Residents are rarely asleep or awake for a continuous hour during the day or night. Residents are usually exposed to less bright light and sunlight than younger community-dwelling adults and require more light to maintain normal circadian rhythm than do younger adults. Many residents who have even mild sleep-wake disturbance have difficulty staying awake during activities, have problems maintaining concentration and memory during the day, and feel overwhelmed with a desire to sleep at inappropriate times (e.g. meals). Thus, we recommend comprehensively addressing even mild sleep-wake disturbance.

Treatment

Sleep-wake disorders are often mismanaged in LTC populations, with excessive focus on pharmacologic approaches and limited use of nonpharmacologic approaches. A variety of evidence-based approaches are available to treat sleep-wake disorders. (See Box 7.8 and Table 7.7.) The choice depends on identified etiology, preferences of the resident and family, comorbidity (including risk of falls), motivation, and cognitive capacity to engage in CBT. Treatment of sleep disorder is treatment of its cause (e.g. OSA or RLS). For many residents (e.g. residents who have advanced MNCD), polysomnography may not be practical. For these residents, tentative diagnosis after observation of their behavior at night, bedside pulse oximetry, and

BOX 7.8 Evidence-Based Approaches to Treat Insomnia

Dietary approaches
- Restrict intake of caffeine and chocolate, particularly in evening
- Avoid heavy meal late at night
- Offer light snack (e.g. glass of milk, crackers) if nighttime awakening caused by hunger
- Avoid fluid intake in evening by resident who has nocturia and encourage maximum bladder emptying before retiring
- Switch from alcoholic to nonalcoholic beverage

Environmental approaches
- Limit time spent in bed
- Remove clock from room (especially if resident repeatedly looks at clock while trying to sleep)
- Increase exposure to natural light in daytime (30–60 minutes or more per day, preferably outdoors [with appropriate use of sunscreen], but sitting next to window [open window if weather permits and resident is agreeable] is also worthwhile)
- Increase exposure to indoor light in daytime on cloudy or rainy days
- Bright light therapy (20 minutes to 2 hours in morning)
- Ensure optimal room temperature and humidity
- Reduce nighttime noise and nighttime exposure to bright light
- Use of low-intensity nightlight for resident who has nightmare and/or other fear may promote sleep and increase safety during nighttime awakening (e.g. to void urine)
- Change room if conflict with roommate or location of room is an issue

Activity-oriented approaches
- Limit daytime napping to short period in morning or early afternoon
- Increase physical activity in daytime (e.g. regular exercise program)
- Increase meaningful activity and socialization in daytime
- Offer warm bath in evening
- Avoid excessive stimulation and exercise after dinnertime

Sleep hygiene
- Regular sleeping and waking times and structured bedtime routine
- Calming bedtime rituals (e.g. soothing music, reading or listening to nonfiction books [such as spiritual and religious books])
- Use bed only for sleep (rather than watching TV, eating, or reading)

Staff-oriented approaches
- Educate and train staff regarding evaluation and treatment of insomnia and other sleep disorders
- Staff address resident's maladaptive beliefs regarding sleeplessness
- Staff teach and assist resident in relaxation strategies
- Staff mediate differences between roommates (e.g. one resident wants to watch TV late at night, thus disturbing roommate who wants to sleep early) or better pairing of residents living in one room
- Minimize staff interrupting resident's sleep
- Offer massage therapy (e.g. back rub, hand massage)
- Aromatherapy

Approaches for motivated resident who has relatively intact cognitive function
- Relaxation training (e.g. deep breathing exercises, visualization exercises, progressive muscle relaxation, listening to soothing music, repeating self-soothing thoughts)
- Cognitive behavioral therapy for insomnia (CBT-I) including Internet-based CBT-I

BOX 7.8 (cont.)

Stimulus control therapy (go to bed only when feeling sleepy, get out of bed if not asleep after 20 minutes)

Sleep restriction therapy (limit time in bed to total perceived sleep time [not less than 6 hours])

Pharmacological approaches

If HCP suspects medication causes or contributes to insomnia, discontinue offending agent, reduce dosage, change timing, or replace medication with better alternative

Restrict use of alcohol and tobacco, particularly in evening

Judicious trial of ramelteon or suvorexant for chronic insomnia

Judicious short-term use of hypnotic (e.g. zolpidem, zaleplon, eszopiclone) for severe insomnia due to acute stress (e.g. resident's spouse is hospitalized)

Tasimelteon for non-24-hour circadian rhythm disorder (classically seen in individual who has congenital blindness but may be seen in individual who acquired blindness late in life)

Antidepressant with sedating properties to treat insomnia (e.g. low-dose trazodone [25-50 mg], mirtazapine)

Atypical antipsychotic with sedating properties to treat insomnia in resident who has severe psychotic symptoms (e.g. quetiapine)

Pharmacological treatment of underlying medical condition (e.g. analgesic to treat pain, CPAP for OSAHS, dopamine agonist for RLS, clonazepam for RBD, antibiotic for infection)

Supplement or herbal remedy (e.g. melatonin, chamomile tea [half an hour before routine sleep time], valerian, lettuce-leaf oil)

trial of appropriate treatment (e.g. CPAP for OSA, pramipexole or ropinirole for RLS, clonazepam for RBD) may be appropriate.

It is apparent that sleep problems are the result of many underlying disturbances. Thus, approaches need to be multifaceted. The first step is to review the resident's medication and discontinue any offending medication(s), reducing its dosage (e.g. reducing the dosage of memantine from 10 mg twice daily to once daily at bedtime [especially for a resident who has moderate to severe kidney insufficiency] may improve EDS) or replacing it with a better alternative agent (e.g. replacing amitriptyline, which has high anticholinergic activity, with nortriptyline, which has much lower anticholinergic activity, may improve EDS). Changing the timing of administration of some medications (e.g. changing donepezil from bedtime administration to morning for a resident who is experiencing insomnia and/or vivid dreams/nightmares) may improve sleep problems. In most situations, more needs to be done.

The next step is a multicomponent psychosocial environmental approach (Box 7.8). Although this may seem daunting for already overburdened staff, a mini-education session with staff, enlisting family or volunteers when possible, and praising staff for making an effort may provide successful outcome. If the resident is not disruptive at night and adequate supervision can be provided, the HCP should consider allowing the resident to sleep in the daytime and be awake at night.

The HCP may consider pharmacological approaches if sleep-wake problems are debilitating, psychosocial-environmental approaches fail, and the potential benefit of a pharmacological approach outweighs the risk of adverse effect. The HCP may consider short-term use of hypnotic (e.g. zolpidem, zaleplon, eszopiclone) for acute-onset insomnia related to a specific stressor (e.g. death of a loved one) or while waiting for antidepressant to improve depressive or anxiety symptoms. The HCP should minimize the use of hypnotic, especially by an ambulatory resident, frail resident, or resident who has severe cognitive impairment, because of the risks of falls and cognitive impairment. When used, hypnotics should be used for the shortest possible duration and following the OBRA or similar governmental guidelines. The HCP may consider prescribing a sedating antidepressant (e.g. low-dose mirtazapine or trazodone) to treat chronic insomnia in some residents (e.g. a resident who has low-grade depression or anxiety). Treatment of psychiatric disorders (e.g. antidepressant for MDD) may improve insomnia without any need for hypnotic. A combination of melatonin given at night and bright-light treatment in daytime may also help manage disturbed circadian

Table 7.7 Evidence-Based Approaches to Treat Sleep-Wake Disorder

Approach	Clinical Pearls	Key Concerns/Limitations
Onsite individual counseling/ psychotherapy (cognitive behavior therapy-insomnia [CBT-I])	Psychotherapy is first-line treatment for motivated resident who has insomnia disorder and has relatively intact cognitive function	Lack of availability of counselors trained in providing psychotherapy to LTC populations Lack of availability of counselors visiting LTC facilities to provide psychotherapy services Resident may need to visit local mental health clinic for such services
Internet-guided or telepsychiatry treatment	Cognitive restructuring (to address cognitive distortion) and relaxation training (CBT-I) can be effectively administered via Internet or telepsychiatry by psychiatric nurse or other mental health professional to treat insomnia disorder	Resident needs to be motivated and have relatively intact cognitive function Technophobia (in resident as well as staff) may be a difficult barrier to overcome
Psychoeducation and self-management	Providing pamphlets and other educational material on sleep-wake disorder and relaxation strategies	Cognitive deficit in resident may limit its benefit
CPAP, BiPAP	First-line treatment for sleep-wake disturbance due to OSA	Resident who has advanced MNCD may not comprehend importance of these approaches and hence may not adhere to treatment
Melatonin (1–9 mg daily at bedtime)	First-line treatment for Non 24-hour circadian rhythm disorder May be tried for sleep-onset insomnia disorder May be tried for sundowner syndrome May be tried for RBD	It is important to ensure that melatonin is from reliable source and pharmaceutical grade, as many formulations may not have the amount of melatonin claimed on label
Zaleplon (5–10 mg daily at bedtime)	Nonbenzodiazepine hypnotic May be considered for short-term (1–7 days) treatment of acute insomnia (due to known precipitant)	May increase risk of falls Potential for dependence (especially psychological but also physical), tolerance, and abuse
Zolpidem (2.5–5 mg daily at bedtime) Zolpidem controlled release (6.25 mg daily at bedtime) Zolpidem sublingual (1.7–5 mg daily at bedtime) Zolpidem oral spray (5 mg daily at bedtime)	Nonbenzodiazepine hypnotic May be considered for short-term (1–7 days) treatment of acute insomnia (due to known precipitant)	May increase risk of falls Potential for dependence (especially psychological but also physical), tolerance, and abuse; next-morning sedation
Eszopiclone (1–2 mg daily at bedtime)	Nonbenzodiazepine hypnotic May be considered for short-term (1–7 days) treatment of acute insomnia (due to known precipitant)	May increase risk of falls Potential for dependence (especially psychological but also physical), tolerance, and abuse
Suvorexant (5–20 mg daily at night)	Orexin-receptor antagonist May be considered first-line treatment for sleep-maintenance insomnia disorder	Not well studied in LTC populations; cost

Table 7.7 (cont.)

Approach	Clinical Pearls	Key Concerns/Limitations
	Preferred over other hypnotics because of better risk-benefit ratio (including no reports of dependence, tolerance, or abuse potential) May be used long term	
Ramelteon (4–8 mg daily at bedtime)	Melatonin 1 and 2 receptor agonist hypnotic May be considered first-line treatment for insomnia disorder Preferred over other hypnotics because of better risk-benefit ratio (including no reports of dependence, tolerance, or abuse potential) May be used long term	Not well studied in LTC populations
Doxepin (3–6 mg daily at bedtime)	Tricyclic antidepressant used as hypnotic in low doses Many residents may have been taking doxepin for insomnia disorder for years or even decades before coming to LTC facility For some residents who have been taking doxepin for years, benefit of continuing it may outweigh risks associated with its use	Strong anticholinergic effect and cardiac toxicity limit its use with LTC populations
Tasimelteon (20 mg daily at bedtime)	Melatonin receptor agonist Only FDA-approved medication for Non-24-hour sleep-wake disorder	Limited experience of its use with LTC populations; cost
Temazepam (7.5–15 mg daily at bedtime)	Benzodiazepine hypnotic Many residents may have been taking temazepam for insomnia disorder for years or even decades before coming to LTC facility For some residents who have been taking temazepam for years, benefit of continuing it may outweigh risks associated with its use	Increased risk of falls Potential for dependence (especially psychological but also physical), tolerance, and abuse Should be avoided with LTC populations, as risks are high and safer alternatives are available
Trazodone (25–50 mg daily at bedtime)	Enhances serotonergic neurotransmission May be used to treat insomnia for resident who has MDD	Increased risk of orthostatic hypotension and falls
Mirtazapine (7.5–15 mg daily at bedtime)	Enhances noradrenergic and serotonergic neurotransmission and alpha 2 antagonist May be used to treat insomnia for resident who has MDD	Increased risk of orthostatic hypotension and falls Weight gain associated with its use may be concern for resident who has obesity
Modafinil (50–200 mg daily in morning), Armodafinil (25–250 mg daily in morning)	Wake-promoting agents that HCP should consider for treatment of excessive daytime sleepiness (EDS) for resident who has OSAHS (especially if CPAP has not reduced EDS)	Not well studied in LTC populations May cause insomnia

Table 7.7 (cont.)

Approach	Clinical Pearls	Key Concerns/Limitations
Rational deprescribing (geriatric scalpel) with input from consultant pharmacist	Discontinuation of unnecessary or inappropriate medication (based on Beers list) and reducing anticholinergic burden may improve resident's cognitive and emotional functioning and reduce adverse drug–drug interaction with medication used to treat sleep-wake disorder	None
Optimizing control of pain and other comorbid physical health problem (e.g. diabetes) and correction of reversible physical health problem (e.g. dehydration, constipation, vision or hearing impairment, thyroid disorder)	Recommended for all residents	None

Note: Any medication used for insomnia may cause daytime sedation and increase risk of falls.

rhythm in a resident who has MNCD. We do not recommend prescribing tricyclic antidepressant, antihistaminic agent (e.g. diphenhydramine), certain sedative hypnotics (e.g. triazolam, flunitrazepam, flurazepam, barbiturate, chloral hydrate), or antipsychotic medication to treat insomnia in LTC residents due to the high risk of adverse effect (e.g. falls, daytime sedation, and decline in cognition and functioning). The HCP may consider prescribing modafinil, armodafinil, or methylphenidate for a resident who has MNCD and disabling EDS and does not have OSA or narcolepsy. OSA is a relative contraindication to the use of benzodiazepine and other agents that suppress respiratory drive. In situations where sleep-wake disturbances are due to other psychiatrist disorder (e.g. MDD), treatment of the underlying psychiatric disorder usually improves sleep-wake symptoms.

Insomnia Disorder

The resident who has insomnia disorder has persistent difficulty falling asleep, difficulty staying asleep (intermittent awakening), and/or early-morning awakening with subsequent difficulty going back to sleep (at least three nights per week for at least three months) (American Psychiatric Association 2013d). There is significant subjective distress, low energy/fatigue, difficulty concentrating, memory problems, irritability, verbal and physical aggression, decrease in daytime functioning, and increased risk of falls (Winkelman 2015). Prolonged (chronic) insomnia is an independent risk factor for MDD and suicide (independent of depression). Additionally, prolonged insomnia increases the risk of cardiovascular and cerebrovascular disease. Typically, the resident who has insomnia disorder has a long history of insomnia. The resident may also have a history of taking hypnotics for long periods of time. Even for a resident who has long-standing insomnia, we recommend a thorough evaluation for secondary causes of insomnia and comorbidity (e.g. MDD, pain). Treatment follows general principles mentioned before. Staff education and training in instituting sleep hygiene and other interventions listed in Box 7.8 is key to successful outcome.

Non-24-Hour Sleep-Wake Disorder

The diagnosis of non-24-hour sleep-wake disorder is made when a person has insomnia and/or EDS due to disruption in synchronization of 24-hour light-dark (day-night) cycle and the endogenous circadian rhythm. Residents who have congenital blindness or acquired blindness accompanied by loss or decrease of light perception often have or develop this disorder. Residents who have TBI are also at risk of developing this disorder. Treatment involves the use of melatonin to help align the endogenous cycle with the light-dark cycle. For severe cases, we recommend a trial of tasimelteon. Residents who have some light perception may respond to timed exposure to sunlight and bright light therapy.

Nightmare Disorder

Nightmare disorder is characterized by recurrent well-remembered nightmares (scary dreams involving threats to survival and security) that cause daytime distress and fear of going to sleep. Nightmares may be part of manifestations of PTSD. Some medications used to treat depression (e.g. SSRI, venlafaxine, bupropion), PD (e.g. levodopa, dopamine agonists [ropinirole, pramipexole, rotigotine]) can impair sleep by causing vivid dreams and nightmares. Any traumatic event that can cause PTSD can also cause nightmare disorder without PTSD. Nightmare disorder can be acute (duration less than one month), subacute (duration one to six months), or chronic (more than six months) (American Psychiatric Association 2013d). Psychosocial environmental approaches (e.g. removal of triggers such as news involving violence on TV, calming bedtime rituals, exercise) are the first line. The HCP may prescribe prazosin judiciously for disabling symptoms, although it carries a risk of orthostatic hypotension.

REM Sleep Behavior Disorder

REM sleep behavior disorder (RBD) is prevalent in LTC populations, and the diagnosis is often missed due to lack of awareness. RBD is a condition in which the central nervous system (CNS) mechanisms that cause muscle paralysis during REM sleep cease to function properly and the person experiences recurrent episodes of vocalization and complex motor behaviors during REM sleep ("acting out" dreams). It is typically seen in males older than 50 years. RBD precedes or accompanies many neurodegenerative disorders, especially synucleinopathies (e.g. DLB, PD, multisystem atrophy [MSA]) and less frequently tauopathies (e.g. AD, corticobasal degeneration [CBD], progressive supranuclear palsy [PSP], FTD). RBD is also described in amyotrophic lateral sclerosis (ALS), limbic encephalitis, epilepsy, and PTSD. In younger populations, RBD may be due to narcolepsy or induced by medication. RBD is confirmed with a sleep study in which the patient has dream enactment behavior associated with a loss of muscle atonia during REM sleep on polysomnographic electromyogram recordings. Muscle atonia is not only normal but necessary during REM sleep. The main concern associated with RBD is safety. A resident can fall out of bed or engage in dangerous behavior during the night as a result of acting out dream-related behaviors while asleep. Treatment involves securing the sleep environment to ensure safety. Treatment of RBD with a small dose of clonazepam (0.25–0.5 mg at night) is usually effective. High-dose melatonin may be tried before trial with clonazepam.

Restless Legs Syndrome

Restless Legs Syndrome (RLS, also called Ekbom syndrome) is common in LTC populations. RLS is defined as an irresistible desire to move one's legs, usually associated with paresthesia, other uncomfortable sensation in the legs, and motor restlessness. For diagnosis, symptoms need to be present for at least three nights per week for at least three months. The symptoms start or worsen at rest and improve with activity. Additionally, the symptoms worsen in the evening and/or night, which often results in disturbance of sleep with daytime tiredness. Other symptoms and signs of RLS include pacing/walking excessively, complaints of leg discomfort, flexing, stretching and crossing legs repeatedly, rubbing legs, and general restlessness. Diagnosis is clinical. In atypical presentations, polysomnographic evidence of periodic limb movements during sleep can help clarify the diagnosis. The pathophysiology of primary RLS is associated with a deficiency in dopaminergic neurotransmission. Secondary RLS occurs in association with iron-deficiency anemia, uremia, and polyneuropathy. The prevalence of primary RLS is twofold greater in women than men, and onset may occur in up to 45 percent of persons before the age of 20. Prevalence increases with age. People who have primary RLS often have a positive family history of RLS. Individuals who have poorly controlled RLS may develop depression. RLS may be responsible for some of the wandering, pacing, restlessness, agitation, and sleeplessness that occurs in residents who have MNCD. A resident whose insomnia and agitation improve with ambulation should be screened for RLS. For a resident who has intermittent RLS, we recommend nonpharmacologic therapy (e.g. scheduled walking, sleep hygiene, avoiding drugs that may worsen RLS [e.g. SSRI], and avoiding factors that provoke symptoms [sedentary lifestyle]). A resident who has daily RLS symptoms may need pharmacologic treatment. The pharmacologic treatment is iron supplementation if iron deficiency is present and/or a small dose of gabapentin, pregabalin or a dopamine agonist (e.g. pramipexole, ropinirole). We do not recommend using levodopa to treat RLS due to the risk of augmentation, in which the symptoms of RLS begin appearing earlier during the day and involve new parts of the body with increasing severity. In severe or refractory cases, we recommend referral to a movement disorder specialist (neurologist). In secondary RLS, the HCP should first treat the underlying illness, although gabapentin, pregabalin or a dopamine agonist may also be useful.

Obstructive Sleep Apnea/Hypopnea Syndrome

Obstructive Sleep Apnea/Hypopnea Syndrome (OSAHS) is a condition in which airflow during respiration is interrupted. This can occur because the airway collapses during sleep or because CNS signaling is impaired. These respiratory events can involve a complete cessation of airflow (apnea) or a partial reduction in airflow (hypopnea). Disturbed nocturnal breathing, such as snoring or snorting/gasping, is typically present. Events are considered clinically significant when they occur five or more times per hour of sleep. This can lead to decreased oxygen saturation, interruption of nighttime sleep, and daytime fatigue and sleepiness. Prevalence of OSAHS increases with age, reaching 20 percent in adults age 65 years or older. After age, obesity is the strongest risk factor. It is more common in males than females. OSAHS is prevalent and an under-recognized cause of insomnia, daytime sleepiness, and cognitive impairment in LTC residents. The HCP should suspect OSAHS in any overweight resident who has a history of snoring and/or daytime sleepiness. OSAHS can be screened by simple overnight oximetry. After sleep study (polysomnography) confirms the diagnosis, treatment with continuous positive airway pressure (CPAP) to deliver nasal oxygen at night may improve cognitive impairment as well as improving sleep and reducing daytime sleepiness. The HCP may consider prescribing armodafinil or modafinil to treat disabling excessive daytime sleepiness that persists despite the use of CPAP.

Sleep Disorders among Individuals Who Have Major Neurocognitive Disorder

Nighttime behavioral abnormalities and sleep disturbances affect up to half of all people who have MNCD. The severity of the disordered sleep and daytime napping tends to parallel that of the MNCD as it progresses. Sleep changes seen in MNCD (especially AD) appear to be an exacerbation of normal age-related changes (e.g. increased number of nighttime awakenings [sleep fragmentation], lowered sleep efficiency, increased daytime napping, difficulty initiating and maintaining sleep, decrease in both slow-wave sleep and rapid eye movement [REM] sleep, and decrease in total sleep), which increase in magnitude with the progression and severity of the disease. Nighttime awakenings are more disturbing to caregivers, but daytime napping and early morning awakening are usually not. Some residents who have MNCD may sleep up to 16 hours a day. Others may sleep only two to four hours a night. The cycle of sleep and wakefulness may be reversed. Disruptive nighttime behaviors often develop in residents who have moderate to severe MNCD, including nocturnal wandering, agitation, and even combativeness. High rates of OSAHS (typically undiagnosed) in residents who have MNCD may also contribute to the daytime sleepiness and agitation in people who have MNCD. RLS and RBD are more serious sleep-wake disorders that commonly occur in residents who have MNCD (especially DLB and PDD).

"Sundowner syndrome" refers to increased confusion usually accompanied by agitation "after the sun goes down" in a resident who has MNCD. It occurs mostly in the afternoon and evening. Sundowning is associated with disruption in circadian rhythm. Sundowning, in contrast to general agitation during other times of the day or night, correlates highly with rates of cognitive decline in affected persons. MDD may also manifest as sundowner syndrome, but other clinical signs of depression are usually present.

Treatment of disturbed sleep in a resident who has MNCD follows the principles and recommendations listed in Box 7.8 and Table 7.7. ChEI (e.g. donepezil, rivastigmine, galantamine) can improve daytime alertness in a resident who has AD, DLB, or PDD but may cause or contribute to insomnia.

Medication-Induced Sleep-Wake Disorder

A variety of medications can cause sleep-wake disorder (Kotlyar et al. 2011; American Geriatrics Society 2015). (See Boxes 7.4 and 7.5.) Some specific medications, such as sympathetomimetics and bronchodilators, can be particularly problematic when taken near bedtime. Also, the use of sedating medication listed in

Box 7.5 during the daytime can contribute to disrupted sleep-wake cycle by causing daytime drowsiness and tiredness leading to daytime sleeping. Sleep attacks (sudden, irresistible onset of sleep without awareness of falling asleep) have been described in people taking dopaminergic medication.

Sleep-Wake Disorder Induced by a Medical Condition

Insomnia, hypersomnia, circadian rhythm disorder, and nightmares are four most common sleep-wake disturbances induced by a medical condition. Due to a decrease in slow-wave deep sleep with aging, even low-intensity pain or discomfort caused by symptoms of a medical condition, as well as other stimuli (full bladder), may disturb sleep. Nightmares and EDS are seen in up to 32 percent of people who have PD. Pain (e.g. from arthritis), paresthesias, nighttime cough, dyspnea, and gastroesophageal reflux (GERD) are common causes of insomnia in LTC residents. Loss of vision accompanied by loss of light perception can cause circadian rhythm disorder. Treatment of the underlying medical condition usually improves sleep. For some conditions (e.g. PD), a combination of approaches listed in Box 7.8 and Table 7.7 is necessary. For many medical conditions, the effect may be bidirectional (e.g. pain causes insomnia, and insomnia worsens pain). Efforts to improve sleep may also promote recovery from the underlying medical condition. For example, with a resident who has persistent pain, improving sleep may reduce pain and lower the need for analgesic. Nocturia and urinary incontinence are a common cause of insomnia and fragmented nighttime sleep. Nocturia is typically seen in males who have prostate problem and people taking diuretic (especially near bedtime) but can be seen in any resident. Treatment involves prompt voiding protocol in the daytime, avoiding caffeine intake, and adjusting diuretics. In individuals who have ESRD, a variety of sleep disorders are prevalent. These include, but are not limited to, insomnia (69 percent), OSAHS (23 percent), RLS (18 percent), and EDS (12 percent). We recommend screening all LTC residents on dialysis for sleep-wake disorders and instituting appropriate treatment.

Summary

Physicians often inadequately recognize anxiety disorders, trauma- and stress-related disorders, obsessive-compulsive and related disorders, and sleep-wake disorders, making it difficult for the resident to receive effective treatment to help the resident cope with these highly prevalent and disabling disorders. These disorders often co-occur with mood and psychotic disorders and are common causes of treatment-resistant mood and psychotic disorders. They are a common cause of agitation and verbal and physical aggression in LTC populations. Even after diagnosis, they are often inappropriately treated (e.g. with long-term use of benzodiazepine). We recommend a comprehensive assessment for accurate diagnosis, identification of reversible etiological factors (e.g. medication), and institution of a combination of evidence-based treatments. A combination of relaxation strategies, soothing activities, psychosocial environmental approaches, psychotherapeutic approaches (e.g. CBT, TFCBT, ERP), and psychotropic (e.g. SSRI, SNRI) can effectively treat these disorders.

Key Clinical Points

1. Generalized anxiety disorder is prevalent in LTC populations, is often treated inappropriately with long-term use of benzodiazepine, and can be effectively treated with a combination of relaxation strategies, soothing activities, CBT, and psychotropic medication (e.g. SSRI, SNRI, buspirone).
2. The prevalence of PTSD in LTC populations is growing due to the aging of the population of military combat veterans and is eminently treatable with a combination of psychosocial environmental approaches, TFCBT, and psychotropic medication (e.g. SSRI, SNRI, prazosin).
3. OCD, hoarding disorder, and excoriation disorder are underdiagnosed in LTC populations, are disabling, and can be adequately treated with a combination of psychosocial environmental approaches, ERP, CBT, and SSRI.
4. Medication-induced sleep-wake disorders and MNCD-related sleep-wake disorders account for the majority of sleep-wake disorders in LTC populations and are often misdiagnosed and inappropriately treated.
5. A combination of psychosocial environmental approaches, sleep hygiene, CBT-I, melatonin, ramelteon, suvorexant, and short-term use of hypnotic (e.g. zaleplon, zolpidem, eszopiclone) can effectively treat insomnia disorder and other sleep-wake disorders.

References

American Psychiatric Association. 2013a. Anxiety Disorders. In *Diagnostic and Statistical Manual of Mental Disorders*, 5th ed., pp. 189–234. Arlington, VA: American Psychiatric Association Press.

American Psychiatric Association. 2013b. Trauma and Stressor-Related Disorders. In *Diagnostic and Statistical Manual of Mental Disorders*, 5th ed., pp. 265–290. Arlington, VA: American Psychiatric Association Press.

American Psychiatric Association. 2013c. Obsessive-Compulsive and Related Disorders. In *Diagnostic and Statistical Manual of Mental Disorders*, 5th ed., pp. 235–264. Arlington, VA: American Psychiatric Association Press.

American Psychiatric Association. 2013d. Sleep-Wake Disorders. In *Diagnostic and Statistical Manual of Mental Disorders*, 5th ed., pp. 361–422. Arlington, VA: American Psychiatric Association Press.

American Geriatrics Society. 2015. 2015 Updated Beers Criteria for Potentially Inappropriate Medication Use in Older Adults. American Geriatrics Society Beers Criteria Update Expert Panel. *Journal of the American Geriatrics Society* **63**:2227–2246.

Barak, Y. 2011. Posttraumatic Stress Disorder in Late-Life. In M.E. Agronin and G. J. Maletta, eds., *Principles and Practice of Geriatric Psychiatry*, 2nd ed., pp. 515–522. Philadelphia, PA: Lippincott Williams & Wilkins.

Campbell Burton, C.A., J. Murray, J. Holmes, et al. 2013. Frequency of Anxiety after Stroke: A Systematic Review and Meta-Analysis of Observational Studies. *International Journal of Stroke* **8**:545–559.

Chen, J.J. and L. Marsh. 2014. Anxiety in Parkinson's Disease: Identification and Management. *Therapeutic Advances in Neurological Disorders* **7**(1):52–59.

Desai, A.K., and G.T. Grossberg. 2017. Psychiatric Aspects of Long-Term Care. In B.J. Saddock, V.A. Saddock, and P. Ruiz (eds.), *Comprehensive Textbook of Psychiatry*, 10th ed., pp. 4221–4232. Virginia: American Psychiatric Press Inc.

Lenz, E., J. Mohlman, and J.L. Wetherell. 2015. Anxiety, Obsessive-Compulsive, and Trauma-Related Disorders. In D.C. Steffens, D.G. Blazer, and M.E. Thakur (eds.), *The Textbook of Geriatric Psychiatry*, 5th ed., pp. 333–372. Arlington, VA: American Psychiatric Publishing.

Grant, J.E. 2014. Obsessive-Compulsive Disorder. *New England Journal of Medicine* **371**: 646–653.

Kotlyar, M., S.L. Gray, R.L. Maher Jr., J.T. Hanlon. 2011. Psychiatric Manifestations of Medications in the Elderly. In M.E. Agronin and G. J. Maletta, eds., *Principles and Practice of Geriatric Psychiatry*, 2nd ed., pp. 721–733. Philadelphia, PA: Lippincott Williams & Wilkins.

Krystal, A.D. and M.E. Thakur. 2015. Sleep and Circadian-Rhythm Disorders. In D.C. Steffens, D.G. Blazer, and M.E. Thakur (eds.), *The Textbook of Geriatric Psychiatry*, 5th ed., pp. 435–458. Arlington, VA: American Psychiatric Publishing.

Neikrug, A. and S. Ancoli-Israel. 2010. Sleep Disturbances in Nursing Homes. *Journal of Nutrition, Health and Aging* **14**:207–211.

Pachana, N.A., G.I. Byrne, H. Siddle, et al. 2007. Development and Validation of the Geriatric Anxiety Inventory. *International Psychogeriatrics* **19**:103–114.

Sorathia, L.T. and U.K. Ghori. 2016. Sleep Disorders in the Elderly. *Current Geriatrics Reports* **5**(2):110–116.

Streim, J. 2015. Clinical Psychiatry in the Nursing Home. In D.C. Steffens, D.G. Blazer, and M.E. Thakur (eds.), *The Textbook of Geriatric Psychiatry*, 5th ed., pp. 689–748. Arlington, VA: American Psychiatric Publishing.

Winkelman, J. 2015. Insomnia Disorder. *New England Journal of Medicine* **373**:1437–1444.

Wood, S., J.L. Cummings, M. Hsu, et al. 2000. The Use of the Neuropsychiatric Inventory in Nursing Home Residents. *American Journal of Geriatric Psychiatry* **8**:75–83.

Chapter 8 Personality Disorders, Somatic Symptom and Related Disorders, Substance Use Disorders, and Intermittent Explosive Disorder

Psychiatric disorders that need to be considered in the differential diagnosis of behavioral and psychological symptoms in long-term care (LTC) populations include personality disorders, somatic symptom and related disorders, and substance use disorders (Desai and Grossberg 2017; Streim 2015). In residents who exhibit violent behavior, the health care provider (HCP) should consider intermittent explosive disorder in the differential diagnosis. Having a high index of suspicion is required for the HCP to diagnose these disorders, as they usually go unrecognized until multiple complications and failure of treatment response has led the team to look for them. These disorders are more prevalent in LTC populations than is usually recognized, are debilitating, and cause considerable stress to the LTC staff.

Personality Disorders

It is important to assess the resident's personality characteristics, as personality problems and disorders are risk factors for a host of medical and mental disorders (e.g. coronary heart disease, major depressive disorder [MDD], late-life suicidal behavior). Myths associated with personality and aging are prevalent among staff and family members of residents and need to be corrected. It is not true that most older adults become stubborn, resist change, and are dependent. Quite the contrary: people tend to become more open and less impulsive with age (Vaillant 2012). Small increases in obsessive-compulsive traits with aging reflect efforts to adapt to failing health or environmental changes rather than a personality problem. It is also not true that most personality disorders "burn out" with age. Some personality disorders (e.g. borderline personality disorder, antisocial personality disorder) may have sufficient reduction in symptoms by middle age, so as many as half may not meet the full criteria for the disorder. Due to maturational effects, there may be some quantitative changes (reduction in the frequency of emotional crises, self-destructive behaviors, less paranoia during stress) and qualitative changes (reduction in behaviors leading to legal problems but continued interpersonal difficulty) in personality, but serious maladaptive behaviors usually persist (see Table 8.1).

A resident is diagnosed with a personality disorder if she or he has shown an enduring pattern of inner experience and behavior involving ways of perceiving and interpreting self that deviate markedly from the resident's culture (American Psychiatric Association 2013a). This manifests as an inappropriate and intense emotional response to ordinary stresses, pervasive challenges in interpersonal functioning, and/or severely impaired impulse control across a broad range of personal and social situations. The initial signs of personality disorder can be recognized in adolescence or earlier. The symptoms become obvious in young adulthood and usually persist into late life. The prevalence of personality disorders in older adults is essentially equivalent to that of younger groups and approximates 10 percent (Oxman 2015). Some 10 to 20 percent of older persons who have MDD have a personality disorder as well. An even larger percentage of older adults who have chronic depression (chronic MDD and/or persistent depressive disorder) have comorbid personality disorder. Obsessive-compulsive personality disorder, dependent personality disorder, and mixed personality disorder (personality disorders with more than one type of personality trait) are the most frequently diagnosed personality disorders in older adults receiving treatment at mental health clinics. In general, detailed

Table 8.1 Age-Related Personality Changes, Personality Problems, and Personality Disorders in Long-Term Care Populations

Personality	Key Clinical Features	Therapeutic Pearls
Age-related personality changes	Reduction in impulsivity Improved openness to different opinions	Emotional resilience and less likelihood of MDD despite multiple losses than younger adult
Five Factor Model	Extraversion versus introversion Agreeableness versus antagonism Openness versus closedness to experience Conscientiousness versus impulsivity Neuroticism (tendency to experience negative emotions [negative affectivity]) versus emotional stability	Traits of agreeableness and openness help resident adjust to living in LTC facility Neuroticism predisposes resident to mood and anxiety disorders in response to entering LTC facility Conscientiousness may protect against development of MNCD
Personality disorders	Symptoms and dysfunction exacerbate following major stressor (e.g. move to LTC, loss of spouse) HCP should expect dissatisfaction with care, multiple accusations of mistreatment and abuse by staff, and nonadherence to treatment	Involvement of ombudsman early in course of stay in the LTC facility is strongly recommended
Personality change	Overall personality traits do not change with age	HCP should thoroughly evaluate any new onset of change in personality in middle age or later life to identify a medical / neurological cause (e.g. MNCD, brain tumor)
Paranoid personality disorder	Staff should expect waxing and waning of paranoia, distrustfulness, and self-centered thinking that is exacerbated due to frequent changes in staff and frequent errors in care by staff	Staff keep sufficient emotional distance that resident does not feel staff are trying to manipulate or trick him/her with kindness
Schizoid personality disorder	Have particular difficulty participating in group activity	Individualized activities or activities in small groups recommended
Schizotypal personality disorder	Have particular difficulty having staff respect resident's odd ideas and experiences	Staff education that odd ideas and experiences do not reflect psychotic disorder and should be respected
Antisocial personality disorder	Some decrease in full spectrum of antisocial behavior (especially criminal behavior)	Lack of empathy and callous behavior toward other residents and staff need to be addressed promptly, and vulnerable residents need to be protected
Borderline personality disorder	Stress related to aging-related illness often triggers crisis in identity, mood instability (emotional rollercoaster), and recurrence of impulsive, acting out, and self-harmful behavior after years of stability	Give resident who has this disorder a lot of structure and clearly state rules and boundaries Manipulative and splitting behavior (viewing some staff as *all good* and others as *all bad*) needs to be promptly addressed with consistent unified staff approach
Histrionic personality disorder	Excessive emotionality and attention-seeking behavior may lead to undertreatment of legitimate health problem and overtreatment with psychotropic medication	Staff education and avoiding unnecessary psychotropic medication recommended
Narcissistic personality disorder	Have particular difficulty adjusting to age-related decline in physical health, sensory health, and skin changes Strong desire to be treated as special (better than others)	Judiciously giving resident who has this disorder special status (e.g. serving his/her meals first) may reduce anger and bolster fragile self-esteem

Table 8.1 (cont.)

Personality	Key Clinical Features	Therapeutic Pearls
Avoidant personality disorder	May become less evident with age	Avoid prescribing SSRI to treat social anxiety related to this disorder
Dependent personality disorder	Have particular difficulty coping with interpersonal loss (e.g. loss of spouse)	Individual psychotherapy (especially interpersonal psychotherapy) for motivated resident who has relatively good interpersonal functioning may prevent complications (e.g. MDD, separation anxiety disorder) in response to significant loss
Obsessive-compulsive disorder	Have particular difficulty coping with life in LTC facility and rules and regulations facility has to follow	Individual psychotherapy (especially cognitive behavioral psychotherapy) for motivated resident who has relatively good interpersonal functioning may prevent complications (e.g. MDD) in response to stress of living in LTC facility

history from a knowledgeable informant (e.g. spouse, child, close friend, sibling) is crucial for accurate diagnosis of a personality disorder, as cognitive impairment and physical health concerns pose barriers to diagnosis based on history obtained from only the resident. See Box 8.1 for clinical cues to the presence of a personality disorder.

A pre-existing personality disorder needs to be differentiated from personality change due to a major neurocognitive disorder (MNCD) or another medical condition (e.g. stroke, traumatic brain injury [TBI], brain tumor). In the latter, a persistent personality disturbance represents a change from the individual's previous characteristic personality. Damage to orbitofrontal lobe is associated with reduced empathy and disinhibited behavior. Damage to dorsolateral frontal lobe is associated with apathy, and damage to temporal or parietal lobe is associated with misperception of stimuli and paranoia. Changes in personality due to MNCD or another medical condition include anger outbursts and aggressive behavior that are disproportionate to the stressor, chronic irritability, impulse control problems, apathy, mean and/or cruel behavior, loss of empathic behavior, social and interpersonal insensitivity, asociality, overcautiousness, suspiciousness, childishness, and emotional lability. MNCD may exacerbate a pre-existing personality disorder, which in turn may result in severe behavioral disturbance (e.g. verbal aggression).

A personality disorder may predispose an individual to anxiety and/or mood disorder. A personality disorder in an older adult is associated with poor or partial response to antidepressant used to treat MDD or anxiety disorder, refusal of or nonadherence to medical care (including rehabilitative therapy [physical therapy, speech therapy, occupational therapy]), increased disability, disruption of interpersonal relationships, and suicidal behavior.

Despite challenges, personality disorders are treatable psychiatric conditions, and treatment may improve the resident's quality of life and reduce family and professional caregivers' stress. Box 8.2 lists a variety of evidence-based approaches that, in combination, can help a resident who has personality problems. Treatment involves education of staff and family regarding the diagnosis so that expectation for the resident to "change" is lowered. Treatment of symptoms (depression, anxiety, hostility) that are part of the personality disorder and treatment of superimposed comorbidity (e.g. MDD, generalized anxiety disorder [GAD]) are key. Residents who have personality disorders may generate strong negative emotions in the staff and may cause the staff to split (some staff taking the resident's side and other staff strongly opposed to the resident). Despite such challenges, treatment should be respectful and relevant to the resident to relieve symptoms, allow interdependence, accommodate change, and support healthy narcissism. In general, residents who have personality disorders

BOX 8.1 Clues Indicating the Presence of a Personality Disorder

- Staff develop strong negative countertransference toward resident (e.g. staff express that resident is hateful, manipulative, help-rejecting, toxic)
- Resident rejects multiple roommates (e.g. resident is on fifth roommate), as he/she cannot get along with anyone
- Resident has estranged relationships with all or almost all family members
- Family members do not want to be involved in resident's life or care
- Resident has no close friends
- Resident has history of pitting his/her children against each other
- Family considers resident always to have been "high maintenance"
- Resident has history of multiple short-lived emotionally intense relationships
- Resident held a variety of jobs, each for only a short time
- Resident generates strong emotions in staff (generally negative or negative in some staff and positive in others)
- Resident's behavior causes staff to split (some staff taking resident's side and others strongly opposed to resident)
- Multiple changes of HCP due to resident's dissatisfaction
- Resident misuses medication (e.g. self-medicating, adjusting dosage of high-risk medication without input of HCP who prescribed medication)
- Resident cannot tolerate many or most psychotropic medications
- Resident makes recurrent threats of suicide
- Resident has history of self-injurious behavior (e.g. making cuts with a small knife to the wrists/forearms, sticking pins into the thigh)
- Resident's mood and/or anxiety disorders do not respond to multiple trials of psychotropic medication
- Resident's demanding behavior accompanied by help-rejecting behavior

BOX 8.2 Strategies to Help a Resident Who Has Personality Problems

General

- Form a therapeutic alliance (a trusting, nonjudgmental, and supportive relationship)
- Seek to understand resident's life story (including any history of abuse or trauma) without any intention to manipulate or control resident
- Develop positive regard for resident's strengths
- Enhance resident's social support (through family meetings, help of volunteers and chaplains, etc.)
- Validate resident's experiences, emotions, and perspectives
- Nonpunitive confrontation and limit setting
- Avoid reflexively reacting to resident's provocation and other negative behavior
- Establish boundaries and provide choices within boundaries
- Reward appropriate behavior with attention and appreciation
- Respond to underlying distress, not content of complaints and grievances
- Do not judge resident's family and friends harshly

Psychological strategies for motivated resident who has relatively intact cognitive function

- Help resident who is bitter (overly critical, blaming others, harsh) by making efforts to show that no one is trying to take advantage of her and that being overly critical may push staff away
- Help resident who is acquiescent (blaming self, not assertive, overly trusting) slowly to become assertive (by practicing with staff, counselor, psychiatrist) and reassuring that one can be assertive without being harsh
- Help resident who is overly anxious (brooding, pessimistic) with mind-body approaches (e.g. relaxation, breathing, meditation, other mindfulness-based strategies) and reassuring that worrying less does not mean being careless

BOX 8.2 (cont.)

- Help resident who is hedonistic (careless, chaotic, never plans) by helping her realize potential benefits of thinking about a problem and solving it and costs of solving any difficulty by seeking pleasure (risk of injury, poorer health)
- Help resident who is "fiercely independent" (avoiding intimacy, avoiding help from family and friends) by reassuring that one can be close to others without being engulfed or controlled
- Help resident who is overly dependent (always seeking nurturance from others) by addressing fear of abandonment
- In an empathetic manner, enhance resident's capacity for balanced reflection of her own behavior and its potential consequences

Psychotherapeutic approaches for motivated resident who has relatively good cognitive function

- Establish and maintain collaborative therapeutic alliance with experienced psychotherapist
- Implement written behavioral contract
- Therapeutic encirclement by treatment team (close coordination among staff, medical team, mental health team, allied health care professionals)
- Therapeutic splinting (augment traditional services with creative psychosocial support)
- Provide individual and group psychotherapy
- Use combination of various psychotherapeutic techniques (e.g. psychodynamic, cognitive-behavioral, mindfulness-based, interpersonal, dialectical-behavioral)
- Crisis management to ensure safety
- Consistent therapeutic process with clearly defined and realistic treatment goals and roles and responsibilities of resident and treatment team members
- Nidotherapy (systematic manipulation of physical and social environment to help achieve better fit between individual who has persistent mental disorder and environment)

Pharmacological strategies

- Antidepressant for co-morbid mood and/or anxiety disorder
- Low-dose atypical antipsychotic for transient distressing psychotic symptoms and/or recurrent rage and aggression
- Mood stabilizer for recurrent rage and aggression
- Judicious use of low-dose benzodiazepine for acute anxiety attack or behavioral emergency

Staff education

- Origins of personality disorder (e.g. traumatic childhood, neurological insult)
- Healthy ways for staff to manage their own strong negative emotions
- Potential for abuse of resident by staff (typically through neglect but also verbal abuse) and ways to prevent abuse (e.g. better management of their own negative emotions, staff support from leadership team and supervisors, rotation of staff, team approach)
- Importance of identifying emotional strengths and resilience that all residents, including resident who has personality disorder, have that are not being recognized and can be tapped into, to further improve resident's psychosocial well-being
- Importance of compassion and setting limits in caring for all residents, especially for resident who has personality disorder
- Importance of staff rotation in caring for resident who has personality disorder to avoid staff burnout, because caring for resident who has personality disorder can be emotionally draining
- Vigilance for pitfalls of making resident who has personality disorder overly dependent/reliant on or emotionally close to staff, as this may meet emotional needs of staff but harm resident in long run

have a history of traumatic and difficult childhood, and awareness of such a history by the staff may enable them to have compassion for the resident despite the resident's hostile behavior.

Clinical Case: "I cannot wait to get out of this miserable place"

Ms. L was a 64-year-old woman admitted to a nursing home for rehabilitation after a prolonged hospital stay (three months) for nephrectomy and postnephrectomy complications (infection, bleeding, and delirium with agitation). The psychiatrist was consulted to help manage the resident's hostile and aggressive behavior toward staff. The staff expressed anger and resentment at having to provide personal care to Ms. L because of her persistent name calling, yelling at the staff, and demeaning them almost daily. Some staff members had started to call in sick if they found out that they had to care for Ms. L, and some refused to care for her. The psychiatrist found Ms. L to be an intelligent person who had relatively intact cognitive function (Montreal Cognitive Assessment score 26) and was quick to take offense but also willing to accept help from "competent" professionals. She repeatedly expressed, "I cannot wait to get out of this miserable place." Ms. L was taking sertraline, 100 mg daily, for MDD. After interviewing Ms. L, the psychiatrist met with the staff to explain that, in his opinion, Ms. L had been experiencing moderate to severe depression (MDD) (Patient Health Questionnaire-9 score was 20) with underlying long-standing personality disorder. Ms. L had confided in the psychiatrist that she had been severely physically and emotionally abused as a child and had had three "horrible" marriages. She had expressed to the psychiatrist that she "hate[d] everyone," liked animals more than people, had lots of pets that she took care of, and helped the Humane Society in caring for sick pets. The psychiatrist provided emotional support to the staff, validated their feelings related to dealing with Ms. L's negative behaviors, discussed specific therapeutic ways the staff could respond to these negative behaviors, and explained the treatment plan (increase in antidepressants and individual psychotherapy). The psychiatrist (with Ms. L's permission) shared minor details about her abusive childhood and spousal relationships and the good volunteer work she was doing with the Humane Society. This helped the staff feel supported, improved their compassion for Ms. L, and enabled them to be more patient with her so that treatment could be given time to help. The psychiatrist increased the dosage of sertraline from 100 to 150 mg and encouraged the staff to tell Ms. L that she was being disrespectful when she used foul language or yelled at them. Staff was also encouraged to respond calmly (without resentment) and appreciatively when Ms. L talked respectfully. The psychiatrist gently helped Ms. L understand that her hostile behavior put her at much higher risk of prolonged stay in the nursing home because the staff would be less likely to meet her needs diligently or promptly. Ms. L agreed to go to an outpatient clinic once a week for counseling with a social worker. Over the next few weeks, the frequency and intensity of hostile comments by Ms. L decreased modestly, the staff was able to meet more of her needs, and Ms. L made significant progress in physical therapy.

Teaching Points

Depressive disorders are common among residents who have personality disorder and often underrecognized and undertreated. Also, a resident who has personality disorder generates strong negative feelings in others that may result in staff being less likely to meet the resident's needs. Approaches (e.g. antidepressants, staff education, counseling for the resident) should be designed to make at least a modest change in behavior (e.g. reduction in name calling by the resident toward the staff) possible to achieve the desired result (e.g. increased likelihood that the staff will be able to meet the resident's needs). Psychotherapy is useful for residents who have personality disorder and relatively intact cognitive function. Optimization of treatment of comorbid mental disorder (MDD in this situation) and specific guidance to staff in therapeutic ways to respond to negative behaviors are also crucial for a successful outcome.

Somatic Symptom and Related Disorders

Somatic symptom and related disorders (SSRDs) involve distressing somatic symptoms accompanied by negative thoughts, feelings, and excessive behaviors devoted to address the somatic symptoms (Agronin 2015). If any physical disorder is present, it is insufficient to explain the severity of symptoms or the resident's distress. (See Table 8.2.) For diagnosis,

Table 8.2 Somatic Symptoms and Related Disorders in Long-Term Care Populations

Assessment	Key Diagnostic and Clinical Features	Therapeutic Pearls
Comprehensive assessment	History of childhood trauma and/or serious childhood illness Temperamental trait of neuroticism (tendency to experience negative emotions) Learned sick role Review of previous psychiatric records indicates multiple unexplained somatic symptoms with multiple tests, procedures, and treatments without significant benefit	Early accurate diagnosis is key to avoiding unnecessary or even harmful tests, procedures, and treatments
Somatic symptom disorder	One or more somatic complaints accompanied by significant negative thoughts and feelings related to symptoms and excessive behavior devoted to seeking relief Underdiagnosed in older adults Typically accompanies diagnosable medical condition(s)	High index of suspicion and early diagnosis can avoid unnecessary tests and treatments
Illness anxiety disorder (hypochondriasis)	Preoccupation with having or developing serious medical/neurological condition accompanied by significant anxiety about staying healthy In older adults, fear of Alzheimer's disease and other MNCD is the most common condition involved in illness anxiety disorder	High index of suspicion, early diagnosis, and repeated reassurances can avoid unnecessary tests and treatments and provide some relief
Conversion disorder (functional neurological symptom disorder)	One or more neurological symptoms (e.g. limb paralysis, seizure-like event) with clinical examination findings that are incompatible with neurological complaint(s) Many residents who have epilepsy may have co-occurring conversion disorder with pseudoseizure	High index of suspicion and early diagnosis can avoid unnecessary tests and treatments

conversion disorder requires the absence of medical explanation in addition to neurological complaints. The trait of neuroticism, defined in part as the tendency to experience negative emotion, is a better predictor of somatic complaints than age. A history of childhood abuse and/or a serious childhood illness is the most common risk factor for later development of SSRD (American Psychiatric Association 2013b). A learned sick role in childhood may predispose an individual to SSRD later in life. Gender (more common in females than males), education (more common in individuals who have lower education than individuals who have higher education), and socioeconomic class (more common in lower socioeconomic class than higher socioeconomic class) also influence the development of SSRD. With some residents, SSRD may reflect aging-associated conflict such as fear of irrelevance or abandonment, sexual decline, and repressed expression of helplessness and anger. Individuals who have SSRD may not express anger easily. Personality characteristics such as alexithymia, the impaired ability to describe emotions, also are seen frequently with SSRD.

Mood disorders (e.g. MDD) and/or anxiety disorders (e.g. panic disorder) may present with somatic symptoms but can be accurately differentiated from SSRD by the presence of typical mood and anxiety symptoms accompanying somatic complaints. Comorbid SSRD and MDD are highly associated with suicide. If the degree of somatic preoccupation is severe, the HCP should consider delusional disorder (somatic type) in the differential diagnosis.

Up to 50 percent of illness anxiety disorders are of short duration, typically after a stressor (e.g. sibling had a heart attack and now the individual is worried he has heart disease) or a minor problem (e.g. mild age-related memory lapse causes the individual to worry that this may be the start of Alzheimer's disease). In others, illness anxiety disorder is chronic, waxes and wanes, and is usually present for years before the individual enters a LTC facility.

The most important consideration in the treatment of any resident suspected to have SSRD is to accurately diagnose SSRD and treat comorbid anxiety and/or depressive disorder aggressively. We recommend building a strong therapeutic alliance and avoiding unnecessary or excessive testing to clarify the etiology of multiple somatic complaints. It is equally important to avoid excessive medical treatments and surgical procedures to treat somatic symptoms for an individual who has SSRD. We recommend cognitive behavioral therapy (CBT) for a motivated resident who has relatively intact cognitive function. Psychotropic medications play a role only in the treatment of co-occurring mood and/or anxiety disorders.

Substance-Related and Addictive Disorders

Substance-related and addictive disorders are clinical syndromes that occur as a result of using substances that trigger intense activation of the brain reward networks and hijack motivational networks. *DSM-5* classifies these substances into 10 categories: alcohol, caffeine, cannabis, hallucinogens (phencyclidine and other hallucinogens), inhalants, opioids, sedatives/hypnotics/anxiolytics, stimulants, tobacco, and others (American Psychiatric Association 2013c). Substance use disorders (SUDs) are the most common substance-related and addictive disorders in LTC populations, followed by substance withdrawal. Diagnosis of SUD can be applied to all 10 classes except caffeine and requires that the individual develop one or more of the following: impaired control (e.g. failed attempts to cut down); impaired social functioning (e.g. estrangement from family members); risky use (e.g. using substance despite documented health problems caused by the substance [e.g. nicotine smoking despite having developed chronic obstructive pulmonary disorder {COPD}]); tolerance (requiring higher amounts of the substance to elicit the desired effect); and withdrawal syndrome. SUD is more prevalent in men than in women, but it is more likely to be overlooked in women than in men. Currently, the prevalence of SUD in LTC populations is low (see Table 8.3). Significantly higher rates of illicit drug and alcohol use and related mental disorders are expected in future LTC residents because of the higher prevalence

Table 8.3 Substance Use Disorders in Long-Term Care Populations

Assessment	Key Clinical Tips	Key Therapeutic Implications
Detailed history	Clarify at-risk use (use that does not yet cause problems but has high potential to cause serious adverse event), problem use (use that has caused serious adverse event but does not meet criteria for substance use disorder), and substance use disorder (mild, moderate, severe) Many residents may report much lower amounts of intake (intentionally due to stigma or unintentionally) than actual use	Intensity of treatment needs to be appropriate to severity of problem In complex cases, referral to a psychiatrist or specialty center for older adults is recommended
Standardized screening tools	Drug Abuse Screening Test (DAST) to screen for substance use disorder (except alcohol use disorder) CAGE (Cut down, Annoyance, Guilt, Eye-opener) useful to screen for alcohol use disorder Short Michigan Alcoholism Screening Instrument – Geriatric Version (SMAST-G) Alcohol Use Disorder Identification Test (AUDIT) and its abbreviated version AUDIT-C Nicotine dependency assessment Caffeine consumption questionnaire	Staff training required

Table 8.3 (cont.)

Assessment	Key Clinical Tips	Key Therapeutic Implications
Standardized withdrawal assessment tools	Clinical Institute Withdrawal Assessment for Alcohol (CIWA-A) to assess for alcohol withdrawal symptoms Clinical Institute Withdrawal Assessment for Benzodiazepines (CIWA-B) to assess benzodiazepine withdrawal symptoms Clinical opiate withdrawal scale to assess for opioid withdrawal symptoms Minnesota Nicotine Withdrawal Scale to assess for nicotine withdrawal symptoms	Staff training required
Alcohol use disorder	Usually there is history of alcohol addiction Modest elevation or high-normal level (>35 units) of gamma-glutaryltransferase (GGT) and elevated level (>20 units) of carbohydrate-deficient transferrin (CDT) can help identify person who drinks heavily	HCP should consider prescribing FDA-approved drugs for alcohol use disorder to reduce risk of relapse
Benzodiazepine use disorder	At-risk use and problem use of BZD is prevalent in LTC populations Most residents who chronically use BZD do not have BZD use disorder	Slow taper (over weeks to months) and discontinuation of long-acting BZD (e.g. clonazepam, diazepam) is recommended Switching short-acting BZD (e.g. alprazolam) to long-acting BZD (e.g. clonazepam) may be necessary before instituting slow taper and discontinuation
Nicotine use disorder	Prevalent in LTC populations (5–20%), with prevalence higher in younger residents than older residents Prevalence is high (30–50%) in residents who have serious mental disorder (e.g. schizophrenia, bipolar disorder)	Harm-reduction strategy (goal is to reduce amount of substance used [e.g. lowering number of cigarettes smoked per day]) is recommended if resident is not motivated for total abstinence, as even a small reduction in substance use can have significant health benefit
Cannabis use disorder	Prevalence is low but will increase in coming decade as more Baby Boomers enter LTC	High index of suspicion is necessary for early diagnosis Urine drug screen may be helpful, as cannabis stays in urine for few weeks
Opioid use disorder	At-risk use and problem use of opioids is prevalent in LTC populations Most residents who chronically use opioids do not have opioid use disorder	Comprehensive pain management and slow taper and discontinuation of opioid is recommended
Caffeine use related disorder	Under-recognized as cause of anxiety symptoms and insomnia	Limiting caffeine intake to morning or replacing caffeinated beverage with decaffeinated beverage is recommended
Substance use related mental disorder (e.g. anxiety, depression, psychoses, insomnia)	Common examples: opioid use related mood disorder and neurocognitive disorder, benzodiazepine use related neurocognitive disorder, alcohol use related psychotic disorder	High index of suspicion and resident and family education are key to successful outcome

of these disorders in the Baby Boomer generation (Taylor and Grossberg 2012). Due to high medical and psychiatric comorbidity, residents are at risk of serious adverse events with even modest use of these substances. Hence, the HCP should consider any use of these substances in LTC populations at-risk use (even if it does not meet the criteria for SUD). Substance use in LTC populations can result in accelerated cognitive and functional decline, falls and injury, lack of response to treatment for co-occurring mental disorders (e.g. MDD, GAD, insomnia disorder), harmful drug interaction, liver disease, cardiovascular disease, and increased mortality. Thus, comprehensive evidence-based treatment of SUD is important to improve residents' safety and psychosocial well-being (Mavandadi and Oslin 2015).

Many alcohol drinkers maintain steady consumption levels into later life. Evening or nightly cocktail hour ("happy hour") is a growing trend at many LTC facilities. According to the US Department of Health and Human Services 2015–2020 Dietary Guidelines, individuals should not drink alcohol if they are consuming medication that may adversely interact with alcohol and/or if they have a medical condition that can worsen with alcohol (US Department of Health and Human Services and US Department of Agriculture 2015). Based on these guidelines, the HCP should recommend that almost all LTC residents not drink alcohol. The standard definition of a unit of alcohol (one standard drink) is that contains 8 grams of ethanol. Typically, one unit is contained in a 12-ounce bottle of beer (5 percent alcohol content), 8 ounces of malt liquor (7 percent alcohol content), one 5-ounce glass of wine (12 percent alcohol content), or 1.5 ounces (a shot) of 80 percent proof distilled spirits or liquor (whiskey, vodka, rum, gin) (40 percent alcohol content). Daily consumption of 0.5–2 standard drinks of alcohol or weekly consumption of 1–14 standard drinks of alcohol may be more prevalent than is usually recognized in LTC populations, and its negative health consequences are under-recognized. Therefore, all residents should be screened for alcohol consumption and related problems. Although such consumption does not constitute SUD, it should be considered at-risk drinking and discouraged, especially with a resident who has cognitive impairment or behavioral and psychological symptoms. Residents and their family should be educated regarding harmful effects of even modest intake of alcohol (0.5–1 drink per day). Each visit to the resident who consumes alcohol regularly can be an opportunity to provide education. Polypharmacy is highly prevalent among LTC populations. Alcohol reacts negatively with more than 100 prescriptions and over-the-counter medications as well as many herbs and supplements. Therefore, alcohol-medication interactions are possible among residents who drink even 1 or 2 standard drinks regularly. Most residents who have alcohol use disorder have a long history of alcohol addiction problems, typically with onset before age 40, although 10 percent have onset after age 40. Residents who have a history of alcohol use disorder have high comorbidity of nicotine use disorder, sleep-wake disorder, mood disorder, and anxiety disorder. The HCP should routinely inquire into these comorbidities during assessment.

Many residents have used prescription benzodiazepine (BZD) chronically (daily use for more than a year, typically for several years or even decades). They usually do not have a history of taking more than the prescribed dosage of BZD, do not have a history of using other substances (e.g. alcohol or street drugs), and have a history of regularly seeing a physician. They have a high prevalence of comorbid anxiety disorder (especially GAD and/or panic disorder) and sleep disorder (especially insomnia disorder). By the time they enter a LTC facility, they have significant cognitive deficits and physical health problems, making continued use of BZD a serious concern. These residents usually do not meet the criteria for benzodiazepine use disorder.

Nicotine use disorder (typically with cigarette smoking but also chewable tobacco, electronic cigarettes, and snuff), like alcohol use, is under-treated in LTC populations. Residents typically have consumed large amounts of nicotine over their lifetime and as a result have developed serious complications (e.g. COPD due to cigarette smoking). Smoking tobacco is associated with many deleterious health outcomes besides COPD, such as cardiovascular disease, a variety of cancers (especially lung cancer), abdominal aortic aneurysm, peripheral arterial disease, nicotine-drug interaction, and accelerated cognitive and functional decline. Smoking is associated with induction of cytochrome P450 1A2 liver enzymes, which in turn can lower levels of drugs metabolized by this enzyme system (e.g. clozapine, olanzapine). Almost all residents who use nicotine usually meet the criteria for nicotine use disorder.

Residents who have cannabis use disorder before entering LTC often continue to use marijuana. Staff may not be aware of such use. Residents who use marijuana may also have co-occurring alcohol use disorder, nicotine use disorder, or other drug use disorder. Older adults who have cannabis use disorder are at risk for MDD and suicide. With a resident who has MDD, the use of marijuana can precipitate a psychiatric crisis involving suicidal ideas, attempts, and/or severe agitation.

Residents who have opioid use disorder usually have a history of opioid addiction (e.g. use of heroin) and treatment. Many residents develop opioid use disorder after being prescribed opioid medication for pain management, but this problem typically goes unrecognized. The majority of LTC residents taking opioids chronically do not have opioid use disorder but have or are at risk of serious adverse consequences (especially falls and cognitive impairment) associated with opioid use. Caffeine use may cause or exacerbate insomnia and/or anxiety. Residents who have a history of drug use (e.g. cocaine, methamphetamine, heroin) may engage in an occasional use (e.g. after visiting a friend) or may relapse following a stressful event (e.g. loss of a key support person). Awareness of the resident's history of drug use and high index of suspicion of relapse with any acute change in mental status is key to early diagnosis and successful outcome.

A variety of approaches are available for treating SUD in LTC populations (see Table 8.4). Integrating routine SUD screening and brief therapy (changing substance use behavior by raising awareness and sharing knowledge) at the LTC facility form the backbone of treatment. It is important that the HCP proactively and directly acknowledge issues of stigma and ambivalence, as well as cultural issues that may affect the resident's feelings about substance use behavior and treatment. It is equally important to address negative health consequences in a consistent but nonjudgmental manner. We recommend referral to a psychiatrist or a specialty center for older adults for a resident who has moderate to severe SUD, as the resident needs more intensive rather than brief treatment. Complex SUD (e.g. opioid use disorder in a resident who has chronic pain) is best managed by an interdisciplinary team involving a primary care physician (PCP), psychiatrist, addiction counselor, and other specialists (e.g. pain management specialist). Effective treatment of MDD, insomnia disorder, GAD, schizophrenia, or other co-occurring mental disorder may prevent relapse of substance use in a resident who has SUD, and treatment of SUD may prevent relapse of co-occurring mental disorder.

In general, the goal of treatment is total abstinence, and the substance use needs to be reduced slowly to avoid significant withdrawal symptoms. In situations in which substance use needs to be stopped right away (e.g. alcohol, methamphetamine), we recommend monitoring for emergent withdrawal symptoms and

Table 8.4 Evidence-Based Approaches to Treat Substance Use Disorders

Approach	Key Features	Limitations
Brief treatment	Educate resident about risks of continued use Educate resident about benefits of quitting Provide emotional support	None
Motivational interviewing	Involves four general strategies: roll with resistance (avoid confrontation), express empathy, develop discrepancy (between resident goal to quit and current behavior), and support self-efficacy (strength of belief in ability to reach goal)	Staff training required
FRAMES model	Feedback (regarding risks of substance use), change as a personal Responsibility, specific Advice to reduce use, offering Menu of options, expressing Empathy, and validating resident's Self-efficacy	Staff training required
Five A's Approach	Ask about substance use, Advise to quit Assess willingness to quit, Assist in attempt to quit, and Arrange follow up	Staff training required

Table 8.4 (cont.)

Approach	Key Features	Limitations
Substance use agreement	Useful to establish daily limit of substance use (especially alcohol, cannabis, cigarettes)	Needs motivated resident who has relatively intact cognitive function
Daily substance use card	Useful to monitor daily substance use between follow ups	Needs motivated resident who has relatively intact cognitive function
Pharmacotherapy for alcohol use disorder	Naltrexone (FDA-approved opioid-receptor antagonist) (pill form and long-acting injectable form) Acamprosate (inhibitory effect on GABA/NMDA) (FDA approved) Topamax (not FDA approved) for treatment-resistant cases Gabapentin (not FDA approved) for alcohol withdrawal if benzodiazepine cannot be used	Needs to be part of comprehensive treatment plan Dose reduction of acamprosate required for resident who has moderate to severe chronic kidney disease, as acamprosate is excreted unchanged by kidneys Topamax may impair cognition
Nicotine replacement therapy	Use of one or more nicotine products (e.g. gum, patch, inhaler, nasal spray, lozenge, sublingual tablet)	Needs monitoring for potential adverse effect (e.g. insomnia)
Varenicline	Partial agonist at alpha 4 beta 2 nicotinic acetylcholine receptors Use for nicotine use disorder	Small increased risk of suicidality, and thus should be used with caution by resident who has MDD and avoided by resident who has suicidal ideas
FDA-approved medication for opioid use disorder	Buprenorphine (partial opioid agonist) Buprenorphine-naloxone combination (partial opioid agonist/antagonist) Naltrexone (injectable) (opioid antagonist)	Involvement of psychiatrist with expertise in opioid addiction is recommended Methadone is approved by FDA for opioid use disorder, but due to high risks associated with its use (e.g. QT prolongation, drug–drug interactions), HCP should avoid prescribing it for LTC populations
Management of withdrawal symptoms	In most cases, can be safely done in LTC facility For severe symptoms (e.g. delirium) or moderate symptoms in frail resident, hospitalization is recommended	Staff education and training to monitor withdrawal symptoms is necessary

prompt treatment. Moderate to severe withdrawal symptoms are best managed in a hospital setting. Some residents may be allowed continued use of small amounts of daily consumption of alcohol, if, after comprehensive assessment, use of alcohol is deemed critical for the resident's quality of life and the resident and/or family have been educated about potential risks of continued use of these substances. Continued use of BZD in the LTC setting may pose a high risk of falls and injury (e.g. hip fracture), cognitive impairment, and functional decline. Most residents tolerate gradual dose reduction (done over a few weeks to several months) without worsening of anxiety symptoms or impaired sleep and may even show cognitive and functional improvement. Some residents may be able to be weaned off BZD completely by slow taper over weeks to months. Distressing insomnia is a common reason for a resident to ask to resume use of BZD. Comprehensive treatment of insomnia with exercise, relaxing bedtime routines, sleep hygiene, and other psychosocial environmental strategies instituted early in the course of BZD taper usually are sufficient to improve sleep. Many residents who have nicotine use disorder or cannabis use disorder do not want to quit but often can be persuaded to reduce the amount of use (harm reduction). Residents who have insomnia and/or anxiety may need to reduce their caffeine intake or limit caffeine intake to morning. If insomnia and anxiety symptoms persist despite reduced caffeine intake, it is preferable to eliminate caffeine intake completely before instituting any psychotropic medication therapy for insomnia and/or anxiety symptoms.

Intermittent Explosive Disorder

Intermittent explosive disorder (IED) is characterized by impulsive recurrent aggressive behavior (verbal [e.g. temper tantrum, tirade] and/or physical) that is disproportionate to the stressor or situation (Coccaro 2012). Following the episode, the individual may experience regret, embarrassment, and/or guilt for the action. For diagnosis, at least three episodes of violence (destruction of property and/or physical assault) over 12 months is needed or at least two less-severe episodes per week for three months. Residents who have IED usually have a long history of aggressive behavior. New onset of impulsive aggression in LTC populations are usually in the context of pre-existing MNCD, delirium, stroke, traumatic brain injury, or mood or psychotic disorder. Damage to the frontal lobe and the presence of executive dysfunction are commonly seen in residents who have recurrent impulsive aggression. Treatment involves staff education, identification and avoidance of triggers, and staff training in de-escalation. We recommend anger management, mindfulness-based therapy, and CBT for a motivated resident who has relatively intact cognitive function. We recommend a trial of an SSRI or an SNRI for the treatment of IED, and in refractory cases, the HCP may consider a trial of an antipsychotic or valproate or propranolol.

Summary

Personality problems and disorders, somatic symptoms and related disorders, and substance use disorders are prevalent in LTC populations, are associated with increased morbidity, and are common causes of treatment-resistant MDD. Having a high index of suspicion is necessary for early, accurate diagnosis. A comprehensive assessment can accurately diagnose these disorders. Despite challenges, these disorders are treatable psychiatric conditions, and treatment may improve the resident's quality of life and reduce family and professional caregivers' stress. For complex cases, we recommend referral to a psychiatrist or a specialty center for older adults. The HCP should consider intermittent explosive disorder in the differential diagnosis of recurrent severe aggressive behavior. It can be treated with staff training in de-escalation, psychotherapeutic strategies (e.g. anger management, CBT), and if necessary SSRI or SNRI.

Key Clinical Points

1. Personality change due to MNCD or another medical condition and personality disorders are prevalent in LTC populations and frequently contribute to aggressive behavior, agitation, and treatment resistance of MDD.
2. Somatic symptom and related disorders are underdiagnosed in LTC populations, typically accompany a diagnosable medical condition, and are often mismanaged by unnecessary or harmful tests, procedures, and treatment.
3. At-risk and problem use of benzodiazepine and opioids and nicotine use disorder are prevalent in LTC populations, and the prevalence of substance use disorders (especially alcohol, cannabis) is growing in LTC populations.
4. The HCP should consider intermittent explosive disorder in the differential diagnosis of recurrent severe aggressive behavior.
5. Despite challenges, these disorders are treatable psychiatric conditions, and treatment may improve the resident's quality of life and reduce family and professional caregivers' stress.

References

Agronin, M.E. 2015. Somatic Symptom and Related Disorders. In D.C. Steffens, D.G. Blazer, and M.E. Thakur (eds.), *The Textbook of Geriatric Psychiatry*, 5th ed., pp. 373–388. Arlington, VA: American Psychiatric Publishing.

American Psychiatric Association. 2013a. Personality Disorders. In *Diagnostic and Statistical Manual of Mental Disorders*, 5th ed., pp. 645–684. Arlington, VA: American Psychiatric Association Press.

American Psychiatric Association. 2013b. Somatic Symptom and Related Disorders. In *Diagnostic and Statistical Manual of Mental Disorders*, 5th ed., pp. 309–328. Arlington, VA: American Psychiatric Association Press.

American Psychiatric Association. 2013c. Substance-Related and Addictive Disorders. In *Diagnostic and Statistical Manual of Mental Disorders*, 5th ed., pp. 481–589. Arlington, VA: American Psychiatric Association Press.

Coccaro, E.F. 2012. Intermittent Explosive Disorder as Disorder of Impulsive Aggression in *DSM V*. *American Journal of Psychiatry* **169**:577–588.

Desai, A.K. and G.T. Grossberg. 2017. Psychiatric Aspects of Long-Term Care. In B.J. Saddock, V.A. Saddock, and P. Ruiz (eds.). *Comprehensive Textbook of Psychiatry*, 10th ed., pp. 4221–4232. Virginia: American Psychiatric Press Inc. In Press.

Mavandadi, S. and D.W. Oslin. 2015. Substance-Related and Addictive Disorders. In D.C. Steffens, D.G. Blazer, and M.E. Thakur (eds.), *The Textbook of Geriatric Psychiatry*, 5th ed., pp. 459–490. Arlington, VA: American Psychiatric Publishing.

Oxman, T.E. 2015. Personality Disorders. In D.C. Steffens, D.G. Blazer, and M.E. Thakur (eds.), *The Textbook of Geriatric Psychiatry*, 5th ed., pp. 491–506. Arlington, VA: American Psychiatric Publishing.

Streim, J. 2015. Clinical Psychiatry in the Nursing Home. In D.C. Steffens, D.G. Blazer, and M.E. Thakur (eds.), *The Textbook of Geriatric Psychiatry*, 5th ed., pp. 689–748. Arlington, VA: American Psychiatric Publishing.

Taylor, M.H. and G.T. Grossberg. 2012. The Growing Problem of Illicit Substance Abuse in the Elderly: A Review. *Primary Care Companion CNS Disorders* **14**(4): PCC.11r01320. doi:10.4088/PCC.11r01320

US Department of Health and Human Services and US Department of Agriculture. 2015. *2015–2020 Dietary Guidelines for Americans*. 8th ed., Washington, DC.

Vaillant, G.E. 2012. *Triumphs of Experience: The Men of the Harvard Grant Study*. Cambridge, MA: Harvard University Press.

Chapter 9

Nutritional Medicine and Long-Term Care Psychiatry

There is growing evidence that well-balanced diet rich in brain-essential nutrients may improve cognition and reduce the risk of a variety of psychiatric disorders (especially mood, anxiety, sleep-wake, and cognitive disorders) (Sarris et al. 2015). The Mediterranean diet may reduce the risk of major neurocognitive disorder (MNCD; e.g. Alzheimer's disease) and major depressive disease (MDD). The DASH (Dietary Approaches to Stop Hypertension) diet may reduce the risk of MNCD. Healthy dietary patterns are related to decreased total mortality and disease-specific mortality, especially in older adults. Besides providing nutrients and neurotropic factors required for optimal brain function (e.g. adequate vitamin B_{12}, omega-3 fatty acids), nutrition can influence mental health by modulating the immune system (e.g. increased inflammation due to intake of more calories than needed to maintain normal weight increases the risk of depression and suicide) and antioxidant activity (protective against synaptic and neuronal loss) (Porter Starr, Bales, and Payne 2015). The majority of residents in long-term care (LTC) do not consume the recommended intake of several brain-essential nutrients, including protein, omega-3 fatty acids, B-group vitamins, zinc, and magnesium. Thus, LTC populations are at risk of developing a variety of psychiatric disorders and exacerbating pre-existing psychiatric disorder due to poor nutrition. Nutritional rehabilitation plays a key role in cognitive and emotional well-being in LTC populations.

Undernutrition

Undernutrition, defined as deficiency of energy (calories), protein, and/or other nutrients, is associated with high morbidity and mortality. (See Box 9.1.) Typically, a resident who has a body mass index (BMI) less than 20 and/or significant unintentional weight loss (loss of 5 percent or more of body weight within six months) is thought to have undernutrition. Loss of 10 percent or more weight within six months and/or BMI less than 18.5 is considered severe undernutrition. More than 50 percent of residents may be undernourished when screened using the Mini-Nutritional Assessment (MNA). Only one in five undernourished residents considers him- or herself undernourished. More than 45 percent of

BOX 9.1 Potential Complications of Undernutrition

- Increased mortality and morbidity
- Decreased quality of life
- Higher health care costs
- Delirium (due to hypoglycemia, dehydration, electrolyte imbalance, drug toxicity due to reduction in serum protein binding, etc.)
- Cognitive impairment
- Functional impairment
- Mood disorder (especially depression)
- Sleep-wake disorder (e.g. insomnia, hypersomnia)
- Frailty
- Sarcopenia
- Cachexia and failure to thrive
- Increased length of hospital stay
- Acute renal failure (due to severe dehydration)
- Falls and injury (e.g. hip fracture, subdural hematoma)
- Pressure ulcer/decubitus and skin failure
- Compromised immune system, leading to recurrent infection (e.g. urinary tract infection or pneumonia) and poor wound healing
- Vitamin deficiency and its complications (e.g. MNCD, peripheral neuropathy, MDD)
- Anemia
- Electrolyte imbalance and its complications (e.g. seizure)
- Oral ulcer
- Exacerbation of chronic medical illness (e.g. diabetes, chronic kidney disease, osteoporosis)

undernourished residents do not receive treatment by a registered dietician. Protein and/or energy malnutrition, dehydration, and micronutrient deficiency are the most common causes of undernutrition.

Undernutrition can manifest in myriad ways. (See Table 9.1.) Self-perception of lack of energy and unintentional weight loss are the two most common manifestation of undernutrition in LTC populations. We recommend asking a screening question, "Did you feel full of energy in the past week?," in addition to MNA-short form to screen for undernutrition in LTC populations. Undernutrition is typically multifactorial. See Box 9.2 for common causes of undernutrition in LTC populations. Depressive disorders are among the most common causes of undernutrition, and unintentional weight loss is one of the most common reasons for psychiatric consultation. Rapid and acute weight loss in excess of 3 percent of baseline body weight is most likely due to reduced total body water from dehydration. Eating disorders in LTC populations are rare, and typically there is a long history of symptoms of an eating disorder (e.g. binge eating, dramatic fluctuation in weight, purging, phobia of weight gain, disturbance in self-image). Disease-related malnutrition (DRM) is a term used to describe undernutrition due to acute and/or chronic disease and/or treatment. DRM causes undernutrition by interfering with ingestion (anorexia) or absorption of nutrients and/or increased energy requirements. We recommend a thorough assessment for any resident who has undernutrition to clarify the type and severity of nutrient deficiency and identify underlying causes. (See Box 9.3.) Some of the key areas for nutritional assessment include but are not limited to: assessment of alertness; cognitive and functional impairment; condition of teeth, gums, and oral health;

Table 9.1 Manifestations of Undernutrition and Mental Health Implications

Nutrient Deficiency	Key Clinical Manifestations	Clinical Relevance and Potential Mental Health Consequences
Protein and/or calorie malnutrition	Anergia (lack of energy), significant unintentional weight loss,* recurrent infection, sarcopenia	Prevalent in LTC populations (especially resident who has MNCD) Risk factor for cognitive impairment and MDD
Dehydration	Lack of energy, falls, dizziness, orthostatic hypotension, acute renal failure	Prevalent in LTC populations (especially resident who has MNCD) Risk factor for cognitive impairment and delirium
Vitamin A (retinoids) deficiency	Xerophthalmia (dryness of conjunctiva and cornea), night blindness	Rare in LTC populations May be seen in resident who has severe celiac disease, pancreatic insufficiency, or terminal ileum disease Along with other co-occurring nutritional deficiency, increases risk of MDD
Vitamin B_{12} (cyanocobalamin) deficiency	Anemia, peripheral neuropathy, fatigue	Prevalent in LTC populations Often causes or exacerbates cognitive impairment and MDD
Folate (vitamin B_9) deficiency	Anemia, fatigue, glossitis	Uncommon in LTC populations due to food fortified with folate May cause or exacerbate cognitive impairment and MDD
Vitamin B_6 (pyridoxine) deficiency	Peripheral neuropathy	May be seen in resident who has alcohol use disorder and severe undernutrition May exacerbate cognitive impairment
Vitamin B_2 (riboflavin) deficiency	Glossitis, cheilosis (fissuring of angles of mouth), anemia	May be seen in resident who has alcohol use disorder and severe undernutrition May exacerbate cognitive impairment

Table 9.1 (cont.)

Nutrient Deficiency	Key Clinical Manifestations	Clinical Relevance and Potential Mental Health Consequences
Vitamin B_1 (thiamine) deficiency	Wernicke encephalopathy (ataxia, diplopia, delirium)	May be seen in resident who has alcohol use disorder If severe, may cause delirium and amnestic disorder (Korsakoff syndrome [anterograde amnesia with confabulation])
Vitamin C (ascorbic acid) deficiency	Bleeding gums, easy bruising, poor wound healing	Resident who has vitamin C deficiency is at increased risk of bleeding with some antidepressants (e.g. SSRI)
Vitamin D deficiency	Recurrent falls, osteomalacia, musculoskeletal pain	Prevalent in LTC populations May exacerbate cognitive impairment and increase risk of MDD
Vitamin E deficiency	Peripheral neuropathy, ataxia, myopathy	Rare in LTC populations May be seen in resident who has severe celiac disease, pancreatic insufficiency, or terminal ileum disease High-dose vitamin E along with antidepressant (e.g. SSRI) may increase risk of bleeding
Vitamin K deficiency	Bleeding	Rare in LTC populations May be seen in resident who has severe celiac disease, pancreatic insufficiency, or terminal ileum disease Resident who has vitamin K deficiency is at increased risk of bleeding with some antidepressants (e.g. SSRI)
Hypocalcemia	Usually asymptomatic In moderate to severe cases, may cause osteomalacia, seizure (severe hypocalcemia), cardiac arrhythmia (severe hypocalcemia)	Resident who does not consume dairy products is at risk of developing hypocalcemia May cause or exacerbate anxiety and insomnia
Hypomagnesemia	Leg cramps Cardiac arrhythmia	Uncommon in LTC populations May cause or exacerbate insomnia
Zinc deficiency	Alopecia, poor wound healing, diarrhea	Underrecognized in LTC populations May exacerbate MDD
Iron deficiency	Anemia, poor wound healing	Prevalent in LTC populations May exacerbate MDD
Selenium deficiency	Low energy	Underrecognized in LTC populations May exacerbate MDD
Copper deficiency	Poor wound healing	Underrecognized in LTC populations Poor healing of pressure ulcer may predispose to depressive disorder
Manganese deficiency	Poor wound healing	Underrecognized in LTC populations Poor healing of pressure ulcer may predispose to depressive disorder

* Significant unintentional weight loss: More than 10 percent over six months or more than 5 percent in one month

BOX 9.2 Common Causes of Undernutrition in Long-Term Care Populations

- Age-related changes in appetite, taste, smell, thirst recognition, and satiation (includes anorexia of aging)
- Environmental causes
  - Inadequate assistance with eating (most important and prevalent cause, especially among residents who have MNCD)
  - Poor mealtime environment (e.g. too much noise, disorganized food service)
  - Trouble getting meals ready on time
  - Interpersonal aspects of food service and meal environment (e.g. lack of prompt help for toileting during meals, which may reduce resident's willingness to consume adequate amount of food and fluid)
  - Financial constraints of LTC facility (e.g. leading to suboptimal staffing [number of staff and adequately trained staff] preventing adequate assistance with eating, inadequate availability of fresh fruits and vegetables)
- Issues with quality of food
  - Unfamiliar food
  - Food not in keeping with resident's ethnic, cultural, and religious background
  - Food not in keeping with resident's personal desires
  - Therapeutic diets (e.g. low salt, low cholesterol, diabetic diet)
  - Poor-quality food (e.g. too mushy, lack of variety, food cooked the same way)
- Psychiatric disorders
  - Alzheimer's disease and other MNCD
  - MNCD-related behavioral and psychological symptoms (e.g. apathy, wandering, pacing)
  - Mood disorder (e.g. MDD, bipolar disorder)
  - Psychotic disorder (e.g. schizophrenia)
  - Anxiety disorder (e.g. swallowing phobia [phagophobia])
  - Eating disorder (e.g. binge eating disorder)
- Medication-induced
  - Medication-induced anorexia, nausea, and/or weight loss (e.g. opioid, metformin, digoxin, amiodarone, cholinesterase inhibitor, antibiotic, stimulant, topiramate, antidepressant [e.g. SSRI, SNRI, bupropion], theophylline, cimetidine, calcium)
  - Medication-induced altered taste (dysgeusia) (e.g. captopril, metronidazole, lithium)
  - Drug-induced micronutrient deficiency (e.g. folate deficiency with use of phenytoin; calcium deficiency with use of tetracycline)
- Physical health conditions
  - Oral problem: ill-fitting dentures, loss of teeth, lesion in mouth, dysgeusia, gingival and periodontal disease
  - Gastrointestinal problem: swallowing problem (dysphagia); gall bladder problem (e.g. gallstones, cholecystitis), protein wasting enteropathy and malabsorption syndromes
  - Cancer
  - Endocrine disorder (e.g. hyperthyroidism, hypothyroidism, hypercalcemia, hypoadrenalism)
  - Chronic infection (e.g. tuberculosis, AIDS)
  - End-organ failure (e.g. heart failure [cardiac cachexia], end-stage renal disease [ESRD], end-stage COPD)
  - Parkinson's disease (PD)
  - Tremor, especially affecting dominant hand (e.g. essential tremors, PD)
  - Multiple sclerosis
  - Huntington's disease
  - Rheumatoid arthritis
  - Lactase deficiency/lactose intolerance

BOX 9.3 Tests and Measurements to Assess Undernutrition

Test/Measurement	Reason
Body weight	Diagnose and monitor loss or gain in weight
Body mass index (BMI)	Diagnose and monitor loss or gain of body fat
Abdominal circumference	Diagnose and monitor abdominal obesity
Waist-hip ratio	Diagnose and monitor abdominal obesity
FoodEx-LTC questionnaire	Assess individual's satisfaction with meals
EdFED-Q	Assess eating needs of individual who has MNCD
Mini-nutritional assessment (MNA)	Identify individual at risk for undernutrition
Serum total protein, prealbumin, albumin	Identify protein undernutrition
Total lymphocyte count	Nonspecific marker for undernutrition
Serum B_{12} and folate levels	Assess vitamin B_{12} and folate deficiency
Serum calcium and vitamin D levels	Assess calcium and vitamin D deficiency
Serum cholesterol level	Marker for undernutrition
Serum blood urea nitrogen and creatinine	Assess for dehydration
Serum sodium and potassium	Assess for electrolyte imbalance
Serum levels of specific micronutrients*	Assess micronutrient deficiency

* Micronutrients: other vitamins, magnesium, zinc, copper, iron, manganese

ability to chew and swallow; ability to see, hear, and follow instructions; ability to speak clearly; presence or absence of saliva in the mouth; ability to seal lips and move tongue in a coordinated way; and ability to cough (Wu et al. 2016). Albumin has a longer half-life (two to three weeks) than prealbumin (two to three days). Serum levels of prealbumin and albumin decline with reduced intake of protein and in catabolic state (increased breakdown of protein) associated with inflammation, stress, or hepatic or renal disease. Assessing reduced serum levels of prealbumin is preferred to albumin levels to detect early protein undernutrition.

A variety of evidence-based approaches can successfully prevent and treat undernutrition in LTC populations. (See Box 9.4.) Best practice requires an individualized plan of care with the dual objectives of providing adequate food and fluid intake and maintaining the resident's self-feeding ability, to the extent possible. A resident's eating behavior may change during an acute illness or with progression of MNCD or other disease(s), requiring staff to assess regularly and adjust the plan as needed. Staff training in assistance with eating is key to successful prevention of undernutrition in LTC populations. We recommend food and fluid fortification as the first-line treatment for prevention of undernutrition in LTC populations, as it is effective and can reduce the need for supplements, thereby reducing the potential for toxicity (e.g. hypervitaminosis D), reducing pill burden, reducing cost, reducing staff time to dispense medication, reducing the need for laboratory testing for nutrient deficiencies, reducing the risk of choking (due to large size of some supplements), and avoiding drug-supplement interaction. A resident who has certain medical conditions (e.g. severe chronic obstructive pulmonary disease, congestive heart failure) may be unable to consume a large meal at one sitting and may do better with multiple small meals. A resident who is at risk of weight loss (has poor appetite, feels full after eating only a small amount, reports that food tastes bad, or eats at most one meal a day) and a resident who already has weight loss should have the MNA done and be treated for reversible causes of weight loss. Health care providers (HCPs) should be aware that medical record documentation overestimates quality of care, assistance with eating, supplements offered, and oral intake of meals. Accurate documentation of oral intake of meals and fluids is a crucial component of staff training.

The amount and quality of assistance with eating provided to a resident is one of the most powerful determinants of daily food and fluid intake. A feeding skills training program for staff increases eating time for residents who have advanced MNCD. HCPs should also note the staffing levels during mealtime. Expert panels recommend a minimum of five residents to one nurse aide or staff eating assistant during

BOX 9.4 Prevention and Treatment Strategies for Undernutrition

- Routinely screen all residents for undernutrition at time of admission and quarterly thereafter
- Implement weight loss and undernutrition prevention strategies for at-risk resident based on Weight Loss Prevention Training Manual (most important approach) (http://geronet.med.ucla.edu/centers/borun/modules/Weight_loss_prevention/wlmod.pdf)
- Institute interdisciplinary team approach led by registered dietician to devise individualized nutritional plan (with input of speech therapist if dysphagia present)
- Discontinue medication that may cause anorexia, nausea, and/or unintentional weight loss (with input of consultant pharmacist)
- Liberalize diet
- Fortify food and fluid with energy (calories) and/or protein
- Fortify micronutrients (e.g. calcium, vitamin D, B vitamins, vitamin E)
- Offer oral nutritional supplements and health shakes
- Increase eating assistance time (includes hand feeding)
- Implement person-centered care practices
  - Offer familiar food that is in keeping with resident's ethnic, cultural, and religious background
  - Allow family to bring resident's favorite ethnic foods
  - Individualized schedule
  - Preferred food and fluids
  - Preferred time
  - Preferred amount
  - Preferred place
  - Preferred frequency, menus, and dining locations
  - Preferred temperature of food
- Strategies to increase physical activity (improve appetite)
- Improve quality of food
  - Fresh fruits and vegetables
  - Freshly cooked food
  - Optimally warm meals
  - Flavor-enhanced foods
- Improve meal environment
  - Residents are able to enjoy aromas of freshly cooked foods nearby
  - Soothing background music
  - Improve lighting
  - Bright and contrasting colors for tableware and placemats
  - Improve opportunity for social interaction during meals
  - Seating in comfortable chairs (not wheelchairs) with good posture
  - Minimize disruption due to excessive noise (e.g. turn off television)
- Staff training for improved eating assistance, problem solving, and documentation
  - Verbal cuing (e.g. "Pick up your spoon," "Take a bite," "Chew," "Swallow"), eating motions so that resident can imitate, and verbal encouragement
  - Hand-over-hand technique to initiate and guide self-feeding
  - Seat staff at resident's eye level
  - Ensure that resident has dentures and/or glasses if needed and can see and reach food plate or tray
  - Simplify meal presentation; serve one food item at a time if necessary; remove unnecessary utensils
  - Provide finger foods if resident experiences difficulty managing utensils
  - Remove items that should not be eaten and hot items that may be spilled
  - Accurately document food and fluid consumed by resident

BOX 9.4 (cont.)

- Assess and manage medical and psychiatric conditions thought to cause anorexia and/or unintentional weight loss (e.g. MDD, pain)
- Provide vitamin and mineral supplements (e.g. vitamins B_{12}, folate, thiamine, vitamin D, calcium, zinc, selenium)
- Use specialized utensils (e.g. weighted spoon, rocker-bottom knife, side-cutter fork) and other assistive devices as recommended by occupational therapy evaluation
- Refer to speech therapist for suspected dysphagia
- Provide separate, smaller eating area for resident who becomes agitated in large dining area
- Offer smaller, more frequent meals for certain residents (e.g. resident who has lifetime history of multiple small meals, resident who has severe COPD, GERD)
- Pharmacological strategies
  - Dronabinol to stimulate appetite in palliative care situations
  - Testosterone for male resident who has testosterone deficiency, sarcopenia, or undernutrition
  - Antidepressant (especially mirtazapine) for resident who has depressive disorder
  - Megestrol (especially for resident who has cancer, AIDS with anorexia and significant weight loss)
- Appropriate palliative care and referral to hospice for resident in terminal stages of MNCD or other progressive disease

mealtime. Staffing below 5–7:1 (one staff person for 5–7 residents) may require targeting residents who are most in need and/or using non-nursing staff (e.g. social worker, volunteer) for some daily mealtime tasks. Increasing eating assistance time (from 10 minutes to 30 minutes), verbal cuing, and social interaction along with adequate staffing can dramatically improve residents' oral intake of food and fluids. Staff or volunteers should offer eating assistance to groups of three to four residents three times per day between meals (10 a.m., 2 p.m., 7 p.m.), for about 15–20 minutes per snack period.

In our teaching nursing homes in St. Louis, all staff, including clerical and administrative staff, receive training in eating assistance and are present in various dining areas in the facility for all meals to assist residents who need help with eating.

Verbal prompts to drink liquids on four to eight occasions between meals, offering beverages of choice, offering enhanced between-meal snacks with appropriate assistance with eating, and actively encouraging residents to eat and drink several times a day are some strategies recommended to prevent and treat dehydration and weight loss. The management should consider offering family-style meals, especially for residents who do not have MNCD. Encouraging residents to take extra food (with verbal prompts, physical assistance) at mealtime over a period of time, rather than having them eat of their own volition, can promote weight gain. Having a social "Happy Hour" with snacks and nonalcoholic beverages helps improve food and fluid intake for some residents and may add an element of fun to their lives. Although offering food and fluids is time consuming and requires special knowledge of physiological changes and empathy for persons whose behavior might be objectionable at times, it may be one of the few times during the day when a resident (especially a resident who has MNCD) receives normalized social interaction.

Staff should offer a variety of foods during each snack period. Morning and afternoon snack periods are more successful than evening snack periods, and snack periods offered three times a day are more successful than those offered twice a day. Staff should present snacks on a moveable attractive cart so that residents can see them. Juices, yogurt, ice cream, fresh fruit, pudding, cookies, pastries, cheese/peanut butter and crackers are good choices for most residents. Snacks for residents who have diabetes or other special diets should also be available. We recommend that staff and family casually converse or otherwise socially interact with the resident throughout the snack period. The HCP should consider liberalizing diet for any resident who has anorexia, poor oral intake, or unintentional weight loss. The HCP should use restricted and specialized diets judiciously with LTC populations and only after thorough discussion among the resident, family, primary care physician, and registered dietician. This is because a restricted diet (e.g. no salt, diabetic diet) can make food so unappealing that the resident won't eat and may become undernourished and even cachectic. The

HCP should recommend it only if it is in keeping with the resident's overall goals of care. Most specialized diets have significant mental health implications, and the HCP should take these into account in the decision to institute such diets. (See Table 9.2.) Many residents are put on specialized diets without explanation or consent, thereby further exacerbating emotional distress related to specialized diet. Additionally, dieticians need to ensure that specialized diets have optimal variety, resident satisfaction, and therapeutic benefit. We recommend ending the practice of restricted diets for LTC populations, with a few exceptions. We recommend liberalizing diets and making them more appealing, and controlling blood pressure or diabetes by appropriate adjustment of medication. Any resident who needs palliative or hospice care should have her diet liberalized, as most specialized or restricted diets have a negative impact on quality of life in this context.

Oral nutritional supplements may not only promote weight gain but also improve immune functioning, and they have other clinical benefits (e.g. less fever, fewer prescribed antibiotics [because of avoiding need for intravenous], cognitive improvement). When given with meals, supplements may have a suppressant effect on the appetite. Glucose in the

Table 9.2 Various Diets and Their Relevance to Mental Health in Long-Term Care Populations

Diet	Description of Diet	Potential Mental Health Consequences
Regular diet	Used for individual who does not require any dietary restrictions	Improves quality of life of many residents who are on special diets when switched to regular diet
Mechanical soft (dental diet)	Modifies consistency of food and is given to individual who has difficulty chewing (typically due to dental problem)	MDD is prevalent in residents who have dental problems, and switching from regular diet to mechanical soft diet may improve food intake, prevent undernutrition, and accelerate response to treatment for depression
Dysphagia level 1 (pureed diet)	Used for individual who has difficulty chewing and/or swallowing	Many residents in last phase of life may prefer regular or mechanical soft diet despite risk of aspiration, as they may find pureed diet unappealing and hence this diet may predispose them to MDD
Dysphagia level 2 (mechanically altered diet)	Used for individual who has difficulty swallowing regular food	Many residents in last phase of life may prefer regular or mechanical soft diet despite risk of aspiration, as they may find mechanically altered diet unappealing and hence this diet may predispose them to MDD
Dysphagia advanced level 3	Used for individual who has difficulty swallowing regular food	Many residents in last phase of life may prefer regular or mechanical soft diet despite risk of aspiration, as they may find this diet unappealing and hence this diet may predispose them to MDD
Thickened liquids	Used for individual who has difficulty swallowing Nectar-thickened liquids will go through straw and glide off spoon Honey-thickened liquids will not go through straw and will flow slowly from spoon Pudding or liquids of pudding consistency (spoon thick) needs to be fed with spoon	Many residents in last phase of life may prefer regular or mechanical soft diet despite risk of aspiration, as they may find this diet unappealing and hence this diet may predispose them to MDD Many residents are not explained reason for such alternation in diet and are not asked for consent, further increasing emotional distress associated with diet using thickened liquids

Table 9.2 (cont.)

Diet	Description of Diet	Potential Mental Health Consequences
Full liquid	Used for individual who is acutely ill or unable to chew or swallow solid food (typically for few days) If used for extended period, nutritional supplements are recommended between meals	Particularly stressful for LTC populations due to comorbid frailty and neurocognitive impairment and often causes significant behavioral and psychological symptoms (including agitation) in resident who has advanced MNCD
Clear liquid	Used for individual who is acutely ill until she can tolerate full liquid diet or regular diet Nourishment between meals is recommended	Particularly stressful for LTC populations due to comorbid frailty and neurocognitive impairment and often causes significant behavioral and psychological symptoms (including agitation) in resident who has advanced MNCD
Restricted fiber/residue	Used for individual who needs stool weight, fecal output, and frequency decreased due to acute gastrointestinal problem (e.g. exacerbation of Crohn's disease)	Particularly stressful for LTC populations due to comorbid frailty and neurocognitive impairment and often causes significant behavioral and psychological symptoms (including agitation) in resident who has advanced MNCD
Increased fiber	Used for individual who has constipation	Recommended for resident who has constipation and needs to take psychotropic medication that may worsen constipation (e.g. antipsychotic)
Pleasure feedings (e.g. ice cream, pudding, cream soup, applesauce)	Recommended for individual receiving enteral feeding or receiving palliative/ hospice care to improve quality of life (need input from speech therapist and registered dietician)	Recommended for resident who has MDD as part of SPPEICE and individualized pleasant activity schedule May reduce agitation in resident who has MNCD
Small portions	Used per individual preference and when caloric and protein needs are lower than what regular diet provides	Many residents who have MDD and poor appetite may feel overwhelmed with regular portions and may eat better with small portions initially
Large portions	Used per individual preference and when caloric and protein needs are higher than what regular diet provides	Many underweight residents who have MDD may be recommended this diet once their mood and appetite improve but their weight has not normalized
Vegetarian	Used per individual preference and is modification of regular diet Lacto-ovovegetarian: excludes meat, poultry, and fish Lactovegetarian: excludes meat, poultry, fish, and eggs Ovovegetarian: excludes meat, poultry, fish, milk, and milk products Vegan: excludes meat, poultry, fish, eggs, milk, and milk products	Residents on this diet are at risk of developing micronutrient (e.g. omega-3 fatty acids, vitamin B_{12}, iron) deficiency and resultant psychiatric complications (especially depressive and neurocognitive disorders) Vitamin D may be deficient in vegan diet Fortified food/fluids, multivitamins, and mineral supplements are recommended to meet nutritional requirements
No added salt	Regular diet, but no salt may be added to food after preparation (salt substitute may be used with physician input) Used for individual who has hypertension	Liberalization of diet recommended for resident on this diet who develops MDD, resident who has MNCD, underweight resident, and resident needing palliative care

Table 9.2 (cont.)

Diet	Description of Diet	Potential Mental Health Consequences
Low salt (2–4 grams/day)	Regular diet with exclusion of highly salted food and table salt Used for individual who has hypertension	Liberalization of diet recommended for resident on this diet who develops MDD, resident who has MNCD, underweight resident, and resident needing palliative care
Cholesterol-restricted and fat-controlled (low-fat diet)	Used for individual who has dyslipidemia and requires diet lower in total fat, saturated fat, and cholesterol	Liberalization of diet recommended for resident on this diet who develops MDD, resident who has MNCD, underweight resident, and resident needing palliative care
Renal	Used for individual who has acute or chronic renal failure	Liberalization of diet (with or without limited potassium) recommended for resident who has advanced MNCD and resident who needs palliative/hospice care
Carbohydrate-controlled	Used for individual who has diabetes Concentrated sweets are not prohibited but are counted in total carbohydrate allowance	Liberalization of diet may reduce agitation for resident who has diabetes and MNCD Liberalization of diet recommended for resident on this diet who develops MDD, resident who has MNCD, underweight resident, and resident needing palliative care
Calorie-restricted (low calorie)	Used for individual who desires to lose weight (e.g. has obesity and wants to achieve normal weight)	With underweight resident, HCP needs to investigate eating disorder if resident expresses desire to lose weight
Limited concentrated sweets	Regular diet with foods high in sugar and other concentrated sweets excluded Used for individual who has diabetes whose weight and blood sugar are under good control	Liberalization of diet may reduce agitation for resident who has MNCD Liberalization of diet recommended for resident on this diet who develops MDD, resident who has MNCD, underweight resident, and resident needing palliative care
Diabetic calculated (1200, 1500, 1800 calories)	Used for individual who has diabetes and obesity	Not recommended for most residents due to risk of lowering quality of life and undernutrition
Lactose-reduced/Lactose-free	Used for individual who has lactose intolerance	For resident who has MNCD and wants to eat milk products, taking lactase tablet before consuming milk product may help prevent agitation caused by restricted diet
Kosher (based on Biblical rules of food for Jewish religion)	Used per individual preference (typically requested by Jewish individuals) Discussion with resident and family to clarify degree of strictness of diet is recommended	Providing this option may improve emotional adjustment to moving into LTC facility for Jewish resident
Gluten-free	Used for individual who has gluten sensitivity (celiac disease/nontropical sprue/gluten-sensitive enteropathy) Discussion with resident and family to clarify degree of strictness of diet is recommended	Resident who has gluten-sensitive enteropathy may also have micronutrient deficiency (e.g. iron, copper, zinc) that may cause psychiatric disorder (especially depressive and neurocognitive disorders)

Table 9.2 (cont.)

Diet	Description of Diet	Potential Mental Health Consequences
Finger food	Regular diet that can be easily eaten without need for utensils	HCP should consider this for resident who has advanced MNCD to prevent undernutrition and agitation
Enteral nutrition	Feeding tube (gastrostomy tube [G-tube], percutaneous endoscopic gastrostomy tube [PEG tube]) used by individual who cannot meet nutritional requirements with oral intake of food and fluids and has functional gastrointestinal tract (e.g. resident who has severe dysphagia after stroke) and such interventions are in keeping with resident's values and wishes	Palliative care/referral to hospice is preferable to tube feeding for resident who has advanced MNCD and cannot receive adequate nutrition with oral intake, as risks of tube feeding in this context are high and benefits absent or limited
Parenteral nutrition (total parenteral nutrition [TPN] and peripheral parenteral nutrition [PPN])	Provides intravenous proteins, calories, fat, vitamins, and other nutrients Used by individual who cannot be provided with adequate nutrition through gastrointestinal tract	Palliative care/referral to hospice is preferable to parenteral nutrition for resident who has advanced MNCD and cannot receive adequate nutrition through gastrointestinal tract, as risks of parenteral nutrition in this context are high and benefits absent or limited
MAOI diet	Used by individual taking monoamine oxidase inhibitor (MAOI) Individual needs to avoid a host of foods containing tyramine to avoid hypertensive crisis, which may occur due to interaction between MAOI and tyramine	Selegiline is most common MAOI used in LTC populations (for MDD [selegiline patch] and for Parkinson's disease) Resident using low-dose selegiline patch (6–9 mg/day) does not need MAOI diet but resident using 12 mg/day does need
Other dietary modifications	Dietary changes for individual who has gastroesophageal reflux disease (GERD) (e.g. multiple small meals, avoiding foods that can worsen heartburn [e.g. orange juice, spicy food]) Dietary changes for individual who has migraine (e.g. reduction of foods that often trigger migraine headache [e.g. dairy products, chocolate]) Individual who follows Hindu religion cannot have any food cooked with meat (especially beef), as cow is sacred animal for him and he is strictly vegetarian Halal diet involves certain dietary restrictions for individual of Muslim faith (e.g. no pork product, no foods that contain alcohol)	Dietary changes for GERD may reduce need for proton pump inhibitor (PPI), and chronic use of PPI is associated vitamin B_{12} deficiency, which in turn can lead to depressive and neurocognitive disorders Dietary changes for migraine may prevent exacerbation of migraine and reduce risk of depressive and cognitive disorders due to recurrent migraine

duodenum increases appetite in older adults but not in younger adults. Hence, oral nutritional supplements are most effective when given an hour before a meal, not with it. Providing nutritional supplements with a wide variety of sweets and carbohydrates may be additionally helpful to treat weight loss. Residents who are less cognitively and physically impaired respond better to between-meal snack programs, and more cognitively and physically impaired residents respond better to improved mealtime assistance with eating.

Inadequate food intake in LTC populations may be due to the type of food served. More than 50 percent of residents are regularly served food they dislike and report lack of variety in the food. Most residents do not voice dissatisfaction or preferences because of cognitive impairment, fear of retribution from the staff, or a belief that complaining in public is socially inappropriate. Some of these barriers can be overcome by assessing resident satisfaction away from the dining room and the food service staff. Financial constraints may prevent the resident from going to a LTC facility that has staff trained and available for optimal assistance with eating. These residents are also more likely to be undernourished before entering a LTC facility than residents who can afford to go to LTC facilities with financial resources to better address the nutritional needs of the residents. Financial constraints of the LTC facility may limit the purchase of fresh fruits and vegetables, and the facility may use outdated preparations and food-storage techniques (resulting in folate undernutrition). Some LTC facilities may have a registered dietician present only for as long as mandated by law (a shorter time than is optimal), making it even harder to meet residents' nutritional needs on a consistent basis.

Dysphagia may be due to medications (e.g. antipsychotic) or to neurological conditions (e.g. cerebrovascular disease). Metoclopramide is often used for gastroparesis and regurgitation or vomiting, but its use is associated with drug-induced Parkinsonism (which may cause dysphagia), apathy, depression, confusion, and daytime sedation. For residents who have anorexia and unintentional weight loss, a trial of discontinuing medication (e.g. metoclopramide, antipsychotics) may be necessary to clarify if the medication is causing more harm than good. The HCP may prescribe megestrol acetate for a resident who has severe anorexia or weight loss in the context of cancer or AIDS, but, due to the risk of deep-vein thrombosis, should avoid prescribing it for a resident who is immobile. Megestrol should be discontinued after 12 weeks to avoid adrenal insufficiency. Cyproheptadine may increase appetite but is not recommended for LTC populations because it has not been found to be effective in promoting weight gain and has significant risk of causing delirium. Parenteral nutrition and tube feeding carry serious risk and should be restricted to residents who are not in the terminal stages of MNCD or other medical condition, such as a resident who had a recent stroke and has difficulty swallowing but otherwise seems to be healthy and benefiting from rehabilitative therapy. The HCP should provide appropriate palliative care and referral to hospice for a resident who has unintentional weight loss in the terminal stages of MNCD or other progressive disease. The HCP may consider judicious use of dronabinol to improve appetite and food intake for a resident receiving hospice care with close monitoring for adverse effect (e.g. anxiety, delirium).

Loss of Appetite/Anorexia

Appetite is crucial to maintaining nutrition. On average, food intake is about 30 percent lower in an older adult than a young adult secondary to aging-associated physiological decrease in appetite. This is called the anorexia of aging, and it may predispose to undernutrition. Anorexia is a common problem among LTC residents and one of the most common reasons for psychiatric consultation. It should be differentiated from reduced oral intake of food and fluids due to factors other than anorexia (e.g. swallowing problem, dental problem, nausea due to adverse effect of medication [e.g. opioid-induced nausea]). Assessment of anorexia needs to address not only depression (the most common reversible cause of anorexia in LTC populations) but also a host of other causes. (See Box 9.2.) Anorexia is of particular concern in a resident who has diabetes (especially brittle diabetes) because of the high risk of potentially serious or even fatal hypoglycemia.

Treatment of anorexia is treatment of its cause(s). Good nutritional practice described in the section on unintentional weight loss may enhance the response to treatment. Because loss of taste and smell are common in older adults, use of flavor-enhanced food may improve appetite. The HCP should consider discontinuing medication that suppresses appetite and address the resident's complaints of meal service and meal quality. Liberalizing the diet and less rigid meal times may also improve appetite. Other strategies to improve appetite include suggesting that family bring favorite meals or snacks and encouraging residents to eat when they want.

Dehydration and Electrolyte Imbalance

Adequate nutritional care includes monitoring for sufficient intake of fluid. Dehydration refers to the loss of body water, with or without salt, at a rate greater than the body can replace it. Although dehydration is a sentinel event thought to reflect poor care, it is rarely due to neglect from formal or informal caregivers, but rather results from a combination of physiological and disease processes. LTC residents are at risk for dehydration because of both reduced fluid intake and increased fluid losses. As a rule, fluid intake among residents is well below the recommended requirement of 1500–2500 ml/day. Body weight and body water decrease with age, which together with the well-known deterioration of thirst perception in old age may give rise to dehydration and its potentially lethal complications (circulatory collapse, acute renal failure). In addition, with increasing age, there is decline in glomerular filtration rate (GFR), which may contribute to impaired ability to conserve water. Reduced skin integrity due to subcutaneous dehydration may result in xerosis, pruritus, recurrent skin infection, and pressure ulcer in the resident who is immobile. Cystitis and urinary tract infection may result from the irritant effect of highly concentrated urine on the vesical mucosa. Thickened oral and gastrointestinal secretions as a result of dehydration can lead to constipation, fecal impaction, xerostomia, periodontal disease, and mouth ulcer. In a resident who is dehydrated, neurological dysfunction may present as delirium, dizziness, recurrent falls, and subsequent complications, such as hip fracture or traumatic brain injury.

Dehydration may be present in up to one-quarter of LTC residents, and residents who have MNCD are likely to have an even higher prevalence. Besides aging-related neurophysiological changes, other common causes of dehydration include infection, delirium, and use of diuretic. During the warmer months and in warm climates, increased ambient temperature should prompt careful attention to fluid intake. In addition, a resident who has fever, burns, vomiting or diarrhea, or a draining fistula may need additional fluid. A resident who has chronic lung disease, decubitus ulcer, excessive tremor, or movement disorder is likely to have an increased amount of insensible fluid loss and thus may need more than usual daily fluid intake. Increased fluid intake may also be necessary for a resident who has poorly controlled diabetes mellitus or is taking laxative therapy. Use of diuretics in LTC populations can often be avoided. For example, amlodipine can cause edema, and instead of adding a diuretic such as furosemide, the HCP may be able to reduce the dosage of amlodipine. Dehydration is a common problem in LTC populations, often due to failures in the detection of dehydration and appropriate management.

The detection of dehydration is largely dependent on the HCP's having a high threshold of suspicion. Clinical diagnosis of dehydration in LTC populations is unreliable. Serum osmolality greater than 300, blood urea nitrogen (BUN) greater than 20, and BUN/creatinine ratio greater than 20 are useful indices to detect dehydration. Dehydration can be accompanied by hypernatremia (typically due to restricted water intake) or hyponatremia (typically due to use of diuretic). Severe hyponatremia may cause seizure, delirium, and even death. Excessive fluid loss due to diabetes insipidus (which in turn could be due to stroke, neurosurgery, etc.) may cause hypernatremia. Hypernatremia in elderly people carries a poor prognosis, with a mortality in excess of 40 percent when plasma sodium exceeds 150 nmol/l.

Treatment of dehydration is treatment of its cause(s). Common causes of dehydration in LTC populations are preventable and easily treatable. However, early diagnosis and treatment are key. We recommend encouraging oral ingestion of at least 1.5 liters of fluid daily, if cardiac and renal status allow. Aggressive and rapid replacement of fluid and electrolytes may lead to fluid overload and cardiac, pulmonary, and neurological complications. The HCP should avoid rapid correction of hyponatremia, as it may cause central pontine myelinolysis, a serious neurological disorder characterized by decreased awareness, dysphagia, and dysarthria. Availability of water fountains, circulating water or juice carts, encouraging fluid intake at medication rounds, and frequent prompts and assistance with drinking are some simple strategies to reduce the prevalence of dehydration in LTC populations. With the availability of recombinant hyaluronidase, subcutaneous infusion of fluid (hypodermoclysis) provides a better opportunity to treat mild to moderate dehydration in LTC populations.

Micronutrient Deficiency

Many residents have micronutrient (vitamin and mineral) deficiency with or without macronutrient deficiency. See Box 9.5 for a list of common causes of micronutrient deficiency in LTC populations. Requirements for vitamins D, B_6 (pyridoxine), B_9 (folate), and B_{12} (cyanocobalamin) are higher in older adults than in younger people. Vitamins B_{12}, folate, and B_6 are needed for homocysteine metabolism, and deficiency results in an elevated level of homocysteine, which has been associated with cognitive decline. Vitamin B_{12} deficiency is highly prevalent (25–35 percent) in LTC populations. Atrophic gastritis (prevalent in older adults) reduces the absorption of several nutrients, which leads, especially for vitamin B_{12}, to a deficiency state. B_{12} levels decline during prolonged use of proton pump inhibitor by an older adult. Pernicious anemia is a rare but serious disorder associated with vitamin B_{12} deficiency. Vitamin B_{12} deficiency may result in cognitive decline, depression, and, in severe cases, peripheral neuropathy, MNCD, and subacute combined degeneration of the spinal cord. These neuropsychiatric complications can be seen in the absence of anemia or an elevated mean cell volume. Folate deficiency is much less prevalent than vitamin B_{12} deficiency in LTC populations, as many foods are fortified with folate. Folate (up to 95 percent) in vegetables is destroyed by excessive cooking and hence lightly cooked vegetables are preferred. Folate deficiency is associated with anemia, fatigue, and glossitis. Folate deficiency may worsen depression and cognition. Vitamin B_2 (riboflavin) deficiency is seen in conjunction with other vitamin B deficiencies. Vitamin B_2 deficiency may manifest as cheilosis, glossitis, or anemia.

A resident who has low intake of fruits and vegetables or who smokes (and is not taking vitamin C supplements) may have low serum levels of vitamin C. Vitamin C deficiency may result in excessive bleeding from minor cuts, bleeding gums, poor wound healing, and, in severe cases, bleeding disorder. Approximately one-third of the required vitamin D can be obtained from the diet; the rest is synthesized in the skin under the influence of sunlight. Vitamin D deficiency is highly prevalent (30–40 percent) in LTC populations because of limited exposure to sun and a fourfold reduced capacity of the skin to produce vitamin D due to aging-related skin changes. Calcium deficiency may develop in a resident who has little or no dairy products in their diet. Vitamin D deficiency and calcium deficiency may result in osteomalacia, fracture, neuromuscular irritability, musculoskeletal pain, neuropathy, cognitive impairment, depression, and hyperesthesia. Older adults should take in at least 800 IU of vitamin D daily, with at least 1200 mg of elemental calcium in the diet or as a supplement, with the goal of serum vitamin D level of 30–40 ng/dl. Other populations at risk of micronutrient deficiency include residents who have partial gastrectomy (vitamin B_{12} deficiency), bacterial overgrowth (vitamin B_{12} and folate deficiency), celiac disease (folate, vitamins A, D deficiency), pancreatic insufficiency (vitamins A, D, E, and calcium deficiency), terminal ileum diseases (vitamins A, D, E, B_{12} and calcium deficiency), alcoholism (folate, thiamine deficiency), and chronic liver and gallbladder diseases (vitamins A, D, E, K deficiency). Medications are an important cause of micronutrient malabsorption (e.g. antacids and H2 blockers may decrease vitamin B_{12}; use of broad-spectrum antibiotic [e.g. neomycin] is associated with decreased absorption of vitamin K and folate due to changes in intestinal bacteria flora).

BOX 9.5 Common Risk Factors for Micronutrient Deficiency in Long-Term Care Populations

- Older adults require more than younger people
- Part of general malnutrition (along with anorexia, weight loss, and/or obesity)
- Diabetes mellitus
- Celiac disease
- Crohn's disease
- Alcohol use disorder
- Nicotine use disorder
- Liver disease
- Chronic diarrhea
- Chronic total parenteral nutrition
- Inflammatory disease of gastrointestinal tract
- Certain medications (e.g. methotrexate, triamterene, phenobarbital, phenytoin, theophylline)
- Certain diets (e.g. vegan, vegetarian)
- Gastric bypass
- Pancreatic insufficiency
- Terminal ileum disease

Other micronutrients that may have psychiatric significance (e.g. increased risk of cognitive impairment and/or depression) include copper, selenium (especially in a resident who has diabetes mellitus or chronic total parenteral nutrition), zinc, and vitamins B_1 (especially in a resident who has diabetes mellitus or alcohol use disorder), B_5, B_6, and B_7. Maintaining normal zinc levels may be an important factor in reducing the risk of pneumonia in LTC populations and reducing the risk of vision loss in older adults at high risk of macular degeneration.

Micronutrient deficiency may present atypically or be masked by coexisting disease or a general failure to thrive. Thus, we recommend that the HCP maintain a high index of suspicion for early diagnosis and treatment. Older adults are often subject to syndromes that present with early manifestation in the oral cavity (e.g. tongue changes due to nutritional anemia, reaction to medication [such as dry mouth], and deficiency disease such as scurvy [vitamin C deficiency causing excessive bleeding from gums]). Low fiber intake may worsen certain gastrointestinal conditions, such as chronic constipation, diverticulosis, gall bladder disease, and celiac sprue.

We recommend that all residents (unless receiving hospice care) be tested for serum albumin, vitamin B_{12}, folate, calcium, and D_3 levels, ideally at the time of admission. Some older adults may have cellular B_{12} deficiency but B_{12} levels may be in the normal range (usually at the lower end of the range). The HCP may consider measuring serum methymalonic acid and homocysteine (both levels are elevated) for a resident who has vitamin B_{12} level at the lower range of normal when the HCP has clinical suspicion of B_{12} deficiency. A resident at high risk of micronutrient deficiency may need additional tests to detect other micronutrient deficiency. Even if folate levels were within normal limits in the past, a recent development of malnutrition should prompt rechecking, as folate levels drop quickly once dietary intake is decreased. This is in contrast to vitamin B_{12} deficiency, which takes months to years to develop because vitamin B_{12} is stored in the liver.

Although food remains the best vehicle for consuming nutrients, vitamin and/or mineral supplements may be necessary for many LTC residents. We recommend oral supplements of vitamin B_{12} (500–1000 mcg/day) for a resident who has vitamin B_{12} deficiency or who has depression and vitamin B_{12} levels at the lower end of the normal range. A resident who has vitamin B_{12} deficiency due to pernicious anemia may need B_{12} injections (1000 mcg subcutaneously once a month). Besides vitamin D supplementation, we recommend increased exposure to sun (20 minutes per day) for a resident who has vitamin D levels below 30 ng/ml. Vitamin D also has a beneficial effect on the risk of falling, explained by improvement of muscle function. We recommend vitamin C supplementation for the resident at risk for vitamin C deficiency. A malnourished resident usually needs a host of vitamin and mineral supplements besides increased intake of nutritious food and fluids. A resident who has depressive disorder and low serum selenium levels may show improvement in mood with selenium supplementation. We recommend involving a registered dietician for any resident at risk of or suspected to have micronutrient deficiency.

We do not recommend routine vitamin E supplements for most LTC residents because of inconclusive data regarding the benefits of vitamin E supplements and potential risks (e.g. increased all-cause mortality, increased risk of bleeding [especially with concomitant use of blood thinner, such as warfarin]) of high-dose (≥400 IU/day) vitamin E intake. For a resident who has mild to moderate AD, 2000 U/day of vitamin E may be appropriate to slow the progression of disease without risking significant toxicity (Dysken et al. 2014). Vitamin A deficiency is rare in the United States and other industrialized countries (although common in poorly developed countries). We discourage vitamin A and beta-carotene supplementation for most LTC residents due to the lack of data indicating clinical benefits and possible adverse effects (e.g. osteopenia and fractures). The HCP should evaluate any resident taking vitamin and mineral supplements for need of these supplements because many residents may not need some or all the supplements they are consuming and because of the risk of adverse effect with vitamins/minerals–drug interaction and increase in pill burden. Also, some residents may be consuming potentially toxic amounts of vitamins and minerals by supplementation. Unnecessary supplements should be discontinued.

Frailty

Frailty is a state of extreme vulnerability to endogenous and exogenous stressors exposing the person to higher risk of adverse health-related outcome (Cesari et al. 2016). Frailty status is based on the presence of three or more of the following: unintentional weight loss (10 pounds or more in one year), muscle weakness as shown by weak grip strength or lower extremity muscle weakness, exhaustion, slow walking speed, and low physical activity level. Exhaustion can be detected by inquiring if the resident felt that anything she did was a big effort or that he could not keep doing things as before. Low physical activity is identified if the resident engages in less than 3.5 hours of leisure activity per week or self-reported low physical activity. A comprehensive geriatric assessment is key to accurate diagnosis and management of frailty. (See Table 9.3.) We recommend the FRAIL-NH (version 1 [I = incontinence] and version 2 [I = illness]) scale to screen for frailty in LTC residents (Kaehr et al. 2015). The FRAIL-NH scale assesses seven key domains: fatigue (present, absent, depressed [PHQ-9 >9]), resistance (strength to transfer; independent, set-up help only, needs physical assistance), ambulation, incontinence (none, urinary, bowel) or illness measured by number of different medications (<5, 5–9, >9) (versions 1 and 2, respectively), loss of weight (none, ≥5 percent in 3 months, ≥10 percent in 6 months), nutritional status (regular diet, mechanically altered diet, feeding tube), and help with dressing (independent, set-up only, physical assistance). Frailty is a form of predisability. A frail resident is at increased risk of becoming disabled, falling, being hospitalized, and dying within a few years. Frailty is present in more

Table 9.3 Assessment and Management of Frailty in Long-Term Care Populations

Intervention	Key Clinical/Practical Tools and Strategies	Team Leader
Comprehensive Geriatric Assessment (CGA) by physician Saint Louis University Rapid Geriatric Assessment is simpler assessment that can be rapidly done by many health care professionals	Chair-stand test (to assess weakness in lower extremity muscles) Hand grip assessment using hand dynamometer (to assess grip strength) Gait speed (walking speed) measurement (cutoff: less than 7 seconds to walk 5 meters [16.4 feet] excluding space used for acceleration and deceleration) Timed-Up-and-Go Test (TUGT) (cutoff score 10 seconds or more to cover distance of 3 meters) FRAIL-NH scale to screen for frailty in LTC populations Edmonton Frailty Scale for resident having elective surgery Clinical Frailty Scale to measure severity of frailty after completion of CGA	Primary care physician leads efforts, with assistance of interdisciplinary team
Optimal treatment of reversible medical and psychiatric conditions	Correction of vision and/or hearing Relief from pain Treatment of MDD Falls precautions Rehabilitation therapy (physical therapy, occupational therapy, speech therapy) to improve capacity for activities of daily living Treatment of Metabolic syndrome (central obesity, elevated triglycerides, low high-density lipoprotein level, hypertension, elevated fasting blood sugar or HbA1 c)	Interdisciplinary team approach with primary care physician ensuring coordinated care and involvement of psychiatrist in complex cases
Nutritional rehabilitation	Fortified foods and fluids Correction of nutritional deficiency (dehydration, macronutrient and micronutrient deficiency)	Registered dietician leads efforts

Table 9.3 (cont.)

Intervention	Key Clinical/Practical Tools and Strategies	Team Leader
Multicomponent exercise and physical activity program	Flexibility and balance training High-intensity progressive resistance training Mind-body exercise (e.g. Tai Chi, yoga [chair yoga]) Aerobic exercise (e.g. brisk walking)	Physical therapist leads efforts
Strength-based, personalized, psychosocial sensory spiritual environmental initiatives and creative engagement (SPPEICE)	Individualized daily pleasant activity schedule Promoting social interactions and increased interactions with family and friends Promoting engagement in cognitively stimulating activities	Facility leadership provides staff with adequate support and resources to increase their abilities to implement SPPEICE on a daily basis (including volunteer-administered programs)
Addressing spiritual/existential needs	Promoting engagement in religious rituals of resident's preference	Resident's preferred member of clergy or facility chaplain leads efforts
Geriatric Scalpel/rational deprescribing	Discontinuation of medication on Beers list Discontinuation of medication with high anticholinergic activity Discontinuation of unnecessary medication (e.g. statin, proton pump inhibitor) Discontinuation of medication causing more harm than good (e.g. significant adverse effect and insignificant benefit)	Pharmacist leads efforts
Palliative and end-of-life care discussions with resident and family	Discussions about Do Not Resuscitate (DNR), Do Not Intubate (DNI), Do Not Hospitalize (DNH) Assessment of capacity to make medical decisions if significant cognitive impairment is present	Primary care physician leads efforts with involvement of psychiatrist in complex cases
Well-being of family members	Addressing family stress and grief	Social worker leads efforts
Staff education and training	Facility leadership to make identification of frailty a priority	Registered nurse leads efforts

than 20 percent of LTC populations, with higher prevalence in women than in men. Prevalence increases with age. Frailty as a syndrome includes falls, delirium, incontinence, immobility, and susceptibility to medication (British Geriatrics Society 2014). The presence of only one or two of the five criteria denotes prefrailty, which often leads to frailty. Frailty is a dynamic process, characterized by frequent transition between frailty, prefrailty, and base-line states over time, making the prevention of frailty possible.

Typically, frailty is due to a variety of conditions. Atherosclerosis contributes to frailty by decreasing blood flow to the muscles and nerves. Atherosclerosis also directly causes cognitive impairment, which in turn can increase the likelihood of decreased food intake and consequent frailty. Many acute (e.g. pneumonia) and chronic (e.g. undernutrition, Alzheimer's disease, chronic kidney disease, Parkinson's disease, heart disease, anemia, diabetes) medical conditions are commonly implicated as causes of frailty. A resident who enters the hospital or emergency department, even for a minor condition or brief stay, may develop frailty by the time he returns. Although some residents will make gradual improvement in frailty status after returning, for others (especially after prolonged hospitalization) frailty (especially if all five criteria are present) may be permanent and a harbinger of more complications (e.g. falls, hospitalization) in the future. Hospitalization and visits to the emergency department are particularly stressful and burdensome for a resident who is frail and has a high risk of subsequent delirium. Frailty contributes to treatment-resistant depressive disorder (especially MDD, persistent depressive disorder), which in turn may contribute to the etiology of frailty. Thus, early aggressive treatment of depressive disorder may reduce the risk of frailty, and comprehensive efforts to manage frailty may improve the success of treatment of depressive disorder.

We recommend a comprehensive approach to the prevention and management of frailty. (See Table 9.3.) Comprehensive treatment strategies may inhibit the downward spiral of disability in a frail resident and improve her quality of life. The quality of time spent with family may also improve with improvement of frailty. Any frail resident should be screened for pain and depressive disorders, be tested for nutritional deficiencies, have a thorough review of medication (adverse drug reaction, inappropriate or unnecessary medication prescription), and be tested for anemia. A frail resident who has comorbid behavioral and psychological symptoms (BPS) is at higher risk than a nonfrail resident of adverse effect from medication, including psychotropic medication. Thus, dosages of psychotropic drugs used need to be even lower than those used for a nonfrail older adult and increased even more slowly than for a nonfrail resident. When in doubt whether medication may be causing BPS or physical symptoms (tiredness, anorexia), the HCP should err on the side of caution and initiate a trial of dose reduction and/or discontinuation of the suspected offending drug. Testosterone replacement therapy for a hypogonadal male (free testosterone levels below normal range) who has frailty and sarcopenia may improve muscle strength and lead to functional improvement. Testosterone may cause liver dysfunction. Comprehensive treatment strategies for a resident who has prefrailty may prevent the development of frailty. We recommend that all LTC facilities make identification of prefrailty and prevention of frailty a priority for all residents. Even small improvement in frailty status may result in improved mobility and reduced disability in activities of daily living. With comprehensive treatment, the frail resident often shows improvement in cognition, ability to do activities of daily living, ability to participate in leisure activities, strength, stamina, flexibility, and balance. Many frail residents in LTC populations may be in advanced stages of MNCD or other chronic disease. For these residents, we recommend appropriate palliative care and referral to hospice rather than comprehensive assessment and treatment of all factors contributing to frailty.

Sarcopenia

Sarcopenia is characterized by generalized and progressive loss of skeletal muscle accompanied by decline in muscle strength and performance (Argiles and Muscaritoli 2016). It is prevalent in LTC populations and is multifactorial, with a variety of causes (especially undernutrition, prolonged immobility, peripheral vascular disease, testosterone deficiency in a male resident) superimposed on aging-related muscle loss. Sarcopenia puts the resident at risk of physical disability, decline in quality of life, and death. Sarcopenia with limited motility is defined as sarcopenia accompanied by the inability to walk more than 400 meters in six minutes. Computed tomography (CT) scan measurements of body composition can reliably detect skeletal muscle loss and help diagnose sarcopenic obesity (obesity along with sarcopenia) by showing myosteatosis (intramyocellular lipid accumulation). Sarcopenic obesity has been associated with depressive disorder. Sarcopenia is one of the major modifiable causes of frailty in LTC populations. Sarcopenia is a risk factor for MNCD. Co-occurrence of sarcopenia and MDD is prevalent in LTC populations. Sarcopenia may predispose to MDD, and MDD may worsen sarcopenia through its symptoms of lack of motivation and inactivity. Hence, we recommend screening a resident who has sarcopenia for MDD and screening a resident who has MDD for sarcopenia. Sarcopenia is a prefrailty state and requires the same comprehensive assessment and management recommended for frailty. We recommend a trial of testosterone replacement for a male resident who has testosterone deficiency. A combination of testosterone and mirtazapine may be particularly useful for a malnourished male resident who has anorexia, unintentional weight loss, and sarcopenia. Other anabolic steroids (besides testosterone), such as oxandrolone and nandrolone, may increase muscle mass, but we do not recommend them, as they may not improve function and pose significant risk (e.g. liver dysfunction).

Cachexia

Cachexia is a complex syndrome associated with serious diseases (especially cancer but also chronic heart failure [cardiac cachexia], advanced COPD, chronic systemic infection, and renal failure) causing more than 5 percent weight loss, anorexia, and wasting of muscle and adipose tissue (Argiles, Anker, and Evans 2010). It is also called wasting disease and is associated with inflammation, insulin resistance, increased mortality, deterioration in activities of daily living, and increased breakdown of muscle protein. Up to half of residents admitted from the hospital to a skilled nursing facility may have cachexia. Cachexia is often misdiagnosed as a depressive disorder (e.g. MDD) and predisposes to delirium. Any resident who has significant weight loss and MDD should have cachexia in the differential diagnosis.

Cachexia is a serious condition and requires prompt attention by an interdisciplinary team to optimally manage underlying diseases and undernutrition. Eating alone has little effect on the outcome of cachexia. The cornerstone of managing cachexia is a comprehensive nutritional approach and optimal treatment of underlying disease. The initial approach to treatment involves caloric nutritional supplements rich in amino acids and creatine given twice a day between meals along with multivitamins, omega-3 fatty acids, and probiotics. We recommend vitamin D replacement therapy if vitamin D levels are below 30 ng/dl. After ruling out other treatable causes, the HCP may consider treatment with an appetite stimulant (e.g. mirtazapine) for a resident who has weight loss due to cachexia. Comorbid depressive disorder (e.g. MDD) is common in residents who have cachexia and may be treated with mirtazapine. The HCP should consider electroconvulsive therapy if the resident has severe MDD and cachexia, as it can be life saving. A resident who is not eating or is eating less than 25 percent of daily caloric and fluid needs may need short-term peripheral parenteral nutrition. A resident who has cachexia and sarcopenia may be treated with testosterone enanthate or nandrolone. The HCP should consider co-occurrence of cachexia and delirium and cachexia and moderate to severe MDD a psychiatric and medical emergency that is best managed in a hospital setting unless palliative care is more appropriate for the resident (due to advanced MNCD and/or limited life expectancy) and in keeping with the resident's values and wishes. Cachexia during end-of-life care may be treated with dronabinol to improve food intake.

Obesity

Obesity is defined as a body mass index (BMI) of 30 or greater (normal range between 18.5 and 25; overweight between 25 and 29.9), moderate obesity is BMI from 35 to 40, and morbid obesity is BMI above 40. A person who has BMI below 18.5 is said to be underweight. BMI is a measure of body fat and is based on the person's height and weight. Obesity is excess body fat. Excess fat in the abdomen (visceral fat) (central obesity) carries an even higher risk of heart attack and stroke than excess fat in other parts of the body (e.g. around the hips [subcutaneous fat]). Central obesity is identified if the person has a large waist circumference (≥40 inches in men, ≥35 inches in women) or high waist-to-hip ratio (>0.95 in men, >0.85 in women). Accurate diagnosis of central obesity usually requires computed tomography (CT) or magnetic resonance imaging (MRI) to measure visceral fat.

At least 33 percent of the adults in the United States older than age 60 are obese (Porter Starr, McDonald, Bales 2014). Rates of moderate to severe obesity in LTC populations increased from 14.6 percent to almost 24 percent in the last decade. Some 25–30 percent of newly admitted residents have obesity. Nearly 30 percent of residents who have a BMI of 35 or more are younger than 65. Today's older adults who are obese experience more impairment in functional abilities related to movement and activities of daily living than those from previous generations because of higher comorbidities. Obesity not only increases the likelihood of entering a LTC facility but also dramatically compounds the demands put on the nursing staff. Staff may need more than an hour to bathe a resident who is obese. Many LTC facilities lack the infrastructure to care for obese individuals optimally and thus refuse to admit them (especially individuals who are morbidly obese). The cost of care is also higher for a resident who is obese, as he needs more health services and has a longer LTC stay than a resident who is not obese. This is because residents who are obese are typically younger than residents who are not obese. Paradoxically, once the acute situation resolves, a higher BMI is associated with a lower risk of mortality in LTC populations.

In LTC populations, excessive food consumption and sedentary lifestyle contribute to increasing rates of obesity. Residents identified as obese have a higher likelihood of comorbid conditions (e.g. diabetes mellitus, arthritis, hypertension, depression, chronic pain, allergies). Obesity can occur with protein malnutrition, sarcopenia, and micronutrient deficiency or in their absence. Many residents who have psychiatric disorder (especially with frontal lobe impairment [such as a resident who has FTD]) are not able to adjust their food intake after a period of overfeeding and will continue exceeding their caloric needs and thus increase in weight.

Obesity is associated with poor perception of health, poor physical functioning, and poor social functioning. Older adults who are obese are more likely to become disabled and to enter a nursing home. Obesity in older adults is a major predictor of loss of independence and exacerbates age-related decline in physical functioning. Residents who are obese may reduce or stop ambulating (due to pain or need for increased effort), may have chronic pain due to osteoarthritis, and pose a risk of injury to staff during the staff's efforts to help with activities of daily living (e.g. personal care, transfer). Special equipment (e.g. chair lift, Hoyer lift) may be needed for a resident who is obese (especially morbidly obese) to be transferred safely, for ambulation, bathing, and physical therapy. A slight excess of weight may be helpful when a resident is ill and in a catabolic state, when the immune system faces increased wear and tear. By stressing the skeleton, excess weight reduces the loss of bone mass, and overweight older adults are less likely to sustain hip fracture. However, in general, the health risks of overweight and obesity in older adults are greater than any advantages. Residents who are obese may increase the risk for workplace injury among LTC staff, who already face high workplace injury rates. LTC facilities may not have the specialized supplies (e.g. blood pressure cuff to accommodate a resident with larger arms) and equipment (e.g. larger bed and wheelchair to accommodate a person weighing more than 300 pounds) or adequate space (e.g. larger room with wider doorway to accommodate larger equipment and wider wheelchair) to provide care for residents who are obese.

The primary purpose of the treatment of obesity in LTC populations is to increase physical functioning and quality of life and achieve stable weight. Depending on the resident's life expectancy, significant weight loss and disease prevention may or may not be a goal of the treatment of obesity. The focus of treatment should be on prevention of further weight gain (weight maintenance) and preservation of muscle mass and strength without contributing to frailty. This is achieved through increased physical activity (exercise and increased leisure activity) and nutritional strategies (isocaloric but nutrient-rich dietary plan). We recommend progressive resistance training (which helps conserve lean body mass, strengthen bone, and increase energy expenditure) and low-intensity physical activity (e.g. walking) for the treatment of obesity for the resident who does not have medical contraindications to exercise. The HCP should remind residents and their families that most popular diets are not nutritionally balanced, are high in calories, and thus promote weight gain and worsen obesity-related complications if consumed regularly. The goal is to reduce caloric intake, not nutrients. A decrease of 500 calories daily will cause a loss of one pound of body weight weekly. Simple dietary modifications include decreasing saturated fat intake, using lean cuts of meat and low-fat or skim milk, and limiting (as much as possible) or avoiding candy, ice cream, pastry, pie, nuts, and cake. We recommend fruit for dessert. Broiling or baking instead of frying is also helpful. Residents should be encouraged to increase the proportion of fruits and vegetables in their diet, especially dark green leafy vegetables. Portion size should be controlled, and residents should feel under no obligation to "clean their plate." Intake of beverages with high caloric and sugar content (e.g. soda, alcoholic beverage) should be limited as much as possible. All of these changes need to be individualized, implemented at the level that does not significantly compromise existing quality of life, and in keeping with the overall goals of care.

Older adults who are obese and intentionally lose weight may not have the risks of weight loss (e.g. increased morbidity and mortality) seen in older adults who have unintentional weight loss. FDA-approved medications used to treat obesity (e.g. phentermine-topiramate combination therapy, bupropion-naltrexone combination therapy, orlistat, and lorcaserin) are usually not recommended for residents who are obese because they have not been studied in this population and because of the high risk of adverse effect (e.g. insomnia, agitation, cognitive dulling). Long-term quality of life is expected to improve with weight reduction in many residents who are obese due to improved physical and cognitive function, decrease in musculoskeletal pain, and other potential benefits of weight reduction. The HCP should carefully consider whether or not to institute a weight-loss treatment for a resident who is obese with special attention to each resident's preference, life expectancy, weight history, and medical condition. We recommend that the HCP offer residents who are obese and in advanced stages of MNCD or other disease state appropriate palliative care and referral to hospice rather than weight-reduction strategies. If a resident who is obese has a limited life expectancy (less than 1 year), we recommend discontinuing all dietary restrictions and allowing the resident to eat whatever he likes.

Clinical Case: "I like food"

Mr. W was an 81-year-old resident living in an AL home for two years. He was doing well taking 20 mg daily escitalopram for the treatment of MDD-like symptoms and anxiety symptoms secondary to MNCD due to Alzheimer's disease (AD). Over the last two years, he had gained 50 pounds, and in the last three months he had gained 14 pounds (for a final BMI of 42), primarily due to a sedentary lifestyle and excessive eating during and between meals. Mr. W had struggled with obesity for most of his life and intermittently went to Weight Watchers to reduce weight and eat healthier. Due to AD, he had stopped going to Weight Watchers. A psychiatrist was consulted, as Mr. W had become irritable, had expressed feeling "upset" about gaining weight, and his wife felt his depression was coming back and antidepressants should be adjusted. The psychiatrist found Mr. W to be social but upset about his weight gain. Mr. W told the psychiatrist, "I like food." The psychiatrist shared with Mr. W, his wife, and staff that he did not think antidepressant needed to be adjusted. The psychiatrist recommended a program of exercise (five minutes of strength training and 15 minutes of assisted ambulation daily) and nutritional strategies. Nutritional strategies involved portion-controlled diet (smaller portions given during the three meals), replacing consumption of unhealthy snacks (crackers, candy, ice cream) with fruits and vegetables Mr. W liked (blueberries, mangoes, carrots, celery with a vegetable dip), and replacing intake of soda and coffee with diet soda and water. Mr. W initially resisted this change in diet but with the staff's support and his wife's encouragement, he acquiesced. Over the next eight weeks, not only did Mr. W lose four pounds but also he seemed to have more energy, started getting out of the chair on his own (previously he needed one-person assistance to do this), and began walking around the facility. Staff also noticed that Mr. W seemed to carry on longer conversations and showed less irritability.

Teaching Point

For some residents who are obese, simple nutritional changes with modest increase in physical activity and lots of support and encouragement can lead to not only modest but significant weight loss but also improvement in mood, cognition, and function.

Nutritional Disorders Associated with Major Neurocognitive Disorder

Nutritional disorders (anorexia, unintentional weight loss, odd eating habits, hyperphagia, obesity) are common among residents who have MNCD because cognitive impairment and behavioral disturbance can prevent residents from meeting their nutritional needs or from being able to express them to staff. In fact, inability to maintain adequate nutritional status may be one of the reasons for entering a LTC facility. In addition, neurotransmitter abnormalities may play a role in that levels of neuropeptide Y and norepinephrine (potent stimulators of food intake) have been found to be reduced in various brain regions of individuals who have AD. Weight loss in late life may be an early manifestation of MNCD as well as a risk factor for MNCD. Individuals who have advanced cognitive impairment may also be at risk of dehydration due to loss of the protective thirst responses. For this reason, dehydration may be harder to recognize in a resident who has MNCD, as typically there is no subjective feeling of thirst despite the presence of dehydration (Albert et al. 1994).

Approximately 90 percent of individuals who have AD lose weight at some point in the course of the illness. In the early stage of AD, the person may forget to eat and appetite may diminish as a result of depression. Affected individuals may become distracted and leave the table without eating. In the middle stages of AD, the person may have difficulty initiating the eating process or may start eating, become distracted, and fail to finish. The person may not be able to sit long enough to finish a meal or may forget that she has just eaten. At this stage, additional calories may be required for a resident who has AD and develops wandering, pacing, and motor restlessness. In the severe and terminal stages, the person may fail to recognize food, eat things that are not food, no longer have oral-motor skills for chewing and swallowing, or not be able to coordinate activities to self-feed. Thus, a resident who has MNCD in advanced stages needs to be given adequate assistance during eating and adequate increase in calorie intake. Residents who have stroke, Parkinson's disease, or MNCD with Lewy bodies often develop slowing of motor function (bradykinesia) and slowness in thinking (bradyphrenia) and hence may require assistance with eating for a much longer time (30–60 minutes) to achieve adequate intake of nutrients. In severe and terminal stages of MNCD, advanced neurodegeneration may severely impair the person's ability to maintain adequate food and fluid intake to sustain life and may continue to lose weight despite adequate eating assistance, food fortification, administration of oral nutritional supplements, and treatment of reversible factors contributing to weight loss. These individuals are essentially in the process of dying. Tube feeding does not improve the quality or quantity of life in such situations and may worsen the quality of life due to complications associated with tube feeding (e.g. pain, discomfort, aspiration) (American Geriatrics Society 2014). We recommend hand feeding to address anorexia and weight loss in the severe to terminal stages of MNCD. Cachexia and dehydration are common causes of death among residents who have terminal-stage MNCD. We recommend the Edinburgh Feeding Evaluation in Dementia Questionnaire (EdFED-Q), an observational instrument, to identify eating difficulties and determine the level of assistance needed. Residents who have MNCD and eating difficulties may have swallowing disorder that is unrecognized. These residents are sometimes labeled as combative, uncooperative, and difficult to feed when they try to refuse food they cannot swallow. If assessment suggests an undiagnosed swallowing disorder (e.g. resident is coughing or choking during food intake), the HCP should refer the resident to a speech therapist for further evaluation.

Obesity, central obesity, and overweight in middle age are associated with increased risk of all causes of MNCD, including AD and MNCD due to cerebrovascular disease, independent of diabetes and cardiovascular-related morbidity. Many residents who have MNCD develop abnormal eating or appetite behaviors. These behaviors include odd eating habits, tendency to place nonfood objects in the mouth, increase in appetite, overeating (including compulsive overeating [hyperphagia]), eating between meals, preferring sweets and soft drinks, a desire to eat at the same time every day, and a decline in table manners. These are seen more often with frontotemporal MNCD (FTD) but can also be seen with AD. The presence of irritability, agitation, and disinhibition may result in shifts in eating patterns toward carbohydrate and away from protein, placing these residents at increased risk for protein malnutrition. Research has shown shifts in circadian patterns of intake in residents who have MNCD, with lower food intake consistently observed at lunch and dinner, but not breakfast, in individuals who have higher levels of functional disability. These behavioral problems are best managed with psychosocial environmental approaches, such as redirection, replacing high-calorie food items (e.g. dessert) with low-calorie food items (e.g. fruits and vegetables) to prevent obesity due to hyperphagia, and encouraging residents to eat in smaller groups with greater monitoring.

Major Depressive Disorder and Malnutrition

Weight loss is more prevalent in older individuals who have MDD than in younger ones. Loss of appetite is one of the most common symptoms of MDD in LTC residents. Death by starvation can be a method by which a resident who has MDD may try to end her life. Most antidepressants (except mirtazapine and TCAs, which usually are associated with increased appetite and weight gain) have the potential to cause anorexia and even weight loss, although more often antidepressant improves appetite and weight by improving symptoms of MDD. Possible causes of high mortality in residents who have severe MDD and severe undernutrition include protein needs not being met at a time of increased nitrogen turnover (stress) and/or increased release of tumor necrosis factor (cachexin) with an increase in lipoprotein lipase and subsequent weight loss. Convergence of MDD and severe undernutrition is a psychiatric and medical emergency because these individuals are also immune-compromised and susceptible to potentially life-threatening infection. Treating undernutrition (with nutritional rehabilitation) and MDD (with antidepressant and/or electroconvulsive therapy [ECT]) aggressively may be life saving. MDD often leads to poor fluid intake, resulting in dehydration. If the resident is also taking diuretics, dehydration can quickly become severe, lead to orthostatic hypotension and falls, and become potentially fatal.

In such situations, eliminating drugs that may cause or exacerbate dehydration and anorexia (e.g. diuretic, calcium [it may cause constipation and nausea]) and treatment of MDD, as well as improving oral intake of fluid (or even a short course of intravenous fluid) is necessary for successful outcome. Many antidepressants (e.g. SSRI) may cause a syndrome of inappropriate secretion of antidiuretic hormone (SIADH) and consequent hyponatremia, especially for a resident who is already taking a diuretic. The HCP should consider these risks and discuss them with the resident and family at the time of prescribing antidepressant.

Medications, Nutrition, and Mental Health

A variety of medications can cause or worsen undernutrition by causing anorexia and/or nausea, resulting in decline in oral intake of food and fluids. (See Box 9.2.) Medications with anticholinergic activity can cause nutritional problems by causing dry mouth and anorexia, and dry mouth is a symptom also of anxiety symptoms. Certain psychiatric medications (e.g. lurasidone, ziprasidone) need to be taken with food for optimal absorption (at least 500 kcal), as on an empty stomach, only 50 percent of these medications are absorbed. Food also increases absorption of carbamazepine and diazepam. Cholinesterase inhibitors (ChEIs) are best taken on a full stomach to avoid anorexia and nausea associated with their use. ChEIs may cause diarrhea leading to dehydration. Many psychotropic medications (e.g. antipsychotics [olanzapine, clozapine, quetiapine], mood stabilizers [e.g. valproate, lithium], antidepressants [e.g. mirtazapine, TCAs]) may cause significant weight gain and cause or worsen obesity. Weight gain due to psychotropic medication is a growing problem in residents, and the HCP should minimize their use by residents who are already overweight or obese.

Brain-Healthy Nutrition

We recommend that residents who have relatively preserved cognitive function and are interested in eating a brain-healthy diet and residents who have MNCD for whom family members would like healthy nutritional strategies (as compared to a diet with no restrictions) to promote cognitive wellness and reduce the risk of cognitive decline pursue a variety of evidence-based brain health nutritional strategies. (See Table 9.4.) These recommendations need to be adjusted for the resident's medical condition and personal preferences. In addition, we recommend omega-3 fatty acids, calcium, vitamin D, and B_{12} supplements, as typically even a balanced diet may not provide adequate amounts of these nutrients. Caloric restriction has been associated with increased longevity and reduction in age-related illness in community-dwelling middle-aged adults but is not recommended for LTC populations due to the risk of undernutrition.

Summary

There is growing evidence that a well-balanced diet rich in brain-essential nutrients may improve cognitive function and reduce the risk of a variety of psychiatric disorders (especially mood, anxiety, sleep-wake, and cognitive disorders). Psychiatric disorders such as MNCD, MDD, and delirium predispose to nutritional disorder and frailty, and the latter two predispose to a variety of psychiatric disorders. Medications are a common cause of undernutrition and obesity in LTC populations, and the HCP should review all medications taken by a resident who is undernourished or obese and discontinue offending medication. Frailty, sarcopenia, and cachexia are prevalent in LTC populations and should be vigorously treated with comprehensive geriatric assessment, nutritional rehabilitation, and other evidence-based strategies. Convergence of MDD and severe undernutrition is a psychiatric and medical emergency that should be treated in a hospital setting. The prevalence of obesity is increasing in LTC populations, dramatically compounds the demands of nursing care, and increases the risk of workplace injury among staff. We recommend that residents interested in improving cognitive wellness and reducing the risk of cognitive decline pursue a variety of evidence-based brain-healthy nutritional strategies.

Key Clinical Points

1. A well-balanced diet rich in brain-essential nutrients may improve cognitive function and reduce the risk of a variety of psychiatric disorders (especially mood, anxiety, sleep-wake, and cognitive disorders).
2. Undernutrition is prevalent in LTC populations and is eminently preventable with staff training in

Table 9.4 Brain-Healthy Nutrition

Brain-Rich Foods	Specific Examples	Therapeutic Pearls
Food rich in omega-3 fatty acids	Fatty fish* (three or more ounces twice a week)	Omega-3 fatty acids may be obtained through supplements if adequate consumption of fish is not feasible Fatty fish is also high in selenium, vitamin D, and protein
Vegetables (1–4 servings per day)	Green leafy vegetables (e.g. spinach, broccoli)	Fresh vegetables and freshly cooked vegetables that resident prefers may promote increased consumption
Legumes (1–2 servings per day)	Black beans	Particularly beneficial for resident who has sarcopenia and/or low BMI, as they are high in protein and micronutrients brain needs (e.g. folate) Particularly beneficial for resident who has constipation, as they have high fiber content
Fruits (1–4 servings per day)	Berries (e.g. blueberries)	Fresh fruits that resident prefers may promote increased consumption
Whole grains (3–5 servings per day)	Cereals rich in whole grain	Cereals that resident prefers may promote increased consumption
Monounsaturated fats	Avocados Olive oil Nuts (e.g. walnuts)	Particularly beneficial for resident who has low BMI, as they are high in calories
Spices	Turmeric	Help of facility cook is recommended to make addition of turmeric to food more palatable for resident not used to consuming food with turmeric
Food and/or fluids to maintain gut microbiome	Probiotic yogurt with active bacterial culture Probiotic drinks	Nondairy foods/fluids with active bacterial culture recommended for resident who has lactose intolerance

* Fatty fish: e.g. salmon, sardine, herring, anchovy.

assistance with eating, fortified foods and fluids, and a variety of other evidence-based approaches.

3. The HCP should review all medications taken by a resident who is undernourished and/or obese and discontinue offending medication.
4. Frailty is often comorbid with MDD and should be vigorously treated with comprehensive geriatric assessment, nutritional rehabilitation, and other evidence-based approaches.
5. The prevalence of obesity is increasing in LTC populations, dramatically compounds the demands of nursing care, and increases the risk of workplace injury among staff.

Additional Resources

Weight loss Prevention Training Manual. The Anna and Harry Borun Center for Gerontological Research, University of California Los Angeles and The Jewish Home for the Aging, Greater Los Angeles. The manual presents instructions and protocols for implementing an effective weight loss prevention program for nursing home residents. Available at: http://geronet.med.ucla.edu/centers/borun/modules/Weight_loss_prevention/wlmod.pdf

References

Albert, S., B.R. Nakra, G.T. Grossberg, and E.R. Caminal. 1994. Drinking Behavior and Vasopressin Responses to Hyperosmolality in Alzheimer's Disease. *International Psychogeriatrics* **6**(1):79–86.

American Geriatrics Society Ethics Committee and Clinical Practice Models of Care Committee. 2014. American Geriatric Society Feeding Tubes in Advanced Dementia Position Statement. *Journal of the American Geriatrics Society* **62**(8): 1590–1593.

Argiles, J.M., S.D. Anker, and W.J. Evans. 2010. Consensus on Cachexia Definitions. *Journal of the American Medical Directors Association* **11**:229–230.

Argiles, J.M. and M. Muscaritoli. 2016. The Three Faces of Sarcopenia. *Journal of the American Medical Directors Association* **17**:471–472.

British Geriatrics Society. 2014. Fit for Frailty – A Consensus Best Practice Guidelines for the Care of Older People Living in the Community and Outpatient Settings – A Report from the British Geriatrics Society. http://www.bgs.org.uk/campaigns/fff/fff_full.pdf (accessed December 12, 2015).

Cesari, M., M. Prince, J.A. Thiyagarajan, et al. 2016. Frailty: An Emerging Public Health Priority. *Journal of the American Medical Directors Association* **17**:188–192.

Dysken, M., M. Sano, S. Asthana, et al. 2014. Effect of Vitamin E and Memantine on Functional Decline in Alzheimer's Disease. A Team-AD VA Cooperative Randomized Study. *Journal of the American Medical Association* **311**(1):33–44.

Kaehr, E., R. Viswanathan, T.K. Malmstrom, and J.E. Morley. 2015. Frailty in Nursing Homes: FRAIL-NH Scale. *Journal of the American Medical Directors Association* **16**: 87–89.

Porter Starr, K.N., C.W. Bales, and M.E. Payne. 2015. Nutrition and Physical Activity. In D.C. Steffens, D.G. Blazer, and M.E. Thakur (eds.), *The Textbook of Geriatric Psychiatry*, 5th ed., pp. 617–648. Arlington, VA: American Psychiatric Publishing.

Porter Starr, K.N., S.R. McDonald, J.A. and C.W. Bales. 2014. Obesity and Physical Frailty in Older Adults: A Scoping Review of Lifestyle Intervention Trials. *Journal of the American Medical Directors Association* **15**:240–250.

Sarris, J., A.C. Logan, T.N. Akbaraly, et al. for The International Society for Nutritional Psychiatry Research. 2015. Nutritional Medicine as Mainstream in Psychiatry. *Lancet Psychiatry* **2**(3):271–274.

Wu, B., G.G. Fillenbaum, B.L. Plassman, et al. 2016. Association between Oral Health and Cognitive Status: A Systematic Review. *Journal of the American Geriatrics Society* **64**:739–751.

Chapter

10 Resident Abuse and Ethical Issues in Long-Term Care

How beautifully leaves grow old. How full of light and color are their last days.
John Burroughs (American naturalist and author, 1837–1921).

Integrating the unity of one's life and experiences is one of the tasks of living that begins in adulthood and continues in old age. The majority of the residents living in long-term care (LTC) facilities are disabled and diminished due to multiple medical and psychiatric disorders and thus need help to achieve this task with integrity. The health care provider (HCP) should strive to ensure that all residents are cared for with respect and love. Ageism (discrimination based on age) should not be a factor in allocating resources, and when attempting to evaluate the quality of a resident's life, the HCP must be aware of the limitations of purely professional assessment. Resident abuse is prevalent in LTC populations and may cause serious setbacks to a resident's efforts to live with dignity. Ethical issues, if not negotiated well, may pose barriers to a resident's ability to live the last years of life meaningfully. Efforts to prevent abuse and unethical professional conduct are necessary first steps to ensuring that all residents find life in LTC filled with dignity, meaning, happiness, and comfort.

Resident Abuse

Abuse includes psychological, physical, and sexual abuse, neglect, and financial exploitation (Dong 2015). *Abuse* refers to an intentional act of commission or omission which results in harm or threatened harm to the well-being (physical, psychological, spiritual) and/or welfare of the person. Abuse of a resident in LTC (resident abuse) typically involves willful infliction of injury, unreasonable confinement, intimidation, or punishment with resulting physical harm, pain, and/or mental anguish. Resident abuse also includes the deprivation of goods or services necessary to attain or maintain physical, mental, and psychosocial well-being. Withholding of necessary food, clothing, monetary resources, and medical care to treat the resident's physical and mental health needs by a person having responsibility for the resident constitutes abuse. Undue influence that harms the resident should also be considered a form of abuse. This presumes that instances of abuse of any resident, even one in a coma, cause physical harm, pain, and/or mental anguish. *Elder abuse* is another term used for abuse of individuals older than age 65. (See Table 10.1.)

Verbal abuse and neglect are the most common forms of resident abuse, while physical abuse is the most visible; psychological abuse and neglect and financial exploitation are more easily missed. Neglect is the most common form of resident abuse by staff or family member. Often other types of abuse are concurrent with verbal abuse and neglect. Neglect may be intentional or unintentional due to caregiver (family and professional) stress, burnout, and/or limited health literacy. The abuser can be another resident, resident's spouse, family member, friend, facility staff member (includes all staff and HCP), volunteer, family or friend of another resident, resident's guardian, member of the clergy, or any other visitor.

Interpersonal violence (especially resident-to-resident aggression) is especially prevalent in LTC populations. Resident-to-resident abuse (verbal, physical, sexual) is much more common than physical abuse of the resident by a staff member (Lach and Pillemer 2015). A common form of sexual assault is one resident who has hypersexual behavior (typically due to MNCD) assaulting or attempting to assault another resident, who may or may not have cognitive impairment. There may be more than one abuser (e.g. multiple family members verbally abusing or financially exploiting the resident). Approximately 10 percent of older adults in the community have experienced some form of abuse (typically from a spouse or other

Table 10.1 Types of Resident Abuse

Abuse	Description and Manifestations	Therapeutic Pearls
Physical abuse	Intentional infliction of physical pain and/or injury Includes hitting, slapping, punching, kicking, putting resident in physical restraint Manifestations: cuts, abrasions, lacerations, bruises, fractures, burns, avulsion of teeth, pain, depression, agitation, aggression, delirium, nightmares, flashbacks	Resident-to-resident physical abuse more common than physical abuse by staff or family member Most visible form of abuse Bruises due to accidental fall need to be differentiated from bruises due to physical abuse
Psychological/mental abuse	Intentional infliction of psychological pain and/or injury Includes threatening behavior, threat of abuse, harassment, verbal assault, humiliation Manifestations: deferring questions to caregiver or potential abuser, depression, social withdrawal, anxiety, insomnia, nightmares	Often unrecognized Resident-to-resident psychological abuse is more prevalent than psychological abuse by staff or family member Stress and burnout of staff and/or family members often causes them to be psychologically abusive toward resident
Sexual abuse	Nonconsensual touching or sexual act or activity with resident when resident is unable to understand, unwilling to consent, or threatened or forced into it Includes sexual harassment, sexual coercion, sexual assault Male (including staff) is more likely to be abuser than female (including staff) Manifestations: depression, anxiety, nightmares, social withdrawal, insomnia, sexually transmitted disease, UTI	Often unrecognized Sexual abuse by another resident (typically resident who has MNCD and hypersexuality) is more common than sexual abuse by staff or family member Resident's spouse, other family member, or friend may also be abuser Sexually inappropriate verbal behavior toward staff and other residents and sexual abuse of staff (typically during personal care) often accompany sexually abusive behavior by resident who has hypersexual behavior
Neglect (caregiver neglect)	Failure of staff and/or family member to provide resident with necessities of life (e.g. food) when resident is incapable of doing so Manifestations: unattended symptoms, undernutrition, decubitus ulcer, poor personal hygiene, delirium	Improper handling of resident during personal care and lack of care planning can be considered forms of neglect Should be differentiated from self-neglect (e.g. resident ignores personal hygiene needs despite being capable of doing personal hygiene)
Financial exploitation	Misusing or withholding resident's resources to resident's disadvantage and abuser's advantage HCP should consider screening for financial abuse if there is abrupt change in resident's financial circumstances and/or resident is inaccurately deemed lacking capacity to manage own finances	Unexplained change in resident's will, power of attorney, or other legal document, excessive payment for goods or services, missing checks or valuable belongings should raise concerns about resident being financially exploited
Verbal abuse (a form of psychological abuse)	Use of oral, written, or gestured language (including sexual language) that willfully includes disparaging and derogatory terms	Often witnessed by staff or family (typically resident's spouse or other family member

Table 10.1 (cont.)

Abuse	Description and Manifestations	Therapeutic Pearls
	to resident or family, or within resident's hearing, regardless of resident's age, ability to comprehend, or disability Includes, but is not limited to, threats of harm; saying things to frighten resident, such as telling resident that he/she will never be able to see family again	or friend verbally abusing resident) but often unreported or unaddressed
Involuntary seclusion	Separating resident from others or from resident's room or confinement of resident in room against resident's will	Often unrecognized Constitutes type of psychological abuse and, if there is physical pain or injury, additional physical abuse
Domestic violence	Abuse (typically physical and/or psychological) of resident by family member (e.g. spouse) Late-onset domestic violence by resident's spouse may be because spouse has developed MNCD	Abuse by family caregiver may indicate caregiver burnout (caregiver is emotionally drained) Domestic violence occurring in facility may be continuation of long-term abusive behavior by resident's family member

family member [domestic abuse] or paid caregiver). The prevalence of abuse of LTC residents is even higher and is increasing with the growth of LTC populations, making it a major public health problem. More than 50 percent of nursing home staff reported mistreating (physical violence, mental abuse, neglect) residents within a year before the study; more than two-thirds involved neglect (Ben Natan and Lowenstein 2010). Despite such high prevalence, only a small fraction is reported to the Adult Protective Services (APS). This is because most HCPs consider abuse to be a family or social problem and, despite mandatory legal reporting requirements, do not report. Clinical and time pressures are additional reasons for failure on the part of HCPs to identify and/or report resident abuse. Residents may be unwilling to disclose mistreatment out of embarrassment, especially because HCPs make short visits. Incidents of neglect are underreported due to difficulties inherent in defining and recognizing this type of mistreatment. All HCPs (especially physicians) should make prevention of resident abuse a priority, take suspected abuse seriously, and address it comprehensively (Mosqueda et al. 2016). This is because abuse has potentially devastating effects on the victim's physical, mental, and spiritual well-being and financial security.

Resident abuse is predictable, sometimes fatal, and eminently preventable. Residents are vulnerable to abuse primarily because of their significant dependence on others for their care and well-being. See Table 10.2 for key risk factors for resident abuse. Resident abuse is a common problem with serious consequences for the health and well-being of a resident as well as severe negative impact on the emotional and spiritual well-being of the family. Abuse may cause the resident to be anxious, fearful (especially in the presence of or in anticipation of a visit by the abuser), hopeless, resigned, demoralized, or withdrawn. Residents of all socioeconomic and ethnic backgrounds are vulnerable to abuse and neglect. A key reason older adults are fearful of residing in LTC facilities is concern over becoming a victim of abuse. The HCP should have a high index of suspicion for abuse in a resident at risk. For early detection of abuse, we recommend that the HCP routinely ask a few screening questions during each assessment. See Box 10.1 for a list of key questions to detect resident abuse. Indirect questions are less threatening and should be used before direct questions.

Differential Diagnosis

Self-neglect by a resident should be distinguished from neglect related to abuse. Neglect is caused by others, but self-neglect is self-imposed. Individuals older than 75 years of age, African Americans, and individuals from lower socioeconomic classes are at higher risk of

Table 10.2 Risk Factors for Resident Abuse

Risk Factor	Clinical Significance	Therapeutic Pearls
Neurocognitive disorder (especially MNCD)	Prevalence of abuse is in range of 40–50% in residents who have MNCD Caregiver stress is most important modifiable risk factor for abuse of resident who has MNCD MNCD is biggest risk factor for financial abuse	Early education of person who has MNCD, family, and HCP about what constitutes abuse and impact of caregiver stress on risk of caregiver developing abusive behavior is key to prevention
Behavioral and psychological symptoms (BPS) (especially agitation and aggression) of MNCD	Increases risk of abuse	Staff education, staff support, giving staff resources and time to implement SPPEICE can reduce BPS and thus reduce risk of abuse
Resident receiving palliative and hospice care	Increases risk of abuse	Having high index of suspicion is crucial, as these residents are most vulnerable in LTC populations
Frailty	Increases risk of abuse	Prefrailty and frailty are reversible conditions, and their prevention should be part of abuse prevention programs
Multimorbidity*	Presence of three or more vulnerability factors increases risk of abuse fourfold, and presence of five or more vulnerability factors increases risk of abuse 26-fold	Comprehensive Geriatric Assessment is recommended for all residents at time of admission to identify vulnerability to abuse and institute individualized abuse prevention care plan Effective treatment of underlying reversible problem and appropriate involvement of family (and other interpersonal-social resources of resident) are recommended
Psychiatric disorder	Presence of MDD, schizophrenia, or other psychiatric disorder increases risk of abuse	Prevention of MDD and optimal effective treatment of psychiatric disorder for all residents as soon after admission as possible is recommended to reduce risk of abuse
Sensory deficit	Impaired hearing or vision increases risk of abuse	Correction of hearing and/or vision deficit and ensuring appropriate use of hearing and/or vision aid is recommended for all residents as part of comprehensive abuse prevention plan
Age	Oldest old (older adults age 85 and older) are the group most at risk of abuse and neglect	Staff education on risk factors is key to prevention efforts
Sex	Older women more likely to be abused than older men	Staff education on risk factors is key to prevention efforts
Race	Financial abuse is three times higher and psychological abuse four times higher in older adults of African American descent than peers	Staff education on risk factors is key to prevention efforts
LGBTQ**	Prevalence of LGBTQ residents is increasing	Staff education on risk factors and sensitivity training are key to prevention efforts
History of abuse	If resident was victim of abuse in childhood, he is at increased risk of being victim of abuse in late life	HCP needs to inquire sensitively into history of abuse

Table 10.2 (cont.)

Risk Factor	Clinical Significance	Therapeutic Pearls
Lack of family advocate	Prevalence of residents who lack family advocate is high	At least one member of team should be designated as advocate for each resident who does not have family member or friend advocating for resident Early involvement of ombudsman to advocate for resident's rights is recommended
Caregiver stress	Stress and burnout are prevalent in both professional and family caregivers	LTC facility should routinely offer stress management programs for caregivers (both family and professional [facility staff])
Substance use disorder in caregiver (drug and/or alcohol addiction)	Substance use disorder (especially alcohol) is prevalent in both professional and family caregivers	Having high index of suspicion is required to promptly identify this risk factor
Personality disorder (especially presence of antisocial personality trait) in caregiver	Maladaptive personality trait and disorder are prevalent in both professional and family caregivers	Having high index of suspicion is required to promptly identify this risk factor
Legal problem in caregiver	Legal problem in family member (e.g. adult child) associated with increased risk of abuse	Staff should have high index of suspicion of resident abuse if there is known history of legal problem in adult child (or other family member)

* Multimorbidity: Presence of two or more chronic diseases or disorders

** LGBTQ: Lesbian, gay, bisexual, transgender, or queer/questioning individual

self-neglect (Mosqueda and Dong 2011). Cognitive impairment and physical disability also increase the risk and severity of self-neglect. Other terms used for self-neglect in older adults are Diogenes syndrome (DS) and squalor syndrome. Primary DS involves maladaptive personality traits and personality disorders and precipitant factors. Secondary DS may be due to MNCD, MDD, or schizophrenia. Bruises due to falls may be mistaken for physical abuse, and vice versa. Fractures may be due to osteoporosis rather than abuse, but fractures due to abuse may be misattributed to osteoporosis. The HCP should have a high index of suspicion for the coexistence of abuse with accidental falls and self-neglect. Cultural and language barriers may create challenges to accurate differentiation of sequelae of abuse (e.g. pressure ulcer) from common medical conditions in LTC populations.

Prevention

Resident abuse is eminently preventable. It should be considered the seventh vital sign. (Heart rate, respiratory rate, blood pressure, and temperature are the first through fourth vital signs; pain and acute change in mental status in LTC populations should be considered the fifth and sixth vital signs.) Medical directors of LTC facilities are best suited to lead facility-wide efforts to institute resident abuse prevention programs, including routine screening for abuse (at the time of admission and quarterly thereafter), high-quality education and training of staff, and identifying at-risk residents for more intensive monitoring and intervention. See Tables 10.2 and 10.3 for key prevention strategies. Comprehensive geriatric assessment can identify predisposing and precipitating factors that can guide an individualized abuse prevention care plan.

The HCP should integrate screening for resident abuse into routine clinical practice (during each clinical encounter along with monitoring for the other vital signs). Another important strategy to prevent resident abuse is to increase opportunities for bonding between residents and caregivers (professional and family). The facility leadership should consider

BOX 10.1 Screening Questions to Detect Abuse of a Resident

Indirect (Nonthreatening/Nonalarming) Questions

Are your needs being met?
Is your family being supportive?
Is the staff treating you well?
Do you receive help when you call for help?
Do you have to wait a long time before you get help?
Does someone handle your checkbook for you?
At the end of the month, do you have enough money left to spend for yourself?

Direct Questions

Do you feel safe at this place?
Is anyone bothering you?
Is anyone unkind to you?
Is anyone giving you a hard time?
Has anyone mistreated you?
Has anyone hurt you?
Is anyone taking advantage of you?

Physical Abuse

Does anyone hit you?
Are you afraid of anyone at this place?
Have you been struck, slapped, or kicked?

Psychological Abuse

Does anyone tease you?
Has anyone scolded or threatened you?
Does anyone yell or curse at you?
Are you prevented from seeing your friends or family?

Sexual Abuse

Has anyone touched you without your consent?
Has anyone made you do things you didn't want to do?

Neglect

Are you alone a lot?
Has anyone failed to help you take care of yourself when you needed help?
Do you lack aids such as eyeglasses, hearing aids, or dentures?
Are your needs being neglected?

Financial Abuse/Exploitation

Have you signed any document that you didn't understand?
Has anyone taken anything of yours without asking?
Has anyone taken your money or property without your consent?
Have your money or belongings been stolen from you?
Has your credit card or automated teller machine (ATM) card been used without your consent?

Table 10.3 Management of Suspected Resident Abuse by an Interdisciplinary Team

Clinician	Interventions	Therapeutic Pearls
Physician	Perform comprehensive geriatric assessment (includes screening questions) Conduct interview alone with resident to understand resident's experience of abuse and perspectives Conduct interview of abuser (when feasible) in nonjudgmental manner Review resident report, report from family and staff, and facility notes Identify risk factor(s) for abuse Correct reversible risk factor(s) and adverse physical and psychological health consequences of abuse (e.g. MDD) Ensure reporting of resident abuse to appropriate government authority as required by law Follow up to monitor safety and improved well-being Assess decision-making capacity if necessary	Each case is opportunity to educate staff regarding lessons learned to improve prevention of other cases of resident abuse Co-leader with social worker of interdisciplinary team to create individualized safety plan for resident Be role model for responsive, victim-defined advocacy that honors resident's values, life experience, and culture Gather team with diverse background in formulating and implementing state-of-the-science resident abuse prevention programs and initiatives Advocate for increased government funding for Ombudsman Program, for resident abuse prevention research, and for innovative resident abuse prevention programs in LTC
Nurse practitioner, physician assistant, clinical nurse specialist, other healthcare provider	Conduct interview alone with resident to understand resident's experience of abuse and perspectives Conduct interview of abuser (when feasible) in nonjudgmental manner Review resident report, report from family and staff, and facility notes Identify risk factor(s) for abuse Correct reversible risk factor(s) and adverse physical and psychological health consequences of abuse (e.g. MDD)	Be role model for responsive, victim-defined advocacy that honors resident's values, life experience, and culture Advocate for increased government funding for Ombudsman Program, for resident abuse prevention research, and for innovative resident abuse prevention programs in LTC
Social worker	Perform comprehensive social assessment, including interpersonal, social, and cultural context Report suspected resident abuse to appropriate government authority on behalf of facility Recruit resident's support network (family, friends, members of resident's faith community) for assistance Alleviate psychosocial stressors Provide (or refer for) individual psychotherapy (with trauma-aware approach) for resident who has relatively preserved cognitive function to address depression and anxiety Inform banks and financial service organizations about fraud related to financial abuse	Co-leader with physician of interdisciplinary team to create individualized safety plan for resident Lead efforts for resident support and education Lead efforts for staff, volunteer, and family education and support Guide abuser (family member or friend) (especially if resident wants to continue to maintain relationship with him) to seek mental health help

Table 10.3 (cont.)

Clinician	Interventions	Therapeutic Pearls
Nurse	Report directly observed abuse by another staff to team Perform comprehensive nursing assessment Monitor safety Address sensory deficit, pain, constipation, and other reversible symptoms	Lead efforts to implement safety plan Provide support and education to resident Provide support and education to family Teach resident skills to soothe self, manage anxiety better, and cope using mindfulness-based strategies
Nursing assistant	Report directly observed abuse by another staff to team Monitor safety Provide emotional support to resident	Lead efforts to engage resident in social activities, exercise, and other simple strategies to cope with negative psychological effects of abuse
Other LTC staff (e.g. dietician, housekeeping)	Report directly observed abuse by another staff to team Monitor safety	Facility leadership educate and empower all staff to help protect resident's rights and prevent abuse
Ombudsman	Ensure that resident's rights are protected and resident receives comprehensive prevention and intervention services if desired	Facility team work closely with ombudsman and consult in difficult situations
Adult Protective Services (APS) caseworker	Receive report, investigate allegations, and develop case plan if allegations are confirmed	Facility team work closely with APS staff
Elder law attorney	Identify need for and provide (or refer for) legal services (e.g. guardian or conservator, depending on resident's severity of impaired decision-making capacity; inform district attorney's office for possible prosecution of abuser[s]; remove abuser as durable power of attorney for resident)	May also need to involve attorney from state's office of rights for individual who has disability as necessary and appropriate
Chaplain and other member of the clergy	Address resident's spiritual/existential distress	Spiritual/existential distress is especially a concern when abuser is spouse, other close family member or friend, or member of resident's faith community
Psychiatrist, gerontologist, and geriatrician	Help interdisciplinary team in complex situations (e.g. resident's decision-making capacity is difficult to assess due to comorbid MDD) Assess need for neuroimaging and neuropsychological evaluation to clarify etiology, severity, and pattern of neurocognitive deficit Clarify presence of psychiatric disorder (e.g. MDD, PTSD)	Guide interdisciplinary team to create and implement state-of-the-science abuse prevention programs and initiatives Lead efforts to resolve complex conflict between resident, family, and team members Ensure that negative psychological effects and complications of abuse (including psychiatric disorder) are being treated effectively and assist if symptoms are not improving

consulting a team involving an elder-law attorney, geriatrician, gerontologist, and geriatric psychiatrist to help develop rigorous, high-quality hiring practices and staff training programs for the prevention, early detection, and prompt treatment of resident abuse. We recommend screening all employees (e.g. criminal background check), verifying credentials, and ongoing staff training in areas such as language, communication, and sensitivity. The staff are encouraged to be vigilant about problems in the facility and to report these problems. Communication among staff, residents, and family members is important. Everyone needs to know what abuse is and how to initiate an internal complaint. Residents and their family should have a way to lodge complaints with multiple levels of staff, not just the direct care provider. LTC staff members commonly conceal medication in food or beverage without the resident's knowledge or consent. Medication is concealed more frequently for a resident who has severe cognitive impairment and/or aggressive behavior. The HCP should discourage this practice because it can be construed as abuse and encourages both secrecy and poor documentation. No effort to prevent resident abuse is complete without adequately addressing staff concerns about workplace stress, insufficient staffing, education, training, and support.

A resident who has MNCD may be particularly at risk of abuse. HCPs are usually not aware of special vulnerabilities of the resident who has MNCD and fail to recognize abusive care practices. A resident who has advanced MNCD may not be able to report abuse and may express distress caused by abuse in the form of agitation, aggression, or depression, which in turn puts the resident at risk for additional abuse. Nursing assistants report low confidence in their ability to prevent a resident's agitation or aggression and even lower confidence in their ability to decrease a resident's agitation or aggression once the resident becomes agitated or aggressive. This issue may be one of the key reasons that predisposes residents who express needs through aggressive behavior to be victims of abuse by other residents and staff. Another resident may respond to a resident's agitation (e.g. yelling) by slapping the resident. A staff member may respond to a resident's anger, verbal abuse, or physical aggression with anger, disrespect, hostile distancing, or passive-aggressive behavior (not responding to the resident's yelling or calling). Thus, the HCP should have a high index of suspicion for abuse in a resident who has MNCD. To reduce abuse in residents who have MNCD, we strongly recommend education of caregivers regarding clinical manifestations of MNCD, interventions to prevent agitation, and improved support of professional and family caregivers.

The Long-Term Care Ombudsman Program

The Long-Term Care Ombudsman Program is a free, confidential service available to all residents of LTC facilities in the United States, to help safeguard residents' rights, resolve the complaints of individual residents, help with the prevention, early detection, and prompt treatment of resident abuse, and represent residents' needs and interests to public officials. The Administration on Aging, of the US Department of Health and Human Services, is responsible for the national program. Each state has a LTC Ombudsman Program operated through, or by, the area's agency on aging and headed by a state LTC ombudsman. Throughout the state, paid staff and volunteer ombudsmen serve residents. Thus, a LTC ombudsman is an advocate for residents of nursing homes, board and care homes, and assisted living homes.

The ombudsman plays an important role in educating consumers and LTC providers about residents' rights and good care practices. The ombudsman addresses many concerns related to violation of residents' rights or dignity, such as physical, verbal, or mental abuse, poor quality of care, unethical conduct, and inappropriate use of chemical or physical restraint. We recommend early referral to an ombudsman for any resident who has personality disorder and expresses a complaint of receiving poor care to ensure that the resident's rights are protected and the staff are protected from unfounded accusations and allegations. However, unlike social workers, nurses, and other HCPs, LTC ombudsmen are not mandated reporters, so can take action on abuse only with the resident's consent. Most ombudsman programs are inadequately funded, and robust funding is needed to tackle the growing public health problem of resident abuse.

Treatment

Resident abuse is multifactorial and needs individual medical, psychiatric, and social approaches, preferably in the context of an interdisciplinary team (IDT). Interdisciplinary collaboration among physicians, physician assistants, nurse practitioners, clinical nurse specialists, social workers, nurses, nursing assistants, administration, elder law attorneys, and mental health professionals is crucial. See Table 10.3 for key strategies for comprehensive management of resident abuse by an IDT. A comprehensive approach not only helps protect residents' rights, autonomy, and self-determination but also improves residents' emotional well-being, strengthens family ties, and bolsters trust in the health care system. The HCP should document observations of changes in a resident's behavior, a resident's reaction to questions, and resident-caregiver (family and HCP) interactions and conflict. A thorough physical examination can help identify specific findings that may further indicate abuse, and the HCP should document these findings. Laboratory tests and imaging studies to further corroborate findings from history and examination are key to making a case for resident abuse. Convincing evidence is not needed to report, but only reasonable suspicion.

Decision-making capacity (DMC) should be presumed until such time as the HCP or the legal system deems the person lacking such capacity. However, in some situations of abuse (e.g. a resident is refusing psychological help and other services to treat sequelae of abuse and prevent further abuse), the HCP may need to evaluate DMC. It is important that the HCP recognize that capacity can be present for simpler decisions and, as the complexity increases, the capacity can be increasingly compromised (a gradient rather than binary relationship). Despite gray areas, when the resident needs a guardian or conservator, the HCP may need to make black-or-white decisions to protect the resident's rights and prevent further abuse (especially in situations of abuse by a family member).

Physicians must be visible frequently in the LTC facility and available to residents, families, and staff for questions about resident care. Although there are many gray areas in suspected abuse cases, much of the obvious abuse is still being missed. A HCP who suspects abuse needs to report the incident to the treatment team immediately so that one of the team members (typically the social worker) makes a formal report (as mandated by law) to the appropriate local, state, and/or national governmental agency (APS). Police may need to be involved in certain circumstances (e.g. a resident has accused a staff member of sexual assault). When there is potential for psychological harm to the resident from such reporting (e.g. the alleged abuser is a spouse), especially if the resident did not want abuse to be reported, reporting should be done along with steps to minimize the psychological harm to the resident (e.g. provide the resident with emotional support, inform the spouse [the suspected abuser] that the HCP [not the resident and despite the resident's objections] did the reporting). Close monitoring for resident safety is crucial after reporting, as resident abuse by the spouse (or another family member) may paradoxically increase in this context. The HCP should identify and promptly treat all potential modifiable factors that predisposed the resident to abuse and complications of abuse (e.g. MDD, pressure ulcer). In complex cases, we recommend a thorough assessment and discussion by an IDT involving the resident, family, primary care physician, nurse practitioner, physician assistant, clinical nurse specialist, psychiatrist, nurse, nursing assistant, social worker, ombudsman, and elder law attorney.

Ethical Issues in Long-Term Care

Autonomy (self-rule, self-determination), beneficence, nonmaleficence (*primum non nocere,* or first do no harm), and distributive justice are four core principles of clinical medical ethics (Borenstein and Goodman 2011). The principle of beneficence involves intention and acts to do good, and the principle of nonmaleficence involves intention and acts to do no harm and to prevent harm. Distributive justice involves equitable treatment and distribution of resources so that patients are treated fairly, free of bias, and based on medical need.

Autonomy is fundamental in residents' daily lives. Attention to small details may make a big difference in a resident's sense of autonomy. For example, a resident's life-long habit (and joy) of reading the morning newspaper with a cup of coffee may not fit with the staff's regimented schedule but could be accommodated relatively easily. The principle of autonomy is at the center of residents' rights to receive treatment only after valid (informed) consent and an opportunity to refuse care. The dignity of the resident is promoted through valid consent and opportunities for choice and taking risk. Valid consent has two main components: the resident is given adequate information, and the voluntariness (lack of coercion or trickery) of the resident's decision to accept or refuse recommendations. When there are concerns about a resident's DMC, it may be necessary to assess that capacity. Assessment of DMC looks for the resident's abilities to understand and appreciate information given, to reason, and to communicate a decision (McSwiggan, Mears, and Porter 2016). Besides tests to assess cognition (e.g. MOCA) and mood (e.g. PHQ-9), we recommend tests to assess capacity more thoroughly (e.g. Hopkins Competency Assessment Test, MacArthur Competence Assessment Tool–Technique [MacCAT-T]) to assist in the determination of decision-making capacity (Janofsky, McCarthy, and

Folstein 1992; Appelbaum and Redlich 2006). If assessment indicates impaired capacity, the HCP should evaluate reversible causes (e.g. medication-induced cognitive impairment) (Sessums, Zembrzuska, and Jackson 2011). Appropriate procedures for obtaining valid consent are not always followed with LTC populations. Residents often sign consent forms without understanding the risks and treatment options, including doing nothing. Thus, a signed consent form is no guarantee that the consent is valid, and it is the role of the HCP to have an in-depth conversation with the resident and/or surrogate decision-maker. A resident who has DMC should be routinely involved in all decision-making, and a resident whose DMC is compromised should be involved in as many decisions as possible to the extent that the abilities allow, even if the HCP does not allow the resident to make the final treatment decision. We recommend that the HCP promptly document the details of a valid consent and the resident's decision so that there is no confusion about the resident's choice and if, at a later time, the resident's cognitive function declines and he or she is not able to give valid consent, the documentation ensures that the treatment team knows what the resident would have wanted.

If a resident does not have DMC, the legally designated surrogate decision-maker should follow the standard of *substituted judgment* to make decisions on behalf of the resident. The standard of substituted judgment requires that the surrogate decision-maker make decisions as the resident would have. This requires not only that the surrogate decision-maker has known the resident well but also that the surrogate decision-maker has had discussions about preferences (e.g. regarding end-of-life care) and values surrounding issues (e.g. what it means to live with dignity). When the standard of substituted judgment cannot be followed due to lack of adequate knowledge of what the resident would have done in a given situation, the standard of *best interest* is followed. This requires the surrogate decision-maker to make decisions that are in the resident's best interest (setting aside the surrogate decision-maker's own preferences, if necessary). This can pose challenges, as many residents face dire situations in which, without knowing the resident's values and wishes, the surrogate decision-maker may not know what would be in the resident's best interest. For example, one choice may lead to shortening of life and another choice may lead to prolonged suffering during the dying process. In such a situation, a third standard, the *reasonable person* standard, can be applied. This standard is based on the belief that most individuals value more or less the same things, and a reasonable person in a given situation would act in a certain way. The surrogate decision-maker needs to be reassured that in some situations there may be more than one reasonable option. Whatever the standard followed and decision made, the HCP needs to assure the surrogate decision-maker that high-quality palliative care will be provided to the resident to ensure that the resident not suffer without respite or experience any indignity in the last days of life. In emergency situations, if the resident does not have DMC and there is no surrogate decision-maker or the surrogate decision-maker is not available, the consent is presumed.

Advance directives are another means to ensure that the resident's wishes are followed in the event that the resident loses DMC. Although a typical advance directive is helpful in many situations (e.g. choice of Do Not Resuscitate [DNR] by a resident if the resident develops advanced MNCD), there are many situations in which it may be difficult to choose a treatment without more explicit instructions from the resident. The HCP should encourage the resident who has DMC to share with the family and treatment team what she values, what gives her life meaning, and what living with dignity means to her. The HCP should also have the resident put these thoughts and conversations in writing. Instructional directives (besides living will) and psychiatric advance directives can be of great help to the treatment team's efforts to ensure that the resident's autonomy is respected at every step. If granting the resident's (or surrogate decision-maker's) choice causes the physician to feel that he or she is violating conscience (conscientious objection) (e.g. a resident requests physician-assisted suicide in a state where it is legal), it is appropriate for the physician to transfer care to another physician who is morally comfortable with the resident's choices. We prefer the term physician-assisted hastening of death to physician-assisted dying or physician-assisted suicide, as it is more accurate (Quill, Back, and Block 2016).

Privacy and confidentiality of personal information are closely related to autonomy, and the HCP should protect them vigorously. The treatment team needs to clarify (with the resident signing appropriate authorization documents), as soon as possible after admission to the LTC facility, with whom the resident would allow the team to share medical information and with whom the resident does not give consent to share. Thereafter, the team should strictly follow the resident's instructions and periodically update them. Older adults who have mental health disorder are often thought to have lower interest in autonomy than others. There is no evidence for such perceptions, and we recommend taking extra steps to preserve the privacy of any resident who has MNCD or other mental health disorder. Genetic testing (e.g. for APOE E4 genes, whose presence signifies increased risk of AD; psychotropic genomic testing) is being increasingly done for older adults, including in LTC populations. Before doing any genetic testing, the HCP should discuss with the resident with whom the resident would like the genetic testing results to be shared, as the findings can have serious implications for not only the resident but also siblings and other first-degree relatives. In cases in which abuse is suspected, it is ethically appropriate (and legally mandated) to share the resident's protected health information (only the absolutely necessary amount and no more) with APS without the resident's consent.

The HCP will frequently encounter ethical dilemmas in LTC, encompassing a myriad of concerns related to end-of-life care (including palliative sedation), rehospitalization, adequate artificial hydration and nutrition (ANH) (nutrition provided through nasogastric tube, percutaneous endoscopic gastrostomy [PEG] tube, intravenous lines [total parenteral nutrition {TPN}, peripheral parenteral nutrition {PPN}]), capacity for decision-making, use of psychotropic medication, use of opioid for noncancer pain, and dealing with conflict that may arise among resident, family members, and staff. It is common to find an HCP struggling to choose an approach that supports autonomy (e.g. a resident wishes to eat food despite swallowing problems) and safety (risk of aspiration). The majority of ethical challenges result from the high prevalence of MNCD and other disorders (e.g. delirium, MDD) that can compromise decisional capacity. The HCP has an ethical responsibility to defend the best interests of the resident at all times and to act as the resident's advocate when required. This may mean, for instance, resisting pressure to provide futile treatment that is not in keeping with the resident's wishes (expressed in a living will) because the family is not ready to "let go."

Beneficence (i.e. doing good for the patient) and nonmaleficence (i.e. doing no harm to the patient) must be balanced against automony (i.e. the resident's right to take risks). Being guided by the principles of nonmaleficence and distributive justice, we strongly recommend the practice of parsimonious medicine but have serious ethical concerns over the practice of rationing. Rationing involves allocating resources to one group of patients and withholding resources from another group for the sake of others. In LTC populations, certain populations (e.g. residents who have MNCD and severe agitation, residents who have morbid obesity) are often declined admission on the basis of rationing of a LTC facility's limited resources. This practice violates the ethical principle of distributive justice. In contrast, parsimonious medicine not only is ethically sound but also reflects the wisdom of prudent medical practice. Parsimonious medicine is practice of medicine that proactively avoids wasteful or futile care (care that does not benefit the patient because it does not fit the patient's needs and circumstances) (Tilburt and Cassel 2013). Many residents are not treated wisely and in fact are treated too much. Thus, parsimonious medicine has an even bigger role in LTC populations than in hospitals and outpatient clinics. Some examples of parsimonious medicine in LTC populations include (but are not limited to) deintensification of diabetes treatment for a resident who develops hypoglycemia, deintensification of hypertension treatment for a resident who develops hypotension, forgoing colonoscopy and mammogram for a frail resident, and discontinuing statin for a resident who has advanced MNCD. In this sense, parsimonious medicine when practiced with integrity honors the ethical principles of nonmaleficence primarily and distributive justice secondarily (by reducing the use of limited resources). What is best for the resident is often not what the resident or family wants. Sometimes the HCP needs to advise residents and their family with compassion and sensitivity that it is in their interest not to undergo a test or treatment. The practice of parsimonious medicine recognizes that, given the high prevalence of MNCD, frailty, multimorbidity, and advanced disability in LTC populations, many tests and treatments are of marginal or no benefit, can impose substantial burden on the resident and cost on the system, and, in some situations, are outright harmful to the resident.

New medical interventions may provide options many residents did not have a few years ago. For example, until recently, the only treatment for severe symptomatic aortic stenosis was open-heart surgery.

Now, an individual who is not a candidate for surgery may benefit from transcatheter aortic valve replacement. Even if new procedures are technically feasible, before offering such options it is important that the HCP properly counsel the resident and family that these new procedures have not been tested with LTC populations and the risks may be much higher in these populations than in community-dwelling age-matched peers. Subjecting a resident to new treatment without due diligence and discussion may put the resident at significant risk of additional morbidity, thus violating the ethical principle of nonmaleficence. All residents who are recommended a surgical procedure should undergo a preoperative comprehensive geriatric assessment, especially to look for the presence of frailty, undernutrition, neurocognitive and mood disorder, and impaired mobility. Many residents are subjected to treatments (especially surgical procedures) without being assessed for comorbidity that would put them at such high risk for severe disability (e.g. accelerated cognitive decline) when, on learning of such risks, they would often opt to decline such interventions.

The HCP needs to keep in mind that the presence of a Do Not Resuscitate (DNR) order may reduce physicians' willingness to order a variety of treatments not related to CPR, and the HCP should elicit additional information about the resident's treatment goals to inform these decisions and ensure that the resident's needs are not neglected. The widely divergent cross-cultural differences and varying religious views in a pluralistic democratic society require that all professional staff (including physicians) approach treatment decisions with openness and sensitivity. In encounters with the patient, the physician should listen to, adapt, and, if possible, adopt the patient's perspective. Such an approach may help resolve many ethical dilemmas that are commonly encountered in caring for frail LTC populations. Every LTC facility is a community, albeit an artificial one, in which strangers come to live together. Ethicists are now giving thought to the nature of such communities and the obligations of people within it to each other. Having a formalized means of sorting through difficult cases is often not readily available in LTC facilities that have limited staffing and lack of access to physicians with geriatric expertise (especially geriatricians and geriatric psychiatrists) and ethicists from tertiary care centers. Some centers (e.g. Center for Health Ethics, University of Missouri–Columbia) provide innovative 24/7 countrywide ethics consultation service on request through video conferencing ("tele-ethics"), telephone conferencing, and email. Telehealth can provide access to services (especially specialty services such as geriatric psychiatry, dermatology) that are otherwise not available. Telehealth also poses unique ethical challenges (e.g. potential for depersonalization of the resident, inequity when distributing benefits of telehealth services) that need to be addressed at the outset and in an ongoing manner.

We recommend that the LTC facility make available a mechanism to effectively address complex ethical issues in a timely fashion. This process can be instrumental in sustaining the dignity of the resident and maintaining the quality and safety of resident care. Such a mechanism involves five steps: (1) clarify the facts that relate to the organizational, medical, and social circumstances of the case (This also includes obtaining as much information as is feasible regarding the resident's personal values and beliefs, degree of suffering, and spiritual and psychological goals.); (2) clearly identify ethical concerns and differentiate them from legal concerns and/or issues related to miscommunication; (3) frame the issue in ethical terms so that it can be critically discussed; (4) identify and resolve the conflict; and (5) make a decision regarding the issue that raised the ethical conflict (Fleming 2007).

LTC facilities can be communities of caring and interdependence. The goal should be not simply to eliminate or minimize dependence whenever possible, but to make a genuinely creative and nurturing use of the dependence that is inevitable for most LTC residents. LTC facilities may be places for rehabilitation and recovery for some, but for most they need to be places of healing – of making whole – of enabling frail and disabled residents who have advanced illness to use their dependence to learn to value interdependence and grow as human beings.

Research Ethics

The position statement of the Alzheimer's Association regarding research on individuals who have MNCD provides reasonable but not excessive protection for research subjects. The threat of medical, psychiatric, and environmental conditions to the well-being of the large and growing LTC populations requires that research efforts not be hampered by excessive restrictions. A diagnosis of MNCD does not render the resident incapable of making decisions. In general, more than 50 percent of residents who have mild MNCD are able to make decisions about participating in research, but residents who have moderate MNCD do not have decision-making capacity for participation in research (Johnson and Karlawish 2015). We recommend adopting the following key features of the Alzheimer's Association position statement on this issue (with minor modifications):

- For minimal-risk research, any resident should be allowed to enroll in a research project (with consent), even if there is no potential benefit to the resident. In the absence of an advance research directive, proxy consent is acceptable for a resident who does not have the capacity to consent for research.
- For research with greater than minimal risk and if there is a reasonable potential benefit to the individual, the enrollment of any resident is allowable, based on consent of the resident or the proxy. The proxy's consent can be based on either a research-specific advance directive or using the principle of substituted judgment.
- For research with greater than minimal risk and if there is no reasonable potential for benefit to the individual, only those residents who are capable of giving informed consent or who have executed a research-specific advance directive are allowed to participate. In the latter case and for a resident who has MNCD and retains the capacity to give consent, a proxy must be available to help monitor the resident's involvement throughout the duration of the research.

Truth-Telling

Truthfulness is the foundation of all relationships. Without honesty and truthfulness, trust cannot be established and established trust can be quickly eroded. Without trust, caregivers (family and professional) may not be able to meet the emotional and physical needs of a resident and may even cause emotional harm. Most residents do not have the ability or resources to find a different environment in which caregivers are honest and truthful. Truth-telling, especially to a resident who has moderate to severe MNCD, causes ethical dilemmas for many caregivers (family as well as professional). All methods of discourse with residents should be truthful, with rare exceptions. Residents (those who have MNCD and those who don't) are often more resilient than we realize, and even a cognitively impaired resident can quickly detect a lie (e.g. a caregiver tells a resident who wants to go home that the resident is at the facility "only for a few days" and soon will be able to go home). "Benevolent deception" (therapeutic exception, therapeutic lie) should be an exception rather than the rule in caring for vulnerable LTC populations.

Truth-telling is not synonymous with being "bluntly honest," nor does it mean that the staff should constantly correct statements made by a resident who has cognitive impairment. Blunt honesty and repeatedly correcting a resident's beliefs and memory in most situations may actually be harmful to the resident. Strict adherence to the virtues of truthfulness and candor in some situations (e.g. a resident who made a recent serious suicide attempt is given the diagnosis of a terminal illness [e.g. metastatic cancer]) risks violation of the core ethical principles of beneficence and nonmaleficence. In daily practice, such situations are rare but the frequency of lying and dishonesty in dealing with LTC populations (especially those who have MNCD) is far from rare. This culture of dishonesty is fueled more by the irrational fears of caregivers (professional and family) and by the discomfort of caregivers in addressing a resident's grief and loss than by a rational and compassionate approach to care. Truth-telling needs to be done with utmost sensitivity to the resident's emotional state, the individual circumstances, and efforts to understand what the resident is trying to express (e.g. a resident asking when he can go home may be reacting to unrelieved pain; a resident asking for her small children may be feeling a lack of purpose in life; a resident who is looking for her parents is seeking validation, security, and unconditional love). Truthfulness may hurt (e.g. telling the resident that this is her new home), and caregivers need to anticipate the resident's emotional pain and take steps to relieve it. Ultimately, being truthful is about honoring the resident's dignity, and thus is each resident's right and our obligation. This is even more important for the residents who are weakest (e.g. residents who have severe MNCD), as their dignity lies in our hands.

Ethical Dilemmas during End-of-Life Care

The HCP will routinely encounter ethical dilemmas during end-of-life care in LTC populations. Examples include dilemmas around futile care, euthanasia and physician-assisted hastening of death, discontinuing medical treatment with high burden, and discontinuing ANH and life-prolonging treatment for a resident who has severe or terminal MNCD. Futile treatments are medical approaches that provide no meaningful possibility of extended life, improved quality of life, or other benefit for the patient. Medically futile situations can stimulate tremendous ethical conflict, both within an individual and between individuals involved in the medical situation. For example, conflict can arise in the LTC setting when family or surrogates demand treatment that the clinical staff view as excessively burdensome and futile for the resident. Situations (e.g. terminal MNCD) involving futile treatment commonly stimulate intense guilt in family members, who may go to great lengths to avoid actions that make them feel guilty. Prompt involvement of a physician (especially an experienced physician, preferably with geriatric expertise [e.g. geriatrician, geriatric psychiatrist]) is critical to address ethical dilemmas in such situations and reduce the emotional suffering (in residents, family, and clinical staff) that accompanies such issues. The HCP with expertise in addressing such situations (e.g. psychiatrist) can often assist families and residents to bear grief, guilt, and disappointment and understand that physical helplessness does not imply psychological helplessness. Medically futile situations may in fact promote the development of psychological mastery. Physicians too can experience psychological growth as they turn from action at any cost to empathetic care of the whole patient, including psychological care. In such situations, we recommend that the HCP address family misunderstanding about suffering during end-of-life care and address their guilt and grief with patience and compassion. Listening to staff concerns and helping the staff understand the family's fears, guilt, and grief is helpful in reducing the staff's concerns and distress.

Determining the benefit of a particular treatment to a resident who has one or more terminal conditions is often difficult. In the LTC setting, the special relationships often established between staff and residents may make the issue more ethically challenging. Sometimes members of the direct care staff feel (often rightly so) that they understand the resident better than anyone else. In working through these issues with the staff, the HCP should distinguish between futile medical treatment and futile care. Although a particular medical treatment may be considered to produce no benefit to the resident, staff members often need to be reassured that their caring is never futile, never in vain. The decision to forgo a particular treatment must never be confused with abandoning the resident.

It is not uncommon for residents or even family members to request euthanasia and physician-assisted hastening of death. Euthanasia and physician-assisted hastening of death can raise serious ethical conflicts among not only professional caregivers but also residents and their family. We have serious concerns about the possibility of a "slippery slope" phenomenon following legalization of euthanasia (in Netherlands, Belgium, Ireland, Colombia, and Luxembourg) and physician-assisted death (assisted suicide) (in Germany, Switzerland, Canada, Albania, Japan, and in the US states of Montana, Washington, Oregon, Vermont, and California), even under restricted conditions. Physician involvement in euthanasia and physician-assisted hastening of death may cause patients to distrust physicians who are administering medication for palliation (e.g. a patient who becomes sedated with morphine may fear that the physician's intention is not to relieve pain but to hasten death). In addition, physicians who work more closely with terminally ill patients are more likely to oppose physician-assisted hastening of death (Rostin and Roberts 2016). The American Medical Association also opposes physician-assisted hastening of death. We strongly advocate palliative care (including palliative sedation) and hospice care in place of euthanasia and physician-assisted hastening of death.

The pre-eminence of autonomy as an ethical principle in the United States can sometimes lead HCPs to disregard other moral considerations and common sense when making clinical decisions. Emphasis on individual autonomy reflects values deeply held in many societies: fierce individualism and self-sufficiency. Many societies and cultures (especially Western cultures) do not value interdependence as much as autonomy. We respect many patients' belief and wish to anticipate and "overtake" death by administering it oneself (i.e. respecting patients' wishes for autonomy) but strongly feel that the role of the medical profession is to understand but *not* support such wishes. Every person's life is valuable, irrespective of physical and mental state, even when the person has ceased to deem life valuable. The HCP should accept death as one of the conditions of human freedom. Valuing and promoting interdependence is crucial to providing dignity-conserving care to LTC populations and helping residents overcome the wish to end life.

Discontinuing medical treatment with high burden often causes considerable ethical dilemmas, especially in caring for residents who have advanced MNCD. For example, decisions regarding when to discontinue dialysis for a frail resident who has multiple disabling comorbidities are difficult, especially if the resident does not appear to be suffering between dialysis sessions. Usually there is no guiding directive. Family or surrogates may be called on to decide on the basis of their impressions of the resident's wishes or their estimate of the resident's best interest whether it would be inappropriate to continue dialysis. If the resident's mental state leads her or him to interpret each dialysis as a threatening event that requires restraint or sedation or both, the decision to give up dialysis is clearly in the resident's interest. We recommend an IDT meeting with the physician as the team leader and the family present to better understand and make decisions that are in keeping with the resident's values.

Withholding and withdrawing ANH also commonly raise ethical dilemmas. Because food and water are basic to human survival and feeding is an expression of caring for another person, the decision to withhold or withdraw a PEG tube may be seen not as the withholding of medical treatment but rather as the denial of basic human care. Even our language can add to ethical challenges. For example, the term *feeding tube* connotes something essential and nurturing (akin to placing a spoon in a resident's mouth) rather than a device (PEG tube), and thus depriving a resident of a feeding tube or removal of a feeding tube causes more discomfort than withholding insertion of or removal of a medical device (PEG tube). Psychiatrists can be key in the efforts of the treatment team to inform and educate the resident's family that providing ANH through PEG tube is a medical intervention that in many situations may cause more harm (e.g. more suffering, infection, aspiration) than good (e.g. increased quantity of life) and hence should not be undertaken. Additionally, family members need to be educated that the resident in these situations is not experiencing hunger and distress due to hunger. In fact, providing ANH via PEG tube in these situations may cause distress (e.g. pain at the site of the tube), exacerbate suffering caused by other processes, and prolong the dying process. Ethical issues are raised in such situations often because of the manner in which the decisions are made and the lack of capacity of the resident to make her or his wishes known. When residents are able to choose and express choice, the decision to withhold ANH may be more comfortable for the staff. In the absence of an advance directive addressing ANH, some LTC staff may believe that there is a moral and legal obligation to do everything medically possible for the resident. Such ethical concerns of staff should be addressed gently, with compassion for the staff, and promptly with interdisciplinary staff meeting and sharing recommendations from reputable organizations and journals.

One area in which there is still controversy is whether antidementia drugs reduce mortality in individuals who have MNCD. There is preliminary evidence that they may reduce mortality. Until further research clarifies this issue, we recommend including potential benefits of antidementia drugs (e.g. reduction in future agitation and ability to maintain some current function [e.g. eating on one's own] for a few months longer than without the medications) for some residents in deciding the risks and benefits of continuing antidementia drugs on an individual basis.

Restricting Resident Autonomy in Different Cultures

In times of crisis and when facing one's own mortality, religious and familial/cultural values are sources of strength and comfort. Western civilization's concept of personal autonomy and self-determination are at the core of health care decision-making, but other cultures do not always share that value system. Sensitivity to multicultural diversity in this context is imperative to maintain individual self-esteem and respect, for both the patient and the patient's family. Emphasis on autonomy and full disclosure may not be respectful of dying residents from certain cultural traditions. In the Asian, Hispanic, and other traditions, autonomy must be balanced against such values as respect for the family and community support. For example, the family may make life support decisions rather than the resident who belongs to one of these cultural backgrounds. Many HCPs from American society may have ethical issues related to restricting a resident's autonomy (e.g. not telling the resident about a terminal prognosis as requested or insisted by the family) while caring for the resident who comes from one of these cultural traditions. Full disclosure may be at variance with cultural beliefs about hope and wellness, and autonomous decision-making may counter family-centered values. In our opinion, the resident's values should dictate whether it is beneficial or burdensome to be fully informed. The challenge to US physicians will be to understand and bridge the gulf between their own values on dying and those of their patients. Although some differences may not be resolvable, residents and their families deserve a meaningful and dignified process of death and dying that is in keeping with their cultural and religious values.

Distributive Justice

An ethical dilemma arises when one has limited resources and multiple groups are trying to access those resources. How does one decide which resident should be given a single room, as single rooms are scarce? How does one decide which new resident to admit when a bed becomes available? Such ethical dilemmas are routine in LTC facilities. For example, a resident who was living in a private room (only one occupant) dies and different staff members want the room for different residents who are currently sharing a room. One staff member wishes the room to go to a resident who is a "yeller" who disturbs every roommate he or she has had. Another staff member wants the room for a resident who is on hospice so that family can stay with the resident in the last days of life. It is important to realize that both options (and others) may be ethically right. Often, there are multiple right solutions. It is best to resolve such dilemmas as a group rather than one person in the leadership team making a unilateral decision.

Ethical Issues in the Use of Restraints

Older persons should be able to enjoy human rights and fundamental freedoms when residing in a shelter, care, or treatment facility, including full respect for their dignity, beliefs, needs and privacy, and for the right to make decisions about their care and the quality of their lives.
Principle 14 of the United Nations Principles for Older Persons

The practice of using restraints to restrict a resident's freedom of movement is prevalent in LTC facilities. Freedom of movement is any movement the person is capable of and wishes to perform (e.g. attempts to access parts of the body, to ambulate). Physical restraint involves using physical means to restrict freedom of movement (e.g. physically holding the person, using material equipment) and not to treat any medical or psychiatric condition or symptom. Chemical restraint involves administering one or more psychotropic medications with the primary intention of restricting the person's freedom of movement, rather than to treat any specific medical or psychiatric condition or symptom. Although the use of physical restraint has declined in the last decade, use of chemical restraint is still prevalent in LTC facilities.

Use of restraints raises serious ethical concerns, the most important being violation of the resident's autonomy. See Table 10.4 for common examples of ethically appropriate and inappropriate use of restraints. Restraints (physical and chemical) are often dehumanizing, are psychologically traumatic to the resident and family, and do not increase safety (the most common reason for using restraints). Use of restraints has also been linked to increased agitation and aggression, especially in a resident who has MNCD. People have unconditional worth and dignity that supports a strong argument for the maintenance of autonomy (e.g. by not restraining them to prevent falls), even in the event of possible harm from an injury (e.g. falls and injury). Use of restraints should be restricted to exceptional situations in which their use is absolutely necessary because there is imminent risk of serious harm to self or others. Their use should be for the shortest possible time and in accordance with the best professional practices. Residents in restraints need to be continuously monitored for any concern related to the use of restraints (e.g. skin breakdown due to improperly placed physical restraint, adverse effect of chemical restraint) and to monitor the situation that required restraints in the first place. A decade ago, lap buddies and other restraints to prevent residents in wheelchairs from ambulating were routinely used in LTC populations to prevent falls, but fortunately their use has been reduced dramatically over the last decade with improved awareness of the harms of use of restraints, regulations to limit their use, and more effective ways to manage the risk of falls (e.g. lowering the bed and surrounding it with soft mats, using alarm devices to monitor a resident's attempt to rise).

Moving from Standard of Care to State-of-the-Science Care

Physicians and other HCPs should try to provide state-of-the-science care, although for medico-legal

Table 10.4 Ethically Appropriate or Inappropriate Use of Restraints in Long-Term Care Populations

Restraint	Description and Common Examples of Ethically Appropriate Use of Restraint	Description and Common Examples of Ethically Inappropriate Use of Restraint
Physical restraint	Resident is having behavioral emergency (severe agitation, severe aggressive and/or suicidal behavior that poses imminent risk of serious harm to self and/or others) and physical restraint is used to prevent resident from harming herself and/or others Typically, physical restraint is used only briefly until treatment to address underlying problem (e.g. analgesic for pain, antipsychotic medication for psychotic symptoms) takes effect Sometimes physical restraint may be used briefly (e.g. physically holding resident in behavioral emergency) to administer medication to address underlying medical and/or psychiatric problem/symptom that is causing behavioral emergency (e.g. intramuscular analgesic to address severe pain)	Use of side rails to prevent resident from voluntarily getting out of bed Tucking resident in or using fastener to restrict freedom of movement in bed or chair Use of any chair that restricts freedom of movement Use of tray or other means that the resident cannot easily remove to prevent resident from getting up from chair
Chemical restraint	Resident is having behavioral emergency (severe agitation, severe aggressive and/or suicidal behavior that poses imminent risk of serious harm to self and/or others) and psychotropic is given (orally or parenterally [intramuscularly, intravenously]) to sedate resident to resolve behavioral emergency	Giving psychotropic medication for convenience of caregiver (professional and or family), not to treat any medical or psychiatric condition or symptom Giving psychotropic medication to prevent resident from ambulating, yelling, or expressing distress in a way that caregiver (professional and/or family) considers disturbing or distressing Giving psychotropic medication to prevent resident from making effort to leave facility

purposes they are required to provide only the standard of care. The standard of care is generally defined as what a reasonable physician or another HCP would have done in the same set of circumstances at the same time. Communication, education of residents and family, and documentation of treatment are critical. Communication with the interdisciplinary team is important. Communicating with the resident and family and educating them about the resident's treatment should involve explanation of the care plan to the family to ensure that they understand the resident's condition and the limitations of treatment. Documenting this conversation is important.

Medical directors have many more responsibilities to ensure that standard of care is being provided to all residents. Medical directors are expected to have regular meetings with department heads at the facility, be aware of trends or problems identified by facility personnel, and be aware of the policies and procedures that need to be implemented about a problem (e.g. physical abuse of a resident by a staff member). Understanding proper reporting procedures can reduce the risk of government sanctions and criminal penalties for those working in LTC. It is incumbent on medical directors of nursing homes to familiarize themselves with criminal mistreatment laws in their own state in order to ensure residents' well-being, promote staff integrity, and assist the facility to manage the risk of criminal liability for resident abuse. Through modeling, medical directors can inspire other physicians and HCPs to move beyond standard-of-care practices and continuously update their knowledge and skills in optimal ethical management of geriatric syndromes and practice state-of-the-science evidence-based care that follows common-sense geriatric principles.

Summary

Resident abuse is a major public health problem, and physicians play a crucial role in the prevention of and comprehensive approach to resident abuse. Verbal abuse and neglect are the most common forms of resident abuse in LTC populations. Physical abuse is the most visible, and neglect and financial exploitation are most often missed. Resident-to-resident abuse (verbal, physical, sexual) is much more common than resident abuse by staff or family. Neglect is the most common form of resident abuse by a staff member or family member. Resident abuse is eminently preventable, and comprehensive geriatric assessment is the first step in identifying risk factors and instituting an individualized abuse prevention care plan for an at-risk resident. During each encounter, the physician should screen every resident for possible abuse. Addressing resident abuse includes assessment by an interdisciplinary team, reporting to the appropriate governmental agency, institution of an individualized safety plan, monitoring safety, and management of the negative health consequences. HCPs who provide care for LTC populations are regularly challenged by ethical issues. Most ethical issues can be resolved by guidance from an experienced physician. Adhering to the ethical principles of autonomy, beneficence, nonmaleficence, and distributive justice requires routine practice of obtaining valid consent, parsimonious medicine, and minimizing therapeutic lying and use of restraints.

Key Clinical Points

1. Resident-to-resident abuse is the most common form of abuse and is predictable, sometimes fatal, and eminently preventable.
2. Every clinical encounter provides a critically important opportunity for the health care provider to recognize resident abuse and intervene.
3. Every facility should institute a facility-wide program to prevent abuse for residents at high risk for abuse (e.g. a resident who has advanced MNCD).
4. A comprehensive approach to prevention and effective early intervention require a diverse interdisciplinary team working together.
5. Adhering to the ethical principles of autonomy, beneficence, nonmaleficence, and distributive justice requires routine practice of obtaining valid consent, parsimonious medicine, and minimizing therapeutic lying and use of restraints.

Additional Resources

Fact Sheet: Abuse of Residents of Long-Term Care Facilities. http://www.centeronelderabuse.org/docs/Abuse_of_Residents_of_Long_Term_Care_Facilities.pdf

Working with Older Survivors of Abuse: A Framework for Advocates. National Clearing House for Abuse in Later Life http://www.ncall.us

National Center on Elder Abuse: Maintains a website with contact numbers and a directory of ombudsmen offices in each state in the United States of America for this purpose. https://ncea.acl.gov

Center for Excellence on Elder Abuse and Neglect at the University of California, Irvine. http://www.centeronelderabuse.org

References

Appelbaum, P. and A. Redlich. 2006. Impact of Decision-Making Capacity on the Use of Leverage to Encounter Treatment Adherence. *Community Mental Health Journal.* **42**(2):121–130.

Ben Natan, M., and A. Lowenstein. 2010. Study of Factors That Affect Abuse of Older People in Nursing Homes. *Nursing Management* **17**(8):20–24.

Borenstein, J., and K.W. Goodman. 2011. Ethical Issues in Geriatric Psychiatry. In M.E. Agronin and G. J. Maletta (eds.), *Principles and Practice of Geriatric Psychiatry*, 2nd ed., pp. 279–288. Philadelphia, PA: Lippincott Williams & Wilkins.

Dong, X.Q. 2015. Elder Abuse: Systematic Review. *Journal of the American Geriatrics Society* **63**:1214–1238.

Fleming, D. 2007. Addressing Ethical Issues in the Nursing Home. *Missouri Medicine* **104**:387–391.

Janofsky, J.S., R.J. McCarthy, and M.F. Folstein. 1992. Hopkins Competency Assessment Test: A Brief Method to Assess Patients' Capacity to Give Informed Consent. *Hospital and Community Psychiatry* **43**(2):132–136.

Johnson, R.A., and J. Karlawish. 2015. A Review of Ethical Issues in Dementia. *International Psychogeriatrics* **27**(10):1635–1647.

Lach, M.S., and K.A. Pillemer. 2015. Elder Abuse. *New England Journal of Medicine* **373**:1947–1956.

McSwiggan, S., S. Mears, and M. Porter. 2016. Decision-Making Capacity in Adult Guardianship: A Systematic Review. *International Psychogeriatrics* **28**(3):373–384.

Mosqueda, L. and X. Dong. 2011. Elder Abuse and Self-Neglect: "I Don't Care Anything about Going to the Doctor, to Be Honest . . ..". *Journal of the American Medical Association* **306**(5):532–540.

Mosqueda, L., K. Burnight, M.W. Gironda, et al. 2016. The Abuse Intervention Model: A Pragmatic Approach to Intervention for Elder Mistreatment. *Journal of the American Geriatrics Society* **64**:1879–1883.

Quill, T.E., A.L. Back, and S.A. Block. 2016. Responding to Request for Physician-Assisted Death. Physician Involvement at the Very End of Life. *Journal of the American Medical Association* **315**(3):245–246.

Rostin, L.A. and A.E. Roberts. 2016. Physician Assisted Dying: A Turning Point? *Journal of the American Medical Association* **315**(3):249–250.

Sessums, LL., H. Zembrzuska, and J.L. Jackson. 2011. Does This Patient Have Medical Decision-Making Capacity? *Journal of the American Medical Association* **306**(4):420–427.

Tilburt, J.C., and Cassel, C.K. 2013. Why the Ethics of Parsimonious Medicine Is Not Ethics of Rationing. *Journal of the American Medical Association* **309**(8): 773–774.

Chapter 11

Psychiatric Aspects of Palliative and Hospice Medicine

Unless we are occupied in our own search for meaning, we may not create the climate in which patients can be helped to make their journeys of growth through loss.

Dame Cicely Saunders, founder of St. Christopher's Hospice, from Journal of Palliative Care, *vol. 4, no. 3 (1988).*

More than 25 percent of individuals dying in the United States die in a long-term care (LTC) facility (Institute of Medicine 2014). Some 30 percent of all LTC residents die within 1 year of admission. It is projected that approximately 40 percent of Americans will die in a LTC facility by the year 2020. Some 80 percent of LTC residents die at the facility and 20 percent are transferred to a hospital immediately before death. The majority of residents have one or more terminal illnesses (an illness from which there is little or no chance of recovery and that will most likely cause death in months to a few years). Thus, death and dying are central features of the practice of medicine in LTC.

Advances in medicine have had an unexpected and unwanted outcome for many individuals who have terminal illness: prolongation of the dying process. This is especially true for many LTC residents. Inappropriate hospitalization, prolonged time spent in the intensive care unit, prescription of inappropriate medication, inadequate relief of symptoms, and undergoing life-prolonging treatment that is not in keeping with an advance directive are prevalent among residents during the last year of life. Many family caregivers feel that their loved one did not experience a good death in the LTC facility. Hence, it is imperative that residents and their family discuss with each other and their primary care physician (PCP) what "a good death" means to them, what prudent choices they would make to ensure that the dying process is dignified and comfortable, and how health care providers (HCPs) can help them achieve these goals.

Palliative medicine is a branch of medicine that focuses on helping patients who have terminal illness avoid harmful and futile medical treatment and live the rest of life with dignity and comfort. Palliative medicine is different from other branches of medicine in its equal focus on the well-being of the family and friends involved in caring for the patient. The practice of palliative and hospice care, research, education and training of HCPs, and public policy are the pillars of palliative medicine. Palliative and hospice care has been found not only to improve quality of life but also at times to positively influence the course of illness (Volicer 2011).

Palliative and End-of-Life Care

Palliative care is a popular buzzword in LTC these days but often the concept is misunderstood among staff working in LTC. The World Heath Organization defines palliative care as an approach that improves the quality of life of patients and their families facing the problems associated with life-threatening illness, through the prevention and relief of suffering by means of early identification, assessment, and treatment of pain and other problems – physical, psychosocial, and spiritual (World Health Organization 2002). Table 11.1 lists various terms used in palliative care. The ultimate goal of palliative care is to help the individual make the best of every day remaining. Achievement of this goal rests on the recognition that each person has inherent value, and autonomy and uniqueness need to be acknowledged and respected at every step. The decision to intervene with active palliative care is based on an ability to meet stated goals (e.g. enhancing quality of life, maintaining function, maximizing comfort, achieving a timely, peaceful, and dignified death) rather than affect the underlying terminal disease. All treatment options are explored and evaluated in the context of the individual's values and symptoms. The individual's choices and decisions regarding care are paramount and must be followed. Palliative

Table 11.1 Terms Used in Palliative and End-of-Life Care

Term	Description	Therapeutic Pearls
Palliative care	Care for resident who has life-limiting illness that focuses on improving quality of life, maintaining function, and maximizing comfort	Ideally suited for LTC populations, as most residents have one or more advanced illnesses and less than two years life expectancy
Hospice care	End-of-life care provided to individual deemed by a physician to have six months or less to live Focus is on improving quality of life, maximizing comfort, and addressing family grief Individual has to forgo curative treatment	Prediction that a resident who has noncancer terminal illness (e.g. advanced MNCD) has six months or less to live is difficult for physician
End-of-life (EOL) care	Palliative care given in the last few days to months of life (includes hospice care)	Many facilities can provide high-quality EOL care without having to refer resident for additional hospice services
Restorative care	Care that provides rehabilitation services to restore lost function (e.g. physical therapy after hip fracture surgery to restore ability to ambulate)	Many residents are admitted to LTC facility for rehabilitation but have such poor health due to one or more terminal illnesses that they are unable to participate in rehabilitation and need palliative care
Curative care (also called life-prolonging treatment; includes life-saving treatment, such as cardiopulmonary resuscitation [CPR])	Care that cures underlying illness (e.g. antibiotic for pneumonia, some surgical treatment for cancer)	Treatment aimed at curing an illness (e.g. pneumonia) may prolong the dying process for a resident who has end-stage condition (e.g. end-stage heart failure)
Euthanasia	On explicit voluntary request by a mentally competent patient, a physician administers a medication intentionally to end that patient's life	Legal in Belgium, Canada, Colombia, Luxembourg, and Netherlands Choice of euthanasia is driven more by issues surrounding fear of loss of dignity, independence, and control; and fear of being a burden than by fear of pain and physical suffering
Physician-assisted hastening of death (physician-assisted dying, physician-assisted suicide)	On explicit voluntary request by a mentally competent patient, a physician provides that patient medication or a prescription to obtain medication that the patient intends to use to end life	Legal in Switzerland, Germany, Japan, Albania, and in the following US states: California, Montana, Oregon, Vermont, Washington Choice of physician-assisted hastening of death is driven more by issues surrounding fear of loss of dignity, independence, and control and fear of being a burden than by fear of pain and physical suffering
Palliative sedation	Intentional lowering of awareness toward and including unconsciousness to relieve suffering due to severe and refractory symptoms Can be intermittent or continuous sedation	Midazolam is typically used because it can be easily titrated

Table 11.1 (cont.)

Term	Description	Therapeutic Pearls
	Has a sound ethical basis when used in appropriate situation with valid consent from individual and/or family	
Continuous sedation until death (CSD)	A type of palliative sedation in which consciousness is reduced until death	A combination of benzodiazepine and opioid is typically used
Nontreatment decisions (NTD)	Withholding or withdrawing treatment from a patient either because of its medical futility or on explicit voluntary request by a mentally competent patient Does not intend to hasten death but accepts death as a natural phenomenon by forgoing futile, burdensome, or unwanted life-prolonging treatment	Declining treatment of pneumonia by a resident who is imminently dying due to cancer or terminal MNCD is an example of NTD Many residents and/or their family may persist in wanting futile treatment out of desperation, and it is up to the physician to help them come to terms with medical reality
Medical futility	Treatment that is not expected to have any benefit for the patient	Medically futile treatment is prevalent in LTC populations receiving EOL care
Appropriateness of treatments	Appropriate treatment is a treatment in which the expected health benefit exceeds the negative health consequences by a sufficiently wide margin that the treatment is worth doing	Inappropriate treatment is prevalent in LTC populations receiving EOL care
Advance care planning	Process of engaging a patient who has a life-limiting illness and the family in discussions about their preferences regarding future care, including EOL care	Should occur before admission to LTC facility or as soon after admission as possible and periodically thereafter
Advance directives	Individual describes future preferences for EOL care in a document (includes living will, durable power of attorney for health care)	PCT should strongly encourage resident who has decision-making capacity (DMC) to have an advance directive
Advance directive for euthanasia	Individual describes a desire for euthanasia in advance and the circumstances under which the individual would want euthanasia	Most popular advance directive in the Netherlands
Do Not Resuscitate (DNR)	Individual forgoes CPR by medical team CPR is a life-saving intervention when an individual goes into cardiac and/or respiratory arrest	Should be a rule for frail LTC populations with a few exceptions because risks are high and benefits minimal
Do Not Intubate (DNI)	Individual forgoes life support with a mechanical ventilator Treatment with a mechanical ventilator is a life-saving approach for respiratory failure	Should be a rule for frail LTC populations with a few exceptions because risks are high and benefits minimal

Table 11.1 (cont.)

Term	Description	Therapeutic Pearls
Do Not Hospitalize (DNH)	Individual forgoes hospitalization for treatment of acute severe medical condition (e.g. pneumonia) Intensive treatment in a hospital for acute severe medical condition can be life saving	Should be a rule for residents receiving EOL care with a few exceptions because risks are high and benefits minimal
Physician Orders for Life-Sustaining Treatment (POLST)	Enacts legally valid medical orders for current treatment based on patient's wishes to have or to forgo life-sustaining medical treatment (e.g. CPR) Most useful when patient or surrogate decision-maker is unlikely to change decisions in response to changes in context (e.g. resident who has advanced MNCD)	POLST orders for withholding antibiotics and orders regarding artificial nutrition are commonly violated in LTC populations Not designed to address context-specific decision-making (e.g. resident who has respiratory distress allows short-term mechanical ventilation if chance of returning to previous level of functioning is high but declines mechanical ventilation if chance of recovery from acute respiratory problem is low) and thus may curtail patient-centered decision-making

care is provided to the individual up until death and to the family even after death and is by definition never futile. Allowing death to occur naturally by forgoing or withdrawing life-prolonging treatment (e.g. cardiac defibrillator, mechanical ventilator) may shorten survival but is ethical (honoring the patient's right to self-determination [ethical standard of autonomy]) if it is in keeping with the patient's wishes.

Palliative care should be offered to all the LTC residents. Many residents entering a LTC facility for postacute care (e.g. rehabilitation) may also need palliative care, regardless of their status as "terminally ill" or not. Any resident who has a life expectancy of two years or less should be offered palliative care (Morley, Cao, and Shum 2016). A resident who has a terminal illness that has a protracted course (e.g. advanced major neurocognitive disorder [MNCD], end-stage renal disease [ESRD], advanced multiple sclerosis) should be offered palliative care even earlier. LTC facilities must be able to provide high-quality palliative care for all residents as an integral part of their mission. Palliative care should be provided by a palliative care team (PCT) that consists of HCPs with training in palliative care. (See Table 11.2.) The primary care team (physicians, physician assistants, nurse practitioners, clinical nurse specialists, nurses, nursing aides, social workers) working with LTC populations should have expertise in providing high-quality palliative care and be key members of the PCT. Specialists (e.g. geriatricians, geriatric psychiatrists, palliative medicine physicians [physicians with fellowship training in palliative medicine]) can be consulted in complex situations and for assistance in the creation and implementation of state-of-the-science palliative care initiatives and high-quality staff training programs. Quality measurement and reporting should include assessment of staff education and training in palliative care, satisfaction of the dying resident and the family, and quality of control of pain and symptoms. We support several measures of palliative and end-of-life (EOL) care endorsed by the National Quality Forum and international palliative care organizations (National Quality Forum 2012; Bausewein et al. 2016). (See Box 11.1 and Table 11.3.) Usual palliative care outcome measures (e.g. Edmonton Symptom Assessment Scale) are not good at screening for MDD in residents receiving EOL care. We recommend that measures for screening and assessing depression (Patient Health Questionnaire–9 [PHQ-9] for a resident who has relatively preserved cognitive function and Cornell Scale for Depression in Dementia [CSDD] for

Table 11.2 The Palliative Care Team in Long-Term Care Facilities

Team Member	Description of Role	Therapeutic Pearls
Resident	Clearly voice wishes, values, concerns, fears, and expectations to PCT	All residents should have a high-quality advance directive (e.g. Five Wishes Document*) that clearly states preferences regarding EOL care
Family/Friend	Clearly voice concerns, fears, and expectations to PCT	Family members should be encouraged to try to balance their wish to be with resident and attend to their own stress and grief
Medical director of LTC facility	Ensure high-quality palliative care for all residents at all times through creation and implementation of facility-wide directives Be role model for other physicians in making inquiries about spirituality and religion a routine part of assessment Create mechanisms in place to address moral distress that staff often undergo while and after witnessing inappropriate use of life-prolonging treatment and promote psychological empowerment	As training for palliative care in medical school and residency is often inadequate, medical director can be role model in concept of "learning by doing"
Primary care physician	Lead discussions about palliative and EOL care with resident and family Create and ensure implementation of individualized palliative care plan in keeping with resident's wishes and values Ensure optimal control of symptoms (e.g. pain, dyspnea, nausea) Be easily available to answer questions and address concerns of resident and family and engage in collaborative problem-solving in situations with uncertain outcome Refer resident to specialist in complicated case	Have low threshold for seeking input of medical director and/or referral to specialist (e.g. geriatric psychiatrist, geriatrician)
Primary care nurse practitioner and physician assistant	Create and ensure implementation of individualized palliative care plan in keeping with resident's wishes and values Ensure optimal control of symptoms (e.g. pain, dyspnea, nausea) Be easily available to answer questions and address concerns of residents and family Refer resident to specialist in complicated case	Have low threshold for seeking input from physician or medical director and/or referral to specialist (e.g. psychiatrist, geriatrician) in difficult case
Psychiatrist (preferably geriatric psychiatrist) and psychiatric nurse practitioner and physician assistant	Help PCT in complicated case (e.g. if DMC is not clear, help differentiate normal sadness from MDD, clarify if depression is impairing DMC, management of severe MDD, resident requesting physician-assisted dying, provide second opinion) Psychiatrist or other mental health professional should be involved in EOL care for any resident who has chronic mental	Psychiatrist can play key role in ensuring that PCT gives psychological distress the same importance regarding symptom control as physical symptoms (e.g. pain, dyspnea)

Table 11.2 (cont.)

Team Member	Description of Role	Therapeutic Pearls
	illness (e.g. schizophrenia, bipolar disorder), LGBTQ resident, and resident who has intellectual disability	
Geriatrician	Help PCT in complicated case (e.g. if DMC is not clear, resident requesting physician-assisted dying)	Geriatrician can play a key role in ensuring that PCT members understand concept of frailty and disproportionately high negative effect it has on prognosis
Social worker	Address psychosocial concerns of resident and family, problem solve practical day-to-day challenges (e.g. concerns about their pets), and help resolve any unsettled issues with family With psychologist, lead efforts to prevent and treat depression, anxiety, agitation, and other mental health symptoms using mindfulness-based strategies and SPPEICE Provide (or refer for) individual and group meaning-centered psychotherapy for resident and grief counseling for family Address caregiver stress and grief using mindfulness-based strategies and support groups Provide relevant up-to-date educational materials and handouts to resident and family With primary care physician, lead PCT efforts to address concerns related to abuse of resident	LTC facility leadership should give social worker adequate time and support to address myriad psychosocial issues that are prevalent in LTC populations receiving EOL care
Nurse	Assess pain, other physical symptoms (e.g. dyspnea, nausea), psychological symptoms, and spiritual/existential distress Help resident and family problem solve practical day-to-day challenges Lead efforts to prevent and treat common physical symptoms (e.g. constipation, nausea) and psychological distress Provide emotional support to resident and family Provide relevant up-to-date educational materials and handouts to resident and family	By virtue of being able to spend more time with resident than other PCT members, nurses are in ideal position to be the voice of resident if PCT has overlooked or misunderstood resident's perspectives
Nursing assistant	Help nurse assess pain, other physical symptoms, and psychological symptoms Provide emotional support to resident and family	By virtue of being involved in providing daily intimate care to resident (e.g. bathing), nursing assistants may have strongest bond with resident among all PCT members and for some residents, the only important relationship they may have

Table 11.2 (cont.)

Team Member	Description of Role	Therapeutic Pearls
		Routinely obtaining input and guidance of nursing assistants who know resident well is essential in order to achieve goals of palliative care
Chaplain	Provide spiritual support to resident and family and help them accept the reality that some suffering is part of our human condition Work with resident's preferred member of faith community (e.g. priest, pastor, rabbi) Conduct spiritual assessment using standardized instrument (e.g. HOPE questionnaire) Address spiritual/religious/existential needs and concerns of resident and family, including helping them find meaning in life and in suffering	Every facility should have in-house chaplain, as chaplain's role is as important as physician's in achieving goals of palliative care
Psychologist (preferably gerontologist)	With social worker, lead efforts to prevent and treat depression, anxiety, agitation, and other mental health symptoms using mindfulness-based strategies and SPPEICE Provide individual and group meaning-centered psychotherapy for resident and grief counseling for family Address caregiver stress and grief using mindfulness-based strategies and support groups Provide relevant up-to-date educational materials and handouts to resident and family	Psychologist (especially gerontologist) is most underused professional in palliative care despite evidence of greatly increased success rate of achieving goals of palliative care when psychologist is involved
Trained volunteer	Provide emotional support to resident and family Help PCT ensure that resident is not alone in last hours to days of life	Volunteers are unsung heroes of PCT and should be recognized for their compassionate help
Allied health professional (speech therapist, music therapist, recreational therapist)	Address specific problems to maximize comfort (e.g. speech therapist helps with choice of favorite food for resident who has dysphagia; recreational therapist helps resident engage in meaningful activities)	PCT should have low threshold for involving allied health professionals
Hospice team	Assist LTC staff in providing EOL to resident receiving hospice care Provide bereavement support to family up to 13 months after death of resident	PCT is still primarily responsible for ensuring that all care given to resident is appropriate and of high quality, and needs to work closely with hospice team to prevent resident distress related to underlying conditions being overlooked due to lack of timely communication between PCT and hospice team and inadequate documentation

* Five Wishes Document: https://agingwithdignity.org/shop/product-details/five-wishes-online

BOX 11.1 Palliative and End-of-Life Care Measures Applicable to Long-Term Care Populations

1. Screening for pain
2. Assessment of pain
3. Bowel regimen for individual taking an opioid
4. Screening for dyspnea
5. Treatment of dyspnea
6. Honoring treatment preferences
7. Discussion of spiritual/religious concerns
8. Comfortable dying
9. Resident evaluation of care
10. Family evaluation of care
11. Survey of bereaved family

Note: Measures endorsed by National Quality Forum

a resident who has significant cognitive impairment) be added to the standard outcome measures mentioned in Table 11.3. We recommend the Palliative Performance Scale and the FRAIL-NH together to improve identification of LTC residents in need of palliative and EOL care.

In many circumstances, PCT members may need to combine elements of palliative care with life-sustaining measures to maximize a resident's quality and quantity of life. No specific therapy is excluded from consideration. This model abandons the "either/or" wall between curative and palliative care and starts addressing quality-of-life and family issues at the time of diagnosis of a terminal illness. In general, as curative treatment become less likely to be effective (and more burdensome), palliative and EOL care should take on greater importance.

The most common causes of death in LTC populations include terminal-stage MNCD (usually with superimposed complicated infection, such as urosepsis or aspiration pneumonia), congestive heart failure, chronic obstructive pulmonary disease (COPD), cancer, and stroke. Pneumonia, cachexia, dehydration, and hip fracture are the most common acute medical events that precipitate death in LTC populations with underlying terminal conditions. Delirium and MDD are the two most common psychiatric syndromes in residents receiving EOL care. LTC residents often develop multiple chronic medical problems and endure complicated medical courses with a variety of disease trajectories. Expertise in the diagnosis and management of a variety of geriatric syndromes (e.g. frailty, MNCD, MDD, delirium, agitation, pain, falls and fractures, urinary incontinence, weight loss, pressure ulcers, dyspnea) in the complexities of LTC settings is essential to providing high-quality palliative care to LTC populations.

EOL care is palliative care in the last days or months of life. Hospice care is EOL care, although many LTC residents receive EOL care without involvement of hospice. Palliative and EOL care in LTC settings is often inadequate because of chronic staff shortages, rapid staff turnover, poor staff training, inadequate reimbursement of palliative care, and limited physician participation. Last but not least, the prevailing societal attitudes and deeply ingrained prejudices against aging, frailty, and MNCD are extremely challenging barriers to providing high-quality palliative care for LTC populations. The EOL care needs of all residents should be reconceptualized to encourage more attention to quality of life and comfort and less active efforts to treat every medical exigency that arises. There is more to medicine than curing disease and/or postponing death. Life in the shadows of death can be immensely rewarding and fulfilling. Palliative and EOL care is one of the most important components of high-quality care for all LTC residents. Many HCPs find palliative care work the most meaningful aspect of their professional life.

A comprehensive geriatric assessment of the resident by a physician is an essential first step in formulating a high-quality palliative care plan. The Saint Louis University Rapid Geriatric Assessment is a simple tool that a nurse can reliably complete. Key factors to ensuring high-quality palliative and EOL care for LTC residents include facilitating choice (allowing the resident or proxy to retain as much control as possible within the limits of belonging to a community), respecting the choice (of the resident or proxy), providing evidence-based palliative care, securing the resident's network of significant relationships, and promoting sensitivity and respect for cultural diversity.

Hospice

The term *hospice* is derived from the Latin word *hospitium*, meaning "hospitality." Many centuries ago, care provided to weak and ill travelers was called hospice care. Dame Cicely Saunders (trained as a nurse, a social worker, and a physician) founded the St. Christopher's Hospice, in London, United Kingdom, in the 1960s. Hospice care is focused on easing the dying process by

Table 11.3 Key Outcome Measures for Palliative and End-of-Life Care with Long-Term Care Populations

Outcome Measure	Description of the Measure	Therapeutic Pearls
Palliative Performance Scale version 2 (PPSv2)	Assesses functioning of five domains (ambulation, disease severity, self-care ability, intake, and consciousness level) to give a score from 0% (lowest) to 100% (highest) at 10% increments Takes 5-10 minutes to complete	Excellent tool for communicating functional level of resident receiving palliative and EOL care to family and other PCT members; also has prognostic value (e.g. estimating life expectancy)
Palliative Care Outcome Scale (POS)	Assesses physical, psychological, and spiritual domains of distress Patient, staff, and family caregiver versions (each takes 6-7 minutes to complete)	Most widely used outcome measure
Edmonton Symptom Assessment Scale (ESAS)	10 symptoms/problems measured Takes 5 minutes to complete	Available in a wide range of languages
Memorial Symptom Assessment Scale (MSAS)–Short Form	Assesses 28 physical and 4 psychological symptoms Takes less than 5 minutes to complete	May be used in place of ESAS
Visual Analog Scale	Used to measure a subjective symptom that ranges across a continuum of values and cannot be objectively measured (e.g. pain, nausea, anxiety, desire to hasten death) Patient makes a mark on a line anchored on one side by a word descriptor (e.g. no pain) and on the other side by another word descriptor (e.g. worst pain imaginable) Takes only a few seconds for each symptom Can be used to measure multiple symptoms	Easy to use Needs less staff time Can be used reliably with resident who has mild to moderate MNCD
Numerical Rating Scale (Likert Scale)	Used to measure a subjective symptom that ranges across a continuum of values and cannot be objectively measured (e.g. pain, nausea, anxiety, desire to hasten death) Patient states or marks the number that most closely reflects the severity of the symptom (e.g. 0=no pain, 10=worst pain imaginable) Takes only a few seconds for each symptom Can be used to measure multiple symptoms	Easy to use Needs less staff time Can be used reliably with resident who has mild to moderate MNCD
Brief Pain Inventory	Assesses location of pain, severity, effect on mood and sleep, and response to treatment	Cannot be used with resident who has significant cognitive impairment

Table 11.3 (cont.)

Outcome Measure	Description of the Measure	Therapeutic Pearls
Pain Assessment in Advanced Dementia (PAINAD)	Five-item observational tool to assess pain, useful with resident who has advanced MNCD (severe and terminal MNCD)	Staff training required for its use
Bereavement Risk Assessment Tool	Assesses risk and protective factors for complicated bereavement for family after patient has passed away Takes 10-20 minutes	Useful tool even for family members experiencing grief while resident is alive (e.g. resident who has MNCD)
Zarit Burden Interview (ZBI)	Assesses caregiver burden in family of individual who has MNCD	Useful tool to assess family burden even for resident who does not have MNCD

Note: All measures listed are copyrighted but free for use.

helping an individual who is terminally ill and has limited life expectancy (few months) live rest of life in comfort and at the same time helping family members pass through this process with support. Hospice plays a key role in the management of terminal illness for LTC residents. Hospice services are increasingly used in LTC populations, primarily for noncancer terminal conditions (e.g. advanced MNCD, heart failure).

One of the key goals of palliative care in the United States is identifying those residents who would benefit from and qualify for hospice care. Hospice care is defined within the context of Medicare benefits as an alternative to other Part A benefits, whereas Medicare and Medicaid do not recognize palliative care as a separate specialized care. To make a referral to hospice, the resident's physician needs to state that the resident's life expectancy is six months or less due to a terminal (progressive and incurable) illness and the individual is willing to forgo life-prolonging and curative treatment. Although many terminal illnesses can benefit from hospice (including end-stage MNCD), except for cancer, it is often difficult to determine when to refer a patient to hospice. Hospice eligibility for a resident who has nonmalignant disease is based on clinical judgment. Hospice also offers a 13-month bereavement benefit following the death of the resident. Although the use of hospice in LTC populations is increasing rapidly, there is concern for both underuse of hospice services for many residents who may benefit from it and inappropriate overuse for many residents (especially residents who have MNCD). Residents and their families may benefit from services that hospice provides, such as better management of pain, dyspnea, and feeding tube, increased satisfaction of the family regarding quality of end-of-life care, and lower rates of hospitalization. After a resident enrolls in hospice, the care plan must document and designate which services the hospice will be responsible for and which services the LTC facility will provide.

Palliative and End-of-Life Care for a Resident who Has Major Neurocognitive Disorder

The prevalence of MNCD in LTC populations is high (50–90 percent). Alzheimer's disease (AD) is the sixth leading cause of death in the United States. Recognition that most MNCDs (e.g. AD, vascular MNCD, MNCD due to Lewy bodies, MNCD due to Parkinson's disease, frontotemporal MNCD) in LTC populations are inevitably progressive, shorten life, and eventually lead to death should provide impetus to delivering high-quality palliative care to all residents who have MNCD as soon as possible after admission. Palliative care goals are appropriate even at early stages of MNCD (van der Steen et al. 2014). A resident who has MNCD and the family need substantial guidance from the physician at every stage, as goals are expected to change as the MNCD progresses and cognitive impairment becomes more severe. For example, maintaining function is important in early stages of MNCD, but maximizing comfort is of primary importance in severe and terminal stages. PCT members may need to address a host of questions and concerns of family

BOX 11.2 The Five Components of Palliative Care

1. Dignity-conserving care
2. Spiritual care
3. Advance care planning: Includes customized care that reflects the individual's preferences and respects that person's wishes, thoughtful use of personal and family resources, and ongoing discussion of wishes regarding various medical emergencies
4. Relieving symptoms to ensure maximal comfort: Includes symptoms in the following domains
    a. Physical (e.g. pain, dyspnea, incontinence, fatigue, cough, dry mouth, seizures, constipation, nausea)
    b. Psychological (e.g. depression, anxiety, loneliness, illusions, psychotic symptoms [delusion, hallucination])
    c. Spiritual/existential (e.g. loss of meaning in life remaining, despair, demoralization)
    d. Behavioral (e.g. agitation, aggression)
5. Caring for the caregiver: Includes caring for family and professional caregivers, bereavement counseling, stress-reduction strategies, and empowerment of staff

members before a palliative care plan that is in keeping with the resident's values and wishes can be agreed on and implemented. (See Box 11.2.)

The disease trajectory of advanced cancer is usually well defined and involves rapid decline in the last few months of life. The disease trajectory of advanced MNCD involves a slower decline often punctuated with acute illnesses (e.g. severe weight loss, sepsis) and multiple hospitalizations over one to three years (Mitchell 2015). Severe disability may persist for years. Life expectancy after diagnosis is variable and ranges from less than 3 years (especially for an individual older than age 85) to 20 years (for an individual younger than 60). A resident who has MNCD and other advanced disease (e.g. congestive heart failure) may die of complications associated with that disease rather than advanced MNCD-related complications. Thus, prognostication is much more complex, challenging, and uncertain for MNCD than for metastatic cancer. This uncertainty is one of the key stressors for a resident who has MNCD and even more so for the family. In addition, as the MNCD progresses, residents frequently develop significant behavioral and psychological symptoms (especially depression and agitation), further adding to the suffering of the resident and the family. Clinical judgment combined with use of tools to predict mortality can help with prognostication. MNCD usually goes through stages (mild, moderate, severe, terminal), and complications (e.g. difficulty in swallowing leading to aspiration pneumonia, unsteady gait leading to fall and hip fracture) in the severe to terminal stages typically herald the dying process. It is not uncommon for family members to express relief on the loved one's death because of the long and difficult journey both the resident and the family have had in living with MNCD.

MNCD-specific palliative care strategies are different in many ways from palliative care strategies for other advanced disease. (See Table 11.4.) Discussions about palliative and EOL care need to be done early in the course of MNCD, when the resident has sufficient cognitive capacity to clearly understand the nature and complexity of the potential life-limiting events in the future, share his or her perspective of what living with dignity means, and express EOL care choices. Advance directives (especially durable power of attorney for health care and living will) are the most common means of making wishes for EOL care formally known to the PCT. Lack of such directives is prevalent in LTC populations, especially among residents who have MNCD, making palliative care discussions even more challenging. Many residents are in advanced stages of MNCD and have not had these discussions with their PCP when they were diagnosed several years ago. Family members are also often unsure of what the loved one would have wanted, or there may be disagreement among family members regarding what EOL treatment the loved one would have chosen. In other situations, physicians and family have made efforts but many residents in early stages of MNCD do not want to discuss EOL care, as it is emotionally overwhelming. Despite these barriers, the HCP should make every effort to understand as much as possible the values and wishes of the resident who has MNCD. Much of the EOL care of LTC populations has become EOL care for residents who have MNCD. Residents who have MNCD often die with inadequate pain control, with a feeding tube in place, and without the benefit of hospice care. Thus, high-quality palliative and EOL care is crucial for the well-being of the resident as well as family members.

Table 11.4 Differences in Palliative Care for Major Neurocognitive Disorder versus Other Advanced Illness

Major Neurocognitive Disorder	Other Advanced Illness (e.g. metastatic cancer)	Therapeutic Pearls
Palliative and EOL discussions to help individual and family prepare for future need to occur soon after diagnosis, as there is a risk that once cognitive decline progresses, individual may not have medical DMC	The urgency of palliative and EOL discussions to be taken up soon after diagnosis is less, as loss of DMC at later date is usually not a concern	Involving geriatric psychiatrist or geriatrician is recommended if PCT has limited experience of helping individual who has MNCD Other specialist (e.g. oncologist) should be involved in complicated situation (e.g. cancer in resident who has MNCD)
PCT needs to be prepared to effectively address inquiries by individual who has MNCD and family regarding euthanasia and assisted dying (physician-assisted suicide)	Inquiries by individual and family about euthanasia and assisted dying are rare	Involving geriatric psychiatrist or geriatrician is recommended if PCT has limited experience of addressing such concerns in individual who has MNCD
Predicting mortality is challenging, with lots of variability between individuals	Predicting mortality is relatively less challenging and less variable between individuals	Clinical judgment and mortality-prediction tools may help reduce uncertainty Geriatrician and geriatric psychiatrist should be consulted to help with predicting mortality and timely recognition of dying in complicated case
HCP should periodically review continued need for medication for chronic disease (e.g. diabetes) and comorbid condition in light of progressive decrease in life expectancy and progressively increased risk of adverse effect	In majority of situations, medication for chronic disease and comorbid condition can be continued until individual enrolls in hospice care	Consultant pharmacist can play key role in helping PCT implement rational deprescribing and deintensification of care Avoiding overly aggressive, burdensome, and futile care is single most important palliative care approach for individual who has MNCD
Life-prolonging effect of treatment of pneumonia should be considered in decision to treat or not to treat pneumonia for individual who has advanced MNCD even when not receiving hospice care	In general, this is a concern only when individual is receiving hospice care	Physician and other healthcare providers can assure family that high-quality palliative care will ensure that individual who has advanced MNCD and pneumonia is kept maximally comfortable if family decides to forgo antibiotic treatment for pneumonia (using standard of *substituted judgment* or *best interest*)
Permanent enteral tube nutrition is to be avoided for individual who has advanced MNCD; skillful hand-feeding is recommended	Permanent enteral tube nutrition may be appropriate in certain situations (e.g. individual who has severe dysphagia is receiving potentially life-prolonging chemotherapy and/or radiation therapy for cancer)	Educating family and staff is key, as many family members and staff may incorrectly perceive that resident is suffering as result of unaddressed hunger

Table 11.4 (cont.)

Major Neurocognitive Disorder	Other Advanced Illness (e.g. metastatic cancer)	Therapeutic Pearls
PAIN-AD and other pain assessment tools are needed to assess pain in individual who has advanced MNCD	Usual pain assessment tools (e.g. numerical rating scale) are often sufficient, as individual is able to communicate pain	Nurse can lead efforts to accurately assess pain in resident who has advanced MNCD using PAIN-AD and other pain-assessment tools
Management of symptoms frequently involves management of agitation and aggressive behavior	Management of symptoms typically involves physical symptoms (e.g. pain, nausea, vomiting) rather than agitation and aggressive behavior	Psychologist and social worker together can lead efforts by PCT to prevent and manage agitation and aggressive behavior with SPPEICE Involving psychiatrist is strongly recommended to avoid unnecessary or excessive use of psychotropic medication to manage agitation and aggressive behavior and improve use of SPPEICE
Skills for shared decision-making (family and individual who has MNCD as partners) so that cognitively impaired individual is included to extent abilities allow	Skills for communication are less complex, as usually individual has relatively preserved cognitive function	Nurse, social worker, and psychologist can play key role in helping individual who has MNCD communicate perspectives and wishes to family and rest of PCT
Skills to support family of individual who has MNCD in decisions and empathizing with struggles in face of many uncertainties	Skills to support family involve helping them with grief and anxiety	Physician and other healthcare providers need to share their confidence regarding certain options that have excellent research support (e.g. avoiding ANH using PEG tube for individual who has terminal MNCD) and acknowledge uncertainty regarding other options (e.g. when is it best to forgo surgery for hip fracture for resident who has MNCD)
Advance care plans should be revisited periodically, especially after significant change in health condition	Advance care plans usually need relatively fewer periodic updates	Every hospitalization should be seen as an opportunity for discussions about EOL care goals and updating advance care plans based on these discussions if necessary Communication of any updated plan is key during transfer of care (e.g. from hospital to LTC facility)
Supporting children and adolescents of individual who has young-onset MNCD (onset before age 60) and grandchildren of individual who has late-onset MNCD (onset after age 60) cope with individual's not recognizing them and forgetting their names	Supporting children and adolescents cope with grief	Chaplain can play key role in helping children and adolescents cope with unique losses and spiritual/existential issues of witnessing their loved one slowly but relentlessly decline cognitively
Place of care may need to include not only wishes of individual who has	Place of care issues are usually not major concern	Planned move to LTC facility is preferred, as it is less stressful on

Table 11.4 (cont.)

Major Neurocognitive Disorder	Other Advanced Illness (e.g. metastatic cancer)	Therapeutic Pearls
MNCD but also safety concerns and burdens on family		individual who has MNCD than unplanned admission
Supporting health (physical and emotional) of family caregiver is often of as much importance for long-term well-being of individual who has MNCD as addressing health needs of individual who has MNCD	Well-being of individual who has advanced disease is relatively less dependent on health and well-being of family	Support groups, individual psychotherapy, mindfulness and meditation groups, spiritual counseling, and other wellness programs for family caregivers may prevent caregiver burnout and catastrophic effects (e.g. abrupt admission to LTC facility) of caregiver burnout on quality of life of individual who has MNCD
PCT should tell family caregivers that it is okay to experience and express relief after individual who has MNCD passes away	In general, PCT will need to help family members cope with grief after individual passes away	Social worker and psychologist need to begin addressing caregiver grief months to years before the individual who has MNCD passes away
A calm and soothing environment with plenty of natural light is important to maximize comfort for individual who has advanced MNCD	Environment is relatively less important in maximizing comfort	Safe indoor and outdoor wandering paths in LTC facility can improve comfort of resident who has advanced MNCD and reduce need for psychotropic medication

Ethical Issues around Physician Involvement in Euthanasia, Physician-Assisted Hastening of Death, and Palliative Sedation

I will not relinquish old age, if it leaves my better part intact. But, if it begins to shake my mind, if it destroys its faculties one by one, if it leaves me not life but breath, I will depart from the putrid or tottering edifice. If I must suffer without hope or relief, I will depart, not through fear of the pain itself, but because it prevents all for which I would live.
Seneca, 1st century CE

It is not uncommon for residents and even some family members to request euthanasia or physician-assisted suicide (Hendry et al. 2013). (See Table 11.1.) The HCP should address such a request without judgment and with compassion and respect. Questions to residents such as, "Do you often go to sleep hoping that you won't wake up?" and "Do you feel that doctors should do something to end your life?" may help assess these concerns. The PCT should explore underlying drivers of such requests promptly and with careful attention and sensitivity. Determinants of these requests are complex, with issues around loss of dignity and being a burden usually being primary drivers. The HCP needs to explore the voluntariness of such requests. Such requests do not reflect the individual's wish to commit suicide as much as the wish to avoid intolerable pain (emotional, spiritual, and physical) in the context of living with one or more terminal illnesses by controlling when and how to die. We prefer the term physician-assisted hastening of death to physician-assisted dying or physician-assisted suicide, as it more accurately reflects the physician's efforts (Quill, Back, and Block 2016). Euthanasia and physician-assisted hastening of death can raise serious ethical conflicts among not only professional caregivers but also residents and their family. We have serious concerns about the possibility of palliative care being devalued following legalization of euthanasia (in Belgium, Canada, Colombia, Luxembourg, and Netherlands) and physician-assisted hastening of death (in Switzerland, Germany, Japan, Albania, and the US states of Montana, Washington, Oregon, Vermont, and California). Physician involvement in euthanasia and physician-assisted hastening of death may cause patients to distrust physicians who are administering medication for palliation (e.g. a patient who becomes sedated with morphine may fear that the physician's intention is not to relieve pain but to hasten death) (Yang and Curlin 2016). Physicians who work more closely with terminally ill patients are more likely to oppose physician-assisted hastening of death (Rostin and Roberts 2016). The American Medical Association also opposes physician involvement in euthanasia and physician-assisted hastening of death. Furthermore, the European Association for Palliative Care position paper explicitly states that euthanasia and physician-assisted hastening of death should not be included in the practice of palliative care (Radbruch et al. 2016). We strongly advocate palliative care (including palliative sedation) and hospice care in place of euthanasia and physician-assisted hastening of death. Palliative sedation is an accepted ethical practice when used in appropriate situations and after the resident and/or the family is properly informed and the implications and consequences are understood. The HCP should educate any resident requesting euthanasia or physician-assisted hastening of death about what palliative care can offer (including palliative sedation), and the resident should have easy access to high-quality palliative care services.

The opposite is also true. Sometimes a resident and/or family will distrust a PCT member's recommendation that the resident forgo life-prolonging treatment as a veiled effort to hasten death, to which the resident and/or family are morally opposed. PCT members need to reassure the resident and family that the intention is to spare the resident the burden of futile treatment. Many family members perceive recommendations to forgo life-prolonging treatment as meaning that the PCT or the family has "given up." The resident and family should be helped to differentiate between "giving up" and "letting go," that by withholding certain treatments, the team is allowing the natural process of dying to help the resident achieve a timely, dignified, and peaceful death. The HCP can help alleviate the suffering of a resident and/or family by clarifying the difference between actively shortening a resident's life and simply not using medical treatment that is futile or burdensome and not in keeping with the resident's preferences and values. For many other residents and their family, simply informing them that it is time for the resident to forgo life-prolonging treatment (including ANH) and allow a natural death is sufficient for them to feel comfortable about these decisions and can relieve their stress and anxiety.

Key Components of a High-Quality Palliative Care Program in Long-Term Care

The level and types of palliative care services provided vary among LTC facilities. Some facilities have a separate palliative care wing or unit or beds, some focus on pain management as part of palliative care, some are able to administer intravenous medication, and some have access to physicians, nurse practitioners, physician assistants and clinical nurse specialists who can assess an acute medical problem on site within four hours (thus avoiding hospitalization or a trip to the emergency department). Training staff members in bereavement services is another approach to palliative care.

Palliative care has five components, and all five should be integrated into the routine care provided to every resident. (See Box 11.3.) All staff members should be involved in palliative care, rather than just a few staff members on a separate unit. Even housekeepers can be trained to have an eye for pain and other symptoms in residents, informal grief remarks

BOX 11.3 Key Questions and Concerns of Residents Who Have Major Neurocognitive Disorder and Their Family That the Palliative Care Team Needs to Address

- What stage of MNCD am I in? What stage of MNCD is my loved one in?
- How fast does MNCD progress from one stage to another?
- Why is MNCD considered a terminal illness?
- How long will I live with MNCD?
- How does one die because of MNCD?
- Will my wishes for end-of-life care be honored when I can no longer express them?
- Can you ensure a peaceful and dignified dying process?
- What are the benefits and risks of a feeding tube?
- What is physician-assisted dying? Can you provide it?
- What is euthanasia? Can you provide it?

by family, etc. Ideally, palliative care should start before admission or at least at the time of admission. It starts with a review of the resident's and family's expectations of care and education about the philosophy and goals of palliative care. Successful communication among team members is key for effective palliative care, and knowing the residents well and developing close relationships with them is key to successful communication. Talking about death and dying does not need to be morose and devoid of creativity. We support creative efforts, such as the Happy Coffin initiative by the Lien Foundation's Life before Death Campaign (www.lienfoundation.org/sites/default/files/happy_coffins.pdf), that can help alter perceptions of symbols such as coffins and funerals as opportunities to bring out the artist within.

The next level of palliative care is implementing a formal six-step program.

Step 1. Assess each resident for the five components of palliative care and identify one or more areas of focus (e.g. pain, depression or agitation, caregiver grief).

Step 2. Identify measures to track outcomes using standardized tools (e.g. PAIN-AD pain scale for a resident who has advanced MNCD, PHQ-9 depression scale, Cohen-Mansfield Agitation Inventory) and take pretreatment measurements.

Step 3. Optimize routine psychosocial spiritual and environmental approaches (see Box 11.4) to promote well-being and institute specific evidence-based treatments for target symptoms identified.

Step 4. Measure post-treatment outcome (e.g. improvement in pain, reduction in depression or agitation, reduction in caregiver grief).

Step 5. Share results with staff and family and obtain their input.

Step 6. Modify treatment based on post-treatment outcomes and feedback from Step 5.

Specific facility-wide goals can also be set and outcomes tracked. For example, one goal may be 80 percent reduction in symptoms of moderate to severe pain within 72 hours of the initial assessment. In-house training in palliative care for as many staff members as possible (from housekeeping staff to physicians) by in-house palliative care leaders (e.g. medical director, consulting psychiatrist, director of nursing, social worker) who have themselves received advanced training in palliative care is ideal. See Box 11.5 for key topics of training in palliative care.

Dignity-Conserving Care

Upholding, protecting, and restoring the dignity of all patients is the duty of every HCP and the essence of medicine. Every resident is worthy of honor, and there is meaning in the life of every resident, irrespective of cognitive, physical, and/or emotional condition. Kindness, humanity, and respect – the core values of the medical profession, often overlooked in our time-pressed culture – can be reinstated by dignity-conserving care (Chochinov 2007). How residents perceive themselves to be seen is a powerful mediator of their dignity, as dignity is closely associated with a sense of being treated with respect. Factors that have been identified as fracturing the sense of dignity include but are not limited to: loss of independence, fear of becoming a burden, not being involved in decision-making, lack of access to high-quality care (especially palliative care), and some attitudes (e.g. dismissiveness) of HCPs, especially when a patient feels vulnerable and lacks power. The HCP can uphold a resident's dignity by seeing him for the person he was before MNCD or stroke altered him, rather than seeing just the illness he has. We recommend the "A, B, C, D" approach to dignity-conserving care described by Dr. Chochinov (Chochinov 2007). (See Box 11.6.) Ensuring dignity thus involves spending more time with the resident and family. This quality of professionalism and connectedness also increases the likelihood that the resident and family will be forthright in disclosing personal information, which so often has a bearing on ongoing care. Every LTC facility should have a written policy of "zero tolerance" for lack of dignity in the care of every resident.

Spiritual Care

Addressing spiritual needs is vital to achieving the goals of palliative care. For some residents, coming to peace with God, not being a burden to others, having funeral arrangements in place, and being mentally aware are some of the most important factors determining emotional well-being during EOL care. A chaplain or other appropriate spiritual care provider can greatly assist in adequately addressing a resident's spiritual needs. Even a resident who has severe cognitive impairment can respond to religious rituals, familiar prayers, religious songs, and symbols. Deep into

BOX 11.4 Key Examples of Strengths-Based Personalized Psychosocial Sensory Spiritual Environmental Initiatives and Creative Engagement (SPPEICE) during End-of-Life Care

Psychological
- Life review
- Reminiscing over happy, humorous, and meaningful events of one's life
- Frequent reassurances

Social–Interpersonal
- Spending time with family and friends
- Engagement in meaningful conversation and activity
- Playing games (e.g. board games, card games, Wii) with the resident
- Spending time with pets

Environmental
- Calm and serene environment
- Optimal lighting (not too bright, not too dark)
- Encourage ambulation and wandering in safe areas
- Addressing safety (e.g. falls precautions)

Sensory: Music
- Interventions by a music-thanatologist*
- Soothing background music
- Personalized music several times a day or as often as the resident wishes
- Sing-alongs

Sensory: Touch and Aromatherapy
- Hand and neck massage using soothing lotion several times a day
- Back rub using soothing lotion several times a day

Sensory: Taste
- Offering favorite delicious foods and fluids several times a day

Sensory: Visual
- Spending time in favorite places (e.g. favorite lake, favorite park)

Spiritual
- Singing religious songs
- Reciting familiar prayers
- Meditation
- Contemplative practices
- Spiritual discussions with a chaplain and/or members of one's faith community

Creative Engagement
- Reading, listening to, writing poems
- Visiting art museums

* Music-thanatologist uses harp and voice to ease emotional distress and promote psychological and spiritual well-being of individual receiving EOL care. Music-Thanatology Association International (www.mtai.org/index.php/what_is)

BOX 11.5 Topics for Training in Palliative Care

- Basic principles of palliative care
- Perceptions of death and dying
- Concept of dignity-conserving care
- Standardized tools to assess pain
- Appropriate approaches (pharmacological and nonpharmacological) to prevent and manage pain
- Care for bereavement
- Psychosocial spiritual environmental approaches (SPPEICE) to prevent and manage challenging behavior (e.g. agitation, aggression)
- Differentiating sadness and grief from MDD
- Standardized tools to assess depression and agitation
- Appropriate psychotropic medication to prevent and manage MDD, anxiety symptoms, psychotic symptoms, and delirium
- Strategies to reduce stress (e.g. mindfulness-based stress reduction,* relaxation response**)
- Advance care planning
- Palliative sedation (and how it differs from physician-assisted dying and euthanasia)
- Spiritual care

* MBSR: Center for Mindfulness in Medicine, Healthcare and Society (www.umassmed.edu/cfm/stress-reduction)
** *Relaxation Response,* by Herbert Benson, M.D., Harvard Medical School (www.relaxationresponse.org)

the progression of MNCD, continuities with the past usually exist amid discontinuities. The need for spiritual care varies greatly not only from resident to resident but also by race, gender, economic status, and ethnic heritage. Meaning-centered group therapy (offered to the resident who has relatively intact cognitive function) is a novel approach that may successfully integrate themes of meaning and spirituality into EOL care. Professional caregivers need to realize that besides keeping the resident clean and comfortable, they should feel comfortable helping a resident transport herself beyond the physical diminishment. This can be done in several ways, such as by reading the resident her favorite poem, singing a favorite song, or just spending time with her. The term *holistic suffering* was recently introduced in palliative care literature to reflect severe distress related to existential crises that some individuals experience during the dying process (Best et al. 2015). PCT members need to recognize that a resident who has relatively preserved cognitive function may experience holistic suffering when given a new diagnosis of a terminal illness (e.g. metastatic cancer), that it is a debilitating condition and requires team approach with chaplain, social worker, and psychologist working together to provide relief through spiritual and psychosocial approaches.

BOX 11.6 The A, B, C, and D of Dignity-Conserving Care

A = Attitude: The HCP has utmost respect for all residents at all times (during life and after death).

B = Behavior: The HCP shows respect and kindness to all residents through verbal and nonverbal behaviors at every interaction.

C = Compassion: The HCP has compassion (a deep awareness of the suffering of another person coupled with the wish to relieve it) for all residents at all times.

D = Dialogue: The HCP has an ongoing dialogue with self (e.g. "Am I making ageist assumptions?"), with other HCPs (e.g. "Are we withholding life-sustaining treatment because of our assumption that the resident has poor quality of life?"), with the resident ("What do you value? What gives your life meaning? What is your attitude toward suffering? What is your identity?"), and with the resident's family ("What are the most important things in your loved one's life? Is there a hierarchy?") to know and value every resident.

Clinical Case: "I saw the heavenly gates"

Mr. U, a 78-year-old male in severe stages of MNCD, had developed acute bleeding from the rectum, and his wife was not sure if she should admit him to the hospital or opt for hospice care. The psychiatrist involved in Mr. U's treatment helped Mrs. U understand the futility of hospitalization and that Mr. U would have wanted only comfort care at this point. Mrs. U agreed that her husband would have wanted comfort care only but she wanted to be sure that she was not "giving up" on him. The couple's daughter and son felt sure that their father would want comfort care only. After their children's input, Mrs. U decided to forgo hospitalization and opted for hospice care. Her dilemma was understandable because just three months ago, Mr. U was walking, seemed to enjoy his wife's company, and could feed himself with assistance although he could not recognize family members (including his wife) by name. He had developed pneumonia and Mrs. U had opted for hospitalization and treatment at that time. Although pneumonia was treated successfully, Mr. U developed severe agitation and delirium in the hospital and needed antipsychotic to control agitation. When he returned to the nursing home, he used a wheelchair, had lost the ability to feed himself, had severe speech problems (was extremely difficult to decipher), and was able to articulate only some words but not full sentences. After Mr. U was enrolled in hospice, the family and staff were surprised to learn that two staff members on different occasions had heard Mr. U clearly state, "I saw the heavenly gates" and "I was told to come back later." Mrs. U asked their pastor to come for spiritual support and to help her understand Mr. U's statements. The pastor suggested that maybe Mr. U was waiting for his wife to say goodbye and to say that it was okay for him to go. Mrs. U followed the pastor's advice, and three days later Mr. U died peacefully with his wife holding his hand and their children present at the bedside.

Teaching Points

Even in the terminal stages of MNCD, an individual may be able to say complete sentences on rare occasions. Spiritual needs are more important than ever in the care of a resident in severe and terminal stages of MNCD. Help of chaplains, members of the clergy, and fellow members of the resident's faith community is crucial for the well-being of many residents and their family. Also, family may need guidance to say "goodbye" and understand that allowing nature to take its course (and thus allowing a natural dying process) is not "giving up" but "letting go."

Advance Care Planning

Atul Gawande, M.D., Ph.D., a Harvard surgeon and professor of health policy, in recounting the experiences of his father's end-of-life care, shared that "he was a person and not a patient in the last four months of his life" and gives credit to his father's having written "the best living will ever" with clear instructions for the family regarding his preferences for EOL care (Gawande 2014). Unfortunately, this is not the experience of the majority of residents and their families during the last months of their lives.

Advance care planning documents (advance directives) ensure that a resident's wishes will be carried out when he is no longer capable of making decisions about care (Abele and Morley 2016). Advance directives should be conceptualized as an extension of the fully autonomous patient. All HCPs have the responsibility of upholding advance directives in the care of the resident. We recommend the "Five Wishes Document" (available at www.agingwithdignity.org) for advance care planning. The Five Wishes Document addresses not only who would make decisions for the person when she cannot and what kind of medical treatment she would want at the end of life, but also how comfortable she would want to be (e.g. pain control even at the cost of impaired cognition or consciousness), how she would want others to treat her (e.g. to talk to her periodically even if she is in coma), and what she would want her loved ones to know (e.g. wish for two family members who have grown apart to make amends).

Medical decision-making about a resident who has complex health problems requires careful application of the best medical evidence combined with clinical judgment that is balanced by resident-specific information based on that individual's life circumstance and personal values. PCT members in any area of health care (nursing, social work, medicine, psychology) can take a leadership role in counseling residents and their family to discuss EOL wishes and what "quality of life" means. PCT members should encourage residents and their family to discuss the pros and cons of the following treatments on an ongoing basis and in the context of the resident's gradually increasing disabilities: do not resuscitate (DNR), do not intubate (DNI), do not hospitalize (DNH), do not insert feeding tube, do not do laboratory tests, do not give antibiotic or IV fluid unless the reason is to improve comfort. PCT members should discuss the risks and benefits of DNR with every resident or, more commonly, surrogate decision-maker. In general, because of severe and multiple comorbidity (especially MNCD), the risks of DNR (e.g. severe cognitive impairment, accelerated cognitive decline, rib fracture, need for mechanical ventilation) outweigh the benefit (prolonged survival). In addition, the success rate (defined as discharge from the hospital) of CPR for LTC residents is very low (0.1–5 percent). Hospitalization for hip fracture may be appropriate for a resident who has mild to moderate-stage MNCD and is otherwise healthy and may be inappropriate for a resident who has severe MNCD and has lost the ability to comprehend spoken language and thus is unable to participate in intensive rehabilitation after surgery. The HCP should counsel family members that if surgery is foregone, the resident's pain can be adequately managed with medication and the risks of hospitalization outweigh its benefit.

Communication about death and dying is vital, but the difficulty and stress involved in bringing up the subject is so great that the discussion may be "postponed" for a "better opportunity," which seldom arrives. The HCP should remember that, besides honoring the resident's wishes, an important goal of holding such a discussion is to ease the stress of both the resident and the family and help them cope with the terrifying notions involved with the thought of impending death.

Anticipating the potential loss of decision-making capacity (DMC), PCT members should engage the resident early in advance care planning, such as exploring the resident's values and goals and discussing advance care planning documents (e.g. living will and durable power of attorney for health care). The HCP should assure residents that such planning is a routine part of the admission process. With more intense communication occurring up front, the resident's and family's emotional and spiritual needs become an integral part of care.

PCT members can trigger a dialogue about EOL care by asking questions such as, "Would we be surprised if this resident died in the next few months?" "Is this resident sick enough to die soon?" and using each episode of an acute illness, visit to an emergency department (ED), or hospitalization as a "rehearsal" regarding EOL care discussions. Asking the resident and/or family if goals of care would change if "this happens next time" is also helpful to clarify the type of EOL treatments.

Racial, ethnic, and sex groups differ significantly in EOL health care wishes. In some cultural groups (e.g. Asians, Arabs), families may be reluctant to tell the resident "bad news" and may avoid using words such as *death* and *cancer*. The HCP needs to be truthful with the resident but also sensitive to the wishes of the family and communicate with the resident and family in the least threatening manner possible. Also, PCT members should not generalize about all individuals as being in one group. It is important to be respectful of the resident's preferences while considering the influences of race, ethnicity, and gender.

PCT members need to understand the resident's religious or spiritual beliefs and financial circumstances and the potential impact of any medical treatment on these. Some residents and their families wish to participate actively in discussion of treatment choices, whereas other residents and their families may defer most of the decisions to the physician after only a brief discussion. Also, PCT members need to communicate that for many end-of-life situations and treatments, benefits and burdens may be uncertain. They need to help residents and families emotionally negotiate this uncertainty.

Many family members may not follow the advance directives of the resident who has MNCD if they feel that the resident, though cognitively severely incapacitated, appears "happy." The HCP should advise a resident who has MNCD and DMC to incorporate explicit metadirective (directive of the advance directive) to prevent such possible future conflict.

Estimating Life Expectancy (Prognosis)

For a LTC resident who does not have cancer, the terminal phase is difficult to predict and, once diagnosed, the survival time is short (one to two weeks). Estimating the life expectancy of residents in the last stages of life typically involves estimating the life expectancy of residents who have severe or terminal-stage MNCD. The failure to recognize MNCD as an incurable and progressive disease may result in inadequate EOL care, including late referral to hospice. Hypoactive delirium is a marker of poor prognosis in advanced MNCD. The Functional Assessment Staging for Alzheimer's Disease (FAST) scale (also called Global Deterioration Scale [GDS]) can help the HCP decide which resident who has AD to refer for hospice services (Reisberg 1988). In general, a resident in terminal stages of MNCD (especially stage 7 c or higher using the FAST scale) or in severe stages with acute medical issues (e.g. pneumonia, hip fracture, acute heart failure) would qualify for hospice services, and the HCP should refer the resident for hospice care if such a referral is in keeping with the resident's values and wishes. Stage 6 of the FAST scale corresponds to severe MNCD, and stage 7 corresponds to terminal-stage MNCD. Estimating the life expectancy of a resident who has terminal illness other than MNCD (e.g. congestive heart failure, ESRD) is also challenging. Residents who have ESRD tend to have short life expectancies (one to two years), multiple comorbidities, and a high burden of symptoms (e.g. presence of itching, dry skin, fatigue, bone and muscle pain, muscle cramps, anxiety, psychotic symptoms, depression). A resident who has ESRD may choose to stop dialysis (or the family may decide to stop dialysis) when he feels that the burden of dialysis is high and the benefit in terms of relief of day-to-day symptoms is low. Predictors of poor prognosis for a resident who has a terminal condition (e.g. advanced MNCD, terminal heart failure, terminal COPD, ESRD) include advanced age, frailty, reduced functional ability (e.g. dependence on staff for basic activities of daily living, such as bathing, dressing, toileting), poor nutritional status (e.g. low serum albumin level), and the presence of multiple comorbid illnesses.

Psychiatric Aspects of Hospitalization

Hospitalization and visits to the emergency department (ED) are extremely stressful for most LTC residents, especially frail, cognitively impaired residents. The majority of residents develop delirium and pressure ulcers in the hospital and after return from the hospital often develop frailty, accelerated cognitive decline, and MDD. This is especially true for residents who have a life expectancy of only six months to a year. Poorly executed discharge from the hospital (e.g. poor coordination and communication between the hospital, the patient, the family, and the LTC staff) may result in repeat hospitalizations of residents transferred from hospital to LTC facilities for postacute care (typically for rehabilitation). Hospitalization stemming from a medical condition thought to be largely avoidable or manageable with timely access to a physician and other medical support services has been termed ambulatory care-sensitive hospitalization (ACSH). Issues pertaining to hospitalization in relation to palliative care include reducing ACSH, preventing futile hospitalization, and recognizing the potential benefits of hospitalization for certain medical conditions and palliative care needs. Hospitalization for hip fracture surgery for a resident who has relatively preserved cognitive function may significantly improve the resident's quality of life. Hospitalization to an acute inpatient psychiatric unit (preferably a geriatric psychiatry unit) for the treatment of severe MDD during EOL is also appropriate. Admission to a palliative care unit within a hospital for high-level and complex palliative care treatment (e.g. palliative sedation for severe and refractory pain, delirium with severe aggression and agitation), when available, may be necessary to relieve suffering for some residents during the last days of life.

There is some evidence to suggest that low registered nurse (RN) staffing levels and poor quality-of-care practices significantly increase a LTC resident's risk of experiencing ACSH. A resident who has MNCD is at higher risk of ACSH than a resident who does not have MNCD. Increased RN staffing levels and on-site physicians and/or other HCPs (e.g. nurse practitioner, physician assistant, clinical nurse specialist) may reduce the risk of ACSH. The availability of highly trained nursing staff may improve timely identification of subtle changes in a resident's symptoms (especially a resident who has advanced MNCD and may not be able to communicate physical symptoms), allowing for prompt medical attention. Other strategies to reduce hospitalization include improving the hospital-to-facility transition and aligning reimbursement policies such that providers do not have a financial incentive to hospitalize. More than 50 percent of patients who have advanced MNCD admitted to the hospital with a diagnosis of hip fracture or pneumonia died within 6 months of discharge, compared to 12 percent of patients who did not have MNCD, suggesting that hip fracture and pneumonia are end-stage markers. Some 30 percent of hospital deaths of frail residents occur within five days of admission from a nursing home. Discussions of palliative care based on the resident's wishes for expected medical emergency (e.g. chest pain in a resident who has unstable coronary artery disease or acute neurological deficit in a resident who has a history of multiple strokes) may avoid unnecessary or accidental transfer to the ED for evaluation of possible myocardial infarction or stroke because hospitalization for these problems has been deemed to be not in the best interest of the resident. Avoiding futile hospitalization and providing palliative care and, if indicated, referral to hospice may substantially reduce suffering for many residents. The HCP should discuss "do not hospitalize" orders as part of the treatment plan for any resident in severe or terminal stages of MNCD or other disease.

Reviewing the Appropriateness of Medication

Polypharmacy, defined as concomitant use of more than five different medications, is common in LTC residents receiving palliative and EOL care, frequently resulting in adverse effect (e.g. agitation, depression, delirium) and unwanted drug–drug interaction. To prevent inappropriate use of medication, the HCP should question the usefulness and necessity of each drug taken by the resident receiving palliative and EOL care and discontinue any medication that may not benefit the resident in the short term. Determining the appropriate time to discontinue antidementia medication (e.g. cholinesterase inhibitor [donepezil, galantamine, rivastigmine] and memantine) is a complicated decision. Stopping medication may result in a spectrum of family responses, from significant psychological distress to great relief. In general, antidementia medication should be discontinued when the resident reaches the terminal stage of MNCD. In moderate to severe stages of MNCD, some residents may benefit from discontinuation without any adverse outcome, whereas some may show increased cognitive impairment or behavioral symptoms and may need to have the antidementia medication reinstated. The HCP should discuss the necessity of other medication (e.g. statin, vitamins, medication for osteoporosis, insulin, digoxin, antihypertensive medication) and discontinue any medication that is deemed unnecessary (i.e. does not promote quality of life). An additional benefit of discontinuing a drug used for diabetes for a resident receiving EOL care is that the resident may no longer require daily monitoring of blood glucose by finger sticks (which for many residents with diabetes is monitored two to four times daily). Certain drugs (e.g. anticoagulant [warfarin]) carry a high risk of adverse effect and/or frequent need for blood tests. Their prescription may pose a high burden for a resident in the last phase of life and have few benefits. Hence, the HCP should also consider discontinuing these drugs. Discontinuing certain medication (e.g. antihypertensive) may need to be done slowly to avoid withdrawal symptoms (e.g. rebound hypertension and tachycardia after abrupt discontinuation of antihypertensive). Some medication (e.g. diuretic) may be appropriate to control symptoms (e.g. improve dyspnea due to pulmonary edema) but may be inappropriate for the management of a comorbid condition (e.g. hypertension).

LTC residents who have advanced MNCD frequently have extensive exposure to antimicrobial drugs, often administered parenterally, and the use steadily increases toward the end of life, reaching 42 percent in the last two weeks of life (Rosenberg et al. 2013). Use of antibiotic imposes considerable burden on a resident (e.g. adverse effect, prolongation of life that is not in keeping with the resident's wishes), especially a resident in the last stages of life. The HCP should consider every decision to prescribe antibiotic for a resident who is in the last stages of life only after discussion about whether the antibiotic would serve the resident's interests (e.g. increased comfort by treating urinary tract infection) despite the burden imposed by its use. Treatment of pneumonia with antibiotic for a resident who has terminal-stage MNCD is often not recommended because it may not prolong life and may adversely affect the quality of life. The HCP should inform the resident and family that infections are expected near the EOL, are commonly a terminal event, and may be considered a friend rather than a foe.

Anticipatory prescribing ("just in case" medication) is appropriate for a resident who, based on underlying medical and psychiatric conditions, will probably need symptom control in the last days to weeks of life.

Relieving Symptoms

Burdensome symptoms and inappropriate care practices in efforts to relieve symptoms are prevalent in LTC populations receiving EOL care. Prevention and effective relief of distressing symptoms are core goals of palliative care. Residents in the last days to months of life may experience many distressing symptoms, such as pain, dyspnea, nausea or vomiting, anorexia, seizures, delirium, agitation, aggressive behavior, psychotic symptoms, depression, anxiety, and suicidal ideas. (See Table 11.5.) The burden of symptoms for a resident during terminal stages of MNCD is similar to that of other terminal conditions (e.g. advanced heart failure, cancer), although relief is suboptimal (Perrar et al. 2015). A resident who has chronic mental illness (e.g. schizophrenia, bipolar disorder) or intellectual disability is also at risk of receiving suboptimal palliative and EOL care (especially inadequate relief of symptoms). Intensive management of symptoms is imperative, and the HCP should consider rapidly worsening symptoms a palliative care emergency requiring immediate treatment. The terminal disease phase for most LTC residents is marked with distressing symptoms, low fluid and food intake, general weakness, and dyspnea. Direct causes of these conditions are diseases of the respiratory system (mainly pneumonia) and general disorders

Table 11.5 Key Distressing Symptoms and Syndromes among Residents Receiving End-of-Life Care

Symptom	Diagnostic/Assessment Pearls	Therapeutic Pearls
Pain	Nociceptive pain as well as neuropathic pain can be present In cognitively impaired resident (e.g. resident who has MNCD, delirium, aphasia), agitation (including moaning, groaning) and aggression may be key manifestation of pain	There is considerable variation in individuals' responses to analgesics Rational polypharmacy is appropriate for management of severe and complex pain syndromes
Dyspnea	Death rattle can be extremely distressing symptom for family and staff to witness	Morphine with or without short-acting BZD with or without oxygen is recommended Nondrug approaches (e.g. facial fan, open window) should also be tried
Nausea, vomiting	Common cause of decreased intake of food and fluid	Low dose of antipsychotic can reduce nausea and is preferred over other antinausea agents (e.g. metoclopramide) for resident who has nausea and agitation
Anorexia	Loss of appetite often accompanies severe weight loss	HCP may consider prescribing dronabinol for this symptom
Constipation	Opioid often causes constipation despite resident's being on bowel regimen	Methlynaltrexone or naloxegol may be used to treat opioid-induced constipation
Urinary incontinence	Usually is chronic but can be new onset	UTI is a common cause of acute symptoms or worsening of chronic symptoms
Fecal incontinence	Usually new onset	Fecal impaction with leakage around impaction should be differentiated from true fecal incontinence
Seizures	Generalized tonic clonic seizure, partial complex seizure, and myoclonic seizure may be seen during last weeks to months Seizures are often cause of agitation and aggressive behavior (usually in postictal state)	BZD with or without anticonvulsant (e.g. valproate) is recommended Antipsychotic can lower seizure threshold and may precipitate seizures
Delirium	Fluctuating consciousness, inattention, disorientation, disorganized thinking, day-night reversal, illusions, visual hallucination, delusion, dramatic and intense mood change Delirium is great source of distress not only for resident but also for family	HCP should look for easily reversible cause (e.g. medication, fecal impaction, urinary retention) and treat it Antipsychotic may be needed to relieve symptoms of severe agitation, aggressive behavior, and severe distress related to psychotic symptoms
Depression	Can range from normal sadness about EOL situation to MDD (severe and pervasive depressive symptoms [e.g. tearfulness, feelings of helplessness, hopelessness])	Two key determinants of choice of antidepressant are (1) likely prognosis (e.g. stimulant preferred if resident has only few days to weeks to live), and (2) anticipated beneficial side

Table 11.5 (cont.)

Symptom	Diagnostic/Assessment Pearls	Therapeutic Pearls
	MDD is not normal part of dying process Agitation, resistiveness to care, and aggressive behavior may be manifestations of MDD in resident who has advanced MNCD	effect of antidepressant (e.g. resident who has insomnia and loss of appetite is given mirtazapine because of its sedation and weight gain effects) besides other factors
Suicidal ideas and attempts	Expressions and efforts by resident to end life (usually part of syndrome of MDD when accompanied by other depressive symptoms)	Should be considered a psychiatric emergency, and prompt intervention to ensure safety and appropriate assessment and treatment is recommended
Wish to hasten death	Requests for euthanasia and/or physician-assisted hastening of death (physician-assisted dying/ physician-assisted suicide)	PCT should address this request with sensitivity and education about palliative care and what it can offer to relieve suffering, including palliative sedation
Anxiety	Excessive worries, tension, restlessness, insomnia, palpitations, hyperventilation, tachycardia Death anxiety (self-reported anxiety related to reflection of one's mortality and imminent death) can cause panic attack	Psychosocial environmental approaches (e.g. hand and neck massage, repeated reassurance) with or without BZD recommended
Psychotic symptoms (delusion, hallucination)	Mild symptoms may not be distressing Moderate to severe symptoms can be distressing and can cause severe agitation and physically aggressive behavior	Mild symptoms are best managed with psychosocial environmental approach (e.g. reassurance, family education and support, distraction) Antipsychotic is appropriate to reduce distress due to moderate to severe psychotic symptoms if no reversible cause (e.g. medication-induced psychotic symptoms) is identified
Existential/spiritual distress	Severe distress related to existential crises (*holistic suffering*) may be seen in resident during EOL care Resident struggles with loss of dignity in life remaining, feelings of demoralization, feelings of being a burden, EOL despair, and/or difficulty finding meaning in suffering and in diminished state	Chaplain, social worker, and psychologist need to work collaboratively with each other and with other team members to vigorously address this distress, which is often debilitating
Terminal agitation	Severe restlessness, moaning, groaning, and agitation in last hours or days before death	Combination of morphine, antipsychotic, and BZD* may be necessary to maximize control of symptoms HCP should consider palliative sedation for refractory cases

* BZD = benzodiazepine

(e.g. cachexia). The four main underlying diseases of the terminal phase are MNCD, cardiovascular diseases, COPD, and ESRD. Cancer is the underlying disease in only 12 percent of residents. Residents who have cancer show a different pattern of symptoms (e.g. higher prevalence of pain) from those without cancer. The HCP should use a combination of nondrug treatments and appropriate medication to relieve symptoms if the underlying cause cannot be promptly corrected. If the resident is naïve to the medication, a low dose should be given initially and titrated as clinically appropriate with close monitoring. The use of physical restraint to manage symptoms (e.g. to prevent falls, to prevent the resident from harming others) is prevalent among LTC residents receiving EOL care but should not be used for this most vulnerable of all LTC populations. Physical restraints are an assault to the resident's dignity and can worsen aggression. The six most common symptoms or syndromes seen in the terminal phase (pain; dyspnea; agitation and aggression; delirium; nutritional problems; depression, anxiety, and suicidal ideas) are discussed below.

Pain

Assessment and management of pain is a key aspect of palliative care. Although pain is prevalent in residents receiving EOL care, not all residents in the last days to weeks of life experience pain. Pain can lead to depression, decreased quality of life, decreased socialization, decreased wish to live, wish to hasten death, and insomnia. A LTC resident who has severe cognitive impairment is particularly vulnerable to inadequate pain control. Musculoskeletal pain (e.g. due to osteoarthritis, chronic back pain) is the most common source of chronic pain in LTC residents. Residents who have hip fracture, pressure ulcer, or a diagnosis of cancer often experience excruciating pain. Residents who have MNCD have higher rates of pressure ulcer than residents who do not have MNCD. Residents who experience excruciating pain often have been recently hospitalized (e.g. for surgery), have experienced weight loss, and/or have a terminal illness. Many residents may report pain during pain assessment but may not report it spontaneously and may not request pain medication. This may be because they perceive that persistent pain has little potential for change, stoicism, they voice ability to handle the pain, concern about medication in general and pain medication in particular, and concern about the expected staff response to the request (e.g. fear of being labeled a "bad" resident).

Pain is eminently treatable with evidence-based pharmacological and nonpharmacological treatments. A comprehensive pain-management program is critical to improving pain management in the LTC setting. A comprehensive pain-management program involves staff education, changes in pain policies and procedures, and identifying pain management as a quality indicator. The best way to relieve the pain of a resident who has severe cognitive impairment is to have an attentive and consistent caregiver who notices that the resident is in pain and then observes the resident's response to treatment. Nursing care together with physical therapy and occupational therapy can help prevent contracture and increase mobility in residents who have terminal-stage MNCD.

The HCP may need to prescribe analgesic on a trial basis to manage pain. For a resident who does not have hepatic dysfunction, acetaminophen is a reasonable first choice and is safer than a nonsteroidal anti-inflammatory drug (NSAID). The use of NSAID with LTC populations carries a significant risk of gastrointestinal bleeding and renal toxicity, especially if prescribed on a chronic basis. The HCP may consider prescribing short-term use of NSAID for a resident who has acute musculoskeletal pain and low risk of gastrointestinal bleeding and renal toxicity. The use of NSAID with acid suppressant (e.g. proton pump inhibitor or histamine 2 receptor antagonist) may reduce the risk of gastrointestinal toxicity. Antidepressants (preferably antidepressant with norepinephrine and serotonin reuptake inhibition activity, such as venlafaxine, duloxetine, desvenlafaxine) may have a substantial beneficial effect on chronic pain, and the HCP should consider prescribing it for any resident who has moderate to severe chronic pain, even in the absence of depression.

The next group of medications in the analgesic ladder include tramadol and codeine. Tramadol acts on opioid receptors and is appropriate for use on moderate to severe pain but carries a risk of drug-drug interaction with antidepressant (e.g. serotonin syndrome and seizures risk). Tramadol also has weak serotonin and norepinephrine reuptake inhibitor activity and thus may help improve depressive symptoms besides pain. We do not recommend prescribing codeine because of a lack of efficacy data in older adults, risks of severe constipation, requiring conversion to morphine via cytochrome P450 2D6 hepatic enzyme system, and risks of drug–drug interaction with other medication requiring the 2D6 enzyme system. The HCP may consider prescribing an opiate that is more potent than codeine (e.g. hydrocodone, oxycodone, morphine, and fentanyl) for moderate to severe pain. Opioids are drugs of choice for the management of pain in a resident receiving EOL care. Their use carries a substantial risk of cognitive toxicity, constipation, delirium, fecal impaction, respiratory suppression, and death. Thus, the dosages should be low and increased slowly with close monitoring of adverse effect. When used judiciously, opiates have a potential to dramatically improve pain and thus quality of life for a resident who has moderate to severe pain and is receiving EOL care. The HCP should avoid concomitant use of benzodiazepine (BZD) and opioid with LTC populations, but in the context of EOL care combination use may be necessary if the resident is in severe distress due to pain and anxiety. For a resident who cannot swallow pills, alternative routes of administration of opioid are useful and effective. For quick pain relief, transmucosal fentanyl can be as fast as intravenous administration. The HCP should avoid prescribing opiate with anticholinergic property (e.g. meperidine, pentazocine) because of the high risk of cognitive and cardiac toxicity. Any resident taking opioid should be on a bowel regimen (e.g. use of senna and/or polyethylene glycol) to prevent opioid use-related constipation and intestinal obstruction. Opioid may not adequately control pain in up to a third of residents receiving EOL care. Addition of other medication to opioid (e.g. an SNRI, a muscle relaxant, a BZD, dronabinol, cannabis, topical analgesic) may relieve pain. This kind of rational polypharmacy for pain management is appropriate to ensure that the palliative goal of maximal comfort during EOL care is achieved. The HCP should consider prescribing a muscle relaxant for a resident who has pain due to muscle spasticity (e.g. baclofen pump for the management of severe pain in a resident who has advanced multiple sclerosis and severe muscle spasticity).

Dyspnea

In LTC populations, dyspnea rather than pain may be the most prevalent symptom during the final 48 hours of life because most residents die of noncancer causes. Its differential diagnosis is important to elucidate because palliative treatments may differ considerably. Substantial reduction of distress associated with dyspnea in LTC facilities is achievable. Opioids are effective in treating dyspnea by relieving feelings of suffocation. For acute exacerbation of dyspnea, a dose as low as 25 percent of the equivalent every four-hour pain dose can provide substantial relief. Supplemental oxygen can also have a beneficial effect when dyspnea is related to hypoxia. BZDs also aid in the management of dyspnea, even for a resident who does not have prominent anxiety or who has terminal COPD. The HCP may also consider prescribing bronchodilator if the HCP suspects dyspnea due to airway obstruction. Noisy respiratory secretions may benefit from repositioning and suctioning. For many residents, the onset of dyspnea may signal a transition to the final stage of disease. PCT members should pay extra attention to educating family members that this is a normal manifestation of the dying process and that death is expected in hours to days, correct any misperception (e.g. that the resident will have this problem for weeks or even months), and help them with grief.

Agitation and Aggression

Agitation and aggression are common among residents receiving EOL care, especially residents who have MNCD. Aggression is often the only manifestation of delirium, depression, an undiagnosed acute reversible medical condition (e.g. urinary tract infection, acute urinary retention), medication toxicity, or a painful condition. Knowing the resident well is key to prompt and accurate diagnosis. We recommend psychosocial environmental approaches listed in Box 11.4 for the prevention and treatment of agitation and aggression along with treatment of potentially reversible causes of agitation or aggression. If psychotropic medication is needed for severe agitation and aggression, an atypical antipsychotic is usually the drug of first choice (haloperidol being second), unless the HCP suspects depression, in which case antidepressant should be used first. BZD is usually not recommended for the treatment of agitation and aggression due to the risk of worsening cognitive impairment and paradoxical increase in aggressive behavior but may be added if the resident is not responding to antipsychotic. During the last hours or days of life, agitation associated with delirium may also be treated by adding BZD to antipsychotic, as antipsychotic may lower the threshold for seizure and precipitate seizure and BZD may prevent this problem.

Delirium

Periods of confusion and delirium are common during the last days to weeks of life. Many residents may develop delirium as part of the syndrome of imminent death (terminal delirium). Physical disability and mood instability in a resident who has delirium can lead to family distress, and perceptual disturbances and severity of delirium can lead to staff distress. Restlessness and mood lability are the most upsetting for family members. Although delirium may be an inevitable part of dying from most terminal illnesses, efforts to minimize its impact are important.

If delirium is associated with severe agitation, treating reversible causes of delirium (e.g. dehydration [with gentle hypoderoclysis {subcutaneous infusion of fluids} or intravenous fluid if oral intake is not feasible], urinary tract infection, untreated pain) may reduce agitation. PCT members should educate family and staff that delirium is usually a normal part of the dying process and take time to answer questions (e.g. can he/she hear me?) and concerns (e.g. is he/she suffering?), thus reducing distress. Illusions, delusions, and hallucinations (especially visual) are common during delirium. The HCP should encourage family members and staff not to correct the resident's delusional statements and try to perceive some illusions and hallucinations (e.g. heavenly gates) as the resident's adaptive efforts to make meaning of the strange experiences. Aggressive behavior and mood fluctuations are also common during delirium. If the resident is being aggressive, it is important for the family and staff to understand that this is a manifestation of the underlying disease process and does not reflect the essence of the resident. Opioids can cause delirium. Delirium-associated agitation and restlessness are often misinterpreted as symptoms of worsening pain. This interpretation may lead to excessive use of opiate, which may worsen delirium unnecessarily. EOL delirium in LTC populations is typically multifactorial. PCT members should practice parsimonious medicine and guide family members that, in general, it may not be worthwhile to pursue a thorough delirium work-up, as the burdens of any work-up are substantial and will accrue with every test. The HCP may facilitate decreasing or stopping drugs that contribute to delirium. For opiate-induced delirium, we recommend rotating to an equipotent or slightly less than equipotent dose of another opiate. Anticholinergic medication (e.g. TCA) used to treat neuropathic pain, antisecretory agents (e.g. scopolamine) or antinausea drugs, BZD, and corticosteroid are among the most frequently implicated as deliriogenic.

Delirium often progresses to coma and then death. Distressing psychotic symptoms and severe aggression may require the use of antipsychotic along with psychosocial environmental approaches. Before using antipsychotics, the HCP should ensure that, during the last hours or days of life, agitation associated with delirium is also treated by adding a BZD to antipsychotic. BZD is also appropriate for the treatment of agitation accompanied by severe anxiety associated with delirium during the last hours or days (especially for a resident who has myoclonus or seizures or who has severe dyspnea not responding to opiate).

Nutritional Problems

Severe nutritional problems, such as unintentional weight loss usually associated with poor or absent food and/or fluid intake resulting in cachexia and dehydration, are common and fatal complications of many terminal diseases in LTC populations. The HCP should look for easily fixed causes of not eating (e.g. ill-fitting dentures, a sore in the mouth, a toothache, medication-induced anorexia) and correct them before proceeding to diagnose and treat depressive symptoms, as undernutrition can cause depressive symptoms. The HCP may consider prescribing dronabinol to treat anorexia in the context of palliative and EOL care, as it may also improve nausea and pain and enhance mood and general well-being. With advanced MNCD, residents may reach a point when they are neurologically incapable of eating. In fact, at the end of any long and terminal illness, people often stop eating; this seems to be part of the "wisdom of the body" and is one of the most peaceful and comfortable ways of dying. Decreased fluid intake leads to drying of oropharyngeal and bronchial secretions, which in turn reduces the risk of *death rattle*, a distressing symptom (not only to the resident but also to the family witnessing it) that can occur in more than 50 percent of individuals in the last days of life. Death rattle is often treated with anticholinergic drugs (e.g. hyocyamine subcutaneously), and use of these drugs carries significant risk of hallucinations, agitation, and delirium. Drying of oropharyngeal and bronchial secretions due to reduced fluid intake during EOL also reduces the risk of aspiration pneumonia. Severe dehydration due to poor intake at the EOL usually leads the resident gradually to become sleepy and slip into coma and eventually death, without developing physical pain or agitation. Assisted feeding (including hand feeding) instead of feeding through percutaneous endoscopic gastrostomy (PEG) tube is a better alternative for a resident who has advanced MNCD and stops eating despite the potential serious complications of undernutrition (e.g. pressure ulcer, acceleration of the dying process) and oral intake of food (e.g. aspiration) (American Geriatrics Society 2014). Assisted feeding should be gentle and not overly aggressive. PEG tube feeding is usually not beneficial for a resident who has advanced MNCD. Tube feeding usually does not change the survival of a resident who has MNCD and is unable to eat orally. Moreover, for a resident who has severe or terminal MNCD, providing nutrition through a PEG tube does not reduce aspiration or pressure ulcers or improve markers of malnutrition; rather, a PEG tube can lead to increased infections, more discomfort, increased oral secretions, and use of physical restraint (as the resident often attempts to pull out the tube). One reason that many families and physicians continue to opt for ANH is that the case for a feeding tube is moral and not scientific. What may be at issue for families is how best to demonstrate caring. PCT members should acknowledge the symbolic value of nutrition for a resident in terminal stages of MNCD or other illness and seek an alternative means of satisfying the need to feed, such as hand feeding or giving sips of water. MDD can cause anorexia and weight loss, and treatment of MDD can improve anorexia and nutrition status, giving the resident improved capacity to make the most of life remaining.

Depression, Anxiety, and Suicidal Ideas

Positive Psychiatry is a branch of psychiatry that focuses on the prevention of mental disorders and the promotion of psychological and spiritual wellness and growth. Preventing depression and anxiety during EOL care and promoting psychological and spiritual growth are eminently possible for residents receiving high-quality palliative care. Effectively controlling physical symptoms (e.g. pain) is the first step in preventing psychological distress. Discontinuing unnecessary medication, avoiding futile and/or inappropriate care (including futile and/or inappropriate hospitalization and life-prolonging treatment), aggressive use of strength-based personalized psychosocial sensory spiritual and environmental initiatives and creative engagement (SPPEICE), guiding the family in ways they can help the resident make the most of life remaining, and providing spiritual support can go a long way in preventing depression and anxiety and keeping psychological distress to a mild level. PCT members need to inquire whether there are any financial matters that could be causing stress and creating barriers for the resident to obtain optimal palliative care. Addressing financial concerns is a key component of the prevention of depression and anxiety among residents receiving EOL care.

Authentic listening to the resident's wishes and emotional distress in a nonjudgmental manner can be tremendously healing for the resident and can prevent worsening of depression and anxiety. Being mindful of the resident's situation and one's own emotional response to requests for hastening death, although difficult, can be profoundly healing to the resident because of the compassion it can generate. Simple practices, such as holding the resident's hand and commitment to presence (being available in person to the resident and family when needed), are central to the role of PCT members as caring and compassionate HCPs (Kleinman 2013).

Four simple statements, "Please forgive me. I forgive you. Thank you. I love you," are powerful tools for easing suffering as well as promoting psychological and spiritual growth of a resident facing life's end – and the resident's family. These four statements also help prepare the resident and family to say, "Goodbye." The key message the resident and family need to hear from the treatment team is that dying does not have to be agonizing, that physical suffering can always be alleviated, and that the resident will not die alone. Also, it is important to share with the resident and family that this last stage of life holds remarkable possibilities for personal and spiritual growth, for strengthening bonds with people they love, for repairing broken ties and making amends, and for creating profound meaning in the final passage. For a resident in terminal stages of MNCD, providing comfort through use of all five senses (touch [soothing massage], smell [aromatherapy], taste [delicious food and fluids], sight [seeing natural surroundings, family], and hearing [listening to favorite soothing music]) and spiritual activities (e.g. saying prayers, listening to religious songs) may improve mood and prevent agitation and insomnia.

Life review and reminiscence therapy is also helpful in preventing depression and anxiety and promoting feelings of life well lived for a resident who has relatively preserved cognitive function. Life review is an important part of bringing life to a close. As life ends, many people express a wish to know that they have truly been seen by someone and that their life has had value and meaning. Reminiscence is common at the end of life, and many people find it helpful to reflect on their lives. This can be done in structured ways, to recall and sometimes document a life that is coming to an end. During this last phase of life, music often offers a special medium for healing and growth. It allows experiencing, sharing, and communication of feelings that otherwise would not be experienced, shared, or communicated. A music thanatologist can help transport the resident to a place of peace, beauty, and joy. A music thanatologist uses harp and voice to ease emotional distress and promote the psychological and spiritual well-being of individuals receiving EOL care.

Occasional thoughts of suicide or a desire for death are fairly common in residents who have relatively preserved cognitive function receiving EOL care. A resident who has relatively preserved cognitive function or mild to moderate MNCD may make an explicit request or give a hint for a hastened death. For example, the resident may ask, "Doctor, I would like you to help me die. I am ready to die. Would you help me?" Other expressions reflecting suicidal ideas and emotional suffering include but are not limited to: "Just shoot me [verbally expressed or by pointing to the temple with a hand as if the resident had the gun]"; or inquiring about the Hemlock Society (an organization that supports euthanasia in the United States). Certain diagnoses (e.g. amyotrophic lateral sclerosis [ALS, or Lou Gehrig's disease]) are particularly associated with a request for physician-assisted hastening of death. Typically, such statements express a fear of loss of dignity during EOL rather than a fear of death. Other fears that trigger the wish to hasten death include fear of pain, loss of control (not knowing when and how one will die), loss of independence, fear of dying alone, fear of alteration in personality and cognitive function, and fear of being a burden to family. Often, such expressions are a way to elicit assurance from PCT members that suffering will be aggressively treated and comfort maximized with a symptom-directed treatment plan using all available therapeutic strategies, including palliative sedation. Lack of trust on the part of the resident and family that PCT members will deliver what they promised is another barrier that PCT members should expect and take steps to overcome by having regular discussions and updates. Fear of pain can be addressed by making it explicit to the resident and the family that a detailed pain management plan has been put in place, with contingencies in case pain gets out of control. Suicidal ideas in the context of MDD may involve feelings that the resident is a burden and family members would be better off if the resident ended her own life or that family members want the resident to die because she is a burden. Other symptoms of MDD are also present. Psychotic symptoms accompanying MDD increase the risk of suicide dramatically. The HCP should consider preoccupation with a wish to die, a suicide attempt, and/or request for a hastened death a psychiatric emergency and immediately institute appropriate safety measures until a detailed assessment is done. The HCP should consider formal consultation with a psychiatrist for any resident who is terminally ill and voices suicidal ideas and plans or requests a hastened death.

Most residents experience at least some psychological distress (anxiety, fear, sadness, anger, agitation). Mild psychological and behavioral symptoms may require only brief assessment (e.g. medication review for medication-induced symptoms) and fine tuning of SPPEICE (e.g. increasing music-based activities if the resident seems to find great relief). (See Box 11.4.) Severe symptoms need comprehensive psychiatric assessment to look for potentially reversible causes and appropriate treatment. Many residents use denial to cope with a diagnosis of terminal illness. Denial doesn't respond to reason, so it is best to honor the resident's psychological position and focus on providing comfort, rather than confrontation. Efforts to force residents to overcome denial may do more harm than good. Denial is one of the stages of loss, and thus the HCP needs to anticipate it and respond with compassion. A resident in denial may nevertheless accept a comprehensive palliative plan of care the family agreed to, without feeling stressed by medical decisions that the resident is not emotionally prepared to make.

Major depressive disorder (MDD) is common among residents receiving EOL care. Residents and family members need to know that MDD is not a normal or inevitable part of the dying process. Many of the somatic symptoms of MDD (e.g. fatigue, anorexia, loss of energy, sleep disturbance, cognitive impairment) are common in terminal illness. Hence, psychological symptoms (e.g. hopelessness, worthlessness, guilt, helplessness, loss of meaning, preoccupation with death and suicide) are more useful in identifying MDD (Desai, Lo, and Grossberg 2013). When MDD during EOL is severe, different methods of diagnosing MDD (e.g. replacing physical symptoms with psychologically oriented criteria) identify depression equally well. The presence of hopelessness correlates highly with suicidal ideation in these patients. Symptoms of MDD can be reliably diagnosed using PHQ-9 with a resident who has relatively preserved cognitive function and by CSDD with a resident who has advanced MNCD. A resident in the terminal stages of MNCD may also develop MDD, but manifestations are mostly behavioral (e.g. depressed affect, tearfulness, vocalizations such as "Help me, help me," irritability, agitation, aggression, insomnia, poor oral intake, weight loss, social withdrawal, poverty of speech, absence of smile, anxious or fearful affect). MDD is an important risk factor for requests to hasten death or for euthanasia. A history of MDD may indicate that current depressive symptoms may be a relapse of a depressive illness. A resident who has MDD and chronic pain needs simultaneous treatment of pain and depression.

We recommend combining psychological (e.g. meaning-centered psychotherapy, life review, dignity-conserving therapy, creative expression), behavioral (pleasant activities, social and physical activation when feasible), sensory (music, therapeutic touch [e.g. massage]), environmental (exposure to nature, sunlight), and spiritual approaches with psychotropic medication therapy to treat MDD.

We recommend referral to a mental health specialist (e.g. geriatric psychiatrist) in any complicated and high-risk situation (e.g. resident is suicidal, depression is accompanied by severe agitation/aggression, psychotropic medication therapy is indicated). The HCP should institute treatment of pain and/or other physical symptoms before or with initiation of specific antidepressant treatment. The HCP should consider prescribing an antidepressant for any resident who has MDD, and antidepressant medication is the first-line treatment for moderate to severe MDD and MDD with psychotic symptoms. No one antidepressant is superior to another. Options include stimulants (e.g. methylphenidate), selective serotonin reuptake inhibitors (SSRIs), selective serotonin norepinephrine inhibitors (SNRIs; e.g. venlafaxine, duloxetine, desvenlafaxine), tricyclic antidepressants (e.g. nortriptyline, desipramine), and other antidepressants (e.g. mirtazapine, bupropion, vilazodone, vortioxetine, levomilnacipran). The choice depends on several factors, such as the resident's preference, comorbid condition (e.g. duloxetine preferred for a resident who has diabetic neuropathy, as duloxetine is indicated for both MDD and diabetic neuropathy), beneficial side effect profile in relation to the resident's symptoms (e.g. mirtazapine's sedative effect and effect of weight gain for a resident who has insomnia and weight loss), past response to an antidepressant, and risk of drug–drug interaction. Because of the rapid onset of action, stimulants (methylphenidate, dextroamphetamine) deserve special consideration in treating MDD in the context of EOL care. Therapeutic benefits can be achieved within 24–48 hours of starting medication. Stimulants may also augment opioid analgesia, diminish opioid sedation, and reduce feeling of fatigue. ECT is appropriate for the treatment of MDD for a resident receiving EOL care if the symptoms are severe and refractory or if severe psychotic symptoms are present. ECT remains the most effective treatment for MDD to date and provides quick response (especially important in EOL setting). Relief of MDD can allow the resident to smile again and have memorable and meaningful last days or weeks with family and friends. Relief of MDD also reduces family members' stress and feelings of helplessness. Although there are case reports of intravenous ketamine for the treatment of severe MDD with suicidal ideas in palliative care settings, we recommend avoiding this approach until more research clarifies the benefits and risks.

A resident who has relatively preserved cognitive function may experience *death anxiety* after receiving a diagnosis of terminal illness (e.g. metastatic cancer) (Tong et al. 2016). Many residents develop severe anxiety symptoms along with depressive symptoms during the terminal stages of the illness. Residents who have pre-existing anxiety disorder may have a relapse of the symptoms (e.g. panic attack in a resident who has panic disorder), and comorbid medical conditions (e.g. pain) and medications (e.g. steroids) can also cause intolerable anxiety symptoms. Typically, anxiety symptoms in a resident receiving EOL care are multifactorial. Many residents who have mild anxiety symptoms during EOL respond to SPPEICE. (See Box 11.4.) Moderate to severe anxiety symptoms or anxiety is usually best treated with a BZD, as in this context speed of improvement is of the essence and no psychotropic medication is better than BZD for relieving anxiety symptoms rapidly. Residents receiving EOL care are an exception to the general rule that the HCP should avoid or minimize the prescription of BZD for LTC populations because of serious risks associated with its use (e.g. sedation, falls).

Caring for the Caregiver

The HCP should routinely address the emotional needs of family caregivers as part of palliative and EOL care of all residents. Caregiver stress and grief can be addressed by education, preparation for EOL care of the resident, and counseling. (See Box 11.7.) The bulk of suffering of caregivers of residents who have MNCD occurs in the years before the resident's death. A majority of caregivers experience substantial relief after the loved one who had MNCD has died. Thus, the HCP should institute grief and stress-reduction approaches for all caregivers soon after the resident is admitted to the facility, continue throughout the resident's stay, and consider intensifying them during the last few weeks or months of the resident's life. Family and friends should be allowed to visit as often and as long as they like without set visiting hours. Most caregivers identify religious activities (e.g. going to church, reading sacred texts, etc.) as a major source for coping with the difficulties in caregiving activities. Prayer is a particularly vital source of empowerment for many family caregivers. Praying often gives the family member a sense of peace, strength, and even answers to questions related to the loved one's EOL care. Struggling with and caring for a loved one who is frail and in a LTC facility may increase some caregivers' feelings of spiritual connectedness and emotional stability. Hence, we strongly recommend identifying dimensions of spirituality/religiosity to help family develop effective and appropriate support systems. This in turn may make caregiving less stressful and more rewarding. Support

BOX 11.7 Approaches to Help Family Members Cope with a Resident's Distress during the Dying Process

- Let family members know that the dying process has begun (i.e. the resident is in essence dying).
- Educate family members that what is happening is a normal part of the dying process (normal natural way the body prepares to "call it a day").
- Help family members "let go" and understand that "letting go" is not "giving up."
- Help family members understand that medical treatments can be futile but palliative care efforts are never futile.
- Help family members make meaning of suffering.
- Help family members understand what may be going on with the resident.
- Educate family members that for many, death happens over a series of little good-byes.
- Educate family members that delirium is a normal part of the dying process (brain winding down/brain failure).
- Help family members recognize that some distress (e.g. pain, sadness, anxiety, confusion) is part of the human condition and that in many situations, "fix" (medical treatment) may cause more suffering than the symptoms being addressed.
- Educate family members that the resident's physically aggressive behavior (or other inappropriate behavior) is due to brain disorder and does not reflect the essence of who the person is (e.g. staff telling the daughter of a resident who has been cursing and spitting at the staff who was attempting to administer pain medication, "That was not your mother").
- Help family members verbalize their fears and discuss them.
- Spend time comforting family members and validating their feelings (e.g. validating a family member's angst when he states, "It is so difficult, not knowing what this is like for her").
- Help family reframe hallucinations and delusions as something positive (e.g. deathbed visions can be viewed as something beautiful and comforting that the family members are privileged to witness).
- Share (in as much detail as possible) with family members any and all positive events and moments the resident experienced between visits by family members.
- Educate family members that MDD is not an inevitable part of the dying process, so treatment with antidepressant for the resident is allowed.

groups, bereavement groups, and mindfulness-based stress reduction techniques are also useful in addressing caregiver stress and grief. Life review and reminiscence therapy can help relieve caregiver stress and grief. Some family caregivers (e.g. those who have persistent depression, guilt, severe anxiety) may need referral to a mental health clinician for individual psychotherapy and, if necessary, psychotropic medication. Family caregivers often feel that the loved one did not experience a good death in the LTC facility. The PCT should do all they can to prevent such outcomes, inquire about family members' experience of the resident's EOL care, and address any negative feelings family members have about the care received. It is also important to address grief and stress of professional caregivers who have grown emotionally close to the resident. PCT members should not be afraid to show compassion, respect, and sadness for the resident and family.

Sending a sympathy card is helpful to the family, but a call from the physician inquiring about the family's well-being after the resident's death can have a profound positive impact on the well-being of the family members and should be adopted as the standard of practice. If the HCP suspects complicated grief in a family member, encouraging the family to come for a formal office visit to address grief is also an important aspect of palliative care for LTC populations.

Approximately 20 percent of bereaved family members will experience complicated grief after the death of the loved one. Complicated grief (also called abnormal grief) is characterized as a long-lasting maladaptive response to bereavement that can exacerbate pre-existing psychological, physical, and/or social problems. *DSM-5* proposed the term *Persistent complex bereavement disorder* to describe complicated grief (American Psychiatric Association 2013). Symptoms of complicated grief can include intense longing and yearning for the person who died and recurrent intrusive and distressing thoughts about the absence of the deceased, making it difficult for the family to move beyond an acute state of mourning. Psychosocial treatments designed to decrease caregiver burden and distress and address grief (especially for a resident who has MNCD) before the resident's death may prevent complicated grief after the death. We recommend early identification and aggressive psychiatric treatment of complicated grief with grief counseling (complicated grief therapy) and antidepressant. LGBTQ family members of residents face additional barriers and stressors (e.g. homophobia, failure by LTC staff to acknowledge the relationship) that the PCT should anticipate, proactively prevent, and address with sensitivity and compassion.

Educating and Preparing the Resident and Family for End-of-Life Care

Much of the emotional distress during EOL care is preventable by timely, thorough, and periodic education and preparation of the resident and/or the family regarding EOL care. Residents and their family usually have a host of questions and concerns that the PCT should inquire about and address. (See Box 11.8.) Assessing a resident's and/or family's understanding of the prognosis and course of disease is the first step

BOX 11.8 Key Questions the Palliative Care Team Can Ask the Resident and/or the Family to Clarify End-of-Life Care Wishes and Better Address Concerns

- What are you most worried about? (Especially clarify if worries are related to fears of loss of control, dignity issues, or fear of poor control of symptom [e.g. pain, shortness of breath].)
- Can you give me more specifics?
- Is there a scenario that you envision that is most terrifying?
- Have you witnessed a bad death in your family?
- Would you prefer to be alert even if you are in severe pain, or would you prefer maximal pain control even if it makes you sleepy?
- What are you hoping to receive from me? (Especially clarify if there is any desire for physician-assisted hastening of death [physician-assisted dying, physician-assisted suicide].)
- Are you seeking physician-assisted hastening of death because you fear possible severe pain or abject debility?
- Are you seeking physician-assisted hastening of death because you fear possible alteration in your personality or loss of verbal, cognitive, and physical function?
- What about the current problems is most intolerable?
- What is causing you the most suffering?
- Would you like me to clarify what to expect in the next few hours or days?

in tailoring the education to their needs. Most families of residents who have MNCD are faced with having to make all the decisions regarding EOL care because of the resident's loss of DMC, typically years before the EOL phase. Many family members have a difficult time making EOL decisions because they are not emotionally prepared or informed. Also, family members may not reach a unanimous decision. The key strategies to prepare the resident and family for the EOL care include: promoting excellent communication with the resident and family; encouraging appropriate advance care and decision-making; demonstrating empathy for difficult emotions and conflicts in relationships due to disagreements; and attending to family grief and bereavement. Use of simple, clear language that the resident and family will understand rather than clinical language is important. PCT members should allow the resident and family to control the pace and flow of information whenever possible and let them guide how much detail and how much information they are able to handle at the time. The resident and family may be more satisfied if they have an opportunity to speak while the physician listens. Providing printed materials from reputable organizations (e.g. American Medical Association) for residents and families with key points that will be covered during the discussion is useful. PCT members should plan for repeat visits to readdress difficult issues and view discussion of prognosis as a spectrum from diagnosis to death rather than a one-time event. The HCP should reassure the resident and family that it is normal to be confused or overwhelmed. Encouraging residents and family to write down questions as they arise so that they can be discussed at a later meeting is also a useful strategy. One or more PCT members can summarize the meetings and discussions (especially decisions agreed on and the reasoning behind the decisions) and encourage the resident and family to record this summary for later review and sharing with family members who could not attend the meeting.

If the resident does not have DMC, the legally designated surrogate decision-maker should follow the standard of *substituted judgment* to make decisions on behalf of the resident. The standard of substituted judgment requires the surrogate decision-maker to make decisions as the resident would have made. This requires not only that the surrogate decision-maker has known the resident well but also that he has had discussions about preferences (e.g. regarding end-of-life care) and values surrounding issues such as what it means to live with dignity. When the standard of *substituted judgment* cannot be followed due to lack of adequate knowledge of what the resident would have done in the given situation, the standard of *best interest* needs to be followed. This requires the surrogate decision-maker to make decisions that are in the best interest of the resident (setting aside her own preferences if necessary). This can pose its own challenges, as many residents face dire situations in which, without knowing resident's values and wishes, what would be in the best interest of the resident may not be clear. For example, one choice may lead to shortening of life and another choice may lead to prolonged suffering during the dying process. In such situations, a third standard, the *reasonable person* standard, can be applied. This standard is based on the belief that most individuals value more or less the same things, and a reasonable person in a given situation would act in a certain way. The HCP needs to reassure the surrogate decision-maker that in some situations there may be more than one reasonable option. Whatever the standard followed and the decision made, the HCP needs to assure the surrogate decision-maker that high-quality palliative care will be provided to the resident to ensure that the resident will not suffer without respite or experience indignity in the last days of life. The HCP may need to remind some family members that they have an ethical obligation to make decisions based on one of these three standards irrespective of whether or not they would do the same for their own EOL care.

PCT members should be easily available and accessible to residents and their family, should walk the family through various stages of MNCD or other terminal condition, tell them what to expect, what approaches will replace aggressive medical treatments, how the resident's comfort will be maximized, the risks of treatments that promote comfort, and the differences between palliative sedation, physician-assisted hastening of death, and euthanasia. Because they perceive that they need to be with the resident all the time, some families may need counseling on an appropriate amount of visits from friends and family. The physician and staff must strive to be "on the same page" before approaching the resident and family, because the resident and family may try to reverify what they think they heard at a meeting. The staff often know which family members to contact first, as well as the family's particular preferences for communication with the treatment team. It may also be useful to have the social worker call each of the involved family members (e.g. resident's children) with the same message. Although face-to-face meetings to discuss EOL care are ideal, a telephone conference (or video conference) call may also be arranged to include long-distance family members.

PCT members should understand families' emotional distress, give information regarding steps to keep the loved one comfortable, and encourage families to tell important things to the loved one and treat the loved one as when he was cognitively intact and healthy. PCT members should never say, "There's nothing more to be done" or "Do you want everything done?" Instead, PCT members should talk about the life yet to be lived and what can be done to make it better. Addressing financial planning needs (e.g. adequacy of the resident's finances to meet the desired level of care [at the place of the resident's choice whenever feasible] for the remaining limited time, ensuring that the resident's finances are being used for the resident's care) is also an important part of comprehensive palliative care with LTC populations.

Educating and Training Staff regarding Palliative Care

The PCT can provide leadership in promoting a culture that normalizes death and dying in the facility. As part of a program of continuous quality improvement, PCT leaders should conduct frequent (at least once a month, preferably once a week), one- to two-hour long educational seminars for the staff (tailored to their needs and strengths) based on specific cases in the facility as well as on topics listed in Box 11.5. These sessions should be video and/or audio recorded so that they are available for staff members who did not attend. The goal of such seminars is to increase the comfort level, knowledge, and skills of staff members to discuss advance care issues, normalize the topic of dying for the staff, encourage discussion, and validate concerns. It can also model communication strategies and help prompt shared experiences between older and younger staff members. Use of standardized assessment tools can also help the staff gain a better grasp on different dimensions of a specific problem (e.g. pain, agitation). In general, such case-based seminars and use of standardized tools can help the staff feel more confident in their ability to assess and manage pain, prevent and relieve agitation, and address family grief. Staff also may feel more competent to break bad news to family of residents about illness, discuss families' concerns regarding care, and help decision-making. Addressing grief not only in family members but also in staff who have grown close to the resident is a crucial aspect of palliative care for LTC populations.

Summary

Death and dying are central features of LTC practice. There is more to medicine than curing disease and/or postponing death. Life in the shadows of death can be immensely rewarding and fulfilling. Palliative and EOL care is one of the most important components of high-quality care for all residents in LTC facilities. Key factors to ensure high-quality palliative and EOL care include facilitating choice (helping the resident or proxy retain as much control as possible within the limits of belonging to a community), respecting choice (of the resident or proxy), providing evidence-based palliative care, securing the resident's network of significant relationships, and promoting sensitivity and respect for cultural diversity. One of the goals of palliative care in the United States is identifying those residents who would benefit from and qualify for hospice care. Euthanasia and physician-assisted hastening of death (physician-assisted suicide, physician-assisted dying) should not be part of palliative care. The HCP should educate any resident who requests euthanasia or physician-assisted hastening of death about what palliative care can offer (including palliative sedation), and the resident should have easy access to high-quality palliative care services. The HCP should routinely address the emotional needs of family caregivers as part of palliative and EOL care for all residents.

Key Clinical Points

1. High-quality palliative and EOL care is an essential component of caring for LTC populations.
2. The five components of high-quality palliative and EOL care for LTC populations are conserving dignity, providing spiritual care, advance care planning, relieving symptoms, and caring for family members.
3. One of the key goals of palliative care is early identification of residents who would benefit from and qualify for hospice care.
4. The HCP should routinely educate any resident who requests euthanasia or physician-assisted hastening of death about what palliative care can

offer (including palliative sedation), and the resident should have easy access to high-quality palliative care services.

5. Addressing the grief of family members as well as staff who have grown close to the resident is a key component of palliative and EOL care.

Additional Resources

Care of the dying adult in the last days of life. National Institute of Clinical Excellence (NICE) Guidelines, published December 2915 https://www.nice.org.uk/guidance/ng31

End-of-Life Care. Journal of the American Medical Association, JAMA Patient Page. July 6, 2016. http://jama.jamanetwork.com/collection.aspx?categoryid=6258

Advance Directives. Journal of the American Medical Association, JAMA Patient Page. February 24, 2015. http://jama.jamanetwork.com/collection.aspx?categoryid=6258

Hospice Care. Journal of the American Medical Association Patient Health Page. February 8, 2006. http://jama.jamanetwork.com/collection.aspx?categoryid=6258

Physician Orders for Life Sustaining Treatment (POLST): National POLST Paradigm. http://polst.org

Being Mortal: Medicine and What Matters in The End. Atul Gawande. http://atulgawande.com/book/being-mortal/

Music-Thanatology Association International. http://mtai.org

The End-of-life Namaste Care Program for People with MNCD. www.namastecare.com

The Happy Coffin Initiative, Lien Foundation. www.lienfoundation.org/sites/default/files/happy_coffins.pdf and www.lifebeforedeath.com/happycoffins/

References

Abele, P. and J.E. Morley. 2016. Advance Directives: The Key to a Good Death? *Journal of the American Medical Directors Association* **17**:279–283.

American Geriatrics Society. 2014. American Geriatrics Society Feeding Tube in Advanced Dementia Position Statement. American Geriatrics Society Ethics Committee and Clinical Care and Models of Care Committee. *Journal of the American Geriatrics Society* **62**:1590–1593.

American Psychiatric Association 2013. Conditions for Further Study. *Diagnostic and Statistical Manual of Mental Disorders*, 5th ed., pp. 783–806. Arlington, VA: American Psychiatric Association.

Bausewein, C., B.A. Daveson, D.C. Currow et al. 2016. EAPC white paper on outcome measurement in palliative care: Improving practice, attaining outcomes, and delivering quality services – Recommendations from the European Association for Palliative Care (EAPC) task force on outcome measurement. *Palliative Medicine* **30**(1): 6–22.

Best, M., L. Aldridge, P. Butov, et al. 2015. Treatment of Holistic Suffering in Cancer: A Systematic Review. *Palliative Medicine* **29**(10):885–898.

Chochinov, H. 2007. Dignity and the Essence of Medicine: The A, B, C, and D of Dignity Conserving Care. *British Journal of Medicine* **335**:184–186.

Desai, A.K., D. Lo, and G.T. Grossberg. 2013. Depression in Older Adults Receiving Hospice Care. In H. Laveretsky, M. Sajatovic, C.F. Reynolds (eds.), *Late-Life Mood Disorders*, pp. 516–531. New York, NY: Oxford University Press.

Gawande, A. 2014. *Being Mortal: What Matters In The End.* New York, NY: Metropolitan Books.

Hendry, M., D. Pasterfield, R. Lewis, et al. 2013. Why Do We Want the Right to Die? A Systematic Review of the International Literature on the Views of the Patients, Carers, and the Public about Assisted Dying. *Journal of Palliative Medicine* **27**:13–26.

Institute of Medicine. 2014. *Dying in America: Improving Quality and Honoring Individual Preferences near the End of Life.* Washington, DC: National Academies Press.

Kleinman, A. 2013. From Illness as Culture to Caring as a Moral Experience. *New England Journal of Medicine* **368**(15):1376–1377.

Mitchell, S.L. 2015. Advanced Dementia. *New England Journal of Medicine* **372**:2533–2540.

Morley, J.E., Li Cao, and C.K. Shum. 2016. Improving the Quality of End-of-Life Care. *Journal of the American Medical Directors Association* **17**:93–95.

National Quality Forum. 2012. NQF Endorses Palliative and End-of-Life Measures. www.qualityforum.org/News_And_Resources/Press_Releases/2012/NQF_Endorses_Palliative_and_End-of-Life_Care_Measures.aspx (accessed December 12, 2015).

Perrar, K.M., H. Schmidt, Y. Eisenmann, et al. 2015. Needs of People with Severe Dementia at the End of Life: A Systematic Review. *Journal of Alzheimer's Disease* **43**(2):397–413.

Quill, T.E., A.L. Back, and S.A. Block. 2016. Responding to Request for Physician-Assisted Death. Physician Involvement at the Very End of Life. *Journal of the American Medical Association* **315**(3):245–246.

Radbruch, L., C. Leget, P. Bahr, et al. 2016. Euthanasia and Physician Assisted Suicide. White Paper from the European

Association of Palliative Medicine. *Palliative Medicine* **30**(2):104–116.

Reisberg, B. 1988. Functional Assessment Staging (FAST). *Psychopharmacological Bulletin* **24**:653–659.

Rosenberg, J.H., J.S. Albrecht, E.K. Fromme, et al. 2013. Antimicrobial Use for Symptom Management for Patients Receiving Hospice and Palliative Care: A Systematic Review. *Journal of Palliative Medicine* **16**(12):1568–1574.

Rostin, L.A. and A.E. Roberts. 2016. Physician Assisted Dying: A Turning Point? *Journal of the American Medical Association* **315**(3):249–250.

Tong, E., A. Deckert, N. Gani, et al. 2016. The Meaning of Self-Reported Death Anxiety in Advanced Cancer. *Palliative Medicine* **30**(8):772–779.

van der Steen, J.T., L. Radbruch, C.M.M.P. Hertogh, et al. 2014. White Paper Defining Optimal Palliative Care in Older People with Dementia: A Delphi Study and Recommendations from the European Association for Palliative Care. *Palliative Medicine* **28**(3):197–209.

Volicer, L. 2011. Palliative Care and Hospice. In M.E. Agronin and G. J. Maletta eds., *Principles and Practice of Geriatric Psychiatry*, 2nd ed., pp. 251–264. Philadelphia, PA: Lippincott Williams & Wilkins.

World Health Organization. 2002. Definition of Palliative Care. www.who.int/cancer/palliative/definition/en/ (accessed December 12, 2015).

Yang, T., and F.A. Curlin. 2016. Why Physicians Should Oppose Assisted Suicide. *Journal of the American Medical Association* **315**(3):247–248.

Chapter 12

Psychiatric Aspects of Rational Deprescribing

Will I survive my medications?
Jim Waun, M.D., R.P.H., Journal of American Geriatrics Society, *2014.*

Medication is one of the most common causes of behavioral, neurocognitive, and psychological symptoms (BNPS) in long-term care (LTC) populations. Residents in LTC facilities often do not tolerate medication (prescription or over the counter) well, and even a small dose may cause intolerable adverse effect. This is because of changes related to age and medical illness in the way the body processes medication, altered sensitivity to medication's adverse effect, complicated interactions because of polypharmacy, multiple comorbidities, and impaired ability to compensate physiologically for even minor "nuisance" effect, such as mild sedation or nausea (Mulsant and Pollock 2015). The need to minimize risk and enhance outcome in clinical practice requires the health care provider (HCP) to take into consideration all these complications. There can be tremendous heterogeneity between residents in each of these areas, and there is often a lack of rigorous efficacy and safety data for many of the prescribed medications in LTC populations. Thus, the management of medication for any resident, and particularly for a resident who is frail and/or has major neurocognitive disorder (MNCD), is a complicated and difficult task.

Potentially Inappropriate Prescribing

Finding the right balance between appropriately and adequately treating medical and psychiatric conditions and avoiding medication-related harm is a critical objective for physicians, physician assistants, and nurse practitioners (Scott et al. 2015). Polypharmacy is concomitant use of five or more medications. Polypharmacy is often the norm in LTC populations, and rational polypharmacy may be appropriate to adequately address multiple medical and psychiatric conditions and improve a resident's quality of life. The HCP needs to minimize polypharmacy, as the risk of an adverse drug event (ADE) increases with the number of medications an older adult takes. The risk of ADE is 13 percent with the use of two medications and 58 percent with use of five medications (Patterson et al. 2014). If an individual takes seven or more medications, the incidence of ADE increases to 88 percent.

Polypharmacy is associated with potentially inappropriate prescription (PIP; also called potentially inappropriate medication [PIM]). Table 12.1 lists different forms of PIP. PIP should include not only medication that is unnecessary or that causes more harm than good, but also lack of appropriate medication at an appropriate dosage (underprescribing) (Patterson et al. 2014). Underprescribing is lack of prescription of medication that is indicated for a particular condition (medical and psychiatric) based on up-to-date clinical practice guidelines. Point prevalence of PIP in LTC populations ranges from 20 to 43 percent. Point prevalence of use of psychotropic medication in LTC populations ranges from 50 to 80 percent. Prevalence of PIP is even higher among residents taking psychotropic medication and residents who have MNCD (the most vulnerable of LTC populations). Tools with explicit criteria have been developed to help physicians identify PIP. The most studied tools are the Beers criteria, the Medication Appropriateness Index (MAI), the STOPP (Screening Tool of Older Person's Potentially inappropriate Prescription) criteria, and the START (Screening Tool to Alert doctors for the Right Treatment) criteria (Barry et al. 2007; Gallagher et al. 2008; American Geriatrics Society 2012; Hanlon and Schmader 2013). Use of three or more psychotropic medications and anticholinergic medications has also been defined as PIP (Juola et al. 2016). Despite the availability for more than a decade of such tools and definitions to minimize PIP, inappropriate prescribing in LTC populations has not

Table 12.1 Key Forms of Potentially Inappropriate Prescription in Long-Term Care Populations

Type of PIP	Common Examples	Approaches
Medication given with no clear evidence-based indication	Cholinesterase inhibitor (ChEI) given to a resident who has frontotemporal MNCD Antiplatelet given with anticoagulant therapy	Rational deprescribing (taper and discontinue the medication)
Medication given at higher dose or for longer time than necessary	Antipsychotic given at dosage higher than recommended by APA practice guidelines* for treatment of agitation in resident who has MNCD Iron is given at a higher dosage than what can be easily absorbed, leading to gastrointestinal adverse effect that in resident who has MNCD manifests as agitation	Use published guidelines and evidence-based tools** for appropriate dosing of medication
Medication given in combination with another drug from same drug class	Two SSRIs given to treat MDD Two antipsychotics given to treat psychotic disorder	Discontinue one of the medications that has not helped or has more adverse effect for that resident
Medication given in combination with another drug that leads to drug–drug interaction	Antipsychotic medication (dopamine antagonist) given for psychotic symptoms in resident taking dopamine agonist (e.g. ropinirole) for RLS or Parkinson's disease Anticholinergic medication (e.g. oxybutynin) given to resident who has MNCD and is taking a ChEI and/or memantine, resulting in negating of any potential benefit of ChEI and/or memantine	Consider reducing dosage of dopamine agonist to improve psychotic symptoms rather than adding antipsychotic medication Minimize use of anticholinergic medication for resident who has MNCD
Medication given to a resident resulting in drug-disease interaction	Use of benzodiazepine for resident who has advanced COPD SSRI used for a resident who had recent gastrointestinal bleed Psychotropic medication with potential to cause syncope (e.g. ChEI, prazosin) given to a resident who has a recent history of syncope, resulting in medication-induced syncope	Taper and discontinue BZD and use alternative to BZD (Table 12.3) to manage anxiety symptoms Avoid use of SSRI or SNRI for resident at high risk of bleeding Avoid use of ChEI for resident who has bradycardia and/or syncope
Medication given after incorrect diagnosis	Adjustment disorder with depressed mood diagnosed as MDD and resident given an antidepressant Delirium diagnosed as a psychotic disorder and resident given an antipsychotic Asymptomatic bacteriuria and pyuria diagnosed as UTI and resident given an antibiotic	One of the most common reasons for PIP in LTC populations Residents with adjustment disorder may benefit from psychotherapy

Table 12.1 (cont.)

Type of PIP	Common Examples	Approaches
Medication given for a condition to achieve a goal that is not in keeping with overall goals of care	Resident who has limited life expectancy is being treated with multiple medications for diabetes to achieve hemoglobin A1 c of <7.5 when goals of care have been changed to palliative care goals	Resident who has life expectancy of ≤2 years should receive palliative care if it is in keeping with resident's wishes and values, and aggressive treatment of medical comorbidity can be discontinued
Choice and dosage of medication not adjusted for impairment in renal function	See Table 12.5	Input from consultant pharmacist is recommended for appropriate choice of medication and dose adjustment for resident who has renal impairment (especially moderate to severe renal impairment and end-stage renal disease [ESRD])
Choice and dosage of medication not adjusted for impairment in hepatic function	Dosage of acetaminophen is not reduced for resident who has mild impairment of hepatic function, leading to excessive gastrointestinal distress that may manifest as agitation in resident who has MNCD	Input from consultant pharmacist is recommended for appropriate choice of medication and dose adjustment for resident who has hepatic insufficiency
Choice and dosage of medication not adjusted for pre-existing prolonged QTc interval	Many psychotropics (e.g. ziprasidone, citalopram, mirtazapine) prolong QTc, so HCP should avoid prescribing them for resident who has pre-existing prolonged QTc	Routine review of EKG is recommended for any resident before being started on psychotropic medication
Choice and dosage of medication not adjusted for pre-existing cognitive impairment and anticholinergic load	HCP should avoid prescribing drugs with clinically significant anticholinergic activity for resident who has MNCD	HCP should routinely monitor anticholinergic burden (e.g. at time of every prescription and periodically thereafter) using ACBS***
Medication given to a resident who is susceptible to a particular adverse reaction	BZD given to resident who has falls High-potency antipsychotic medication given to resident who has MNCD due to Lewy bodies	Rational deprescribing (taper and discontinue medication)
Medication given when a more cost-effective medication of equal or better effectiveness is available	Use of newer antidepressant (e.g. vortioxetine) when other generic antidepressants have not been given adequate trial	Physician and other healthcare providers need to be more mindful of high costs of many psychotropic medications and awareness of cheaper medications with equal or better effectiveness
Medication not given due to prejudices related to race or ethnicity (underprescribing****)	African Americans are three times less likely to receive antidepressant for MDD than Caucasians	Physician and other healthcare providers need to be more mindful that conscious and unconscious prejudices may prevent them from appropriately treating resident's medical and psychiatric disorders
Medication not given due to lack of knowledge or prejudices related to ageism or economic reasons or fear	HCP did not consider potential benefits of ChEI and memantine for resident who has moderate to severe MNCD due to AD or resident	Physician and other healthcare providers need to be more mindful of their own prejudices and lack of state-of-the-science knowledge,

Table 12.1 (cont.)

Type of PIP	Common Examples	Approaches
of adverse effect (underprescribing)	age 90 years who has mild MNCD due to AD	preventing them from appropriately treating resident's medical and psychiatric disorders
Medication continued despite lack of evidence of benefit	Antidepressant (adequate dose given for adequate time) continued despite no improvement in depressive symptoms	Most psychiatric disorders often require trials of more than one medication before effective medication is identified
Medication given before adequate trial of nondrug approach	Constipation treated with stool softener rather than discontinuing medication that causes constipation and initiating nondrug treatment (e. g. increase intake of fluids and fiber, increase physical activity)	Staff education and training to treat common medical and psychiatric disorders with nondrug approaches is essential component of LTC

* American Psychiatric Association (APA) practice guidelines for the use of antipsychotics for treatment of agitation in persons with dementia. Recommended daily dose range of antipsychotic: aripiprazole: 2–15 mg; olanzapine: 1–15 mg; quetiapine: 25–200 mg; risperidone: 0.5–2 mg; haloperidol: 0.5–4 mg.

** Published guidelines and tools for appropriate dosing of medications: APA practice guidelines for the use of antipsychotics for treatment of agitation in persons with dementia; Beers Criteria; Medication Appropriateness Index (MAI), STOPP/START criteria

*** Anticholinergic Cognitive Burden Scale (ACBS) available at www.agingbraincare.org/uploads/products/ACB_scale_-_legal_size.pdf

**** Underprescribing: Medication is not given for a medical or a psychiatric condition for which drug therapy is indicated according to up-to-date clinical practice guidelines.

diminished. Residents who receive PIP have a much higher chance of serious ADE and accelerated progression of treatable medical and psychiatric disorders, often leading to hospitalization and even death.

PIP is a major public health problem in the older population in general and in LTC populations in particular, due to its high prevalence and serious negative consequences. (See Box 12.1.) Even intermittent exposure to PIP may increase the short-term risk of death. Early detection of all forms of PIP (including underprescription), discontinuation of inappropriate medication, and institution of appropriate nondrug treatment and safer appropriate alternatives are some of the most important approaches to improve the quality of life of residents in LTC. An approach involving review of medication for appropriateness and discontinuing inappropriate medication is called *rational deprescribing* (also called *geriatric scalpel*). Box 12.2 lists basic principles of pharmacological treatment in LTC populations. Table 12.2 lists approaches to reduce PIP and improve appropriate use of medication in LTC populations. See Table 12.3 for common appropriate indications for the use of psychotropic medication in LTC populations. Box 12.3 lists key pharmacological principles for the prevention and treatment of BNPS in LTC populations. Given the complexities and risks involved in the pharmacologic management of BNPS in LTC populations, the principles of care require the HCP to give serious consideration to routinely involving a specialist such as geriatric psychiatrist, geriatrician, or consultant pharmacist.

Each prescription of medication in LTC populations should be highly individualized. The prescriber, pharmacist, resident's nurse, resident, and family should collaboratively review the risks and benefits of each medication prescribed to a LTC resident. Appropriate and judicious use of medication (including psychotropic drugs) has the potential to dramatically improve the quality of life of many LTC residents who have medical and/or psychiatric disorder and their caregivers. We recommend controlling the use of as-needed medication with education, clear dosing instructions, and monitoring usage.

Many drugs are continued much longer than necessary. This is especially true for drugs used to treat agitation and aggression in LTC populations. In many instances, the HCP can safely discontinue a psychotropic drug (gradual withdrawal rather than abrupt discontinuation) without any worsening of

BOX 12.1 Common Serious Adverse Drug Events and Complications Due to the Use of Potentially Inappropriate Prescription in Long-Term Care Populations

- Delirium
- Seizures
- Intestinal obstruction
- Psychotic symptoms
- Hospitalization
- Falls and serious injury (e.g. hip fracture, traumatic brain injury)
- Treatment-resistant psychiatric disorder (e.g. major depressive disorder, generalized anxiety disorder, insomnia disorder)
- Treatment-resistant medical condition (e.g. chronic obstructive pulmonary disease, coronary artery disease, diabetes)
- Accelerated cognitive decline
- Frailty
- Undernutrition
- Urinary incontinence
- Increased costs
- Increased use of health care
- Poorer health-related quality of life
- Increased mortality

behavior or functional capacity. In fact, discontinuation of a psychotropic may often result in some improvement in the resident's cognitive and functional status, indicating that subtle adverse effect of the psychotropic was adding to the resident's cognitive and functional impairment. When choosing an appropriate medication, the HCP should also recognize the effect of nutritional status and lifestyle on drug metabolism. For example, impaired nutrition may be associated with decreased plasma protein (e.g. low albumin) and result in increased levels of some drugs that are highly protein bound (e.g. valproate). When prescribing certain drugs (e.g. acetaminophen), the HCP needs to pay attention to a resident's misuse of alcohol associated with liver damage. The HCP should also recognize the effect of medical disorders on the likelihood of adverse medication reaction. For example, bowel resection may increase the risk of medication-induced diarrhea by medications that have diarrhea as the usual adverse effect (e.g. SSRI-induced diarrhea).

Multiple factors affect the variability of responses to pharmacological treatment. For example, nicotine smokers clear olanzapine and clozapine faster than nonsmokers or past smokers (due to cytochrome P450 1A2 enzyme induction by nicotine), men clear olanzapine faster than women, and African Americans clear olanzapine faster than other races. African Americans usually require lower dosages of lithium than Caucasians, and a larger proportion of African Americans metabolize drugs more slowly. The FDA issued an alert that people of Asian ancestry (e.g. from China, Thailand, Indonesia, Malaysia, Taiwan, Philippines, India) are at significantly increased risk for fatal skin reaction when treated with carbamazepine and should first undergo genetic testing (looking for the presence of human leukocyte antigen B*1502) to assess their risk before initiating therapy. Genetically determined differences in drug metabolism may cause notable variations in a resident's blood level of most psychotropics. For example, residents who are genetically slow or poor metabolizers via the 2D6 hepatic isoenzyme system may develop toxicity with a low dose of medication metabolized by this enzyme (e.g. codeine, paroxetine). For many residents (e.g. residents who are frail, are old-old [age 85 years or older], or have severe kidney and/or liver disease), microdoses (e.g. one-quarter of the usual optimal dose) may be sufficient for therapeutic response. At the same time, even a resident who is in her 90s may try the usual dosages of antidepressant if she is tolerating a low dose well but not showing any benefit. Drug–drug interactions are also a key factor in the selection of a medication. For example, hypertensive drugs may potentiate psychotropic medication (e.g. quetiapine)-induced orthostatic hypotension, and anticonvulsants with hepatic enzyme induction activity (e.g. phenytoin, carbamazepine [CBZ]) substantially lower the level of psychotropic medication metabolized by the liver (e.g. antipsychotic). Many residents cannot swallow tablets or capsules and need the medications crushed. This may limit the use of certain psychotropics (e.g. duloxetine is available as a capsule and cannot be crushed or capsule opened).

Reducing the Anticholinergic Burden

Anticholinergic drugs block muscarinic receptors in the central and peripheral nervous systems (parasympathetic as well as sympathetic effector cells). Muscarinic receptors are distributed throughout the body (e.g. bladder, bowel, salivary glands, ciliary muscle of the eye, heart) and in regions of the brain

BOX 12.2 Basic Principles of Pharmacological Treatment for Long-Term Care Populations

- Use nonpharmacological treatment before pharmacological treatment for mild to moderate symptoms.
- Ensure comprehensive assessment and accurate diagnosis (especially if considering high-risk medication [e.g. opioid, antipsychotic, BZD, mood stabilizer, stimulant]).
- Consider medication only if in keeping with clinical practice guidelines and benefit is expected to be significantly greater than risk.
- Discuss potential risks and benefits of medication with resident and family.
- Educate staff, resident, and family regarding realistic expectation from any psychotropic medication.
- Clearly identify and document reason(s) for prescribing medication (specific condition, target symptoms) and share with team.
- Select medication and dosage based on side-effect profile, resident's preference, past response, allergies, pre-existing condition (e.g. kidney or liver impairment, orthostatic hypotension, prolonged QTc interval, MNCD), anticholinergic properties, propensity for drug–drug interaction, and cost.
- Adjust selection and dosage of medication based on age, gender, lifestyle (e.g. smoker), and racial and ethnic differences in drug metabolism and tolerance.
- Adjust selection of medication based on formulations available (e.g. tablet, capsule, liquid, transdermal patch) and resident's ability to swallow medication.
- Routinely involve consultant pharmacist (especially for high-risk medication) to help select, initiate, and modify medication therapy; to perform comprehensive review of medication to identify, resolve, and prevent medication errors, adverse drug reactions, use of potentially inappropriate prescription, and drug–drug interaction; and help physicians and other healthcare providers follow governmental regulatory (e.g. OBRA) and other guidelines (e.g. clinical practice guidelines).
- Ensure close collaboration among prescribers to achieve optimal communication and avoid potentially inappropriate prescription and medication error.
- Avoid starting more than one new medication at a time or within a few days of each other (especially medications with central nervous system [CNS] effect and medications with similar adverse effect profile).
- Start low, go slow, and, when appropriate, keep going, to achieve therapeutic levels.
- Use adequate dosage for adequate time.
- Periodically monitor renal function and adjust dosage of renally excreted medication (or active metabolite), as a substantial proportion of LTC populations have chronic kidney disease that may progress over time.
- Monitor response to medication, toxicity, and drug–drug interaction (especially after adding new medication).
- Avoid prescribing more medication simply to treat side effect of previous medication (prescribing cascade).
- Promptly taper and discontinue medication if there is significant adverse effect, drug–drug interaction, or lack of or marginal response.
- Consider periodic taper and discontinuation of medication (especially high-risk medication) if problem is under control for sufficient duration.
- Educate staff to detect overt and subtle adverse effect of prescribed medication.

(e.g. nucleus basalis of Meynert, hippocampus) involved in cognitive function (e.g. attention, memory). The use of anticholinergic drugs is prevalent in LTC populations. Parkinson's disease, irritable bowel syndrome (IBS) with diarrhea, urinary incontinence, and drug-induced Parkinsonism are common conditions in LTC populations for which some drugs have been specifically used for their intended anticholinergic activity. Other medications with significant anticholinergic activity that are commonly used in LTC populations include some antidepressants, antipsychotics, opioid analgesics, muscle relaxants, and antihistamines. The use of anticholinergic drugs is associated with many serious ADEs (e.g. delirium, urinary retention, severe constipation or bowel obstruction, falls and injury, accelerated cognitive decline, agitation, aggressive behavior, visual hallucination, and other psychotic symptoms) as well as other major ADEs (e.g. daytime sedation, constipation, dry mouth, blurred vision, negating the beneficial effect of ChEI and memantine) (Gerretsen and Pollock 2011).

The combined effect of multiple drugs with anticholinergic activity is referred to as the "anticholinergic

Table 12.2 Approaches to Reduce Potentially Inappropriate Prescription and Improve Appropriate Use of Medication

Approach	Examples	Comments
Involve consultant pharmacist	Leads medication review Physician and other healthcare providers routinely consult pharmacist if resident is taking ≥10 medications or ≥2 high-risk medications (e.g. opioid, antipsychotic, BZD, stimulant, warfarin, mood stabilizer, insulin) Consultant pharmacist and nurse review resident's medications before transfer from hospital to LTC facility to clarify details with hospital team (medication reconciliation) Fleetwood model* for improving appropriate use of medication	Involvement of consultant pharmacist should be expanded so that all residents at time of admission and periodically thereafter benefit from their input
Standardized medication reconciliation process	Physician and other healthcare providers work collaboratively with consultant pharmacist, nurse, resident, and family to reconcile medications taken by resident at time of admission (especially after acute hospital stay)	Although aimed at preventing medication errors, medication reconciliation provides ideal opportunity for rational deprescribing for any inappropriate medication resident may be taking
Six-step Geriatric-Palliative Methodology	1. Presence of evidence-based consensus for using medication for the indication 2. Indication seems valid and relevant to particular resident's age group and disability level 3. Benefits outweigh risks for resident 4. Absence of adverse effect 5. Absence of safer alternative 6. Dosage can be reduced without significant risk	Physician and other healthcare providers lead efforts in consultation with pharmacist to use this methodology to safely discontinue multiple medications simultaneously
Computerized Decision Support (CDS)	Electronic alerts guide physicians and other healthcare providers to right treatment Electronic support for risk screening tools to identify PIP	Many CDS systems may not be up to date regarding clinical practice guidelines and risk-screening tools
Involvement of psychiatrist (preferably geriatric psychiatrist)	Consulted regarding psychiatric ADEs of medication for a particular resident and safer alternative (nondrug and psychotropic) Academic detailing**	HCP should routinely consider psychiatric consultation for use of antipsychotic in LTC populations
Geriatrician	Consulted regarding rational deprescription in complex cases (e.g. resident is frail and taking ≥10 medications) Leads case conferences to serve both clinical and educational purposes Academic detailing	Geriatrician can be involved via telemedicine

Table 12.2 (cont.)

Approach	Examples	Comments
Pharmacogenetic testing (pharmacogenomic testing)	Pharmacogenetic testing clarifies choice of antidepressant for resident who has treatment-resistant MDD Pharmacogenetic testing clarifies choice of opioid analgesic for resident who has treatment-resistant severe pain syndrome	Collaboration with consultant pharmacist is recommended for accurate interpretation of genetic testing results
Staff education	All nurses are provided with basic information about risks of PIP and common drugs responsible for PIP	Case-based staff education about PIP should be routinely done for all nurses periodically (e.g. once a month)
Multidisciplinary case conferences	On a monthly basis, primary care team, consultant pharmacist, geriatric psychiatrist, geriatrician, and staff discuss resident cases, with one goal being to reduce PIP Brief review of high-quality studies during case conferences on benefits of reducing PIP and sharing research study article with team	Specialist can be present via video if access to specialist is a barrier
Educational programs aimed at physicians and other healthcare providers	Programs provided by national and international professional organizations*** on PIP and evidence-based tools to identify PIP	Organizations should make such programs available for free on their website with option to obtain free continuing education credits
Educational programs aimed at medical students and residents and students in other healthcare provider training programs	Pharmacogeriatric training provided in medical schools and residency programs as well as other healthcare provider training programs	Pharmacogeriatric training should be essential component of basic training for all future physicians and other healthcare providers
Treatments targeted to resident and family	Education to help recognize that resident's and family's expectations from medications are too high and that they may be minimizing potential risks of medications Provide educational material, leaflets, and handouts from reputable organizations Motivational interviewing to help residents engage better in nonpharmacological strategies to address problems rather than rely on pharmacological strategies	Facility should have routine group medication meetings with resident (especially resident who has relatively preserved cognitive function) and family to improve health literacy regarding PIP
Organizational approaches	Regular audits and feedback related to PIP Facility-wide directives with specific goals related to reduction of PIP (e.g. average anticholinergic burden will be reduced by 25% within six months)	Facility leadership team (e.g. medical director, facility administrator, director of nursing) can play key role in making reduction of PIP a priority

Table 12.2 (cont.)

Approach	Examples	Comments
	Local consensus process in which medical director, physician, other healthcare providers, and consultant pharmacist can agree on specific PIPs (e.g. opioid for chronic noncancer pain) that can be focus of quality-improvement project	
Other approaches	Financial incentives by health insurance companies Changes in government policies or legislation affecting prescribing	Academic institutions and national professional organizations should guide health insurance companies and government to create practical, feasible, and state-of-the-science guidelines regarding PIP in LTC populations
Multifaceted approaches	Combination of above-mentioned approaches tailored to needs and resources of facility	Facility leadership team (e.g. medical director, facility administrator, director of nursing) can play a key role in making reduction of PIP a priority by adopting multifaceted approaches

* Fleetwood model uses medication review by a pharmacist, direct communication with the prescriber, and formalized pharmacotherapy planning for a resident at risk of medication-related problems.

** Academic detailing: A trained professional (usually a specialist such as a geriatric psychiatrist) visits the physician / other healthcare provider in the LTC setting to provide education and guidance

*** National and international organizations that may offer educational programs: American Psychiatric Association, American Association of Geriatric Psychiatry, International Psychogeriatric Association, American Geriatrics Society, Society for Post-Acute and Long-Term Care (formerly known as American Medical Directors Association), Ontario Pharmacy Research Collaboration, American Society of Consultant Pharmacists

burden" or "anticholinergic load." The HCP should closely monitor the cumulative anticholinergic burden of various commonly prescribed drugs that have anticholinergic activity and try to replace some of them with safer alternatives. (See Table 12.4.) We recommend using the Anticholinergic Cognitive Burden Scale (ACBS), developed by Dr. Malaz Boustani and colleagues at the Regenstrief Institute and Indiana University Center of Aging Research, to assess the anticholinergic burden of medications (www.agingbraincare.org/uploads/products/ACB_scale_-_legal_size.pdf). The scale gives one point to each medication that has been found to have anticholinergic activity in the laboratory but no clinically relevant anticholinergic effect has been observed. Two or three points are given to medications that have clinically relevant anticholinergic effect. Zero points are given for a medication with no known anticholinergic activity. In general, the total cumulative score should be as low as possible, preferably below 3. The HCP can also use the Anticholinergic Risk Scale, which uses a similar point system (0–3) to identify anticholinergic medications (Rudolph et al. 2008). Serum anticholinergic activity, a measure of peripheral blood anticholinergic burden, is being used in the research setting and may become available for clinical use. The HCP should avoid prescribing certain highly anticholinergic medications (e.g. tertiary tricyclic antidepressant [amitriptyline, imipramine, doxepin, trimipramine], scopolamine, diphenhydramine, hydroxyzine) for LTC populations.

Adjusting Psychotropic Medication for a Resident Who Has Renal Impairment

Renal impairment can significantly alter the risk-benefit ratio of many commonly used psychotropic medications (Ward et al. 2016). (See Table 12.5.) Some residents who have done well taking certain psychotropics (e.g. bupropion, lithium) and develop renal impairment (or gradually declining renal function) can continue taking these medications at lower

Table 12.3 Common Appropriate Indications for Prescribing Psychotropic Medication for Long-Term Care Populations

Category of Psychotropic Medication	Common Appropriate Indications	Clinical Pearls
Antidepressant	MDD and MDD-like symptoms due to MNCD or another medical condition (e.g. stroke) Persistent depressive disorder Complicated grief reaction Bipolar disorder Schizoaffective disorder PTSD OCD Generalized anxiety disorder Panic disorder Chronic pain syndrome Duloxetine can be used to treat pain related to diabetic neuropathy, fibromyalgia, and chronic low back pain Milnacipran can be used to treat fibromyalgia	HCP should avoid antidepressant monotherapy with individual who has bipolar disorder due to risk of destabilizing bipolar disorder (e.g. switching depression to mania, inducing rapid cycling) Use of citalopram and escitalopram to manage severe and persistent agitation due to MNCD and to manage severe and persistent sexually inappropriate behavior in the context of MNCD may be appropriate in certain situations SNRI (e.g. venlafaxine, duloxetine, desvenlafaxine) is preferred over other antidepressant to manage chronic pain
Stimulant	MDD (especially when rapid response is needed [e.g. resident receiving hospice care]) ADHD Narcolepsy	Stimulants may also be used in certain situations (e.g. EOL care) to reduce opioid-induced drowsiness and fatigue Stimulants may also be used for resident who has severe apathy in the context of MNCD
Antipsychotic	Schizophrenia and schizoaffective disorder Bipolar disorder MDD with psychotic symptoms Treatment-resistant MDD* Delirium with severe agitation and psychotic symptoms Severe agitation in resident who has MNCD**	HCP should prescribe antipsychotic only for a short term (few days to two weeks) to manage severe agitation and psychotic symptoms in the context of delirium
Mood stabilizer***	Bipolar disorder Schizoaffective disorder	HCP should avoid prescribing lithium and carbamazepine in LTC populations due to high risk of toxicity, although for some residents, benefits may be higher than risks because underlying psychiatric disorder is extremely disabling and life threatening without lithium or carbamazepine
Hypnotic****	Insomnia disorder	We recommend only short-term use of zaleplon, zolpidem, and eszopiclone due to limited evidence for long-term use in LTC populations and high associated risks (e.g. falls) HCP may prescribe ramelteon and suvorexant judiciously for long-term treatment HCP should avoid prescribing doxepin (with rare exceptions) in LTC populations due to its significant anticholinergic effect

Table 12.3 (cont.)

Category of Psychotropic Medication	Common Appropriate Indications	Clinical Pearls
Tasimelteon	Non-24-hour Circadian Rhythm Disorder	A resident who is blind (especially congenitally blind) may have disabling sleep disturbance due to this disorder and may benefit from a judicious trial of tasimelteon
Buspirone	GAD and GAD-like symptoms due to MNCD and/or another medical condition (e.g. stroke, ESRD)	Noticeable benefit usually takes six weeks
Dextromethorphan-quinidine combination	Pseudobulbar affect	Use of dextromethorphan-quinidine to manage severe and persistent agitation due to MNCD may be appropriate in certain situations
Pimavanserin	Parkinson's disease psychosis (PDP)	Pimavanserin is the only FDA approved medication for the treatment of PDP
Benzodiazepine (BZD)	GAD Panic disorder PTSD Severe anxiety symptoms in the context of another medical condition (e.g. before dialysis)	BZD (along with antipsychotic, mood stabilizer, stimulant) is high-risk psychotropic medication in LTC populations, and HCP should prescribe it at lowest possible dosage for shortest possible time (with rare exceptions [e.g. maximizing comfort during EOL care])
Prazosin	Nightmares in the context of PTSD and other trauma-related disorder	In LTC populations, HCP needs to prescribe prazosin judiciously due to significant risk of orthostatic hypotension (due to alpha-2 blocking effect) and drug–drug interaction with other cardiovascular medication
Modafinil, armodafinil	Excessive daytime sedation in resident who has obstructive sleep apnea not responding to continuous positive airway pressure (CPAP) Narcolepsy	Modafinil and armodafinil may be appropriate to treat fatigue, opioid-induced daytime sedation, and treatment-resistant depression in certain situations
Clonidine, guanfacine	ADHD	In LTC populations, HCP needs to prescribe clonidine and guanfacine judiciously due to significant risk of orthostatic hypotension (due to alpha-2 blocking effect) and drug-drug interaction with other cardiovascular medication

* Aripiprazole, quetiapine, brexpiprazole and olanzapine are the only FDA-approved drugs to treat treatment-resistant MDD (olanzapine approved only when used in combination with fluoxetine).

** Use of antipsychotic to manage severe agitation in a resident who has MNCD should follow the American Psychiatric Association Practice Guidelines for the use of antipsychotics for the treatment of agitation in persons with dementia. No antipsychotic is approved by the FDA for treatment of agitation / severe behavioral and psychological symptoms of dementia in the United States. Risperidone is the only antipsychotic approved for short-term (6 weeks) treatment of severe behavioral and psychological symptoms of dementia (symptoms are unresponsive to psychosocial interventions or there is severe and complex risk of harm) in Australia, Canada, Great Britain and New Zealand.

*** Mood stabilizer: lithium, valproate, lamotrigine, and carbamazepine are the only mood stabilizers approved by the FDA to treat bipolar disorder.

**** Hypnotic: zaleplon, zolpidem, eszopiclone, ramelteon, suvorexant, and low-dose doxepin are the only non-BZD FDA-approved drugs to treat insomnia disorder.

BOX 12.3 Key Pharmacological Principles for the Prevention and Treatment of Behavioral, Neurocognitive, and Psychological Symptoms in Long-Term Care Populations

1. Reduce potentially inappropriate prescription.
2. Improve appropriate prescription (appropriate indication, dose, duration of treatment, close monitoring).
3. Prevent, reduce, and promptly treat adverse drug event.
4. Prevent and promptly treat drug–drug interaction.
5. Reduce burden of medication (i.e., reduce number of medications and/or amount [dosage] of medication consumed).
6. Minimize medication errors (wrong drug, wrong dose of drug, drug not given/taken).
7. Use "start low and go slow" approach when prescribing medication.
8. Taper and discontinue rather than abruptly discontinue or dramatically decrease medication that resident has been taking for months to years.

dosages and lower frequency (e.g. every other day or every third day for a resident who has ESRD) to continue to keep the debilitating mental illness under control. We recommend that the HCP consult with a pharmacist in complicated cases (e.g. a resident who has ESRD or treatment-resistant symptoms).

Reducing the Use of High-Risk Medication

From a mental health perspective, opioids, antipsychotics, BZDs, dopamine agonists, corticosteroids, and stimulants are high-risk medication, as their use is frequently associated with serious ADE (e.g. delirium). Comprehensive geriatric assessment and use of treatments listed in Table 12.2 to reduce PIP and improve appropriate use of medication is the first step in reducing the use of high-risk medication in LTC populations. See Tables 12.6, 12.7, and 12.8 for practical strategies to reduce the use of opioids, antipsychotics, and BZDs in LTC populations. Use of stimulants should be restricted to management of MDD during EOL care and in certain specific situations (e.g. poststroke severe MDD interfering with participation in physical therapy and requiring rapidly acting antidepressant; severe apathy in a resident who has MNCD and does not have significant cardiovascular disease).

Minimizing Medication Errors

A high number of daily medications are administered in LTC facilities. Medication errors are common in LTC populations. Most serious errors occur at the time a resident is admitted after an acute hospital stay. Most common errors involve medication given at the wrong time. Other common errors include wrong dose of medication given, dose of medication was omitted, extra dose was given, unauthorized drug was given, or wrong drug was given. Medication errors carry a potential risk of adverse effect on residents' cognition, behavior, and psychological wellbeing. They may also be fatal. A resident who is taking high-risk medication (e.g. warfarin, insulin, levodopa) or who has a complex health problem is especially at risk for serious adverse consequences of medication error. Standardized medication reconciliation process at the time of admission (especially after an acute hospital stay) by the physician, physician assistant, nurse practitioner, consultant pharmacist, and nurse working collaboratively is a crucial component of overall strategies and initiatives to reduce serious adverse health consequences due to medication error. Every LTC facility should have policies and procedures in place to minimize medication error. We recommend a systems-based approach to medication error that assumes that individuals are doing their best. Such an approach should use proven protocols and processes that ensure effective communication, consistent knowledge and education, and a means of flagging errors and potential problems. We also recommend institutional safeguards to minimize medication error. Reducing medication burden is a key component of reducing medication error. (See Box 12.4.)

Clinical Case 1: "Leave me alone"

Mrs. L, an 82-year-old married woman living in a nursing home who had chronic pain and chronic MDD, had been doing well taking antidepressants (mirtazapine 15 mg at bedtime and duloxetine 30 mg daily) and using fentanyl pain patch (25 mcg/hour every three days) for more than six months but started showing drowsiness and unsteadiness over the last two days. Staff reported that Mrs. L had been shouting to various staff members, "Leave me alone. I don't feel like getting up." The staff called her psychiatrist to request as-needed lorazepam to calm her

Table 12.4 Anticholinergic Drugs and Safer Alternatives

Condition(s)	Anticholinergic Medication(s)	Safer Alternatives
Insomnia	Diphenhydramine	Nondrug approaches to improve sleep Melatonin, Trazodone
Overactive bladder (OAB)	Oxybutynin, tolterodine, solifenacin	Nondrug approaches to reduce some symptoms of OAB (e.g. scheduled toileting, prompted voiding, and biofeedback to reduce urinary incontinence and nocturia) Discontinuing diuretic Mirabegron (beta-3 adrenergic agonist)
Allergy	Diphenhydramine, chlorpheniramine, dimenhydrinate, cyproheptadine	Nondrug approaches (e.g. avoiding allergen, resident education, emotional support to help resident learn to cope with mild to moderate symptoms) Fexofenadine, loratadine
Itching	Hydroxyzine, doxepin	Discontinuing drug that may cause or worsen itching (e.g. opioid, lamotrigine) Nondrug approaches (e.g. moisturizing skin daily, adequate hydration)
Diarrhea	Diphenoxylate, dicyclomine, atropine, loperamide, belladonna, hyocyamine, propantheline	Avoid prescribing antidiarrheal for diarrhea due to infectious cause Discontinue medication causing diarrhea
Nausea	Prochlorperazine, promethazine, metoclopramide, trimethobenzamide	Ondansetron
Gastroparesis	Metoclopramide	Nondrug approaches (e.g. consulting a dietician, resident education, emotional support to help resident learn to cope with mild to moderate symptoms)
Neuropathic pain	Amitriptyline	Gabapentin, pregabalin, duloxetine
Dyspepsia	Cimetidine, ranitidine (H2 receptor blockers)	Famotidine (H2 receptor blocker), PPI*
Muscle spasm, spasticity	Cyclobenzaprine, carisoprodol, metaxolone, methocarbamol	Passive range-of-motion exercise Physical therapy Massage therapy Tizanidine Botulinum toxin injection
Vertigo, dizziness	Meclizine	Nondrug approaches (e.g. vestibular rehabilitation) for motivated resident who has relatively preserved cognitive function Discontinue medication that may cause or worsen vertigo and dizziness
Moderate to severe pain	Meperidine, pentazocine	Tramadol, hydrocodone, oxycodone, morphine, hydromorphone

Table 12.4 (cont.)

Condition(s)	Anticholinergic Medication(s)	Safer Alternatives
MDD	Tricyclic antidepressant (imipramine, amitriptyline, doxepin, nortriptyline, desipramine), paroxetine	SSRI (e.g. citalopram, escitalopram, sertraline), SNRI (venlafaxine, duloxetine, desvenlafaxine), bupropion, mirtazapine, vortioxetine, vilazodone, milnacipran, levomilnacipran, selegiline patch
Psychotic disorder	Thioridazine, mesoridazine, chlorpromazine	Risperidone, aripiprazole, cariprazine, lurasidone, paliperidone, iloperidone, asenapine, brexpiprazole, haloperidol

* PPI: proton pump inhibitor (e.g. omeprazole)

Table 12.5 Psychotropic Medications Requiring Adjustment for a Resident Who Has Renal Impairment

Medication	Renal Impairment*	Clinical Pearls
Risperidone	Mild and moderate impairment: no adjustment Severe impairment and ESRD: use lower dose (0.25–0.5 mg once daily) and increase more slowly (e.g. one-week interval)	Small amount of active metabolite renally excreted
Paliperidone	Mild impairment: start at 3 mg once daily and increase after a week if necessary to maximum of 6 mg Moderate to severe impairment: start at 1.5 mg once daily and increase after one week if necessary to maximum of 3 mg per day Avoid with resident who has ESRD	Primarily renally excreted
Lurasidone	Mild impairment: no adjustment Moderate to severe impairment: start at 20 mg/day on full stomach and increase slowly (20 mg/week) if necessary to maximum of 80 mg/day Avoid with resident who has ESRD	Before increasing the dosage, HCP should ensure that lurasidone is taken right after a meal (350 kcal or more), as only 50% may be absorbed on empty stomach
Ziprasidone	Reduced dosage recommended because of risk of cardiac arrhythmia, as electrographic changes are common in resident who has renal disease (especially moderate to severe and ESRD)	Before increasing the dosage, HCP should ensure that ziprasidone is taken right after a meal (500 kcal or more), as only 50% may be absorbed on empty stomach
Citalopram	Mild to moderate impairment: no adjustment Severe impairment and ESRD: use lower dosage and increase slowly	For resident age 60 years or older, there is FDA advisory to avoid using more than 20 mg daily due to risk of prolongation of QTc interval
Escitalopram	Mild to moderate impairment: no adjustment Severe impairment and ESRD: use lower dosage and increase slowly	Risk of QTc prolongation is about half that of citalopram
Paroxetine	Mild to moderate impairment: no adjustment Severe impairment and ESRD: use lower dosage and increase slowly	HCP should avoid prescribing for LTC populations due to risk of anticholinergic adverse effect and drug–drug interaction due to cytochrome P450 2D6 inhibitory effect

Table 12.5 (cont.)

Medication	Renal Impairment*	Clinical Pearls
Venlafaxine	Mild to severe impairment: use lower dosage and increase slowly ESRD: low dose every other day, given after dialysis	Some amount of venlafaxine and its metabolite O-desmethylvenlafaxine (desvenlafaxine) are primarily renally excreted
Desvenlafaxine	Mild to severe impairment: use lower dosage and increase slowly ESRD: low dose every other day, given after dialysis	Primarily renally excreted
Duloxetine	Mild to moderate impairment: no adjustment Severe impairment and ESRD: avoid use	Active metabolite renally excreted
Bupropion	Mild to moderate impairment: use lower dosage and increase slowly Severe impairment and ESRD: avoid use	Hydroxybupropion is active metabolite of bupropion that is renally excreted Risk of seizure is primary reason to adjust dosage or avoid use
Milnacipran	Mild impairment: no adjustment Moderate to severe impairment: use lower dosage and increase slowly ESRD: avoid use	Use with caution, as it has not been studied in LTC populations
Levomilnacipran	Mild impairment: no adjustment Moderate to severe impairment: use lower dosage and increase slowly ESRD: avoid use	Use with caution, as it has not been studied in LTC populations
Tricyclic antidepressant	Mild impairment: use lower dosage and increase slowly Moderate to severe impairment and ESRD: avoid use	Avoid prescribing for resident who has moderate to severe impairment and ESRD primarily due to risk of cardiac arrhythmia
Monoamine oxidase inhibitor	Mild impairment: use lower dosage and increase slowly Moderate to severe impairment and ESRD: avoid use	Avoid prescribing for resident who has moderate to severe impairment and ESRD primarily due to increased risk of dialysis-induced hypotension
Lithium	Mild impairment: use lower dosage and increase slowly Moderate to severe impairment and ESRD: avoid use (with exceptions)	Primarily renally excreted and has direct nephrotoxic effect For resident who has severe bipolar disorder that has responded best to lithium, it may be appropriate to continue it judiciously with close monitoring and close working with nephrologist despite its risks
Lamotrigine	Mild to moderate impairment: no adjustment Severe impairment and ESRD: use lower dosage and increase slowly	Consultation with pharmacist is recommended for resident who has ESRD
Oxcarbazepine	Mild to moderate impairment: no adjustment Severe impairment and ESRD: use lower dosage and increase slowly	Consultation with pharmacist is recommended for resident who has ESRD

* Renal impairment: mild: creatinine clearance 90–60 ml/min; moderate: creatinine clearance 30–60 ml/min; severe: creatinine clearance 10–30 ml/min; end-stage renal disease (ESRD): creatinine clearance less than 10 mil/min

Table 12.6 Alternatives to Opioid for the Management of Chronic or Persistent Noncancer Pain

Alternative	Clinical Situation	Clinical Pearls
Acetaminophen	Mild to moderate musculoskeletal pain (e.g. arthritis) Combination of acetaminophen with other analgesic (e.g. tramadol) and nondrug approach may help prevent need for opioid	For resident who has MNCD, scheduled dosage is preferred to as-needed
Topical analgesic (over-the-counter* as well as prescription**)	Especially beneficial for localized pain (e.g. shoulder pain, lower back pain) Lidoderm patch is approved by FDA to treat postherpetic neuralgia	Staff education is needed in appropriate use of topical analgesic
Nonsteroidal anti-inflammatory drug (NSAID)	Especially beneficial for acute musculoskeletal (nociceptive) pain (e.g. acute bout of gout)	Short-term use can be safe, but long-term use is not recommended due to significant risks of gastric ulcer, nephrotoxicity, and cardiotoxicity
Cox-2 inhibitor (e.g. celecoxib)	Especially beneficial for acute musculoskeletal (nociceptive) pain (e.g. acute bout of gout)	Short-term use can be safe, but long-term use is not recommended due to significant risks of nephrotoxicity and cardiotoxicity
Nondrug approach	Physical therapy (e.g. after hip surgery, knee surgery) Multisensory stimulation therapy Cognitive behavioral therapy for resident who has relatively preserved cognitive function Meditation and mindfulness practices, such as yoga, Tai Chi (e.g. for cancer pain) Cold compress (e.g. for acute pain and swelling of knee after a fall, for neuropathic pain) Warm compress (e.g. for chronic arthritis in hand joints) Positioning Motivational interviewing (e.g. to avoid opioid, engage in nondrug approach) Distraction (e.g. watching funny video) and relaxation strategies (e.g. visualization exercise) Massage therapy Acupuncture, acupressure	Staff education and training are required for vigorous and appropriate use of these approaches Support from primary care team and facility leadership required for routine aggressive use of nondrug approaches Handouts on nondrug approaches can be helpful for motivated resident who has relatively preserved cognitive functioning
Antidepressant	Serotonin-norepinephrine reuptake inhibitor (SNRI) (e.g. venlafaxine, duloxetine, desvenlafaxine) useful for chronic pain even in absence of depression Duloxetine is approved by FDA to treat diabetic neuropathy, fibromyalgia, and chronic low back pain Milnacipran is approved by FDA to treat fibromyalgia	Antidepressants are underused for management of chronic pain in LTC populations No resident should be prescribed opioid for chronic noncancer pain without discussion of potential benefit of SNRI

Table 12.6 (cont.)

Alternative	Clinical Situation	Clinical Pearls
Anticonvulsant	Gabapentin and pregabalin are recommended to treat neuropathic pain (e.g. diabetic neuropathy) Pregabalin is approved by FDA to treat fibromyalgia	Neuropathic pain and nociceptive pain are often co-occurring and hence rational polypharmacy for pain management may be appropriate for resident who has moderate to severe chronic pain

* Topical over-the-counter (OTC) analgesic: methyl salicylate, menthol, capsaicin

** Topical prescription analgesic: diclofenac gel, lidocaine 5% patch

Table 12.7 Approaches to Reduce the Use of Antipsychotic to Manage Agitation and Aggression in a Resident Who Has Major Neurocognitive Disorder

Alternative	Key Examples	Practical Pearls
Staff education, training, and support	Training in therapeutic communication (especially with resident who has MNCD) Providing specific guidance to staff regarding countertherapeutic interactions they are engaging in with a specific resident who is severely agitated and coaching them in therapeutic interactions using role play Facility leaders routinely appreciate staff in a visible way	Countertherapeutic interaction (e.g. arguing with resident who has MNCD, repeatedly correcting resident who has MNCD) is common cause of agitation Staff who feel supported are more likely to use their education and training to more effectively identify reversible causes of agitation and engage in therapeutic ways with resident Facility administrator cooks once a week for staff members whose birthdays fall in that week as a demonstration of staff appreciation
SPPEICE*	Continuous activity programming	Boredom and loneliness are two most common causes of depression, anxiety, and agitation in LTC populations
Effective pain management	Empirical trial with analgesic (e.g. acetaminophen) before initiating psychotropic medication to treat agitation	Staff education and training in detection of pain in resident who has advanced MNCD is a key component of effort to reduce use of antipsychotic in LTC populations
Early identification and treatment of medical condition(s) causing agitation	Delirium, medication-induced agitation, constipation, UTI, dental problem, electrolyte imbalance, dermatologic condition, undernutrition (including dehydration), hypo/hyperglycemia and over- or undercorrection of thyroid disorder are ten most common medical conditions (besides pain) that cause agitation in resident who has MNCD	Thorough assessment and team discussion to identify one or more reversible medical conditions (especially these ten conditions) is recommended before initiation of any psychotropic to manage agitation

Table 12.7 (cont.)

Alternative	Key Examples	Practical Pearls
Addressing sensory deficit(s)	Correcting reversible cause of sensory deficit (e.g. ear wax) and ensuring appropriate use of sensory aid	Staff education and training is required to ensure that hearing aids are used appropriately
Addressing underlying psychiatric condition(s) causing agitation	MDD and generalized anxiety disorder (GAD) are common causes of agitation in resident who has MNCD and can be effectively treated with appropriate antidepressant	Cornell Scale for Depression in Dementia is recommended for improving accurate diagnosis of MDD-like symptoms in resident who has advanced MCND
Citalopram / Escitalopram	May be used to manage moderate to severe agitation in resident who has MNCD not responding to other approaches	HCP should consider prescribing trial of citalopram or escitalopram before initiating antipsychotic
Dextroamphetamine with Quinidine	Approved by FDA to treat pseudobulbar affect May be used to manage moderate to severe agitation in resident who has MNCD not responding to other approaches	HCP should consider prescribing trial of dextroamphetamine-quinidine before initiating antipsychotic

* SPPEICE: strength-based, personalized, psychosocial spiritual sensory environmental initiatives and creative engagement

Table 12.8 Alternatives to Benzodiazepine for the Management of Chronic Anxiety Symptoms in Long-Term Care Populations

Alternative	Clinical Situations	Practice Pearls
SPPEICE	Especially useful for anxiety symptoms in resident who has MNCD	Knowing the resident well is key to identifying SPPEICE that are effective
Relaxation training	HCP should offer resident who has relatively preserved cognitive function high-quality education and training in relaxation strategies	Staff competency should include knowledge and skills in teaching and helping residents use various relaxation strategies (e.g. deep breathing, visualization, deep muscle relaxation)
Individual and/or group psychotherapy*	HCP should offer resident who has relatively preserved cognitive function individual and/or group therapy	HCP should consider telepsychotherapy or Internet-based CBT if access to trained counselor is a barrier
SSRI and SNRI	Appropriate for treatment of chronic anxiety disorder (e.g. generalized anxiety disorder [GAD], panic disorder) and chronic anxiety related to PTSD	It may take at least six weeks before relief of anxiety is noticeable
Buspirone	Appropriate for treatment of GAD and GAD-like symptoms in resident who has MNCD	It may take at least six weeks before relief of anxiety is noticeable

* Individual and/or group psychotherapy: cognitive behavioral therapy (CBT), mindfulness-based stress reduction (MBSR)

BOX 12.4 **Strategies to Reduce the Burden of Medication**

- Discontinue unnecessary medication.
- Discontinue medication that has been not beneficial or only marginally beneficial.
- Discontinue medication that was effective before but is not expected to provide continued benefit.
- Discontinue medication that was given on a trial basis but found not to be beneficial.
- Reduce the dosage of medication because of significant change in the resident's health (e.g. increasing frailty, advancing MNCD, stroke, decline in liver or kidney function).
- Use a combination of medications (e.g. acetaminophen with oxycodone) when appropriate and feasible.
- Reduce the frequency of medication (e.g. change medication given three times a day to twice a day when pharmacokinetics of the medication allow).
- Switch from short-acting medication formulation to long-acting formulation if there are no adverse side effects or cost issues (e.g. venlafaxine changed to venlafaxine extended release; bupropion changed to bupropion sustained release or extended release).

Note: Burden of medication = total number of medications, total number of pills, and total amount [dose] of medications

or to reduce her "psych medications" due to drowsiness. The psychiatrist recommended an urgent same-day assessment at his office, as this behavior was new, of sudden onset, and uncharacteristic. Mrs. L could not be brought on the same day, but her husband brought her late the next day. Mrs. L was calm and pleasant during the visit. The psychiatrist asked Mr. L if he was aware of Mrs. L's drowsiness and aggressive behavior. Mr. L replied that he had figured out why Mrs. L's condition had changed. He had checked Mrs. L's pain patch and found that the staff had forgotten to remove the previous one when they put on a new patch two days ago.

Teaching Point

Although psychiatric medications often may be responsible for sedation and unsteady gait, we recommend a thorough assessment to identify various other potential causes of an acute change in behavior. The HCP should always keep the possibility of medication error in the differential diagnosis, especially if the patient has been stable for some time. Also, an informed and astute caregiver (the husband in this case) can often help quickly identify the cause of an acute change in behavior.

Improving the Prescription of Appropriate Medication

LTC residents often require complex medication regimens that substantially increase the risk of adverse drug event or suboptimal pharmacotherapy. To improve the prescription of appropriate medication, we recommend the model proposed by the American Society of Consultant Pharmacists, the Fleetwood Model (Lapane et al. 2011). This model includes using consultant pharmacists with demonstrated expertise in geriatric pharmacotherapy, direct resident assessment by the pharmacist, increased interaction between the pharmacist and prescribing health professionals, evidence-based practices, and explicit assessments of patient outcome. Treatment algorithms for pharmacists to use when making clinical recommendations regarding safer alternatives to potentially inappropriate medication in the older population have been developed. One of the key principles of prescribing appropriate medication is the selection of drugs with minimal or no anticholinergic activity. Table 12.2 lists treatments to improve appropriate medication prescription, and Table 12.3 lists appropriate indications for the use of psychotropic medication in LTC populations.

Prevention and Treatment of Adverse Drug Events

Adverse drug events are prevalent in LTC populations, and more than half are of a potentially life-threatening nature. They often masquerade as a new-onset medical or psychiatric syndrome (Kotlyar et al. 2011). Early accurate recognition of ADE improves outcomes and avoids unnecessary testing and costs. ADEs are eminently preventable. Some 80 percent of preventable ADEs – many of them involving central nervous system agents – occur during ordering and monitoring; dispensing accounts for only 5 percent of such errors and administration for 13 percent. The HCP should view ADE (due to prescribing either inappropriate or appropriate medication) as avoidable by altering existing medication regimens rather than an inevitable part of the aging process. ADEs are a serious safety concern and a key part of the larger quality-improvement picture in the LTC context.

ADEs can manifest as physical problems and functional decline, but often the only manifestation may be accelerated cognitive decline and/or BNPS, especially in a resident who has advanced MNCD. Neuropsychiatric events, such as oversedation, confusion, hallucinations, and delirium, are the most common ADE, comprising 24 percent of the total and 29 percent of preventable events. Hemorrhagic and gastrointestinal events follow closely behind. Medications most commonly implicated in producing ADE in LTC populations include anticholinergic, dopamine agonists, steroids, warfarin, conventional and atypical antipsychotic, loop diuretic, BZD, opioid, insulin, digoxin, antiepileptic, and angiotensin-converting enzyme inhibitor. ADEs are common because of a "prescribing cascade" that begins when an ADE is misinterpreted as a new medical condition. Another drug is prescribed and an adverse effect happens, which is again mistaken for a new medical condition. Then a new drug is prescribed, and the resident is placed at risk of developing more adverse effect from the added medication. (See Table 12.9.) Also, we need to do a better job in recognizing the impact that subtle medication-related adverse effects have on residents. A resident may not be able to recognize or communicate adverse effect from medication she is being given. Therefore, physicians, physician assistants, and nurse practitioners should act pre-emptively to select medication with the best adverse effect profile and avoid potentially toxic dosages.

Many drugs may cause or worsen pre-existing vitamin deficiency. For example, the use of methotrexate, phenytoin, and trimethoprim is associated with folate deficiency, and the use of metformin, neomycin, and proton pump inhibitors is associated with vitamin B_{12} deficiency. Anticholinergic drugs are often implicated in drug-induced delirium and drug-induced visual hallucination. Drugs for Parkinson's disease are frequently implicated in drug-induced psychosis. Benzodiazepines and opioids may cause depression. The use of steroids is associated with mania, psychosis, delirium, and depression. Beta-adrenergic agonists (often used to treat asthma) may cause anxiety symptoms. The FDA has issued warnings about the risk of suicide ideation associated with the use of all anticonvulsants, antidepressants, and varenicline (used to treat smoking cessation). The use of varenicline, interferon alpha (used to treat multiple sclerosis), singulair (used to treat asthma), or zanamivir inhalation powder (used to treat acute influenza symptoms) is associated with a risk of depression. Hence, the HCP should caution a resident who has serious psychiatric illness (e.g. schizophrenia, bipolar disorder, major depressive disorder [MDD]) about the use of varenicline for smoking-cessation treatment.

Clinical Case 2: "Get out of my house"

Mr. M, an 82-year-old widowed male who had MNCD due to Alzheimer's disease (AD), was transferred from the hospital to a nursing home for rehabilitation after being treated for syncope due to severe bradycardia with pacemaker implantation and initiation of 200 mg/day of amiodarone. He started developing changes in mental status a week after discharge, including worsening disorientation, agitation, insomnia, aggressive behavior during personal care, and paranoia. Staff at the nursing home requested psychiatric consult to facilitate hospitalization to an inpatient psychiatric unit, as Mr. M was "violent." The psychiatrist found Mr. M to be agitated and repeatedly yelling, "Get out of my house." After emergency assessment, the consulting psychiatrist diagnosed amiodarone-induced delirium. Amiodarone was discontinued (after consultation with the resident's cardiologist) and Mr. M was given risperidone (0.25 mg twice a day increased next day to 0.5 mg twice a day) for agitation and aggression. The aggression improved dramatically after two days and resolved completely after seven days. Risperidone was discontinued soon after.

Teaching Points

Amiodarone (and many other prescription drugs) has the potential to cause significant cognitive adverse effect in older adults, especially those who have MNCD. Also, prompt short-term treatment of severe agitation with low-dose risperidone in the context of delirium may prevent injury to self or others and may avoid hospitalization for severe aggression that cannot be managed in the LTC facility.

Prevention and Treatment of Drug–Drug Interaction

Drug–drug interaction that adversely affects the resident's health (physical, cognitive, emotional) and

Table 12.9 Common Examples of the Prescribing Cascade in Long-Term Care Populations

Example	Potential Negative Consequences	Clinical Pearls
ChEI prescribed, resident who has MNCD develops urinary incontinence (UI), and anticholinergic medication (e.g. oxybutynin) is prescribed for UI	Anticholinergic may negate beneficial effect of ChEI	ChEI can cause new-onset UI; if other causes (e.g. overactive bladder) are ruled out, it may be better to discontinue ChEI and consider memantine, as it does not pose risk of UI
ChEI prescribed, resident who has MNCD develops anorexia, and mirtazapine prescribed to improve appetite	Mirtazapine can cause daytime sedation	It is better to reduce the dosage of ChEI and/or give it after a meal and, if anorexia persists, to discontinue it
High-potency antipsychotic medication (e.g. risperidone, haloperidol) causes Parkinsonism, which is treated with benztropine, which causes constipation, which is treated with docusate sodium	Benztropine is highly anticholinergic and is associated with serious risk (e.g. delirium)	It is better to reduce the dosage of antipsychotic medication or discontinue and switch to another antipsychotic medication with least potential for Parkinsonism (e.g. quetiapine)
Medication causes constipation, which is treated with stool softener	Drugs with anticholinergic activity routinely cause constipation	Nondrug treatment for constipation (e.g. increase fluid and fiber intake, increase physical activity, discontinue drugs that can cause constipation) used proactively can prevent medication-induced constipation
Medication causes diarrhea, which is treated with anticholinergic medication, which causes dry mouth, which is treated with chlorhexidine mouthwash	Certain psychotropic medications started concomitantly or within a few days of each other (e.g. SSRI along with a ChEI) often cause diarrhea	Even mild diarrhea has potential to cause delirium (especially in frail resident or resident who has MNCD) It is better to discontinue offending medication than to treat diarrhea with anticholinergic medication
Medication causes BNPS, which is treated with another medication	Impulse control disorders (e.g. compulsive or uncontrollable urge to gamble, eat, shop, have sex) due to aripiprazole and dopamine agonist (e.g. ropinirole, pramipexole) treated with SSRI	It is better to discontinue offending medication than to treat medication-induced BNPS with another medication
Medication-induced pain treated with analgesic	Fluoroquinolone (e.g. levofloxacin) antibiotic-induced muscle pain or pain due to tendinitis treated with opioid	It is better to discontinue offending medication than to treat medication-induced pain with analgesic
Metformin causes anorexia and weight loss, which is treated with mirtazapine	Mirtazapine can cause daytime sedation	It is better to discontinue metformin after ruling out other causes of anorexia and weight loss
Amlodipine causes edema of legs, which is treated with diuretic	Diuretic may cause dehydration and electrolyte imbalance	It is better to reduce dosage or discontinue amlodipine after ruling out other causes of edema of legs
Amlodipine causes urinary incontinence (UI), and resident is prescribed tolterodine to treat UI	Tolterodine has significant anticholinergic effect and may negate benefit of ChEI	It is better to reduce dosage of amlodipine or discontinue it after ruling out other causes of UI

functional status is prevalent in LTC populations because of the high prevalence of polypharmacy. For example, the addition of fluoxetine, which is a hepatic cytochrome P450 2D6 isoenzyme inhibitor, to nortriptyline, which is a 2D6 substrate, impairs the ability of 2D6 to metabolize nortriptyline, leading to an increase in the blood level of nortriptyline (leading to nortriptyline toxicity [e.g. sedation, falls, urinary retention, hypotension]). Another example is the addition of quetiapine to phenytoin. Quetiapine is primarily a 3A4 substrate, and phenytoin is an inducer of several cytochrome P450 enzymes, including 3A4. Thus, when quetiapine is introduced with phenytoin already present, there may be as much as a fivefold increase in the clearance of quetiapine (leading to a lack of efficacy of quetiapine). If a resident is transitioned from taking phenytoin to control seizure to taking valproate (which is also an effective anticonvulsant), which usually does not induce most liver enzymes, quetiapine may have a better chance of efficacy. Other examples of replacing a drug that poses significant risk of drug–drug interaction with a safer alternative (a drug with less risk of drug–drug interaction) include substituting omeprazole for lansoprozole or substituting azithromycin for erythromycin. Trimethoprim, an antibiotic commonly used in combination with sulfamethoxazole to treat UTI, may interfere with the elimination of memantine, with potential for toxicity (e.g. myoclonus, delirium). Pharmacy computer programs that alert physicians, physician assistants, and nurse practitioners to drug-drug interaction and maintain resident medication lists can assist in the prevention and treatment of many clinically significant drug–drug interactions. We recommend that the HCP maintain a high index of suspicion for clinically significant drug–drug interaction when prescribing any new drug for a resident who is already taking other medication.

Reducing the Burden of Medication

Medication burden consists of the number of medications consumed as well as the total dosages of medications consumed. The burden of medication is high in LTC populations, and it contributes to ADE, medication error, and high workload for the nurses dispensing the medication. Box 12.4 lists several ways to reduce the burden of medication. Reducing the burden of medication may improve a resident's quality of life in several ways. This is an important pharmacological treatment for all LTC residents in general and specifically for the resident experiencing BNPS, the resident who has difficulty swallowing, and the resident who resists taking pills. A resident experiencing subtle adverse effects of these medications may start feeling and functioning better. Additionally, a resident taking less medication will have reduced risk of medication error-related and drug–drug interaction-related ADE. Staff time spent dispensing medication may decrease, thus freeing up time for staff to bond with residents.

Many LTC residents receive medication that is unnecessary because there is no clinical indication and/or because of limited life expectancy (e.g. use of a statin by a resident who has severe or terminal-stage MNCD). A relatively high proportion of LTC residents taking antidementia drugs (e.g. ChEIs, memantine) may not be benefiting enough from these medications to warrant continuation. Discontinuation of antidementia drugs with gradual tapering does not result in adverse outcome for most residents. If there is subsequently a clinically relevant decline that is temporally related to the discontinuation of treatment, then the medication can be reintroduced. A resident who has MNCD due to AD and has ongoing delusions and hallucinations is at significant risk of clinical deterioration on discontinuation of ChEI, and thus postponing the plan to discontinue ChEI may be prudent (Herrmann et al. 2016). Many residents taking antidepressant may have a diagnosis of MDD in their records but on a thorough assessment, it is clear that they have been misdiagnosed, as their symptoms were either normal depressive symptoms due to loss (e.g. loss of health) or adjustment disorder with depressed mood. For these residents, we recommend taper and discontinuation of the antidepressant and redoubling efforts to address distress by emotional support and other psychosocial approaches. Antidepressant can also be tapered and discontinued for many residents who have MDD single episode and have been stable for more than one year and have current low score on PHQ-9.

For LTC residents, the application of geriatric palliative methodology (e.g. presence of evidence-based consensus for using the drug for the indication, indication seems valid and relevant in a particular patient's age group and disability level, benefit outweighs risk for this particular resident; absence of adverse effect; absence of safer alternative and whether the dosage can be reduced with no significant risk) may enable simultaneous discontinuation of several medications (Garfinkel, Zur-Gil, and Ben-Israel 2007). This in turn may improve the quality of life, reduce mortality rates and referrals to acute care facilities, and lower costs and staff workload. A resident who has terminal-stage MNCD is an ideal candidate for a trial of discontinuation of antidementia drug. Medications are often prescribed on a trial basis. For example, a resident is yelling and agitated, severely cognitively impaired, and thus unable to communicate to caregivers the cause of the distress and, after thorough evaluation, is given a trial of an analgesic (e.g. acetaminophen) for suspected musculoskeletal pain or an antidepressant for suspected depression. It is important to discontinue these agents if the target symptoms have not responded to treatment. Often, this is overlooked and the resident continues to receive the medication. The dosage of a medication that is beneficial may need to be reduced because of a decline in the resident's health. For example, the dosage of gabapentin given for peripheral diabetic neuropathy is reduced to avoid sedation because the resident's kidney function has declined due to worsening diabetic nephropathy. Strategies such as simplifying the drug regimen, using combination drugs, extended-release drugs, or other formulations may reduce the number of drug administrations and chances for error. A resident who is taking a high-potency antipsychotic (e.g. risperidone) and medication (e.g. benztropine) for drug-induced Parkinsonism (DIP) may not need medication for DIP once the antipsychotic is discontinued or switched to another antipsychotic with low potential for DIP (e.g. quetiapine).

Psychiatric Aspects of Potentially Inappropriate Prescription Associated with the Management of Constipation

Constipation is prevalent in LTC populations and is associated with significant emotional distress. It is a common cause of agitation in residents who have MNCD, a common symptom of MDD, and many psychotropic medications can cause constipation. In the context of management of constipation, PIP is prevalent, especially in residents who have MNCD. Common forms of PIP involve not discontinuing medication that causes constipation, prescription cascade, inaccurate diagnosis of the cause(s) of constipation resulting in inappropriate treatment of constipation, use of multiple agents (many are unnecessary or ineffective) to treat constipation, and inappropriate choice of pharmacologic treatment for constipation. Inadequate treatment of chronic gastrointestinal disorders with constipation (e.g. irritable bowel syndrome [IBS]) can often lead to MDD. Hence, appropriate treatment of constipation is an important aspect of improving mental health of LTC residents. The HCP should consider eliminating drugs that cause or exacerbate constipation (especially drugs with anticholinergic activity, opioid analgesics) and, if necessary, replacing them with safer alternatives as a first step in treating constipation. Bulking agents (e.g. bran, psyllium, methylcellulose) are typically used first in the treatment of constipation. The next group of agents is stool softeners (e.g. docusate), followed by osmotic agents (e.g. lactulose, sorbitol, polyethylene glycol). The HCP should prescribe osmotic agents cautiously for a resident who has diabetes mellitus and should monitor the resident for electrolyte disorders, especially with prolonged use. The next class of agents is stimulant laxatives (e.g. bisacodyl, senna). The combination of stimulant laxatives and bulking agent usually effectively treats most cases of severe constipation due to medications such as opioid. The HCP may consider prescribing naloxegol or methylnaltrexone to treat refractory opioid-induced constipation for a resident who has advanced disease and is receiving palliative care. The HCP may consider prescribing lubiprostone for a resident who has chronic idiopathic constipation. Any pharmacological treatment of constipation, ideally, must be part of a comprehensive strategy that involves efforts to increase physical activity, slowly increase fiber in the diet, and correct dehydration with increased fluid intake. Change in the pattern of chronic constipation should alert physicians, physician assistants, and nurse practitioners to look for a serious medical condition, such as bowel cancer, hypothyroidism, hypercalcemia, etc.

Enema (e.g. warm water, soapsuds) may be necessary in severe cases of constipation, when rapid response is needed or when medications are not effective. Manual disimpaction may be required when the HCP suspects impending impaction. Magnesium citrate may be useful in urgent situations. All medications used to treat constipation may cause diarrhea, headache, abdominal pain, abdominal distension, flatulence, and nausea. Excessive use of drugs to treat constipation may lead to fluid and electrolyte disturbances, including hypokalemia. The HCP should routinely look for these adverse effects in a resident who is taking one or more medications for constipation.

Psychiatric Aspects of Potentially Inappropriate Prescription Associated with Pain Management

Pain is prevalent in LTC populations and is one of the most common causes of emotional distress, depression, agitation, and poor quality of life. Musculoskeletal disorders (e.g. osteoarthritis, chronic low back pain), diabetic neuropathy, and sciatica are the most common causes of painful conditions in LTC populations (Society for Post-Acute and Long-Term Care Medicine 2012). Inadequately controlled pain often prevents response to psychotropic medication used to manage psychiatric disorder (e.g. MDD), and vice versa (inadequately controlled MDD will prevent adequate relief from analgesic). Undertreatment of pain and PIP (especially inappropriate use of opioid and NSAID and analgesic-psychotropic drug–drug interaction) is prevalent among LTC residents who have pain syndrome (acute and chronic), especially residents who have MNCD (Corbett, Husebo, and Malcangio 2012). For example, acute pain is often undertreated (resulting in a high risk of developing into chronic pain syndrome) and chronic pain is often inappropriately treated with opioid (American Geriatrics Society 2009). Fear of opioid ("opioid-phobia") and fear of undertreatment are both prevalent among residents and family members as well as physicians, physician assistants, and nurse practitioners, further complicating decisions about pain management. Processes and systems for assessing and managing pain in LTC populations are often inadequate. Another common reason for PIP is misdiagnosing neuropathic pain as nociceptive pain, and vice versa. Medications effective for nociceptive pain are different from those found effective for neuropathic pain. Many residents who have chronic severe pain syndrome have a combination of nociceptive and neuropathic pain that is better managed by rational polypharmacy (e.g. duloxetine plus acetaminophen plus topical analgesics). Certain medications may cause or exacerbate pain (e.g. myalgia due to statin, headache due to SSRI). Before prescribing an analgesic, the HCP should routinely consider discontinuing medication that may cause or exacerbate certain painful conditions. To maximize pain relief, a variety of evidence-based treatments are available (Abdulla, Bone, and Adams 2013). (See Table 12.6.) The use of analgesic (e.g. acetaminophen, opioid analgesic) has been associated with a reduction in agitation, inactivity, and increased socialization in residents who have MNCD. We recommend an empirical trial of analgesic for a resident who has severe agitation (e.g. persistent yelling). The goals of pain management should be "no worse than mild pain" rather than more ambitious "no pain."

One of the key principles of pain management with pharmacological treatment in LTC populations (especially for those who have MNCD) is using scheduled dosing rather than as-needed dosing, because a resident who has cognitive impairment may not be able to seek staff when she has pain. Acetaminophen is probably the safest and most appropriate initial medication for a resident who has mild to moderate pain due to osteoarthritis or other musculoskeletal disorder. In LTC populations, acetaminophen can be dosed up to 3 grams/day. If the resident has mild liver disease, this dosage should be reduced to no more than 2 grams/day to avoid hepatotoxicity. A resident who has advanced liver disease should not use acetaminophen. The HCP should order liver function tests before prescribing acetaminophen or other analgesic. For a resident receiving both scheduled acetaminophen (alone or in combination with opioid or tramadol) and as-needed acetaminophen (alone or in combination with opioid), close monitoring of total dosage of acetaminophen is crucial to prevent acetaminophen-induced liver damage. A resident who is taking acetaminophen should avoid drinking alcohol.

For a resident who has moderate to severe musculoskeletal pain, a nonsteroidal anti-inflammatory drug (NSAID) may be superior to acetaminophen for providing relief. NSAIDs carry substantial risks (especially gastrointestinal, cardiac, and renal) when used by LTC populations, but the HCP may consider prescribing an NSAID to treat acute moderate to severe musculoskeletal pain for a resident who does not have a pre-existing medical condition (e.g. chronic kidney disease, recent coronary bypass surgery, peptic ulcer disease, recent gastrointestinal bleeding, taking warfarin) that would increase the risk associated with the use of NSAID. For a resident who has gastrointestinal risk, the HCP can prescribe a proton pump inhibitor (PPI) or misoprostol as co-therapy with NSAID (e.g. naproxen) to reduce this risk. Diarrhea associated with misoprostol may limit its use in LTC populations. Celecoxib (a COX-2 inhibitor) may be preferred over nonselective NSAID (e.g. naproxen, ibuprofen) for a resident who has minimal cerebrovascular risk but has a history of gastric problems. Over-the-counter topical forms of analgesic (e.g. methyl salicylate, menthol, capsaicin) and prescription topical NSAID (e.g. diclofenac gel) may also help reduce pain associated with arthritis. Some residents using topical capsaicin may experience local burning or a stinging sensation when they first apply the agent, but that effect usually resolves after one week of continued use. The nursing staff need to take appropriate precautions while applying capsaicin to the painful area (e.g. use gloves, avoid accidental contact with the eye).

Tramadol is an analgesic medication that has a dual mechanism of action: it possesses weak mu-opioid receptor binding and it inhibits re-uptake of norepinephrine and serotonin. The HCP may consider prescribing tramadol to treat moderate to severe acute or chronic pain in LTC residents. The starting dosage should be low (25 mg once or twice a day) and gradually increased every three days to the lowest therapeutic dosage. Adverse effects include dizziness, drowsiness, confusion, and the risk of serotonin syndrome and seizure when used with SSRI or SNRI. The HCP should prescribe it cautiously for a resident who has significant kidney disease because of the higher risk of toxicity. The HCP should avoid prescribing tramadol for a resident who has seizure disorder, as it can lower the threshold for seizure. The HCP may consider prescribing tramadol plus acetaminophen for moderate to severe musculoskeletal pain that is not responding to NSAID, for a resident who cannot tolerate NSAID, or if NSAID is contraindicated.

Opioids are a mainstay therapy to manage acute moderate to severe pain in LTC populations. They are used for both cancer pain (acute and chronic) and noncancer pain (acute). The evidence base of opioids for the management of chronic noncancer pain is limited at best (Dowell, Haegerich, and Chow 2016). Hence, it is important that the HCP use all available strategies to manage chronic noncancer pain before considering opioids. (See Table 12.6.) Although tolerance and physical dependence may be unavoidable with opioid, psychological dependence or true addiction is extremely rare in current LTC populations. For a resident who has a history of heroin use or prescription opioid abuse, use of opioid may cause a relapse of opioid use disorder. Opioid use by a resident who has other addiction (e.g. alcohol use disorder, cocaine use disorder, stimulant use disorder, cannabis use disorder) can also result in a relapse of addiction disorder.

Common adverse effects of opioid are nausea, constipation, fatigue, and pruritis. In LTC populations, daytime sedation, fecal impaction, and urinary retention are also a concern. The HCP should expect constipation in any resident taking opioid, so we recommend a prophylactic bowel regimen (e.g. combination of senna and polyethylene glycol) to prevent constipation. Common signs of opioid toxicity include severe sedation, myoclonic jerks, insomnia, nightmares, respiratory suppression, and delirium. If the resident is experiencing opioid toxicity, it may be useful to slowly administer one or two liters of fluids to flush out some of the drug and its metabolite besides discontinuing the medication. Methylphenidate, modafinil, and armodafinil may be helpful in treating opioid-induced daytime sedation and fatigue. Opioids should not be abruptly discontinued due to the high risk of serious withdrawal symptoms (e.g. dysphoria, agitation, insomnia, joint and back pain, muscle ache, lacrimation, rhinorrhea, yawning, fever, nausea).

Hydrocodone is typically used before using more potent opioid (e.g. oxycodone, morphine, hydromorphone). Hydrocodone is metabolized by the hepatic cytochrome 2D6 isoenzyme system to active metabolites. Thus, the use of another medication that inhibits 2D6 enzyme activity (e.g. paroxetine, fluoxetine) may reduce its analgesic effect. Long-acting formulations of opioid (e.g. transdermal fentanyl, long-acting morphine, long-acting oxycodone preparations) are commonly used to treat persistent moderate to severe pain but require a great deal of care when titrating to the steady state. They may be started only after pain control with short-acting opioid is achieved. They should not be administered to an opioid-naïve resident. All long-acting opioids must be prescribed on a fixed schedule for maximal efficacy. For breakthrough pain, usually a short-acting opioid (e.g. transbuccal fentanyl) is also necessary initially. Most residents respond to a low starting dosage and slow titration upward. Morphine has clinically active metabolites, which then undergo renal clearance. Thus, the HCP should prescribe morphine cautiously for a resident who has kidney disease. A fentanyl patch works well but needs a subcutaneous fat reservoir to work, so the HCP should avoid prescribing it for a malnourished resident who requires long-acting opioid. Low-dose methadone (2.5 mg every 8–12 hours starting dose) may be preferred over long-acting morphine in certain situations (e.g. history of opioid use disorder with heroin use) to treat severe chronic pain. The advantages of methadone over other opioids include lack of active metabolites and analgesic effect by opioid receptor agonist effect as well as an N-methyl-D-aspartate (NMDA) receptor antagonist activity. One key disadvantage of methadone over other long-acting opioids is that it is highly lipophilic and easily accumulates in tissues. This accumulation can lead to iatrogenic sedation, respiratory depression, delirium, and death. Long-acting opioid usually takes three to five days to attain optimal analgesic effect, so we recommend that the HCP wait at least five to seven days before considering an increase in opioid dosage.

Opioids are available in many forms besides pills (e.g. intensol of morphine, oxycodone; nebulized opioid), which the HCP may consider prescribing for a resident who needs opioid to manage pain but is unable to swallow pills (but can swallow liquids). Other options for a resident who has difficulty swallowing pills include liquid preparation (e.g. liquid morphine) to control acute pain and transdermal fentanyl to control chronic pain. Patient-controlled analgesia (PCA) pump (placed subcutaneously) is effective in controlling pain for a resident who has relatively preserved cognitive function and is experiencing severe pain (e.g. a resident who has metastatic cancer with bone pain) and can reliably self-administer opioid analgesic using the pump. A combination of acetaminophen with opioid to treat severe pain improves analgesia and may require lower dosages of opioid, thus reducing the incidence of adverse effect associated with opioid. On the other hand, routine use of acetaminophen-opioid combination (especially acetaminophen-hydrocodone) by a LTC resident often prevents the ability to titrate opioids up because of concern of acetaminophen-induced liver damage. The HCP may also consider opioid rotation to reduce adverse effect associated with long-term opioid therapy. Due to incomplete cross-tolerance, we recommend a dose reduction of 30 to 50 percent for the new opioid when the resident is rotating to a new opioid. We strongly recommend that the HCP avoid prescribing meperidine, pentazocine, or buprenorphine to treat pain in LTC populations due to the high risk-to-benefit ratio and availability of safer opioids described above. We do not recommend prescribing opioid to treat pain due to fibromyalgia. Buprenorphine-naloxone combination is preferable to long-acting opioid (including methadone) for a resident who has opioid use disorder and severe pain. The HCP should avoid prescribing BZD (with few exceptions [e.g. during EOL care]) for any resident using opioid and vice versa because of the high risk of delirium, respiratory suppression, aspiration pneumonia, and death associated with concomitant use of BZD and opioid. We recommend staff education and training in the use of naloxone and its easy access to promptly treat accidental opioid overdose (e.g. respiratory suppression) and to prevent fatal consequences of opioid overdose.

Neuropathic pain (e.g. diabetic peripheral neuropathy, central poststroke pain, radiculopathy [e.g. sciatica], trigeminal neuralgia, postherpetic neuralgia) is a common but under-recognized cause of agitation and depressive symptoms in LTC residents. We do not recommend prescribing amitriptyline or imipramine, although effective, to treat neuropathic pain due to the high risk of adverse effect (e.g. worsening cognition, cardiac toxicity). Safer alternatives recommended include gabapentin, pregabalin, duloxetine, and, for some residents who have relatively preserved cognitive function, low-dose nortriptyline. Common adverse effects of gabapentin are somnolence, peripheral edema, fatigue, confusion, depression, and ataxia. Gabapentin, if withdrawn abruptly, may cause a withdrawal syndrome that may present with anxiety, insomnia, nausea, pain, and sweating. The starting dose of gabapentin to treat neuropathic pain in LTC populations should be 100 mg before bedtime, and the dosage can be titrated up every three days to the lowest effective dose. One advantage of gabapentin is that it is primarily eliminated by the kidneys and thus has low potential for pharmacokinetic drug–drug interaction and can be safely used by a LTC resident who has hepatic dysfunction. Dosage adjustment is necessary when gabapentin is used for a resident who has renal insufficiency. The HCP may consider prescribing pregabalin for neuropathic pain or fibromyalgia. Adverse effects are similar to those of gabapentin. Duloxetine may be useful to treat chronic low back pain, fibromyalgia, or diabetic neuropathy pain. Milnacipran is also a good option for the treatment of fibromyalgia. Transdermal 5 percent lidocaine (local anesthetic) patch may be useful in the treatment of both neuropathic and localized pain (especially postherpetic neuralgia). The patch should be applied for 12 hours and removed for 12 hours each day to avoid tachyphylaxis. Up to three lidocaine patches per day may be used. Adverse effect of lidocaine patch is uncommon and includes local skin reaction.

Low-dose steroids may be necessary for the treatment of acute and chronic moderate to severe pain due to rheumatoid arthritis or polymyalgia rheumatica. Although most muscle-relaxant medication is ineffective for chronic pain, tizanidine is effective with both the relaxation of muscle spasms and the reduction in chronic pain symptoms. The HCP may prescribe it judiciously for LTC populations (starting at the lowest dose before bedtime) with close monitoring for its sedating effect. The HCP may consider referral to a pain clinic or a pain specialist for local pharmacological treatment (e.g. PCA pump, epidural steroid injection [for spinal stenosis, herniated disc, or single-extremity pain], facet block [for low back pain], trigger point injection [for localized muscle pain], nerve block [for mononeuropathy, radiculopathy, or postherpetic neuralgia]) as well as more sophisticated procedures (e.g. radiofrequency neuroablation, vertebroplasty, spinal cord stimulation [TENS units]) for a resident who has chronic pain. Also, the HCP may consider prescribing neural blockade, neurolysis, or implantable drug delivery system for a resident who is experiencing severe refractory cancer pain. Intrathecal baclofen pump may be considered for severe pain related to spasticity (e.g. spasticity associated with advanced multiple sclerosis). Hospitalization to a palliative care unit may be necessary for a resident who has severe refractory pain requiring highly complex pharmacological treatment for pain relief (e.g. severe postherpetic neuralgia requiring intravenous lidocaine or oral mexilitene; metastatic bone cancer with excruciating pain requiring palliative sedation).

Psychiatric Aspects of Potentially Inappropriate Prescription Associated with Fall, Fracture, and Osteoporosis

Falls are prevalent in LTC populations, and the prevalence is higher among residents who have psychiatric disorder. Falls often result in serious injury (e.g. fracture, traumatic brain injury), and a history of falls is one of the leading reasons for entering LTC. Residents who are 85 years or older and ambulatory and residents who are agitated are at particularly high risk for fall and fracture. An estimated 70 to 85 percent of LTC residents have osteoporosis (a loss of bone density), putting them at high risk for fracture (either after a fall or spontaneous). Yet, fewer than one in 10 newly admitted LTC residents receive medications to treat osteoporosis and/or calcium and vitamin D. Use of psychotropic medication is associated with increased risk of falls, but effective treatment of psychiatric disorder with psychotropic medication can also reduce the risk of falls. BZD and antipsychotic are especially associated with increased risk of falls. All psychotropic medications (including SSRIs) increase the risk of falls and thus the HCP should prescribe it with extra caution for a resident who has osteoporosis. A high percentage of hip fracture is related to the use of psychotropic medication. Besides psychotropic medication, medication with significant anticholinergic activity (e.g. diphenhydramine), anticonvulsant, and analgesic (especially opioid and tramadol) also increase the risk of falls and fracture. The risk of fracture despite fall may be reduced if a resident who has osteoporosis is treated with vitamin D and biphosphonate (e.g. alendronate, risedronate). Long-term use of high-potency antipsychotic (e.g. haloperidol, risperidone, paliperidone, iloperidone) is associated with hyperprolactinemia and potential increase in risk of osteoporosis and related complications. The HCP should prescribe falls-prevention protocols and initiate approaches that would reduce the risk of fracture after a fall for any resident who is taking psychotropic medication. Staff education, training, and support are crucial to ensure that falls-prevention protocols are followed rigorously. Other factors (e.g. improved ambient lighting, high staff-to-resident ratio) that reduce the risk of falls and fractures should also be used.

Psychiatric Aspects of Potentially Inappropriate Prescription Associated with the Management of Seizure Disorder / Epilepsy

PIP is prevalent in residents who have seizure disorder. Residents who have seizure disorder are often prescribed anticonvulsant (e.g. topiramate, phenobarbital) that poses greater risk of worsening pre-existing cognitive impairment (e.g. resident who has MNCD) despite relatively safer alternatives (e.g. valproate, gabapentin) being available. Anticonvulsants that induce liver enzymes (e.g. phenytoin) are often prescribed to LTC residents despite safer equally effective options (e.g. lamotrigine). Leviracetam carries more risk of destabilizing MDD and other psychiatric disorder, and the HCP should avoid prescribing it for a resident who has pre-existing psychiatric disorder (e.g. bipolar disorder), and anticonvulsant with potential mental health benefit (e.g. lamotrigine, valproate) are preferred over levetiracetam for a resident who has pre-existing psychiatric disorder.

Anticonvulsant should be considered high-risk medication due to the potential to cause serious ADE in LTC populations (especially a resident who is frail or who has MNCD). Anticonvulsant is often not closely monitored in terms of adverse effect and whether blood levels are in therapeutic range, thus posing significant risk of unrecognized ADE and toxic or subtherapeutic drug levels. All anticonvulsants have the potential to cause BNPS, so we recommend that the HCP closely monitor any emergence of BNPS after initiating an anticonvulsant. On the other hand, antidepressants and antipsychotic drugs reduce seizure threshold and may precipitate a seizure in a resident who has seizure disorder (clinical or subclinical [EEG evidence of epileptic activity but no overt seizure]). Thus, close monitoring of seizure control after initiating psychotropic medication is also essential. Destabilization of seizure disorder and/or psychiatric disorder should prompt involvement of a specialist (e.g. geriatric psychiatrist, neurologist) and collaborative decision-making so that optimal control of seizure as well as of psychiatric disorder is achieved with better decisions regarding the use of anticonvulsant and psychotropic medication.

Many residents who have MNCD or stroke may develop nonconvulsive or frontal lobe seizure that may present with "agitation" or BNPS (e.g. a sudden onset of anger or fear, unusual movement of head or arms; aimless wandering; appearing in a trance; periods of confusion that begin and end abruptly; sensory experiences [e.g. visual disturbances]). These types of seizure often go unrecognized and untreated because the resident is unable to describe what she is experiencing due to pre-existing cognitive impairment (e.g. MNCD-related cognitive impairment, stroke-related aphasia). Also, manifestation of nonconvulsive seizure may be mistaken for symptoms of underlying MNCD. The HCP should evaluate for possible seizure any resident showing BNPS that begin and end abruptly. The HCP should first address easily reversible causes of seizure (e.g. dehydration, electrolyte imbalance, and medication-induced seizure). Abrupt or rapid withdrawal of many psychotropic agents (e.g. benzodiazepine, sedative-hypnotic, mood stabilizer [e.g. valproate]) may precipitate one or more seizures.

Psychiatric Aspects of Potentially Inappropriate Prescription Associated with the Management of Dermatologic Conditions

Dermatologic problems (especially itching) are often treated with anticholinergic medication (e.g. hydroxyzine) that poses significant risk of BNPS in LTC populations. Dermatologic conditions (e.g. new skin rash) are often misdiagnosed and treated inappropriately (e.g. with steroids), resulting in potential for serious ADE and progression of underlying skin condition. We strongly recommend consultation with a dermatologist (either in the office or through telemedicine) for accurate diagnosis and treatment of dermatologic conditions before initiating any high-risk medications (e.g. steroids). Certain psychotropic medications can cause serious and potentially fatal skin conditions (e.g. Steven-Johnson syndrome due to lamotrigine; DRESS [drug reaction with eosinophilia and systemic symptoms] reported with use of ziprasidone and olanzapine). Hence appropriate management of dermatologic conditions and close monitoring for skin rash in residents taking these psychotropic medications is essential. Before prescribing psychotropic medication associated with significant risk of dermatologic reaction, the HCP should inquire into any history of drug-induced skin rash.

Itching (pruritis) due to dry skin is a common cause of agitation in residents who have MNCD. Dry skin (xerosis) is prevalent in LTC populations and is the most common cause of itching. Low humidity levels greatly increase the risk of dry skin, especially during the winter months. Dry skin occurs most often on the legs of older adults but may be present on the hands and trunk. Residents with generalized dry skin may complain of "itching all over." Pruritis can lead to secondary lesions (e.g. eczema). Other signs and symptoms of dry skin include flaking, chapping, burning, erythema, pain, scaling, stinging, and tightness. If the skin splits and cracks deeply enough to disrupt dermal capillaries, bleeding fissures may occur. Nonpharmacological treatment (e.g. turning down the heat, using a humidifier in the room, using the soap sparingly, correcting dehydration) in combination with pharmacological treatment (e.g. discontinuation of offending agents and use of nonprescription moisturizing lotion, cream, or ointment on hands and all dry areas) usually improves dry skin. Repetitive use of a moisturizing product over a period of time is needed before a resident experiences the maximal benefits. A thorough application of a moisturizer once or twice daily is an appropriate regimen for most residents who have dry skin. Keratolytics (e.g. 12 percent ammonium lactate lotion) for severe dry skin may also be used. Treatment of comorbid depression and/or anxiety disorders may help improve discomfort associated with xerosis, eczema, or psoriasis. For a successful outcome, the HCP needs to address nutritional deficiency (e.g. zinc and essential fatty acid) and other conditions (e.g. thyroid disease, diuretic therapy, ESRD) that make the resident more susceptible to dry skin. In complicated cases (e.g. breakdown of skin due to excessive scratching; dry skin along with severe eczema or psoriasis), the HCP should consider referral to a dermatologist. All residents should be screened for dry skin periodically (at least quarterly) and when they complain of itching and/or are agitated. We recommend routine use of moisturizing products to prevent dry skin in LTC populations (especially during winter months). Residents who have eczema and psoriasis often see symptoms flare up under dry winter conditions. Eczema and psoriasis are commonly associated with depression and anxiety disorder. Appropriate treatment of dermatologic conditions can prevent BNPS for many residents.

Summary

Potentially inappropriate prescription (PIP) is prevalent in LTC populations and is one of the most common causes of behavioral, neurocognitive, and psychological symptoms (BNPS) in this setting. Early detection of all forms of PIP (including underprescription), discontinuation of inappropriate medication ("rational deprescribing" or "geriatric scalpel") and institution of appropriate nondrug treatments and safer appropriate pharmacological alternatives are some of the most important approaches to improve the emotional well-being of residents in LTC. Application of geriatric palliative methodology (e.g. presence of evidence-based consensus for using the drug for the indication, indication seems valid and relevant in a particular patient's age group and disability level, benefits outweigh risks in this particular resident; absence of adverse effect; absence of safer alternative; and whether the dosage can be reduced with no significant risk) in LTC residents may enable simultaneous discontinuation of several medications. Given the complexities and risks involved in the pharmacologic management of BNPS in LTC populations, the principles of care require the HCP to give serious consideration to expanding the role of the consultant pharmacist and routinely involving a specialist such as geriatric psychiatrist or geriatrician.

Key Clinical Points

1. Potentially inappropriate prescription (PIP) is prevalent and is one of the most common causes of behavioral, neurocognitive, and psychological symptoms (BNPS) in LTC populations.
2. Early detection of PIP, discontinuation of inappropriate medication ("rational deprescribing" or "geriatric scalpel"), and institution of safer appropriate alternatives are some of the most important approaches to improve the emotional well-being of residents in LTC.
3. The use of an anticholinergic cognitive burden scale can help identify medication with significant anticholinergic activity and total anticholinergic burden.
4. Reducing the use of opioid, antipsychotic, and benzodiazepine and reducing anticholinergic burden in LTC populations should be indicators for quality of care, as they are often used inappropriately and their use is associated with high frequency of serious adverse drug event.
5. The role of the consultant pharmacist needs to be expanded so that the pharmacist becomes an integral part of care for every resident, specifically to reduce PIP and improve the prescription of appropriate medication.

Additional Resources

Deprescribing Guidelines for the Elderly by the Ontario Pharmacy Research Collaboration (known as OPEN): www.open-pharmacy-research.ca/research-projects/emerging-services/deprescribing-guidelines/

http://deprescribing.org/about/: A website developed by Dr. Barbara Farrell and Dr. Cara Tannenbaum (pharmacist and physician) to share information and research about deprescribing approaches to reducing harm caused by medications to older adults.

CDC Guideline for Prescribing Opioids for Chronic Pain – United States 2016; The Centers for Disease Control and Prevention www.cdc.gov/mmwr/volumes/65/rr/rr6501e1.htm

Australian Deprescribing Network (ADeN): http://w11.zetaboards.com/ADeN/index/

References

Abdulla, A., M. Bone, and N. Adams. 2013. Evidence-Based Clinical Practice Guidelines on Management of Pain in Older People. *Age Ageing.* **42**:151–153.

American Geriatrics Society. 2012. Beers Criteria Update Expert Panel. Updated Beers Criteria for Potentially Inappropriate Medication Use in Older Adults. *Journal of the American Geriatrics Society* **60**:616–631.

American Geriatrics Society Panel on Pharmacological Management of Persistent Pain in Older Persons. 2009. Pharmacological Management of Persistent Pain in Older Persons. *Journal of the American Geriatrics Society* **57**:1331–1346.

Barry, P.J., P. Gallagher, C. Ryan, and D. O'Mahoney. 2007. START (Screening Tool to Alert Doctors to the Right Treatment): An Evidence-Based Screening Tool to Detect Prescribing Omissions in Elderly People. *Age and Ageing.* **36**:632–638.

Corbett, A., B. Husebo, and M. Malcangio. 2012. Assessment and Treatment of Pain in People with Dementia. *Nature Reviews Neurology* **8**:264–274.

Dowell, D., T.M. Haegerich, and R. Chow. 2016. CDC Guidelines for Prescribing Opioids for Chronic Pain – United States 2016. *Journal of the American Medical Association* **315**(15):1624–1645.

Gallagher, P., C. Ryan, S. Byrne, J. Kennedy, and D. O'Mahoney. 2008. STOPP (Screening Tools for Older Person's Prescriptions) and START (Screening Tool to Alert Doctors to the Right Treatment): Consensus Validation. *International Journal of Clinical Pharmacology Therapeutics* **46**:72–83.

Garfinkel, D., S. Zur-Gil, and S. Ben-Israel. 2007. The War against Polypharmacy: A New Cost-Effective Geriatric-Palliative Approach for Improving Drug Therapy in Disabled Elderly People. *Israel Medical Association Journal* **9** (6):340–344.

Gerretsen, P. and B.G. Pollock. 2011. Drugs with Anticholinergic Properties: A Current Perspective on Use and Safety. *Expert Opinion in Drug Safety* **10**(5):751–765.

Hanlon, J.T. and K.E. Schmader. 2013. The Medication Appropriateness Index at 20: Where It Started, Where It Has Been and Where It May Be Going. *Drugs and Aging* **30**(11):883–900.

Herrmann N., J. O'Regan, M. Ruthirakuhan, et al. 2016. A Randomized, Placebo-Controlled Discontinuation Study of Cholinesterase Inhibitors in Institutionalized Patients with Moderate to Severe Alzheimer Disease. *Journal of the American Medical Directors Association* **17**:142–147.

Juola, A., S. Pylkkannen, H. Kautiainen, et al. 2016. Burden of Potentially Harmful Medications and the Association with Quality of Life and Mortality among Institutionalized Older People. *Journal of the American Medical Directors Association* **276**:e9–e14.

Kotlyar, M., S.L. Gray, R.L. Maher, and J.T. Hanlon. 2011. Psychiatric Manifestations of Medications in the Elderly. In M.E. Agronin and G. J. Maletta (eds.), *Principles and Practice of Geriatric Psychiatry*, 2nd ed., pp. 721–733. Philadelphia, PA: Lippincott Williams & Wilkins.

Lapane, K.L., C.M. Hughes, J.B. Christian et al. 2011. Evaluation of the Fleetwood Model of Long-Term Care Pharmacy. *Journal of the American Medical Directors Association* **12**(5):355–363.

Mulsant, B.H. and B.G. Pollock. 2015. Psychopharmacology. In D.C. Steffens, D.G. Blazer, and M. E. Thakur (eds.), *The Textbook of Geriatric Psychiatry*, 5th ed., pp. 527–588. Arlington, VA: American Psychiatric Publishing.

Patterson, S.M., C.A. Cadogan, N. Kerse, et al. 2014. Interventions to Improve the Appropriate Use of Polypharmacy for Older Adults. *Cochrane Database of Systematic Reviews* Issue 10, Art. No.: CD008165. doi: 10.1002/14651858.CD008165.pub3.

Rudolph, J.L., M.J. Salow, M.C. Angelini, and R.E. McGlinchey. 2008. The Anticholinergic Risk Scale and Anticholinergic Adverse Effects in Older Persons. *Archives of Internal Medicine.* **168**:508–513.

Scott, I.A., S.N. Hilmer, E. Reeve, et al. 2015. Reducing Inappropriate Polypharmacy: The Process of Deprescribing. *JAMA Internal Medicine* **175**(5):827–834.

Society for Post-Acute and Long-Term Care Medicine. 2012. Pain Management in the Long-Term Care Setting. Clinical Practice Guideline, Colombia, Maryland.

Ward, S., J.P. Roberts, W.J. Resch, and C. Thomas. 2016. When to Adjust the Dosing of Psychotropics in Patients with Renal Impairment. *Current Psychiatry* **15**(8):60–66.

Waun J. 2014. Will I Survive My Medication? *Journal of American Geriatrics Society* **62**:968.

Chapter 13

A Psychosocial-Spiritual Wellness Care Plan for Residents Who Have Major Neurocognitive Disorder

I am Richard who seeks to live a purposeful and purpose filled life up to and through my last breath.
*Richard Taylor**

Dr. Richard Taylor, a founding member of Dementia Alliance International, would always introduce himself as, "Hello, my name is Richard and I have Alzheimer's disease." Dr. Taylor and many other people who have major neurocognitive disorder (MNCD) have transformed the portrait of life of people who have MNCD from "exuberant life, gloomy descent" to "exuberant life, dignified descent." The forces of person-centered care (PCC), positive psychiatry, and positive psychology are slowly but surely steering long-term care (LTC) toward promoting physical, cognitive, psychosocial, and spiritual wellness, not just managing disease and infirmity. A traditional medical model of care cannot achieve these person-centered goals (Dementia Action Alliance 2016). A holistic, person-centered approach to caring for people who have MNCD that values emotional and spiritual well-being as much as physical and cognitive health is key to ensuring that their lives are filled with dignity, purpose, meaning, and happiness. Psychosocial spiritual and environmental approaches and initiatives are the core component of holistic, PCC practices (Desai and Grossberg 2017). (See Box 13.1.)

BOX 13.1 Key Components of Person-Centered Care

- Knowing resident well (comprehensive understanding of resident and resident's conditions)
- Maintaining dignity and self-hood of resident
- Recognizing purpose in resident's life
- Facilitating inner exploration by resident
- Facilitating spirituality of resident
- Facilitating creativity of resident
- Facilitating adjustment of resident to "new home"
- Facilitating preserved strengths of resident
- Providing healing and therapeutic interpersonal and physical environment
- Facilitating sensitivity to and expression of resident's culture
- Making relationship central to all aspects of caregiving
- Strengthening existing positive relationships and facilitating new relationships
- Caring for family caregiver
- Caring for professional caregiver

Person-centered long-term care communities (PCLTCCs) foster a culture that supports autonomy, diversity, individual choice, and a sense of belonging. PCLTCCs strive to provide opportunities for continuation of normalcy and personal growth. Leadership and community involvement cultivate relationships among residents, families, support systems, and health care personnel. They commit to responsiveness, spontaneity, and continuous learning. Residents and staff celebrate the cycles of life and connect to the local community to continue relationships that nurture the quality of everyday life. In PCLTCCs, residents are experts regarding life in their homes. They participate in decisions about the rhythm of their days, the services provided to them, and the issues that are important to them. Their family and other members of their support systems are welcomed. A PCLTCC is a place where residents want to live, where staff would want to work, and where both choose to stay. The challenge is to transform the institutional culture of efficiency into a home environment that focuses on the individual (American Geriatrics Society 2015).

For residents who have MNCD, relationship with staff is the most important measure of quality. The second measure is choice: in food, in routine, in

* Richard Taylor, speech on receiving the Carter Williams Legacy Award, Pioneer Network annual conference, August 13, 2009.

decorating one's room. Well-planned activities that create meaning and purpose in the lives of the residents are the next measure. Although residents may need the physical support offered in a LTC facility, they have established their own rhythms of daily life. PCC means the resident is at home, and the staff – not the resident – have to adapt their schedule.

Strength-Based, Personalized, Psychosocial Sensory Spiritual and Environmental Initiatives and Creative Engagement

We recommend that every resident have a formal psychosocial and spiritual wellness care plan. Psychosocial and spiritual wellness is reflected in the resident's experiencing frequent positive emotions and experiences (e.g. feelings of being loved, cherished, and honored; experiences of joy, happiness, and contentment; a sense of security, belonging, and connectedness; and a sense of accomplishment and purpose) and infrequent experiences of negative emotions and experiences (e.g. feeling like one is a burden, feeling that no one cares). A formal care plan symbolizes that the care team has given emotional and spiritual wellness of all residents the importance it deserves. Such a care plan needs to be comprehensive, strengths-based, and personalized (individualized), and the staff proactively seeks to promote well-being by asking key questions while formulating a plan of care: What is important for this resident? What are the resident's values and goals? What are the resident's preferences? What will make the resident happy?

We suggest the term strength-based, personalized, psychosocial sensory spiritual and environmental initiatives and creative engagement (SPPEICE) to represent a psychosocial-spiritual wellness care plan. Table 13.1 provides a template for a ten-point

Table 13.1 Ten-Point Psychosocial-Spiritual Wellness Care Plan for a Resident Who Has Major Neurocognitive Disorder

Key Areas	Practical Tips	Pearls and Real-Life Examples
Getting to know resident well	One-page biography written in first person Life-history book Written inventory of resident's strengths and interests	Staff reads aloud Mr. D's one-page biography to new nurse's aide before she helps Mr. D have a bath
Daily schedule of pleasant activities (daily SPA)	Daily schedule that reflects (as closely as possible) resident's normal routine before coming to the *new home* Strengths-based personalized structured activities (e.g. bingo, live music) Strengths-based personalized unstructured activities (e.g. reminiscence activities, reading book, listening to book on CD)	Ms. M likes to get up around 10 a.m. and have coffee and toast Ms. M loves bingo and craft activities and likes to help staff clean up after activities Ms. M has been an avid reader all her life but, due to vision impairment and cognitive decline, cannot read anymore, but likes to listen to stories read by staff Ms. M likes to have light snack at 10 p.m. and watch TV till midnight
Facilitating sense of being part of greater community and providing opportunities to be productive member of community and society	Resident council Community activism (e.g. leading facility team in annual Alzheimer's Association fundraising walk)	Mr. G asks, "Can we do Wii bowling every day?" in a resident council meeting Mrs. G, a former school teacher, is made a "lunch room monitor"
Enhancing physical fitness (endurance, strength, balance, flexibility)	Group stretching exercises daily in morning Chair yoga Tai Chi	Mr. L said, "I enjoy bowling" after engaging in Wii bowling activity

Table 13.1 (cont.)

Key Areas	Practical Tips	Pearls and Real-Life Examples
Cognitive stimulation program	Cognitive stimulation therapy (CST)* Puzzles (e.g. crossword puzzle) Reading aloud Writing letter Lengthy conversation about topics resident is passionate about	Ms. W, a retired nurse in advanced stages of MNCD, would write long letters (often it was hard to decipher) regularly and seemed to enjoy this activity. It was supported by staff, and family would collect letters and "discuss" with Ms. W various "events" Ms. W wrote about
Re-engaging the senses/robust sensory stimulation program	Music-based activities (e.g. personalized music using iPod/MP3 player with headphones) Massage (e.g. hand massage, shoulder massage, neck rub) Aromas (e.g. lavender to soothe and citrus to stimulate) Taste (cooking activities; sweet and savory snacks periodically throughout day) Multisensory room (e.g. Snoezelen)	Mrs. C states, "That smells so good" and is calmer after staff plugged in aromatic diffuser in her room and gave her a hand massage with lavender (her favorite aroma) lotion Mr. H, who has anxiety and restlessness during afternoon (sundowning), finds multisensory room enjoyable and calming
Spiritual engagement and contemplative practices program	Attending religious services several times a week One-to-one visit by chaplain to sing religious songs together Reading or being read aloud familiar and favorite religious scriptures or poems	Mrs. S, who has not responded verbally for several months, starts singing religious songs along with others in a new group singing activity
Enhance connectedness to nature	Spending time on patio admiring birds, leaves, trees, and sunsets Walking or being pushed in wheelchair on nature trail that has been made accessible to individuals using wheelchair	Mr. G, a fishing aficionado, at a once-a-week fishing outing shouts with joy when the staff reels in the caught fish, "That is a big one!"
Bringing out artist within each resident	TimeSlips** Visiting local museum Engaging in coloring and painting activities Poetry reading/writing	Mrs. B, a doll collector all her life, continues her hobby with staff and family support at the facility and has a beautiful display of her collection next to her bed
Deepen existing connections (e.g. with family and friends), develop new friends and relationships (especially with staff and other residents)	Staff makes every encounter an opportunity to connect and get to know resident a little bit more FaceTime, Skype, or other video-chat activities with family and friends Intergenerational activities (e.g. intergenerational life review writing programs) One-to-one interactions Staff share aspects of their own lives with resident (e.g. telling about spouse or children, sharing quirks)	Mrs. C said, "We have to do that again" after chatting with her daughter on FaceTime

Note: SPPEICE: strength-based, personalized, psychosocial sensory spiritual and environmental initiatives and creative engagement
* Cognitive stimulation therapy (CST): www.cstdementia.com
** TimeSlips: www.timeslips.org

psychosocial-spiritual wellness plan. The goal of SPPEICE is to enhance the resident's emotional and spiritual well-being, strengthen resilience, foster psychological and spiritual growth, and prevent and reduce distress due to unmet psychological, social, spiritual, environmental, and cultural needs.

A Strengths-Based Approach

For a psychosocial-spiritual wellness care plan to work most effectively, it needs to be based on strengths. Each resident has a unique repertoire of strengths that throughout life has helped her cope with challenges and enjoy the good things life has to offer. Our current care culture focuses too much on the "problems," "weaknesses," and "deficits" and too little on assessment and preservation of existing strengths and skills. Skill-appropriate activities facilitate engagement, maintain skills, and enhance the enjoyment a resident can get from them. Facilitating preserved strengths may also be considered "restorative care" that focuses on "helping residents do, rather than doing for them" and "abilities-focused care" that focuses on maintaining and strengthening specific abilities during daily personal care. Box 13.2 lists examples of retained strengths and skills in residents who have MNCD, and Box 13.3 lists examples of meaningful activities that are based on the resident's existing cognitive and sensory strengths. For example, many residents have been lifelong readers and retain the ability to read until advanced stages of MNCD. Having a facility library with a collection of books from different past and contemporary authors can greatly facilitate this activity, as can weekly visits from the mobile public library. See Table 13.2 for descriptions of stages of Alzheimer's disease (AD) from the traditional medical model and strengths-based descriptions of stages of AD (Reisberg 1988). In the manner that vision impairment often leads to enhancement of hearing ability through neuroplastic changes in the brain, as the cognitive functions of a resident who has MNCD progressively decline, hidden strengths of creativity and spirituality may flourish. The capacity to be in the moment, to forget recent negative events and "move on," or not to have self-critical cognitive networks inhibit an impulse to sing or share something deeply moving are a few of the many unrecognized benefits of weakened cognitive function.

A Personalized, Individualized Approach

For maximal impact, SPPEICE needs to be personalized. Comprehensive understanding of the resident who has MNCD goes beyond details about physical

BOX 13.2 Retained Strengths and Skills

1. Attitude (e.g. optimistic)
2. Drive (e.g. highly self-motivated, high energy)
3. Language (e.g. retained comprehension of spoken language, capacity to read, capacity to hold conversation)
4. Cognition (e.g. retained social cognition, capacity to empathize)
5. Social/interpersonal (e.g. easily makes friends, initiates conversations)
6. Ambulation (e.g. can ambulate on his or her own, participate in walking program)
7. Physical strength (e.g. can transfer on his or her own, can use and enjoy strength-training equipment)
8. Sense of humor (e.g. great capacity to laugh at self or situation and not take life too seriously)
9. Cooking (e.g. great interest in all aspects of cooking)
10. Musical ability (e.g. able to play musical instrument)
11. Vision (e.g. can see well)
12. Hearing (e.g. can hear well)
13. Gardening (e.g. has a green thumb)
14. Spirituality (e.g. involved in faith activities, regularly prays)
15. Self-care (e.g. able to do some activities of daily living with only minimal assistance)
16. Altruism (e.g. often expresses compassion, tries to help others)
17. Social support (e.g. lots of family and friends come to visit and are supportive)
18. Financial assets (e.g. can afford weekly or twice-weekly massage therapist, can afford paid caregiver to provide one-to-one support and engage resident in activities for several hours a day)

BOX 13.3 Meaningful Activities for a Resident Who Has Major Neurocognitive Disorder

Meaningful Activities for Resident Who Has Mild MNCD

- Book club
- Discussion group (e.g. current events, sports, politics, science, history)
- Book or poetry reading, religious scriptures study group
- Computer games
- Leading exercise group for other residents
- Brainteasers in group setting (e.g. trivia challenges), puzzles individually
- Learning new musical instrument
- Learning to sing
- Learning to dance
- Learning to plant new flowers
- Learning to cook new recipes and make new drinks
- Learning new artistry skills (e.g. making hand-painted yarn)
- Support group

Meaningful Activities for Resident Who Has Moderate MNCD

- Cooking/baking, kneading dough
- Gardening
- Washing, cleaning, helping with dishes
- Singing in group setting
- Playing musical instrument
- Setting the table
- Reminiscing about previous vacations and trips
- Watching movies or travelogues

Meaningful Activities for Resident Who Has Severe MNCD

- Folding towels
- Sealing envelopes
- Shredding paper
- Attending church daily
- Watching or listening to religious TV shows, radio programs, religious music, church services

and mental health conditions. It involves getting to know the resident well, really well. The hands that hold the fork that feeds the resident must belong to someone who has a sense of who the resident is. All of us caring for the residents must remember what we learn about the resident, and our awareness must grow from one encounter to another.

As we get to know a resident well and over time develop a bond, a unique tenderness and love often follows spontaneously, bathing the resident with its light and as a result giving purpose to both the resident and the caregivers (family and professional). Once we take the trouble to know the resident, at some level the resident begins to feel being seen, heard, valued, and respected. In the course of such an interaction, magical things can happen. A resident who has not spoken for a long time may blurt out, "I love you" or "Thank you." A caregiver may suddenly realize that she is receiving a blessing (e.g. an unexpected kiss) as much as giving. These brief moments of intimacy may make both the resident and the caregiver less fearful of the future.

One of the ways to start knowing a person is to read a one-page biography (created by the resident with help from family and friends), written in the first person so that it has a deeper emotional impact on the reader. All health care providers (HCPs), including frontline staff (nurses, nursing assistants), should read (or be read aloud) this one-page biography before their first encounter with the resident and periodically thereafter. Another way to get to know a resident is to review a life history book created by the resident and family. Such a book would chronicle the life of the resident, including passions, travels, achievements, the love of the life, and many other aspects of life that reflect the richness and resilience of the resident to this moment. The resident's primary care team should encourage and guide the family in creating such a biographical page or life history book (ideally before moving to the new home) and take an active role in ensuring that the staff caring for the resident read it, so that they know who the resident is and that the resident is loved. We recommend a facility-wide directive for all staff (including physicians) to know the resident.

Psychosocial Approaches and Initiatives

Psychosocial approaches and initiatives are the glue that binds the resident to a life worth living. A host of such initiatives promote wellness.

Staff-Initiated Positive Relationships and Encounters

A positive relationship is a relationship in which the resident feels valued and loved and compassion flows naturally. A positive encounter is an encounter in which the resident experiences positive emotions

Table 13.2 Strengths-Based Stages of Alzheimer's Disease

Stage	Traditional Description	Strengths-Based Description
1	Presymptomatic (asymptomatic) stage with positive AD biomarkers*	Normal cognitive functions and capacity to live independently
2	Subjective memory and other cognitive complaints may or may not be accompanied by transient mild symptoms of depression, anxiety, and/or apathy; positive AD biomarkers	Normal cognitive function on objective cognitive testing and retained capacity to live independently
3	Mild neurocognitive disorder with objective evidence of cognitive decline (two or more standard deviations) accompanied by varying severity of depression, anxiety, and/or apathy; positive AD biomarkers	Retained capacity to live independently and to drive
4	Mild major neurocognitive disorder with difficulties in living independently due to significant cognitive decline accompanied by varying severity of depression, anxiety, and/or apathy; positive AD biomarkers	In general, retained general intellect and capacity to eloquently express experience of living with MNCD; retained capacity to live in own home with some help; retained capacity to make medical decisions in own best interest in most situations; may be able to drive short distance on familiar route
5	Moderate major neurocognitive disorder with inability to live independently without substantial help accompanied by moderate to severe depression, anxiety, psychotic symptoms; positive AD biomarkers and neuroimaging evidence of obvious temporoparietal cortical atrophy	In general, retained long-term memory and capacity to reminisce past positive experiences; retained conversation skills and capacity for sense of humor; retained capacity to recognize family and friends; retained procedural memory (e.g. dancing, playing a musical instrument); retained reading comprehension, capacity for social interactions, engage in creative activities and enjoy music, being with pets, spending time in nature, and spiritual rituals
6	Severe major neurocognitive disorder with need for 24/7 supervision for safety, difficulty recognizing family and friends; difficulty expressing basic needs; severe apathy, psychotic symptoms, and/or distress expressed as agitation, aggression common; positive AD biomarkers and neuroimaging evidence of extensive diffuse cortical atrophy	In general, retained capacity to show affection and enjoy touch and social activities and interactions; retained capacity to dance, enjoy music, being with pets, spending time in nature, and spiritual rituals; retained capacity to show empathy toward others and express gratitude
7	Terminal-stage major neurocognitive disorder with limited language functions, loss of narrative self; often bed bound and completely dependent on others for all activities, including feeding; distress expressed as agitation is common	In general, retained capacity to enjoy touch, music, show affection, and respond to spiritual rituals

The Grossberg-Desai Staging Scale. Retained Strengths by Stage of AD

* Alzheimer's disease biomarkers include positive amyloid and tau positron emission tomography (amyloid PET and tau PET) imaging, cerebrospinal fluid (CSF) abeta/tau ratio (decreased abeta and increased tau in CSF), temporoparietal hypometabolism seen in flurodeoxyglucose positron emission tomography (FDG PET) and hippocampal atrophy on neuroimaging

(e.g. laughter) or relief of negative emotions (e.g. distress due to feeling lonely). One of the most effective psychosocial approaches is the emotional warmth the staff can offer the resident through verbal and nonverbal behaviors. No tools or fancy equipment are necessary; just one's self. For a resident who has MNCD, a strong positive relationship is the medium in which happiness is experienced and healing occurs. Holding the resident's hand, rubbing the shoulder or back, hugging the resident if done with genuine concern and respect can be immensely healing and yet is not taught in medical and nursing schools. Unexpected embraces, uncharacteristic expressions of feeling – these are only some of the many ways in which relationships can grow through the demands of MNCD and frailty. To accept help, to depend, to embrace attention may satisfy yearnings long suppressed. When the resident's plight is relieved, even for a brief moment, both the giver and receiver gain a lesson in hope.

Even brief frequent encounters can bring lasting comfort. A positive relationship can also motivate a resident to engage in and stay in a new activity. For staff members who like older and disabled adults and who find value in caring for them, these interpersonal skills come easily. Hence, these two characteristics should be necessary factors in deciding which individuals to hire. Even the best staff frequently become wrapped up in efforts to complete tasks and miss the petite opportunities to connect with the resident with a gentle touch, to bring a smile to a sweet face. Staff training in mindfulness practices can teach the skills to pause when such moments arrive and lean into them. Positive relationships and positive encounters are also essential for the staff's well-being and have the power to neutralize stress inherent in working in LTC. A positive encounter can promote hope that more positive encounters await both the resident and the staff in the future. Making the relationship with the resident central to all aspects of caregiving is the central feature of PCC. Positive relationships and encounters can also provide reason for living for many residents. Perhaps one purpose of life is to experience love, and love is experienced only in the context of a genuinely caring relationship.

Following the Lead of the Resident Who Has Major Neurocognitive Disorder

All team members should make every effort to inquire into and understand the experiences and perspectives of the resident who has MNCD, even in advanced stages (Desai et al. 2016). Research has shown that individuals who have MNCD retain a remarkable level of awareness, even in advanced stages (Clare 2010). The resident who has MNCD should be considered expert in what will make her life more meaningful and happy. Professional and family caregivers need to develop the skill to follow the resident's lead (expressed verbally or nonverbally). If a resident seems content spending time not engaged in group activity, pushing her to attend activities may cause distress, which may be expressed as agitation. If a resident is making an effort to push another resident's wheelchair, instead of stopping the resident, it would be better to join the resident in pushing the wheelchair or gently guide the resident to another task that addresses the need to help others. We have witnessed great outcomes when staff members adopted creative ideas and suggestions for activities by residents who have MNCD in place of certain group activities that were not "fun."

Listening to the Resident's Stories and Allowing the Resident to Vent

Hearing and listening to a resident is critical to her psychosocial well-being. Listening nurtures contentment and builds connections. Learning to elicit and listen to a resident's story also serves as a cultural assessment tool. Every resident has one or more stories to tell, and stories build bridges between staff and residents. Staff can help residents cope with stressful situations by providing an outlet for frustration and an opportunity to vent. The conversations at first glance may not make sense and may be hard to follow, but nevertheless are immensely important to the resident and have the potential to be enjoyable to both.

Meaningful Activities

Psychosocial activities have a powerful effect in promoting happiness in a resident's life if they are made meaningful in the context of the resident's past occupation and current strengths and interests. Box 13.3 lists examples of meaningful activities for a resident who has MNCD. Box 13.4 lists activities caregivers (family and friends as well as professional caregivers) can engage in with the resident to promote wellness. Reading aloud funny quotes or asking a resident to read them, sharing cartoons, watching classic television comedies as well as classic comedy movies, sharing jokes (especially one-liners) can be done either in a formal group setting as a

BOX 13.4 Activities Caregivers (Family and Professional) of a Resident Who Has Major Neurocognitive Disorder May Engage in during Visits and Interactions

- Listening to resident, even when speech seems impossible to decipher, and sharing positive events in their life with resident, even when it is unclear if resident comprehends
- Singing songs (e.g. hymns, Christmas carols, favorite songs ["You are my sunshine"]) with or to resident
- Eating together in facility or going out to eat
- Walking together or pushing resident in wheelchair
- Giving hand massage, hugs and kisses, back rub
- Listening to music, watching a TV show or movie together (even if resident seems not to understand or is not interested: as long as visitor is enjoying activity, at some level resident will benefit from companionship and seeing loved one's enjoyment)
- Paging through memory books or photo albums and reminiscing with resident and staff
- Showing resident photos of recent travel by family member (especially involving children, grandchildren, places that resident has visited or liked)
- Watching birds and splendor of nature (e.g. sunset, sunrise, ocean, mountain, river, lake) with resident
- Gardening together (e.g. watering plants)
- Reading passage from religious text or listening to book on tape/CD/iPod/MP3 player
- Spending "quiet time" with resident (physical presence is sufficient for resident to experience companionship). For example, family member can read book or magazine while sitting next to resident
- Going for nature walk with resident
- Taking resident for car ride
- Dancing together
- Playing live or recorded music by talented family member (e.g. grandson playing piano)
- Playing Ping-Pong or any other game (e.g. board game, card game) together
- Reading greeting cards, letters, or emails from family and friends
- Creative activities (e.g. water coloring, coloring by numbers)
- Sharing jokes, reading humorous passages, watching funny movie
- Bringing and arranging flowers
- Playing Wii games (e.g. golf, bowling) with resident

scheduled activity or incorporated into everyday care to enhance joy in the lives of residents. We have been pleasantly surprised time and again by the remarkable sense of humor (especially one-liners) of residents even in advanced stages of MNCD.

Promoting a Sense of Purpose

An essential aspect of psychosocial approaches is promoting a sense of purpose. Helplessness is the pain one feels when one receives but is unable to give. Many residents in LTC experience this. Engaging a resident in activity that gives her purpose (e.g. the resident is in charge of watering plants with supervision as necessary) may provide a new reason for her to get up in the morning and look forward to the day. Charlotte's purpose in life was to take care of her family (spouse after marriage, children until they were grown, and spouse since then), and her behavior of looking for her small children (when she now has grandchildren and great-grandchildren) may be an expression that she needs to take care of someone, to be needed, to be useful. This is what gives her purpose in life!

Facilitating Expression of Sexual and Intimacy Needs

All residents have sexual and intimacy needs that are not going to disappear when they begin life in the new home. Such needs can range from taking extra care every day to look and dress well to looking for a romantic relationship to wanting a sexually intimate encounter with one's spouse or another resident. Facilitating expression of sexual and intimacy needs of a resident who has MNCD using a variety of

BOX 13.5 **Psychosocial Approaches to Better Meet the Need for Sexual Expression of a Resident Who Has Major Neurocognitive Disorder**

- Staff education and sensitivity training
- Detailed sexual history to improve understanding of resident's sexual needs
- Staff openly discuss their attitudes and concerns, pick up cues that may indicate resident's unmet needs for intimacy
- Promote privacy (no room sharing, "Do Not Disturb" sign outside door, knocking on door and calling resident's name and asking permission to enter)
- Allow conjugal visits, home visits
- Individualized high-touch care
- Encourage alternative forms of sexual expression, such as hugging and kissing
- Beauty salons and cosmetic services
- Educate residents and family about their rights and resources to meet sexual needs
- Encourage friendships and relationships
- Transfer care to another staff member if there is conflict between staff member's duty to address resident's sexual needs and staff member's personal value system
- Address physical limitations and poor health (e.g. better pain management, excess disability)
- When appropriate, offer means and encouragement to resident to help meet his/her sexual goals

psychosocial approaches may have a bigger impact on the resident's well-being than any other activity or initiative. (See Box 13.5.)

Clinical Case 1: "I like the way she laughs"

Mr. T, a resident of a LTC facility for 12 months, was increasingly depressed because his wife had reduced the frequency of her visits to once a week and would visit for only a few minutes. His wife reported that visiting him was too depressing, as he was not the active and intelligent person she married. Over time, Mr. T lost weight and stopped going to group activity programs he previously attended. He was about to be put on an antidepressant when his mood started to improve. He began eating better, started taking part in activity, and seemed to be genuinely happy. This was because Mr. T had developed a friendship with another female resident, and they would spend several hours together, watching TV or sharing stories. When asked what he liked about this new friend, Mr. T replied, "I like the way she laughs."

Teaching Point

This case illustrates the power of friendship, attachment, and intimacy in healing emotional pain. It also illustrates the resiliency of Mr. T (and many other residents) in the face of overwhelming adversity.

Facilitating Expression of the Resident's Culture

Facilitating expression of the resident's culture is an essential aspect of psychosocial approaches to promote wellness, especially for residents who are from a culture different from that of the majority of residents in that PCLTCC. Being able to speak one's native language with someone who understands, having an opportunity to eat the sweet and savory foods of one's ethnic origin, being helped to find and dress in clothes that reflect one's heritage, and experiencing the joy of listening to songs from one's country of origin are just some examples of facilitating expression of the resident's culture. One of the authors comes from India, and listening to Hindi music has been and continues to be an essential activity that promotes his emotional and spiritual well-being and helps him de-stress. The second author relishes opportunities to eat poppy-seed cake and chicken paprikash, which remind him of foods his mother used to prepare while he was growing up in Hungary.

As our community becomes more diversified, so will our LTC populations and LTC facility staff. In large metropolitan areas, this has already started. Respecting the residents' cultural beliefs and traditions as well as those of the staff (who often may be from a different culture) is one of the fundamental components of PCC. Some cultural beliefs may even provide emotional relief in dealing with incurable and progressive conditions such as MNCD. For example, many Asian cultures (e.g. residents originally from India) accept hardships of life, including MNCD, as "destiny" and do not resist or fight, whereas Western culture often reacts initially (and even in later stages) with resistance and a wish to "fight" the condition. Aikido, a Japanese martial art, teaches us to go with the force that threatens us, rather than oppose it. Without resistance, there can be no collision. Instead, there is fluid motion, more like rushing water than the intransigence of stone. This philosophy can be helpful in dealing with MNCD, especially for family caregivers.

Strengthening Existing Friendships and Facilitating New Friendships

Strengthening the resident's existing friendships and facilitating the development of new friendships (e.g. with other residents, with family members of other residents, with the facility chaplain) is a core component of all psychosocial approaches (McFadden and McFadden 2011). Friendships have a remarkable effect on our well-being that is just starting to be appreciated. Friendships influence our identity, sooth angst, and fill emotional gaps in relationships with family. Friendships promote a sense of being part of a community. The Alzheimer's Society of United Kingdom's *Dementia Friends* (www.dementiafriends.org.uk) program encourages all of us to learn to understand the perspectives of persons who have MNCD and make efforts to help them in small and big ways. We strongly recommend that all PCLTCCs adopt such a program. It is important for residents to connect in a meaningful way with other residents and caregivers, besides their own family. Genuine friendships can protect residents from the stress of declining health and functional abilities. Involvement of another person (e.g. another resident, a volunteer) as a "wellness buddy" to engage the resident in various activities (e.g. exercising together, dining together) and to provide day-to-day support may be helpful for some residents.

Facilitating Intergenerational Connections

The mere presence of children can bring a smile, laugh, or caress from a resident who has MNCD and seems not to be interested in any activity. Even a resident who has advanced MNCD and is usually silent may initiate conversation in the presence of children. Family are encouraged to visit their loved one in a LTC facility with small children who can color with the resident (or children can color on their own while the resident watches with interest), play with toys, watch TV (cartoons, educational programs) or movies with the resident, or just bring some laughter and joyfulness by their playful presence. Residents can be encouraged to share stories with children from a local school. The children do not necessarily have to interact with the resident (especially someone who has advanced MNCD and has lost the ability to converse). Their mere presence in the room may be sufficient to provide a sense of peace that comes with knowing that loved ones are around.

Facilitating Companionship

A brief companionship is valuable for resident well-being and does not have to lead to a friendship or relationship. Life can be lonely for many residents who have MNCD, and brief encounters with nurses and nursing assistants may be the only human interaction many residents have in a day, especially in the evening and on the weekend, when staffing is at its lowest and group activities (even scheduled ones) often do not occur. Facilitating companionship with visitors, chaplains, other residents, housekeeping staff, and maintenance staff may also enhance the resident's quality of life in unexpected ways. Most residents love having visitors. Indeed, any visitor generates excitement among residents. Even when a resident has lost the ability to comprehend speech and express herself, she can still savor the physical presence of anyone who sits and listens to her, makes eye contact, and responds eagerly with facial gestures. We strongly encourage all family members and friends of a resident to spend some time with other residents and interact with them, even if only for a few minutes. Even a brief alleviation of loneliness can have a lasting positive effect on the resident's mood.

Activities that Promote a Sense of Being Part of a Greater Community

Facilitating a sense of being a part of the greater community should be a key component of SPPEICE. Most residents have been an integral member of a larger community (e.g. religious community, neighborhood community, professional community) but are forgotten by friends and peers once they move to the new home. Friends and other members of the resident's previous community often need some guidance to start visiting the resident, reconnecting with her, and keeping her abreast of some community activities. Efforts to make a new resident feel that he is joining a loving and fun community can begin with the resident's receiving a welcome gift basket, having meet-and-greet activities, and other similar rituals. Attending a concert at a local theater, going fishing with friends or family, participating in a community service project, going to a local museum, or playing with local children through an intergenerational program can be fun and give the resident a sense of being part of the greater community.

Psychosocial Approaches to Avoid

We do not recommend repeatedly correcting the resident who has cognitive impairment regarding the day of the week or the time of the day or the place of living (reality orientation therapy), as it may trigger frustration and lower mood. However, liberal use of calendars and reality-orientation boards showing the date, day of the week, weather, and name of the PCLTCC may be useful. We also recommend using activity boards showing facility activities and times.

It is not okay to treat residents who have advanced MNCD as children, in essence, to infantilize them. All residents have lived a long life and had a wealth of remarkable experiences before entering the LTC facility. Instead, we recommend paying homage to the resident's life and achievements and treating him as an "elder" whose wisdom and intellect may be "hidden" or "imprisoned" by MNCD but is not lost. Every resident would like us not only to honor her but also to support her in her spiritual and emotional journey, especially in her diminished and fragile state.

Sensory Approaches

For the resident who has MNCD, it can be immensely enjoyable and soothing to engage as many senses (olfactory [smell], gustatory [taste], auditory [hearing], visual [vision], tactile [touch], and proprioceptive [movement and position]) as possible based on preserved strengths in the sensory systems.

Music-Based Approaches

Music-based approaches have the potential to have dramatic positive effect on the well-being of a resident who has MNCD, yet they are the most underused sensory approaches. Music is a superb way of maintaining connections to the past and to other people. A resident who has MNCD and can play a musical instrument (e.g. piano) may not know what he ate twenty minutes ago but at the piano may recall, play, and sing dozens of songs by accessing remote and implicit memory. Music-based activities, particularly live and/or preferred music, may reduce distress and improve mood. Slow classical music (e.g. Bach, Vivaldi) has been found to reduce distress and agitation. Calming music (especially during mealtime) may improve intake of food. "Drumming," in which residents bang on different drums, talking about what the sound reminds them of, taking each person's name, breaking it into syllables, and beating them on the drum can be fun and empowering. Group singing activities or "singing for the brain" programs not only can be fun but also may have a positive impact in maintaining the resident's cognitive functioning. For many, music and dancing is part of their culture and so its value goes well beyond pleasure. Soft music may help relieve tension and anxiety; energetic music may help lift a depressed mood. Religious music may elicit active participation from a resident who is not responding to conventional music. *Alive Inside* is an award-winning documentary movie that is a must-see for all staff working in LTC (www.aliveinside.us/#land). The movie will inspire staff to tap into the power of music to transport the resident who has MNCD to new heights of emotional and spiritual wellness.

Physical Activity and Exercise

Evolutionary forces have shaped our proprioceptive sensory system (the system involved in musculoskeletal movement), whenever it is activated, to have a positive effect on neurocognitive and emotional regulation networks. Regular exercise and physical activity play an important role in the maintenance of emotional, cognitive, and functional well-being of LTC residents (Morley 2016). Exercise and physical activity is associated with an increase in opioid receptor-related neurotransmission, directly stimulating pleasure and reward centers, resulting in a sense of happiness and well-being. The release of brain-derived neurotrophic factor during physical activity and exercise promotes a host of neurocognitive functions (especially attention and memory) that promote better engagement in fun and meaningful activities. An individualized simple exercise program (e.g. one hour, two or more times weekly, of walk, strength, balance, and flexibility training) may slow functional decline, decrease the risk of falls, and reduce symptoms of depression and agitation. We recommend extra flexibility training for men and extra strength training for women. Education in the benefits of regular exercise may improve attendance and the likelihood of implementation by staff. Most residents tolerate exercise well without any adverse effect. Exercise programs should involve aerobic activity (walking, swimming), strength training (using "resistance bands" [e.g. latex-free Thera-Bands, endorsed by the American Physical Therapy Association], weights, Pilates), flexibility (Pilates, yoga, flexibility exercises), and balance training (Tai Chi, other balance exercise). Some LTC facilities have an indoor swimming pool for residents, and staff at these facilities have found that a surprising number of residents enjoy swimming, water aerobics, or just playing with water! High-quality exercise programs, particularly whole-body involvement rather than walking alone, should be routinely available in all LTC facilities. Such programs should have a significant element of fun to motivate the resident who would not otherwise want to engage in an exercise program.

Aromas, Massage, Taste, and Other Sensory Approaches

Most residents respond to tactile stimulation: a hug, an arm on the shoulder, a clasp of the hand, a back rub, and/or a hand massage. At many levels, they still need human touch. Massage therapy (e.g. back and shoulder massage) may provide much-needed relaxation and comfort and may reduce anxiety and agitation related to pain. A gentle aromatic neck or shoulder massage may also promote sleep. Combining massage and aromatherapy (e.g. hand massage with a lotion [e.g. lavender for soothing, citrus for activating]) may have an even better effect in calming an agitated resident. Aromas can be administered through inhalation or during bathing or applied during massage and as a skin cream. We support appropriate use of alternative therapeutic touch practices (e.g. Reiki) to promote psychological and spiritual healing. Group activities involving cooking (e.g. freshly baked bread or cookies, popping popcorn) can get even "difficult" residents involved and enjoying the activity.

Spiritual Approaches and Initiatives

Sustained spiritual well-being is one of the most important goals of caring for residents who have MNCD and should receive the same importance as emotional and physical well-being (if not more). Spirituality refers to meaningful connectedness within the self, with other people, with nature, and with the sacred. Spirituality encompasses organized religion (and rituals associated with it) as well as love for nature, volunteer activities, prayer, loving-kindness meditation practices, and any activity that involves making the world a better place. There is a Sufi saying that two veils separate us from the divine: health and security. When we lose them, we may find ourselves dealing with questions that belong to the spiritual realms. Humbling circumstances may enlarge us, in spite of ourselves.

For most residents, spirituality has played an important role in their lives. Spirituality can be an enormous source of comfort, providing hope, meaning, and purpose. It may ward off depression, speed recovery from depression, and increase the quality of life. Better mental health, in turn, may increase motivation toward self-care activities and even help residents view their problems as less disabling.

Often it is at the later stages of MNCD that the spiritual experiences of those who have MNCD are most profound. Accordingly, the decline in cognitive functioning does not reflect a loss of spiritual capacity, and those who have advanced MNCD remain capable of high levels of spiritual well-being and engagement in spiritual activities, rituals, and interactions.

Participating in Organized Religious Activities and Rituals

Many residents are deeply religious and depend on religion as a major way of coping with health problems and other adversities. Many people have been attending religious services regularly all their lives but lose this ritual to spiritual expression after entering LTC. They should be given as much opportunity as possible to express their faith and participate in religious activities and rituals that they have been practicing before coming to the LTC facility. Rituals, prayers, and sacred liturgy from childhood often stay firmly rooted in memory long after MNCD takes its toll. Helping a resident who has MNCD continue to observe faith can be beneficial and rewarding for both the resident and family caregivers.

Residents may sleep and eat better if they say a prayer before bedtime or grace before a meal. Having a ritual of grieving, such as gathering for prayers when a resident passes away, can also provide spiritual satisfaction. The HCP should consider using an old edition of a devotional book or hymnal and asking older relatives what the old standards were when they were growing up. People who have MNCD or stroke and have been mute for months have been observed to sing the words of a religious hymn spontaneously and otherwise participate in religious service. We recommend that ministers design religious services as multisensory experiences that emphasize noncognitive pathways (e.g. visual symbols). The facility should offer religious book study (either one to one or in a group) for residents who have relatively preserved cognitive function. Visits from spiritual counselors may help fill the void left by many residents' inability to attend church or other preferred place of worship due to frailty.

Participating in the Resident's Spontaneous Spiritual Experiences

As we take care of residents, we can help them get in touch with their spirituality. We can share in their expressions and experiences of spiritual moments, such as their commenting on the sunbeam lighting up a crystal saltshaker into all kinds of colors and sparkles.

Nonreligious Spiritual Activities

Spiritual activities such as saying prayers for the well-being of other residents or family or even unrelated people (e.g. people suffering in another country) can make residents feel satisfied that they have reached out beyond themselves to support someone else. Engaging residents in one-on-one or group loving-kindness meditation practices is another spiritual activity that we recommend for residents who have MNCD and are willing to engage in these activities.

Chaplain Services

All PCLTCCs should have at least one in-house chaplain to better meet the spiritual needs of LTC residents, especially residents who have MNCD and otherwise may not be able to advocate for their own spiritual needs. A resident may indicate spiritual distress by a statement such as "God has forsaken me!" "I have no reason to live," or "Is there life after death?" We recommend that a member of the clergy familiar with the resident address the spiritual distress. Hope is the subjective sense of having a meaningful future despite obstacles. Preservation of hope can maximize psychological adjustment to progressive disability. Clergy are best suited among the team members to encourage hope despite the future perils of terminal cancer, advancing MNCD, or other disability.

Facilitating Inner Exploration

Keeping physically active in later years is important, but movement inward may prove even more important. Inner exploration is one of the chief spiritual benefits of slowing down in later life. Facilitating inner exploration is an essential component of spiritual approaches. Although cognitive impairment may make inner exploration difficult, the resident is nevertheless doing so, and we can facilitate this journey. Many residents faced with long stretches of silence turn inward to a silent place inside that brings them closer to their spiritual beliefs. The resident may be ushered by MNCD or stroke into a previously unknown place in him-/herself. In the domain of frailty and immobility, where the commotion of worldly events finally ceases, residents are brought closer to the sacred, a realm that thrives through silence and relinquishment. PCC recognizes and encourages such moments that happen spontaneously and are often expressed by the resident out of the blue. We urge caregivers (professional and family) to respond to such moments with deep awareness that something tender is being shared. Just being with the resident (e.g. squeezing a hand to communicate that you heard him/her) during such moments is sufficient. Such moments may even deepen the caregiver's own connection with life.

Dignity-Conserving Approaches

Upholding, protecting, and restoring the dignity of all patients is the duty of every HCP and the essence of medicine. Every resident is worthy of honor, and there is meaning in the life of every resident, irrespective of cognitive, physical, or emotional condition. Kindness, humanity, and respect – the core values of the medical profession, often overlooked in our time-pressed culture – can be reinstated by dignity-conserving care (Chochinov 2007). How residents perceive themselves to be seen is a powerful mediator of dignity. Dignity is closely associated with a sense of being treated with respect. Factors that have been identified as fracturing the sense of a resident's dignity include but are not limited to: loss of independence, fear of becoming a burden, not being involved in decision-making, lacking access to high-quality care, and some attitudes (e.g. dismissiveness) of HCPs, especially when a resident feels vulnerable and lacks power. HCPs can uphold the resident's dignity by seeing him for the person he was before MNCD or stroke altered him, rather than just the illness he has. We recommend the "A, B, C, D" approach to dignity-conserving care described by Dr. Chochinov (Chochinov 2007). (See Box 13.6.) Ensuring dignity thus involves spending time with the resident and family. This quality of professionalism and connectedness also increases the likelihood that the resident and/or family will be forthright in disclosing personal information, which so often has a

BOX 13.6 The A, B, C, and D of Dignity-Conserving Care

A = Attitude:	all HCPs have utmost respect for all residents at all times (during life and after death).
B = Behavior:	all HCPs show respect and kindness to all residents through verbal and nonverbal behaviors at every interaction.
C = Compassion:	all HCPs have compassion (deep awareness of suffering of another coupled with wish to relieve it) for all residents at all times.
D = Dialogue:	all HCPs have ongoing dialogue with self (e.g. "Am I making ageist assumptions?"), with other HCPs (e.g. "Are we withholding life-sustaining treatment because of our assumption that resident has poor quality of life?"), with resident ("What do you value? What gives your life meaning? What is your attitude toward suffering? What is your identity?"), and with family ("What are the most important things in your loved one's life? Was there a hierarchy?") to know and value every resident.

bearing on ongoing care. Every LTC facility should have a written policy of "zero tolerance" for lack of dignity in the care of every resident.

Truth telling is a key dimension of dignity-conserving care. Truthfulness is the foundation of all relationships and signifies respect for the other person. Without honesty and truthfulness, trust cannot be established and established trust can be quickly eroded. Without trust, caregivers (family and professional) may not be able to meet the emotional and physical needs of the resident and may even inadvertently cause emotional harm. Most residents do not have the ability or resources to find a different environment in which caregivers are honest and truthful. Truth telling, especially to a resident who has moderate to severe MNCD, can cause an ethical dilemma for many caregivers (family as well as professional). All methods of discourse with residents should be truthful, with rare exceptions. Our residents (with and without MNCD) are much more resilient than we realize, and even cognitively impaired residents can quickly detect a lie (e.g. caregiver telling a resident who wants to go home that she is at the facility "for only a few days" and soon will be able to go home).

Benevolent deception (therapeutic exception, therapeutic lie) should be an exception rather than the rule in caring for vulnerable LTC residents who have MNCD. Truth telling is not synonymous with being "bluntly honest," nor does it mean that the staff should constantly correct statements made by the resident who has MNCD. Blunt honesty and repeatedly correcting a resident's beliefs and memory in most situations may be harmful to the resident. Strict adherence to the virtues of truthfulness and candor in some situations (e.g. a resident who made a recent serious suicide attempt is told that he has Alzheimer's disease) risks violation of the core ethical principles of beneficence and nonmaleficence. In daily practice, such situations are rare, but the frequency of lying and dishonesty in dealing with LTC residents who have MNCD is far from rare. This culture of dishonesty is fueled more by the irrational fears of the caregivers (professional and family) and by the discomfort of caregivers in addressing a resident's grief and loss than by a rational and compassionate approach to care.

Truth telling needs to be done with utmost sensitivity to the resident's emotional state and individual circumstances and with efforts to understand what the resident is trying to express (e.g. a resident asking when he can go home may be reacting to unrelieved pain; a resident asking for her small children may be reacting to feelings of lack of purpose in life; a resident looking for her parents is looking for validation, security, and unconditional love). Truthfulness may hurt (e.g. telling the resident that this is her new home), and caregivers need to anticipate the resident's emotional pain and take steps to relieve it. Ultimately, being truthful is about honoring the resident's dignity, and thus is each resident's right and our obligation. This is even more important for residents who are weakest (e.g. a resident who has severe MNCD), as their dignity rests in our hands.

Dignity therapy is an innovative life-review psychotherapy developed to address the legacy needs of individuals receiving end-of-life care. It may be used with some modifications to enhance the legacy of any resident who has MNCD and help him/her feel happy and proud about past accomplishments. It may be done using technologies such as FaceTime, Skype, online chat, or email.

Environmental Approaches and Initiatives

Therapeutic physical environment and environmental design is a core aspect of environmental approaches. The design of a LTC facility can have tremendous effect on the resident's physical (e.g. reduced falls) as well as psychosocial and spiritual well-being, especially for a resident who has MNCD. See Box 13.7 for examples of environmental strategies that may help or hinder physical and/or psychosocial well-being. Therapeutic design of a LTC facility may

BOX 13.7 Key Environmental Designs That May Help or Hinder the Well-Being of a Resident Who Has Major Neurocognitive Disorder

Designs That May Help Well-Being

- Small, homelike environment
- Increased personal space
- All private rooms
- Large windows or skylights that allow plenty of natural light and offer beautiful views of nature outside
- Indoor (continuous well-defined) pathways and secure outdoor walking paths and sheltered gardens to encourage enjoyment of nature outdoors, safe wandering, casual strolling, and exercise in a safe environment (includes walled-in areas, way-finding enhancements, reduced stimulation areas, enhanced environments)
- Therapeutic gardens with nontoxic plants for horticulture programming
- Craft studio
- Privacy rooms where residents can go when they want to meditate, spend time alone, or be sexually intimate with spouse or other loved one
- Family room with a fireplace where residents can spend time with family and hold family functions and holiday celebrations
- Room for staff to "chill." Such a room may have a treadmill, soothing music, comfortable chairs, automated massage chairs, etc., to help staff "destress" and feel they are valued.
- Fitness center and temperature-controlled indoor/outdoor swimming pool with wheelchair ramps and walking rails
- Each bedroom door is a Dutch door (Closed door may agitate resident who has MNCD. With top half open, closed bottom may prevent resident who has MNCD from wandering into or meddling in someone else's room.)
- Putting toilet in view of bed so that resident has fewer incidents of incontinence or toileting in inappropriate places
- Traditional nurses station replaced by nourishment centers that provide opportunity for social interaction besides enjoying ice cream or other delicious food or beverage items
- Photos, shadow boxes, or curio cueing cabinets outside resident bedroom that hold meaningful mementos that trigger long-term memories and may help resident identify his or her room
- Glass-sided refrigerator door showing residents food (resident is free to open refrigerator door and eat food inside even if he no longer knows a refrigerator's significance)
- Food is prepared in facility kitchen, with aromas of food floating around, and served restaurant style, with second helpings encouraged

Designs That May Hinder Well-Being

- Long corridors
- Food delivered on trays
- Glare from lighting or insufficient lighting
- Small amount of natural light
- Dark-colored floors or certain parts of the floor (may be mistaken for a hole by resident who has cognitive impairment)
- Glass walls, which resident may walk into inadvertently
- Audible intercoms, which are often distracting and distressing to both resident and staff

also reduce aggressive behaviors by residents toward others. For example, overcrowding and frequent intrusion of others in one's personal space is a risk factor for physical aggression, and thus increased personal space and private rooms may reduce the risk of aggressive behavior. A LTC facility should be a place that supports healthy aging, active engagement in life, spirituality, and the peaceful last years of a resident's life. A recent trend is to diverge from the traditional medical model (large facilities that focus on providing medical care) to a social model (small home-like environments with terraces, landscaping, windows that make the outdoors relevant). Such social models involve well-designed LTC facilities (e.g. large facilities housing two or more "neighborhoods" [each neighborhood with two to four "houses" and each house having 10–12 residents], as well as small-scale "homes" caring for eight to 10 individuals who have MNCD) that not only are esthetically pleasing but also may be spiritually uplifting (e.g. more contact with nature) and give residents reasons to "get out of bed" and socialize, enjoy outdoors, or just wander safely.

Technological solutions to enhance and maintain the resident's independence and freedom are just starting to be studied and in the future may become affordable and a routine part of living in a LTC facility. For example, if a resident gets out of bed in the middle of the night, the bedroom lights turn on; if a resident is detected exiting through a main door at an inappropriate time, a prompt would encourage him or her to go back to bed; should the resident continue to exit, care staff are alerted.

Lighting in LTC facilities is often insufficient for residents as well as for the staff and may contribute to increased risk of falls. Proper lighting is important, especially in certain areas, such as hallways and bathrooms, where residents are at increased risk for falls and during cloudy days, at dusk, and after dark. Appropriate lighting should be considered primary prevention for depression, sleep disorder, and loss of independence besides falls. In general, light levels should be increased without creating glare. All lighting fixtures (preferably fluorescent light), with the exception of those in day-use-only activity spaces, should be able to be dimmed to evenly lower the overall lighting during the evening and nighttime hours.

The integration of residents who have relatively preserved cognitive function with residents who have MNCD may result in increased distress of residents who have MNCD, as the environment has usually not been adapted to their cognitive challenges. The resident who has relatively preserved cognitive function may also frequently experience distress due to inadvertent invasion of her privacy by residents who have MNCD. A LTC facility specifically for residents who have MNCD or a specific "unit" or "wing" may help address this problem. Such a specialized facility may be able to better help residents' ADL function, decrease anxiety and fear, and increase residents' interest in activities because of the high likelihood that the facility has staff better trained in understanding and caring for residents who have MNCD, besides the unique environmental designs the facility may have adopted. Decorating some areas of the facility with scenes of nature or home life, including recorded sounds and smells, has been associated with residents spending more time in these areas and an increase in their level of pleasure. Having contrasting colors and textures on walls, doors, and furniture as well as signs on doors may help the resident who has MNCD be more independent.

Bright light therapy is a specific environmental approach that has the potential to improve mood, cognition, and sleep for some LTC residents who have MNCD. Bright light therapy uses a light therapy unit that is about 1 foot by 1.5 feet in surface area and uses white fluorescent light behind a plastic diffusing screen that filters out ultraviolet rays. We recommend exposure to bright light (minimum 2,500 lux; preferably 10,000 lux) for 30 to 90 minutes in the morning and/or evening for therapeutic effect, which may start within two to four days. The HCP should consider bright light therapy during winter months (for some, in fall and spring also) for any resident who has a history suggestive of seasonal affective disorder (typically major depression in winter). Six percent of the US population, primarily in northern climates, is affected by seasonal affective disorder in its most marked form. Another 14 percent of the US adult population has a lesser form of seasonal mood change, known as winter blues. Bright light therapy may also improve sleep for a resident who has insomnia (especially sleep phase advancement). The resident usually is required to sit in quiet activity in front of the light box while receiving light. For a resident who will not sit in front of a light box, a uniformly high level of light may improve sleep as well as daytime agitation. Bright lights (10,000 lux or more) can be installed in fluorescent fixtures in the ceiling of the activity room. Emerging data show that exposure to bright light therapy in late afternoon or early evening may abort "sundowning" among residents who have MNCD. Bright light therapy does not benefit residents who go to sleep during the session or have their eyes closed. Adverse effects of bright light therapy include eyestrain, headache (which may manifest as agitation), and potential risk of induction of hypomania or mania in a resident who has bipolar disorder. If a resident is unable to tolerate the treatment, the intensity of the treatment can be reduced by increasing the distance from the light box or reducing the duration of therapy. Some health care insurers may cover the expense of a light therapy device if the indication is seasonal affective disorder.

Creative Engagement

We are all artists, and bringing out the artist within each resident should be a core aspect of any psychosocial-spiritual wellness program. Creativity can be broadly defined as any behavioral or psychological activity that is new and provides spiritual and emotional benefits to the resident and others. By this description, creative activities may include a whole spectrum of activities from artistic expression (e.g. painting, writing poetry) and performance (e.g. dancing, music) to creativity in daily activities (e.g. dressing, cooking) to creative problem solving (e.g. a resident who has MNCD creatively negotiates barriers to going outdoors). For a resident who has cognitive impairment, creative activities can offer excellent ways to express feelings (which may reduce anxiety and depression), experience the joys of using cognitive and motor skills (which may help maintain and even improve cognition, mood, and motor skills), experience delight in solving a problem (which can bolster the sense of mastery, control, and self-esteem), and facilitate personal growth. Thus, facilitating creative expression (which is already occurring spontaneously almost daily in every resident's life) through structured activities (e.g. group storytelling, painting, song writing, reading poems) and during activities of daily living (e.g. during caregiving) is a key component of SPPEICE.

Specific Psychosocial Approaches and Initiatives

Simulated Presence

Simulated presence (also called simulated presence therapy) is an approach that involves playing an audio- or audio-video recording to the resident who has MNCD, personalized by a family member or a friend sharing positive experiences from the resident's life and shared happy memories. Simulated presence may help promote feelings of connectedness and relieve agitation and loneliness often manifesting as wish to "go home." An example of such a recording may be a daughter saying, "Hi, Dad. I'm doing well and I hope you are doing well also. You were so wonderful in teaching piano to my son, your grandson Alex. Alex and I will be seeing you soon, and he is eager to play your favorite tune, 'Fur Elise,' for you. Love, your daughter Faith." A resident who has severe short-term memory loss can hear and view such calming messages dozens of times a day without recognizing the repetition.

Animal-Assisted Approaches

Some form of animal-assisted approaches and companion pet programs has become a norm throughout the LTC system in the United States. Animal-assisted approaches such as using a "resident" and/or "visiting" dog, cat, or rabbit may reduce loneliness as well as promote social interaction for LTC residents who have MNCD. Many residents enjoy the touch of a pet, especially if they had a pet in their earlier life. Seeing a dog or cat walk up can elicit a positive response. The resident is suddenly present, captivated, reaching down to pet the animal. It gives the resident a chance to show love and bask in the memory of something warm. Physical touch, whether by a human or a furry animal, creates a sense of relaxation and of connection. A withdrawn resident may smile and laugh, a "nonverbal" resident may speak to, and about, the pet, and a resident may spontaneously begin to reminisce about a childhood pet. The desire for and potential benefits of animal-assisted approaches are strongly influenced by previous pet ownership. Any resident who has a strong life history of emotional intimacy with a pet and wishes to have a pet should be offered animal-assisted approaches to promote happiness and prevent loneliness and agitation. Local humane society and animal shelters often have volunteers who take dogs, cats, puppies, and kittens to LTC facilities for free. These events can be scheduled as a regular recurring (e.g. weekly) activity or as a special event. We recommend health protocols specific to animal-assisted approaches, and animal welfare and safety protocols and specific criteria for animal selection for all LTC facilities.

BOX 13.8 High-Tech Approaches to Promote a Resident's Psychosocial-Spiritual Wellness

- FaceTime, Skype, online chat, and email to connect and interact with family and friends (especially grandchildren)
- CD/MP3/iPod player or iPad/Tablets (to listen to music, books, family conversations)
- Big-screen TV (especially for resident who has impaired vision or if a large group of residents are watching TV in a group setting)
- DVD//Blu-ray player (to watch favorite family events that are video recorded, favorite shows, movies, games, travel, or cooking shows)
- Computer with Internet capability/multimedia devices (legacy websites storing favorite pictures, movies, music, family and other events; Computer Interactive Reminiscence and Communication Aid [CIRCA], and similar products with simplified interface that can be personalized)
- Videogames (e.g. Wii games by Nintendo)
- Robotic animals (e.g. a robot cat that purrs each time the resident moves hands over cats' body; sophisticated robot seal Paro)
- Toy animals that are soft, can be warmed safely (e.g. in microwave), and release soothing aromas (e.g. lavender)
- High-tech innovative approaches and services to promote dignity and happiness in resident provided by certain organizations (e.g. http://in2l.com [It's Never Too Late])

High-Tech Approaches

Facilities may try a variety of high-tech approaches listed in Box 13.8 to promote happiness and prevent agitation among LTC residents. For example, interactive robotic dogs may reduce loneliness. Often residents become attached to these robotic pets. The safety and autonomy of the residents may improve with the use of technologies to manage the facility's domestic ambient environment (e.g. medical sensors, entertainment equipment, home automation systems).

Cognitive Rehabilitation

Cognitive rehabilitation (CR) is an individualized approach that uses nondrug treatments to improve specific domains of cognitive function. The goal is not to enhance cognition but to improve cognitive function in the everyday context. CR is tailored to the resident's level of cognitive impairment, starting with the easiest tasks and increasing in difficulty as success occurs. CR usually requires a high level of motivation from the resident. Family involvement can help a resident who is hesitant to get involved. Such a program is implemented with an interdisciplinary approach with a neuropsychologist or speech and language therapist as the CR specialist.

CR may focus on several cognitive domains (e.g. attention, memory [episodic, procedural], speech, executive dysfunction) or specific functions (e.g. using procedural memory). A resident who has mild to moderate MNCD usually has relatively intact procedural memory and can be taught new skills or maintain existing skills using procedural memory function. These activities have the potential not only to add fun to the resident's life (e.g. learning to play table tennis [Ping-Pong], maintaining skill at playing piano or any musical instrument) but also to give meaningful social roles (e.g. playing the musical instrument for a group of residents). Performing a comedy routine for staff with or without using cards to read from, serving beverages and greeting the audience as they arrive, enhances and maintains social skills that are often preserved until late stages of MNCD. Special care residents have dressed up as clowns to visit residents who have life-limiting conditions. Taking part in a reading and discussion group is another activity that can help maintain cognition and improve mood through socialization and reminiscence. Many of the activities can be initiated by family and professional caregivers as well as volunteers (after brief training). Other examples of CR include training residents who have MNCD to run activities for residents who have more advanced MNCD and the use of intergenerational groups (residents who have MNCD teaching preschoolers phonics and how to count). Residents who have mild to moderate MNCD and have topographical disorientation (i.e. impaired ability to orient oneself in a real-life environment and navigate through it) may benefit from errorless-based techniques to improve the ability to find their room or other commonly used rooms (e.g. activities room, dining room) and prevent complications related to disorientation (e.g. avoiding social contact or wandering into another resident's room). Errorless-based techniques involve correcting the resident just before he goes the wrong way, asking the resident to go backward a short distance from the target location, and then to advance forward to the target location and gradually increasing the distance on subsequent trials until the resident can complete the whole route forward and repeat it.

CR strategies may also be applied to enhance function for even residents who have moderately severe MNCD. For example, teaching residents how to scoop golf balls into a muffin tin (one of many Montessori techniques) and repetition may help residents who have recently lost the ability to feed themselves regain the ability (Camp 2010). A highly motivated resident who has mild MNCD may benefit from a brain and memory wellness program to improve cognitive function and slow memory decline. (See Boxes 13.9, 13.10, and 13.11 and Table 13.3.) Regular engagement of residents in card games, puzzles (e.g. crossword puzzles, Sudoku, jigsaw puzzles), trivia games, and even computer games (e.g. FreeCell, a computer-based game similar to solitaire, in which the player electronically makes four stacks of cards, one from each suit, from ace to king; *Brain Age* by Nintendo) may also provide cognitive stimulation and may slow cognitive decline (Anderson and Grossberg 2014).

Dance and Movement Therapy

For centuries, dance and rhythmic movement has been used to express and modify emotions. Dance and movement therapy combines music, light exercise, and sensory stimulation and has been found to improve cognitive, social, and emotional well-being in LTC residents who have MNCD.

Activities for Special Populations

Residents younger than age 60 typically have advanced stages of young-onset MNCD. These include MNCD due to AD, FTD, stroke, TBI, alcohol, advanced multiple sclerosis, and advanced Huntington's disease. The psychosocial needs of this population are different from those of the typical older LTC resident. We recommend leading activities devoted to the interests of younger populations in LTC (e.g. a different reminiscence group activity that involves events in the 1960s and '70s rather than 1940s and '50s).

In a typical LTC facility, women outnumber men by three or more to one. Men in LTC often experience isolation and lack of male companionship. It may be helpful to establish a men's group or encourage male staff members – including maintenance personnel – to spend a few minutes with them. Many of the activities (e.g. making cookies or craft activities) may not be suited to the interests or strengths of male

BOX 13.9 A Comprehensive Brain and Memory Wellness Plan

Nutrition: Mediterranean diet, Dietary Approaches to Stop Hypertension (DASH) diet
Physical Activity: Aerobic exercise (e.g. brisk walking), strength training, balance training, exercises to promote flexibility, yoga, Tai-Chi, and leading physically active lifestyle
Intellectual Activity and Cognitive Training: Engaging in stimulating and challenging intellectual activities (e.g. puzzles, computer-based games, rekindling hobbies and passions), cognitive training (see Box 3.3)
Social and Spiritual Activities: Engaging in daily meaningful social activities (especially intergenerational) and spiritual activities and rituals
Sleep: Strategies to promote optimal sleep (not too little, not too much) through sleep hygiene and sleep diary
Stress Management: Relaxation strategies, identifying and correcting cognitive distortion, mindfulness-based stress reduction, meditation and mindfulness exercises, spending time in nature, music-based activities
Treatment of Reversible Causes of Cognitive Impairment: Evaluation and treatment of reversible causes of cognitive impairment (e.g. vitamin deficiency, low thyroid)
Treatment of Cardiovascular Risk Factors: Evaluation and treatment of cardiovascular risk factors (e.g. hypertension)
Medications: Low-dose acetylsalicylic acid (aspirin), omega-3 fatty acids, and cholinesterase inhibitors and memantine as appropriate
Resources: Education about brain and memory wellness (see Box 3.4)

Note: Intensity matters, as brain is neuroplastic but needs engagement in daily and fairly rigorous manner for optimal benefit.

BOX 13.10 The ART of Improving Attention, Memory, and Executive Functions

Attention Training: Attention is the gateway to all cognitive functions. Attention and concentration skills can be improved through simple strategies, such as focused slow breathing (bringing one's attention repeatedly to one's breath [exhalation longer than inhalation] for 5–20 minutes one or more times a day), mindfulness in daily living (e.g. mindful eating, mindful walking), and computerized attention-training exercises.

Repetition and Relaxation: Repetition is a key strategy to improve memory. Repetition can be done by repeating in one's mind, repeating aloud, rehearsing, and visualizing. Adding emotional value and context to information being repeated can enhance consolidation of memory through repetition. We also recommend daily engagement in computerized cognitive-training programs targeting specific neurocognitive functions (e.g. attention, memory, problem solving). It is important to relax by taking some slow deep breaths and making some self-soothing statements if one finds oneself becoming tense in an effort to remember. Spaced retrieval training, in which one repeats information after gradually increasing intervals (10 seconds, 30 seconds, 1 minute, 5 minutes, 15 minutes, 30 minutes, once a day) is useful for remembering information that is important and not likely to change (e.g. new grandchild's name).

Tricks and Tools: Tricks include but are not limited to: mnemonics, acronyms, using cues, verbal elaboration, visual elaboration, and "chunking." ART is an example of using mnemonics to remember different cognitive training strategies. If one has to remember a new number, 3145778000, it can be remembered in three chunks: 314 577 8000. Tools to aid memory and planning (executive function) include use of reminders using smart phone, written list, electronic pill dispenser, sticky note as reminders.

Note: The effectiveness of cognitive training is enhanced by leading a physically, socially, intellectually, and spiritually active life, consuming brain-healthy nutrition, and correcting reversible factors that cause cognitive impairment.

BOX 13.11 Resources for a Brain and Wellness Program

Peer-reviewed journal article

Anderson, K., and G. T. Grossberg. 2014. Brain Games to Slow Cognitive Decline in Alzheimer's Disease. *Journal of the American Medical Directors Association* 15:536–537. This article has excellent list of apps for games that can enhance brain function.

Books

- Small, G., and G. Vorgan. 2012. *The Alzheimer's Prevention Program*. New York: Workman Publishing Company.
- Hartman-Stein, P.E., and A. La Rue. 2011. Enhancing Cognitive Fitness in Adults: A Guide to the Use and Development of Community-based Programs. New York: Springer Publication.
- Doidge, N. 2007. *The Brain That Changes Itself*. New York: Penguin Books.

Audio CD

Weil, A., and G. Small. 2007. The Healthy Brain Kit. Audio CDs, brain-training cards, and workbook. Boulder, CO: Sound True.

Internet resources

- www.lumosity.com (online brain exercise programs)
- www.sharpbrains.com
- www.brainhq.com (online brain exercise programs)
- www.cdc.gov/aging/healthybrain/index.htm (Healthy Brain Initiative by the CDC)

residents. Activities geared more toward the interests of male residents (e.g. activities that involve tools [made of rubber or another safe synthetic material rather than metal], hunting and fishing) need to be part of various activities offered to all residents. The opposite is also true. In Veterans Administration homes and other PCLTCCs specializing in caring for veterans, men outnumber women. In these homes, it

Table 13.3 Brain-Healthy Nutrition

Brain-Rich Foods	Specific Examples of Foods	Therapeutic Pearls
Food rich in omega3 fatty acid	Fatty fish*(three or more ounces twice a week)	Omega-3 fatty acids may be obtained through supplements if adequate consumption of fish is not feasible Fatty fish are also high in selenium, vitamin D, and protein
Vegetables (1–4 servings per day)	Green leafy vegetables (e.g. spinach, broccoli)	Fresh vegetables and freshly cooked vegetables that resident prefers may promote increased consumption
Legumes (1–2 servings per day)	Black beans	Particularly beneficial for resident who has sarcopenia and/or low BMI, as they are high in protein besides micronutrients brain needs (e.g. folate) Particularly beneficial for resident who has constipation, as they have high content of fiber
Fruits (1–4 servings per day)	Berries (e.g. blueberries)	Fresh fruits that resident prefers may promote increased consumption
Whole grains (3–5 servings per day)	Cereals rich in whole grains	Cereals that resident prefers may promote increased consumption
Monosaturated fats	Avocados Olive oil Nuts (e.g. walnuts)	Particularly beneficial for resident who has low BMI, as they are high in calories
Spices	Turmeric	Help of facility chef is recommended to make addition of turmeric in food more palatable and tasty for resident not used to consuming food with turmeric
Food and or fluids to maintain gut microbiome	Probiotic yogurt with active bacterial cultures Probiotic drinks	Nondairy foods/fluids with active bacterial culture recommended for resident who has lactose intolerance

* Fatty fish include salmon, sardines, herring, anchovies

is important to have women's groups and activities tailored to women's interests.

Innovative Psychosocial Well-Being Programs and Approaches

A variety of innovative programs and approaches use PCC to improve residents' quality of life. One of the most important factors in a LTC facility embracing one or more of these programs is having a physician (especially the medical director) and the administrator champion these programs. Also, keeping the staff informed about success stories related to the program and involving family are crucial for the program to be sustainable.

Dementia Care Mapping is an excellent tool for developing PCC practices in LTC settings (Bradford Dementia Group 2005). Behaviors of a resident who has MNCD are mapped (tracked) and the resident's well-being or distress is recorded. Staff behaviors that have the potential to undermine residents' self-hood (personhood) (e.g. staff failing to greet residents properly, staff talking over the resident's head) and staff behaviors that boost residents' self-hood (e.g. getting to the eye level of the resident, holding the resident's hand) are also recorded. After analysis, the findings are discussed with the team to create an action plan to improve PCC practices and processes.

The Eden Alternative has become well known for its efforts to transform the institutional austerity of

LTC facilities into a human habitat by ensuring continued contact with people of all ages (especially children), plants, and animals (www.edenalt.org). The vision is to eliminate loneliness, helplessness, and boredom, the three common determinants of poor quality of life of LTC residents. In the language of the Eden Alternative, residents are referred to as elders, and staff are encouraged to see elders as wise. The philosophy of the Eden Alternative teaches that elders who enter a LTC facility should continue to grow and find meaning in life. Getting staff to respect elders as mature adults regardless of cognitive or physical state is a goal of the Eden Alternative education.

Developed by Anne Basting, Ph.D., TimeSlips (www.timeslips.org) involves a host of creative approaches, including the signature group storytelling process. Many LTC facilities around the world use the creative approaches. The process focuses on residents' imagination and creativity rather than memory and reminiscence. For example, a group of residents led by an individual trained in TimeSlips (online certification available) facilitates story writing based on a picture they all look at.

The Montessori method is based on procedural – implicit – memory, which is activated by repetitive muscle movement and focuses on identifying each person's strengths and building an individualized strengths-based activity program (Camp 2010). Montessori exercises are based on taste, vision, hearing, smell, and touch. The key aspect of this method is to let the resident learn and experience things for herself, and to guide the residents. Thus, all Montessori-based activities have by principle to be meaningful, not just leisure activities or "things to do." Montessori-based activities tap into different skills that are used on a daily basis. For example, arranging flowers emphasizes eye-hand coordination, physical movement, and care of the environment. Dishwashing is designed to continue and strengthen preserved skills required for ADL. Reading roundtable is a group reading activity that focuses on social interaction and cognitive stimulation. Based on Montessori principles, Resident-Assisted Montessori Programming is a novel approach in which residents who have early- to middle-stage MNCD are trained to lead a reading activity for residents who have more-advanced MNCD. Montessori-based programming with preschool children, in which people who have early MNCD develop "lessons," has also been found to be beneficial for both the residents and the children.

The Spark of Life Approach program is a planned playful activity program specifically devised for people who have MNCD by Dementia Care Australia (www.dementiacareaustralia.com) under the guidance and direction of Jane Verity, an occupational and family therapist and an international expert in the care of individuals who have MNCD. The focus is on the quality of the interaction rather than on the activity itself. Staff trained in this approach use spontaneity, joy, humor, fun with words, and body language. One of the key principles of this approach is that for any playful activity not to be demeaning, it has to come from the heart and be done in a respectful manner. The response of the person who has MNCD should be a key factor in deciding whether or not to continue the activity.

Snoezelen is an activity program that uses multisensory stimulation to create a comfortable, safe environment. (Snoezelen is a registered trademark of Rompa, Chesterfield, England; www.rompa.com/snoezelen-for-people-with-dementia.) Sight, hearing, touch, taste, smell, and proprioception are stimulated through the use of reminiscence images projected on the wall, wind chimes, savory snacks, weighted blankets with different-textured fabrics, rocking chairs, vibrating cushions and mattresses, meditative music, and aromatic oils. This provides residents with a stimulating and soothing environment and activity without the need for intellectual reasoning and helps release stress and frustration.

The Enriched Opportunities Program is devised by the Bradford Dementia Group, University of Bradford, Bradford, United Kingdom (Brooker et al. 2011). It consists of five key elements that need to work together to bring about a sustainable activity-based model of care: specialist expertise (the staff role of Locksmith); individualized assessment and casework; an activity and occupation program; staff training; and management and leadership.

According to the Six Senses Framework, proposed by Dr. Mike Nolan, professor of Gerontological nursing, University of Sheffield, United Kingdom, in the best LTC environments, all residents experience all the six senses (a sense of security, belonging, continuity, purpose, achievement, and significance) (Nolan et al. 2006). All nursing interactions are guided by the goal of having the resident experience one or more of the six senses.

Barriers to Implementation of SPPEICE

One of the key barriers to implementation of SPPEICE voiced by staff is that it is time intensive. But this is no different from nondrug approaches to address medical issues such as urinary incontinence, in which implementing evidence-based approaches such as scheduled or prompted voiding takes much more time than cleaning up after an "accident." Leadership, innovation, adequate staffing (in quality and quantity), and training can overcome the barrier of "time intensity."

A significant barrier to implementing SPPEICE is lack of adequate staffing on evenings and weekends. Often a lack of adequate structured activities programming is a significant risk factor for decline in wellness and psychosocial distress, which is expressed as agitation and depression. Also, attendance at activity programs does not guarantee engagement. Lack of personal knowledge of a resident's interest and absence of a good relationship with the resident are also barriers to engaging the resident in activity programs. PCC along with determination and support from the administrative leaders of the facility for unit nurse managers are key to overcoming these barriers.

Medicalization of any distress that a resident who has MNCD experiences and use of stigmatizing words to describe the person who has MNCD and the person's distress are two barriers to implementation of SPPEICE because they overemphasize biological factors and neglect unmet psychosocial-spiritual and environmental needs. We do not need "evidence" that providing a soothing hand massage can relieve "agitation" or that personalized music can provide much-needed comfort from life's daily hassles. Words matter, as certain words and phrases (e.g. "demented," "lost his mind") undermine the dignity of the person who has MNCD. Stigmatizing words reflect the therapeutic nihilism and lack of respect for individuals who have MNCD that pervade our society. Phrases such as "behaviors" and "challenging behaviors" should be replaced by "distress expressed as agitation and aggressive behaviors." "Behavioral and psychological symptoms of dementia" (BPSD) should be replaced by "biopsychosocial-spiritual distress" (BPSD) (Dementia Action Alliance 2016). The term "nondrug interventions for treatment of agitation" should be replaced by "psychosocial approaches and initiatives to reduce distress." Furthermore, just replacing the terms in documentation is not enough. Our actions should reflect this fundamental shift in how we view agitated behaviors of people who have MNCD.

Another barrier is poor quality of traditional medical care. Many residents are taking medication that causes more harm than good, have an undertreated medical and/or psychiatric condition, and could benefit from nondrug approaches that have been proven to address medical and psychiatric conditions better than medication. Comprehensive geriatric assessment combined with rational deprescribing (discontinuation of medication that causes more harm than good), optimal treatment of medical and/or psychiatric conditions (e.g. undernutrition, major depressive disorder), and use of nondrug approaches to optimally manage pain, pressure ulcers, delirium, and insomnia are essential for SPPEICE to be most effective. (See Boxes 13.12, 13.13, 13.14, and 13.15.)

Other barriers include lack of leadership and lack of resources for staff to implement SPPEICE. Comprehensive culture change initiatives, such as intentional transformation of LTC settings to be less institutional and more homelike, care that is increasingly centered on and directed by residents, and empowerment of front-line staff (e.g. nurses, nursing assistants), should be the first three steps to overcome these barriers. SPPEICE is a journey, not a destination, an ever-changing journey as the circumstances and strengths of the resident evolve over time. A trial-and-error mindset, a resolute heart, and mindful partnering with the resident can overcome barriers and ensure that LTC residents live the best life possible. Box 13.16 lists practical strategies the leadership team (medical director, administrator, director of nursing, unit nurse manager) can initiate to overcome barriers to implementation of SPPEICE.

Psychosocial-Spiritual Wellness Specialists

Recreational therapists should be considered specialists in SPPEICE, and every PCLTCC should have one, at least as a consultant if not an in-house member of the team. Recreational therapists (certified therapeutic recreation specialists) are professionals trained to use a wide range of activities and techniques to improve the cognitive, physical, emotional, social, and leisure needs of their clients. They use the framework from the American Therapeutic Recreation Association Dementia Practice Guidelines (Buettner and Kolanowski 2003). Their training is much more vigorous and evidence-based than that of many staff

BOX 13.12 Nondrug Approaches to Manage Pain

- Physical therapy (PT): PT is proven effective in reducing pain and inflammation associated with any number of orthopedic problems (e.g. rotator cuff tendonitis, impingement syndrome, sprains and strains)
- Approaches to promote relaxation (e.g. soothing music, calm environment, unhurried approach, soothing voice, breathing exercises, nature, massage [manual, through massage chair]) are essential because pain often causes muscle to tense and anxiety to increase, which in turn causes experience of pain to worsen, creating a vicious cycle
- Physical activities/exercise as appropriate and tolerated with guidance from physical therapist and physician or physician extender
- Cold touch (especially for neuropathic pain, acute pain due to muscle/tissue swelling)
- Superficial heat (especially for chronic arthritis-related pain [e.g. hands soaked in warm water daily in the morning to reduce arthritis pain], low-back pain, other musculoskeletal pain)
- Repositioning (e.g. if resident has pain related to pressure ulcer)
- Massage (e.g. to relieve muscle tension, muscle spasm, spasticity)
- Cognitive behavioral therapy for motivated resident who has mild MNCD (with appropriate modification to account for neurocognitive challenges)
- Acupuncture (e.g. for knee arthritis pain)
- Brace (e.g. hand brace, knee brace) or sling as appropriate
- Addressing staff, resident, and family misconceptions about pain in older adults
    - Pain is a normal part of aging
    - Older adults are less sensitive to pain
    - Persons who have advanced MNCD do not experience pain

BOX 13.13 Nondrug Approaches to Manage Pressure Ulcers

- Nursing assistants check at-risk resident (e.g. resident who spends hours in wheelchair daily) daily during personal care for changes in skin condition
- Nurses perform head-to-toe skin check periodically (e.g. once a week) on at-risk resident (e.g. resident who has morbid obesity and spends hours in bed daily)
- Specialty wound mattress (e.g. constant low-pressure mattress, alternating-pressure mattress), mattress replacement and pressure-reducing support surface on bed (e.g. "padding pack," a shrink-wrapped package of elbow pads, bolsters, and other padding)
- All residents who cannot reposition themselves have calves and heels floated on pillows at night
- All wheelchairs and geriatric chairs have cushions
- Turn bed-bound resident every two hours, and resident using wheelchair or geriatric chair is repositioned every hour
- Moisture barriers are used routinely for incontinent residents
- Improving fluid, protein, and calorie intake by undernourished resident

members given the title of "activity therapist." Recreational therapists use a whole host of tools and approaches (e.g. air mat therapy, sensory stimulation box) to promote residents' well-being after comprehensive assessment to identify background factors (e.g. cognitive ability) and proximal factors (e.g. psychosocial need states).

Music therapists, art therapists, and activity therapists can also take a leadership role in making SPPEICE a reality for all residents. Music therapists have a bachelor's or higher degree in music therapy from a program approved by the American Music Therapy Association. Music therapists develop clinical skills and do more than 1,200 hours of required fieldwork, including internship at a health care and/or education facility. They may lead group music activity as a part of daily continuous activity schedule as well as provide one-on-one music therapy for a resident who has depression

BOX 13.14 Nondrug Approaches to Manage Delirium

- One-to-one staffing address safety concerns (e.g. falls and injury)
- Family spend more time with resident until delirium clears
- Minimize or eliminate use of physical restraint
- Minimize or eliminate use of urinary catheter
- Reduce inactivity and immobility, avoid bedrest, maintain safe mobility and physical activity, and minimize and/or eliminate medical orders for bed rest
- Institute sleep-enhancing strategies (e.g. soothing bedtime routine, relaxing music)
- Ensure that resident who needs them has glasses, hearing aids, and/or dentures
- Improve nutritional status
- Institute fall precautions as appropriate
- Ensure regular skin care and prevention of pressure sores as appropriate
- Ensure structure and keep to resident's normal routine
- Ensure availability of easy, low-key therapeutic activities program
- Reduce ambient noise
- Encourage self-care
- Increase exposure to outdoors, sunlight, and nature

BOX 13.15 Nondrug Approaches to Treat Insomnia

Dietary

- Restrict intake of caffeine and chocolate, particularly in the evening
- Avoid heavy meals late at night
- Light snack (e.g. glass of milk, crackers) if nighttime awakening caused by hunger
- Avoid fluid intake in the evening for resident who has nocturia and encourage maximum bladder emptying before retiring
- Switch from alcoholic to nonalcoholic beverages

Environmental

- Limit time spent in bed
- Remove clock from room (especially if resident repeatedly looks at clock while trying to sleep)
- Increase exposure to natural light in daytime (30–60 minutes or more per day, preferably outdoors [with appropriate use of sunscreen] but sitting next to window [open window if weather permits and resident agreeable] is also worthwhile)
- Increase exposure to indoor light in daytime on cloudy and rainy days
- Bright light therapy (20 minutes to two hours in morning)
- Ensure optimal room temperature and humidity
- Reduce nighttime noise and nighttime exposure to bright light
- Use low-intensity nightlight for resident who has nightmares and/or other fears to promote sleep and increase safety during nighttime awakening (e.g. to void urine)
- Change room if conflict with roommate or location of room is an issue

Activity-Oriented Approaches

- Limit daytime napping to short period in morning or early afternoon
- Increase physical activity in daytime (e.g. regular exercise program, restorative program)
- Increase meaningful activity and socialization in daytime
- Warm bath in evening
- Avoid excessive stimulation and exercise after dinnertime

BOX 13.15 (cont.)

Sleep Hygiene

- Regular sleeping and waking times and structured bedtime routine
- Calming bedtime rituals (e.g. soothing music, reading or listening to nonfiction books [e.g. spiritual and religious books])
- Using bed only for sleep (rather than watching TV, eating, or reading)

Staff-Oriented Approaches

- Staff education and training regarding evaluation and treatment of insomnia and other sleep disorders
- Staff address resident's maladaptive beliefs regarding sleeplessness
- Staff teach and assist resident in relaxation strategies
- Staff mediate differences between roommates (e.g. one resident wanting to watch TV late in night, thus disturbing roommate who wants to sleep early) or better pairing of residents living in one room
- Minimize staff interrupting resident's sleep
- Massage therapy (e.g. back rub, hand massage)
- Aromatherapy

Approaches for Motivated Resident Who Has Relatively Intact Cognitive Functioning

- Relaxation training (e.g. deep breathing exercises, visualization exercises, progressive muscle relaxation, listening to soothing music, repeating self-soothing thoughts)
- Cognitive behavioral therapy for insomnia (CBT-I)
- Stimulus control therapy (go to bed only when feeling sleepy, get out of bed if not asleep after 20 minutes)
- Sleep restriction therapy (limit time in bed to total perceived sleep time [not less than six hours])

BOX 13.16 Key Strategies to Overcome Barriers to Implementation of SPPEICE

1. Fostering a culture of respect and reverence
2. Access to highly supportive leadership
3. High-quality professional caregiver education and training programs
4. Chance to watch peers model person-centered care (PCC) practices
5. Hands-on training
6. Access to mentor
7. Common psychosocial spiritual wellness care-planning time with colleagues
8. Access to resources (e.g. high-tech and low-tech equipment, training videos)
9. In-house stress-management and resilience-building programs for professional caregivers
10. High-quality traditional medical and psychiatric care

and/or agitation and has been referred by a physician or other healthcare provider.

Art therapists are registered through the American Art Therapy Association on completion of a master's or higher degree and more than 1,000 hours of supervised clinical experience above and beyond graduate internship. Art therapists use a variety of media, including paint, ceramics, natural materials, and fabrics, to guide residents through everything from one-on-one painting sessions to group quilting projects.

Activity therapists usually have short (e.g. one-day) training at the end of which they receive a certification. SPPEICE specialists can also have a role as consultants providing guidance and supervision to facility staff to create and implement SPPEICE for individual residents as well as for facility-wide programming initiatives. Family members may hire a recreational therapist, music therapist, or art therapist to create a more individualized and vigorous SPPEICE program for their loved one that the staff and family can implement together.

Helping Visits by Family and Friends Be Meaningful and Joyful

All psychosocial approaches should strive to help the family caregiver make visits with the resident more meaningful and fun. When the facility staff members become more involved with families of their residents and help them make visits more meaningful, the families feel more satisfied with the visits. Family caregivers have expressed many positive effects in their role: a new sense of purpose or meaning in life, fulfillment of a lifelong commitment to a spouse, an opportunity to give back to a parent some of what the parent has given to them, renewal of religious faith, closer ties through new relationships or stronger existing relationships. By sharing this with family members who are struggling with difficult emotions, staff help them gain a much-needed spiritual boost, making visits with the resident a positive event for both.

Many family caregivers stop visiting their loved one or visit for a short time because they feel that their loved one's MNCD is so far advanced (e.g. cannot recognize the family member) that it makes no difference whether they visit or not. Some family members (especially children and, less often, spouses) may not visit because it is painful to see their loved one in such a diminished state. Primary care team members can play a crucial role in counseling family that all visits have tremendous meaning for the resident (even in advanced stages) in ways that may not be obvious and address their grief so that visits can continue and future feelings of guilt by the family can be prevented.

LTC facilities should offer support groups for family caregivers. A support group can provide social support as well as a space to share and learn creative ways of spending quality time with the resident. Staff may also educate family members regarding factors that may agitate the resident (e.g. directing too many questions to a cognitively impaired resident), help them decide the best times to visit, and give specific suggestions (e.g. please walk with the resident for five to 10 minutes, arrange flowers together, reminisce, listen to music together, read a chapter of a religious book to the resident).

Convening family meetings to address feelings of guilt and other negative emotions may improve not only the emotional well-being of the family members but also the quality and frequency of interaction between the family members and the resident. The latter in turn can have a tremendous positive effect on the resident's psychosocial well-being. Often, the seeds of dissension between siblings were sown when they were children. HCPs can help adult children focus on the resident's well-being by encouraging them to help each other in a polite manner and to avoid trying to resolve long-standing differences. The HCP should encourage family members to keep any criticism of each other to a minimum while in the presence of the resident.

"I want to go home" is one of the most common complaints of residents living in a LTC facility. Family members often may be split in their opinions regarding this issue and may give mixed messages to the resident, worsening the resident's emotional distress. The primary care team can recommend that the siblings not expect other siblings to see the parent as they do, as the experiences and relationship of each child with a parent is unique and influenced by a multitude of factors that are different in each relationship (e.g. birth order, stressful events during birth and later). Facilitating positive relationships between family members can have a direct positive effect on the resident's emotional and spiritual well-being.

The Role of Family Education in Promoting the Resident's Psychosocial-Spiritual Wellness

Family caregivers may unwittingly cause or worsen the distress of the resident who has MNCD during a visit. For example, when one or more family members places excessive demands on the resident, a catastrophic reaction may occur. When the resident and family caregiver have had a poor premorbid relationship, the caregiver may misinterpret agitated behavior as purposefully provocative and worsen the situation with an angry reaction. Family caregivers (especially if they are experiencing significant caregiver burden) often underestimate the resident's functional abilities, which can contribute to or aggravate distress, resulting in behavioral disturbances. The HCP should routinely educate the family about MNCD, the importance of not arguing, and other supportive interactions.

Four simple statements – "Please forgive me. I forgive you. Thank you. I love you" – are powerful tools to ease suffering as well as promote the psychological and spiritual growth of residents and their family members. It is important to share with the resident and/or family that this phase of life holds remarkable possibilities for personal and spiritual growth, for strengthening bonds with people they love, for repairing broken ties and making amends, and for creating profound meaning despite challenges posed by cognitive decline.

Caring for the Family Caregiver

Caregiver grief, burden, and stress are prevalent and have serious negative effects on the physical, psychosocial, and spiritual well-being of both the family caregiver and the resident. Caregivers may reduce their visits as a way to manage their grief and guilt, and during a visit may not have the energy to engage in meaningful and fun activities with the resident. The HCP should institute approaches to reduce caregiver grief and stress soon after the resident enters the facility, continue the approaches throughout the resident's stay, and intensify them as needed during the last few weeks or months of the resident's life. The HCP should encourage the family and friends to visit as often and stay as long as they like and gradually become part of the PCLTCC.

Many caregivers identify religious activities (e.g. going to church, reading sacred texts, etc.) as a major help in coping with the difficulties of caregiving. Prayer is a particularly vital source of empowerment for many family caregivers. Praying may give family members a sense of peace, strength, and even answers to questions related to their own conflicts as well as their loved one's care. Struggling with and caring for a loved one who is frail and in a LTC facility may increase some caregivers' feelings of spiritual connectedness and emotional stability. Hence, we strongly recommend identifying dimensions of spirituality to help family members develop effective and appropriate support systems. This in turn may make caregiving less stressful and more rewarding. Support groups, bereavement groups, and mindfulness-based stress reduction (MBSR) are also useful in addressing caregiver stress and grief. Some family caregivers (e.g. those who have persistent depression, guilt, severe anxiety) may need referral to a mental health clinician for individual psychotherapy and, if necessary, psychotropic medication. Family caregivers often feel that their loved one is not receiving good care in the LTC facility, and this feeling can be heartbreaking. All team members should work together to do all they can to prevent such outcomes, inquire about family members' experiences of the resident's care, and address any negative feelings family members have about the care. The team members should not be afraid to show compassion and respect for the resident and family or to be a loving witness to their sadness.

Clinical Case 2: "This is so hard"

Mr. L, a 90-year-old husband of Mrs. L, an 85-year-old woman who had advanced MNCD, commented during an interview with Mrs. L's physician, "My wife is there, but she is not there. She needs a wheelchair now and her speech is largely gone. She recognizes me by face at times but calls me 'Dad' when she says a few words that I can make sense of. She is starting to be combative. This is so hard. I find myself getting angry even though I know that it is her disease that makes her behave this way. Then I get depressed. This is so unlike her." The psychiatrist treating Mrs. L provided emotional support to Mr. L, suggesting that he see a social worker who specializes in helping spouses adjust to MNCD in their loved one and to their residence to a LTC facility. Mr. L was reluctant but agreed after his daughter promised to accompany him on the first visit to the social worker. After several weekly meetings with the social worker, Mr. L gradually felt less guilty, was able to express his grief and loss, and learned ways to make his visits with his wife meaningful and even fun at times. He also started attending spousal support groups run by the local chapter of the Alzheimer's Association. Mr. L resumed his regular exercise program at a local health club after the psychiatrist indicated to Mr. L that if he keeps himself healthy, the treatment team can better focus on improving Ms. L's emotional well-being. Mr. L also became more mindful of "little" gifts from his wife, such as her breaking into a big smile when she saw him approach.

Teaching Point

Addressing the grief and stress of a family caregiver can have the added benefit of improving the emotional well-being of a resident in LTC.

The Critical Importance of Staff Education and Training in Promoting the Resident's Psychosocial-Spiritual Wellness

Staff training programs and environmental modifications appear to be the most effective strategies in promoting wellness and preventing distress expressed as agitation and aggressive behavior. Table 13.4 lists key education and training programs that every staff member working with residents who have MNCD

Table 13.4 Seven Essential Staff Education and Training Programs to Promote the Well-Being of a Resident Who Has Major Neurocognitive Disorder

Staff Education	Key Benefits	Other Benefits
Person-centered care (PCC) and SPPEICE	Improved psychosocial and spiritual well-being of resident	Reduced agitation and use of psychotropic medication
Alive Inside educational documentary/movie	Staff will see for themselves remarkable effects of music on psychosocial spiritual well-being of resident	Many staff have musical skills (e.g. piano playing) that can be used for benefit of residents as well as staff
*Bathing without a Battle** educational movie	Staff will learn practical strategies to make bathing a pleasant experience for resident who has MNCD	Many person-centered techniques in movie can be applied to other situations (e.g. dressing)
Hand in Hand educational video by Center for Medicare and Medicaid Services (CMS)	Staff learn about PCC practices to address complex needs of LTC resident	Increased confidence of staff to be able to make a positive impact on LTC residents
Therapeutic communication	Improved understanding of resident's experiences and perspectives Improved understanding of countertherapeutic approaches	Prevention of agitation due to countertherapeutic communication (e.g. due to repeatedly correcting resident, arguing with resident)
At least one of three models to understand resident's distress (NDB**, PSLT***, habilitation model)	Improved understanding of common triggers and unmet needs of resident that often cause distress to resident	Prevention of agitation due to easily identifiable triggers and unmet needs (e.g. toileting)
Training experienced staff in how to mentor new staff, hands-on training of new staff, easy access to mentor for all staff	Improved confidence and effectiveness of new staff in promoting resident's psychosocial and spiritual wellness	Improved satisfaction of new staff in their job and decreased staff turnover Experienced staff may find improved satisfaction and sense of value of their work

* Bathing without a Battle: http://bathingwithoutabattle.unc.edu. The website has excellent resources and information on person-centered creative bathing care practices and strategies, innovative bathing equipment, and supplies for purchase.

** NDB: Need-driven Dementia-Compromised Behavior Model

*** PSLT: Progressively Lowered Stress Threshold

should undergo. Involvement of other team members besides nurses in education and training to provide guidance to family members (e.g. the resident is having a "bad" day and the social worker advises whether the family should lengthen, shorten, or avoid their visit; a recreational therapist or activity therapist educates the family regarding the potential benefits of simulated presence to address loneliness and who should make a tape or video recording) can reduce the burden on nurses, who are expected to "do it all."

Staff members who are educated to understand MNCD, the expected progression, and resulting progressively lowered stress threshold are likely to be less judgmental and more caring. Staff members need to be trained in the person-centered approach and towel bath technique to reduce distress during bathing. Staff need to be trained in the "hand-in-hand" technique, in which the caregiver's hand is under or over the hand of the person who has MNCD. This technique is an effective way of leading a resident who has MNCD to participate in daily care (e.g. feeding self, bathing self, changing clothes) even if the resident is not doing the task. This approach can reduce resistance to care. Training caregivers to help residents balance activity with quiet time is also important.

During personal care activities, such as feeding or toileting, many caregivers may act in a task-oriented way, saying, "Open your mouth" and "Swallow." They may not address the resident as a person. This may occur even though caregivers understand that the resident's behaviors are expressions of feelings of anxiety, abandonment, and dissolution. The reason for the discrepancy is that caregivers may feel ineffective, helpless, and powerless. By avoiding eye contact with the resident, they try to avoid these feelings. Caregivers should watch for triggers of distress and do their best to avoid or anticipate them and help the resident cope with the distress better. Both family and professional caregivers need to learn to compromise, to simplify things in the resident's life. Caregivers also need to understand the huge positive impact set individualized routines (e.g. eating meals at the same time each day, going to bed and waking up at the same time) can have on many residents and help residents keep to their routines.

As a part of a continuous quality improvement program, SPPEICE specialists should be given support and resources to conduct frequent (at least once a month, preferably once a week), one- to two-hour educational seminars for staff based on specific cases in the facility. Sharing success stories should be an essential part of such educational programs. These sessions should be video-audio recorded so that they are available for staff members who did not attend. The goal of such seminars is to increase the comfort level, knowledge, and skills of various staff members to understand and implement SPPEICE. It can also help prompt shared experiences between older and younger staff members.

Interactive training has been demonstrated to be effective in shaping more appropriate staff reactions to distress expressed as aggressive behavior. This training can effectively be delivered on the Internet led by a geriatric health care specialist. Staff and physician education regarding SPPEICE and the risks of pharmacological treatment (especially antipsychotic) and restraints has been found to increase the implementation of SPPEICE and reduce antipsychotic prescription and restraints without worsening agitation. Staff need to be taught that tasks are secondary to relationships, and supervisors should be trained not to supervise staff members in a regimented manner that precludes the responsiveness that every resident needs. Staff members who provide personal care to residents need to be given more power and say in decision-making and be seen as doing the most valuable work in the facility. Staff need to be taught that their relationship with the residents is the hub of life in a LTC facility. Staff members need to be rewarded for spontaneous innovative approaches, such as a new staff member who decides to read aloud a resident's favorite poem to lessen that resident's unease.

The success of SPPEICE relies on the quality of caregiving. A resident's "behavior" (e.g. pacing, wandering) is often disturbing to the caregivers (professional and/or family) but not to the resident herself. In such cases, treatment of "behavior" involves educating caregivers that the "behavior" needs not "treatment" but accommodation. In fact, educating and training caregivers so that they can change their approach to a resident who has "behavioral disturbances" is one of the key approaches to prevent and reduce agitation in LTC residents who have MNCD. Also, at times, a caregiver's stress can result in inappropriate interaction with the resident, which in turn may cause the resident to have "behavioral disturbances." Addressing caregiver stress thus may prevent or decrease resident agitation. Last but not least, a caregiver's emotional distress (sadness, anger, anxiety) may "spill over" onto the resident, causing the resident in turn to become emotionally distressed. A resident (especially one who has cognitive impairment) may misinterpret the caregiver's emotional distress as having something to do with the resident and react with agitation. Mindfulness training can help staff members become better aware of their emotional state and take a few moments to "reset" before entering the resident's room.

Cognitively impaired residents may be sensitive to body language and to the tone of a caregiver's voice, especially when it conveys criticism – even when the resident is no longer able to understand the specific content of the message. Residents often sense a caregiver's frustration or anger and may become anxious or angry in response. Relaxed and smiling caregiver behavior during communication can help calm the resident and thus improve the resident's attention. Staff members may need to modify their linguistic behavior (including body language and tone of voice) to accommodate to the declining cognitive abilities of a resident who has MNCD. Use of "yes-no" questions can facilitate communication with a resident who has advanced MNCD by reducing the demand for a response. How the staff speaks and how the resident perceives are also important. The primary goal of the communication should be connecting with the resident rather than testing the resident's memory or obtaining information. When staff genuinely seek information from residents and provide a meaningful context for the question, even a resident who has MNCD may respond successfully to questions that might be difficult to answer from a linguistic standpoint. The staff should avoid commanding, condescending, patronizing, and critical communicative behaviors and instead be patient, respectful, and caring and use rephrasing statements and provide explanations. Staff should also avoid overaccommodating behavior (e.g. simplified grammar and vocabulary, slow speech, withdrawal from conversation) or underaccommodating behavior (e.g. avoiding communication with the resident). We discourage the use of pet names, diminutives (e.g. dearie, sweetie, honey), and exaggerated intonation, although in certain contexts they may be appropriate as they convey qualities of nurturing, endearment, intimacy, and solidarity.

Naomi Feil, M.S.W., developed validation-based relating and communication approaches. This involves acceptance of the reality and personal truth of another person's experience, and it incorporates a range of specific techniques (https://vfvalidation.org). For example, caregivers (professional and family) should validate the emotion the resident expresses instead of trying to reorient the resident to "reality." By not emphasizing the accuracy of "facts," the caregiver is freed to express more empathy and find a meaningful point of connection.

Communication skills to respond to an angry resident or family member include calm tone, open posture, apology when appropriate, reflecting the resident's or family member's feelings ("You look upset, worried, angry, anxious"), validation ("I understand why you feel this way"), empathy ("I would also feel frustrated in this situation"), respect ("I respect and admire your dedication to your loved one's well-being"), support ("I'll be here if you want to talk later on"), and a problem-solving approach ("Let's try to solve this problem together").

Many local chapters of the Alzheimer's Association have affordable programs that provide excellent staff education and training in these areas. Training of staff should involve direct systematic clinical supervision and supervised implementation of individually planned care. Such training can lead to a more positive perception of the residents, less "burnout," increased creativity, increased job satisfaction, and improved interactions between resident and caregiver. Staff training should include the understanding that although there is a significant neurochemical basis for many behavioral disturbances, this does not mean that there is no experience behind the behavior or that the behavior cannot be affected by human interaction. Caregivers must make a genuine effort to find meaning in residents' communication, which is a prerequisite for experiencing caring for residents who have MNCD as meaningful and being able to help residents lead a meaningful life despite advanced MNCD. Caregivers need to train themselves not to personalize any unkind statement voiced by the resident, not to misinterpret the resident's agitated behavior as purposefully provocative, and not to respond with anger. Among the goals of staff training are to reduce ineffective approaches, such as arguing or appealing to a resident's logical thinking when the resident is unable to think logically due to MNCD.

Improving Staff-Family Relationships

A resident's emotional and spiritual well-being depends to a considerable degree on the quality of relationship and interaction between the staff and the family. Staff and family may experience anger during interactions with each other in response to their own experience of the resident's illness, the health care system, or the different expectations and stress the resident's complex health and psychosocial needs create. Staff who cultivate personal awareness, practice mindful self-monitoring during interactions, explore the different possible reasons of their anger toward family member(s), demonstrate specific communication skills, set clear boundaries, and seek personal support can overcome the challenges of these difficult conversations with family and begin to restore trust in the staff-resident-family triad. Mindful self-monitoring is the ability to be in the moment, to be both participant and observer during interpersonal interactions in order to adjust to nuances of information, behaviors, and feelings in oneself and others, and to integrate this with one's professional knowledge and experience. When staff members have developed connections with family members, the staff interact with the resident more respectfully, engage with the resident in friendly conversation more often, and, in general, care for the resident better.

Caring for the Professional Caregiver

A professional caregiver who has not been adequately trained, not been given adequate resources (e.g. adequate staffing) and emotional support and appreciation cannot be expected to engage a resident who has MNCD in SPPEICE in a systematic, mindful, and creative manner. In fact, high caregiver stress can often lead to untherapeutic or countertherapeutic approaches and, not uncommonly, even verbal and/or physical abuse or neglect. Growing research calls for LTC facilities to make every effort to find managers (e.g. administrators, directors of nursing, supervisors) who know that the well-being of the residents is inseparable from the welfare of the professional caregivers and that the needs of the professional caregiver transcend mere bread-and-butter considerations. Such managers fashion a workplace that recognizes the person behind the role of the front-line staff (e.g. nursing assistant, nurse), challenges and supports them, and helps them achieve, relate to, and grow in their professional life and enjoy their work. The engagement of the front-line staff deepens when managers care about them as persons, appreciate their work, evaluate them fairly, and communicate with them on important matters. In fact, managers play a critical role in the satisfaction, loyalty, and commitment of the staff. The front-line staff members usually perceive their managers as exerting a pervasive influence in their work life. Another important area for managers to address is workplace safety. Residents frequently push, grab, or verbally abuse staff members (especially nursing assistants and nurses). Staff members are often asked to handle residents (e.g. transfer, lift) with inadequate assist devices, putting them at high risk for serious injury and even persisting disability. Thus, caring for the professional caregiver is a key component of any effort to improve the psychosocial-spiritual wellness of LTC residents.

The first step in caring for professional caregivers is to provide them with high-quality education and training so that they can not only deliver high-quality care but also enjoy their work and feel proud of their contribution to the well-being of the residents and families. Caring for professional caregivers involves several things: helping them mature; maintaining their motivation to care for frail and vulnerable but challenging LTC populations; helping them be mindful that, for some residents, a professional caregiver may be the only person a resident has a chance to touch and engage in conversation in the entire day; helping them adjust to the realities of working in a LTC facility (e.g. limited resources); helping them balance their personal and professional lives; encouraging them to have a self-care plan (physical, emotional, spiritual); and helping them find and cultivate hidden strengths and successes. Caring for professional caregivers may also involve having a room to "chill" for the staff. Offering professional caregivers onsite services such as yoga, MBSR, relaxation response, deep breathing and other relaxation training exercises, Tai Chi, daycare for children, a healthy and delicious "café," and other amenities may go a long way in improving professional caregivers' well-being.

Psychosocial and Environmental Strategies for Easing Adjustment to the New Home

For most individuals moving into a LTC facility, their new room will become their new home. "Being at home" often means "an existence that offers possibilities" (i.e. choices), whereas "not feeling at home" may be a response to an inability to find meaning and connectedness. Many residents may become agitated after the move and try to leave the facility. Such behavior is a normal expression of the resident's loss of home and thus is to be expected. In general, residents may take two to six weeks to settle into the new home, and a minority may take several months. Most residents adjust sooner or later and soon forget they lived elsewhere. Many residents ask to be taken home. For many residents who have advanced MNCD, that home is the home of their childhood rather than the home before the LTC facility. Many residents may show significant disturbed behavior and disorientation for three months after a move. Sudden or unplanned relocation can increase depressive symptoms and mortality for residents who have MNCD. Conversely, a positive change in the environment, such as a planned relocation from home (and lonely life at home) to a vibrant PCLTCC, can result in improved mood, motor function, and even cognitive function.

Several strategies can be used to ease adjustment of a new resident to the new home. These strategies are guidelines rather than firm recommendations, may not apply to everyone, and should be individualized (e.g. use only a few of the listed strategies). Although at first look the list seems daunting, we have seen time and again that initial hard work pays off great dividends (e.g. the resident is thriving in the new home after only a brief initial period of distress). We have also witnessed disastrous results when the transition was handled poorly (e.g. the resident becomes suicidal or violent because of extreme grief and fear of the new place and new people who do not know her).

Recommended strategies are as follows:

1. Planned admission. Typically, admission to a LTC facility occurs during a crisis (medical, psychiatric, social). Such abrupt change in living circumstances causes immense stress and distress to an individual who has MNCD as well as the family members. This distress is further compounded by the distress of not being involved in the transition process. We strongly recommend planned admission so that the transition is as positive as possible for both the individual who has MNCD and the family members. As much as possible, the family should involve the person who has MNCD in all aspects of the move. The person should be told two to three months before the move, with periodic reminders about the reason for the move. Ideally, this possibility should be discussed soon after the diagnosis of MNCD (several years before the move). We recommend telling the person who does not want to move that it is the physician's recommendation to move into a LTC facility due to medical conditions and medical needs rather than the family's decision, to prevent discord between the resident and the family.
2. Have the individual make several visits to the LTC facility before moving to become familiar with the place and people and even take part in activities in the facility before moving in.
3. The family may encourage the person who has MNCD to volunteer at the LTC facility for months to years before moving in. In fact, all of us should try to volunteer in a LTC facility in order to make helping frail older adults a routine part of life. This may help fundamentally change the part of our culture that tries to deny the existence of frail older adults in order to be in denial of our own future of dependency and frailty.
4. High level of social support and involvement of family and friends. This includes allowing several opportunities for the new resident to vent, expressing grief and anger. Involving small children (e.g. grandchildren), if done judiciously, may be helpful, as they may be more "fun" and "creative" and may help the resident cope with multiple losses involved in moving into a LTC facility. It may be preferable to use the terms "new home," "almost home," and/or "retirement community" rather than "nursing home" or "assisted living home."
5. Family should prepare and bring either a one- to two-page "life story" or a life history book for the staff to know the person better. Family may also bring a list of favorite activities, food and drinks, topics of conversation, music, movies, family members, animals, and spiritual and cultural preferences.
6. Family may make a list of the person's daily routines (sleep time, wake-up time, meal time, bathing ritual) for the staff.
7. Family may make a list of the person's unique personality characteristics (e.g. likes to be touched, likes to be left alone, is easy going, easy to please, assertive, particular about cleanliness), family role (e.g. has always been the decision-maker, a patriarch, a matriarch of the family), and relevant past experiences (e.g. poverty during childhood, resulting in the person's being frugal; experience in World War II resulting in the person's being sensitive to news regarding wars and terrorist attacks).
8. Create a homelike environment, a room filled with memorabilia, personal furnishings, pictures, perfume/aroma that person is familiar with.
9. Family may make a list of the person's strengths (e.g. can play a musical instrument, can sing, good at card games) to share with the staff.
10. Family may bring a list of approaches they have found useful in comforting the person (e.g. responds well to humor, becomes easily distracted by favorite music, leaving the person alone and reapproaching her later always works, calms down easily after talking to a particular family member) to share with the staff.
11. Family may bring a list of common triggers for distress and agitation (e.g. telling the person what to do or not to do instead of giving options, that the person is particular about bed sheets, window shades, air conditioning, and other things in the room being in a specific manner),

and list of Dos and Don'ts they have learned (sometimes the "hard way") while caring for the person.

12. The facility may offer a welcome gift for new residents from residents already living at the facility. This may help the resident feel welcome in a strange place.
13. Prior experience in an adult day center usually helps a person who has MNCD emotionally make the transition from the community to institutional residence less distressful. It may also attenuate the cognitive decline seen in many residents soon after entering a LTC facility. The increased cognitive decline on entry may reflect difficulty adapting to an unfamiliar environment. Adult day programs also help family become accustomed to the idea of LTC. Ideally, the adult day program should be in the same LTC facility into which the person is moving.
14. Family should spend a lot of time with the resident in the first few days to weeks so that the resident does not feel abandoned. Family may gradually reduce their visits if necessary, as the person becomes more adjusted.
15. Family may request staff from the Alzheimer's Association or other appropriate local organization to have a family meeting to gain suggestions and resources (e.g. books, pamphlets, video from the association's own library) to ease the transition. Such meeting(s) should be held weeks to months before the transition date.
16. Family members should consider seeking professional help from a local Alzheimer's center or memory clinic for individual therapy for the family caregiver, family therapy to address family conflict, and if necessary medication for the person (e.g. as-needed low-dose benzodiazepine for a few days around the transition) to emotionally prepare both the person who has MNCD and caregivers for the stress involved in transition and to reduce severe anxiety, depression, and agitation surrounding issues of moving into a LTC facility.
17. Family can attend support groups and learn creative tips from other family caregivers who have "been there, done that." Alternatively, staff at the LTC facility may ask family members of current residents to talk to and help family members of the new resident cope with this difficult time.
18. Family and staff need to have patience, as it usually takes several weeks for a new resident to adjust to a new place of living. Transition into a LTC facility is hard on almost everyone. It is important for the family member to recognize and accept that this stress is normal and avoid trying to fight it, deny it, or "fix" it with drugs or think that only their loved one is "difficult" and other residents have transitioned easily.
19. Family should try to continue as many family rituals and activities as possible after the transition, albeit with necessary modifications (e.g. smaller and shorter gatherings during birthdays, celebrating at the facility rather than the family member's home).
20. Family members need to tap into the power of humor and spirituality to help themselves and the resident negotiate this difficult time. Seeking support from a facility chaplain can be invaluable.

Helping the Resident and Family Make the Most Dreaded Decision

The decision to move to a PCLTCC is one of the most dreaded decisions, for both the person who has MNCD and the family members. Denial and avoidance are typical ways of coping with increasing safety concerns at home and the growing urgency of moving to a safer place. Even HCPs may avoid these discussions until there is a crisis. This is unfortunate, as gentle, compassionate, and creative discussions over weeks to months can emotionally prepare most people to come to terms with the notion that moving to a PCLTCC is possible. Individuals and their families usually have a host of questions and concerns that the primary care team members should inquire into and address. Assessing a resident's and/or family's understanding of safety concerns and care needs is the first step in tailoring the education to their needs. Most families of a person who has MNCD are faced with having to make most of the decisions regarding the move to a PCLTCC because of the resident's loss of decision-making capacity, typically years before the move is even considered. Many family members have a difficult time making such decisions because they are not emotionally prepared or adequately informed. Also, family members may not reach a unanimous decision. The key strategies to prepare the person and the family for the move include: promoting excellent communication with the person and family; demonstrating empathy for difficult emotions and conflict in relationships due to disagreements, and attending to individual and family grief. Use of simple, clear language that the person and family will understand rather than clinical language is important. Primary care team members should allow the person and/or family to control the pace and flow of information whenever possible, and let them guide how much detail and how much information they are able to handle at the time. The person and family may be more satisfied if they have an opportunity to speak while the HCP listens. Assuring the person who has MNCD and the family that the physician, physician assistants, and nurse practitioners will be by their side the entire way is the most important approach to ease anxiety and fears and ensure that the transition goes as peacefully as possible. It is useful for the HCP to provide the 20-point guidelines for easing transition described above as well as printed materials from reputable organizations (e.g. Alzheimer's Association) with key points that will be covered during the discussion. Primary care team members should plan for repeat visits to readdress difficult issues and view the discussion of transition as a spectrum from diagnosis to the move rather than a one-time event. The HCP should reassure the person and family that it is normal to be confused or overwhelmed. Encouraging the person and family to write down questions as they arise so that they can be discussed at a later meeting is also a useful strategy. We strongly recommend encouraging the person and family to attend support groups and hear from peers who have "been there, done that." One or more of the primary care team members can summarize the meetings and discussions (especially decisions agreed on and the reasoning behind the decisions) and encourage the person and the family to record this summary for later review and sharing with other family members who could not attend the meeting.

Primary care team members should be easily available and accessible to the resident and the family, should walk the family through various stages of MNCD, tell them what to expect, what psychosocial-spiritual approaches and initiatives will ease the transition, how the resident's adjustment will be addressed, and the risks of delaying a move to a PCLTCC. A family who feels burdened because they believe that they need to be with the resident all the time may need counseling on an appropriate amount of visits from friends and family. The primary care team members must strive to be "on the same page" before approaching family members, because the family members may try to re-verify what they think they heard for days after a meeting. The primary care team needs to clarify which family member should be contacted first, as well as the family's preferences for communication with the treatment team. It may also be useful to have the social worker call each involved family member (e.g. children of the person who has MNCD) with the same message. Although face-to-face meetings to discuss a move to a PCLTCC are ideal, a telephone or video conference call may also be arranged to include long-distance family members.

Input from all team members can facilitate the family's decision whether a loved one should return home after rehabilitation or make the LTC facility the new home. A realistic appraisal of the resident's needs, available resources, and coming to a compromise that would best meet the resident's needs in the long run are essential. Avoiding a short-term fix despite the strong emotions and wishes of the resident and some family members is vital. The HCP should encourage the family to approach the resident together to inform her that the family has agreed that she needs to stay in the LTC facility on recommendation of the physician instead of having one family member become the "bad guy."

Bathing: From Frustration to Fun, From Stress to Bonding

For many people who have MNCD, bathing has been one of the most enjoyable activities all their lives. They have found a warm bath or shower washes away their troubles and the soothing aromas of soap rejuvenating. With the disabilities and limitations imposed by MNCD and the related requirement for assistance by another person, bathing becomes a stressful event, an activity to be dreaded. This is not surprising. Bathing is one of the most vulnerable times for a resident who has MNCD. The resident may not wish "a stranger" to assist her (e.g. help her disrobe), may feel apprehensive because of past negative experiences during a bath (e.g. inadvertent exposure to cold water), may not comprehend what the staff member is attempting, may misperceive the staff member's attempt as hostile, may not feel she needs the bath, or may be in significant pain so doesn't want to be bathed. Times of personal care provide some of the best opportunities for staff to bond with the resident and provide the resident with a wonderful experience of relaxation and fun. Table 13.5 lists a variety of simple and practical practices that can flip the experience of the resident as well as the staff from frustration to fun, from stress to bonding.

Most episodes of physical aggression occur during personal or hands-on care for a resident who has MNCD and are expressions of distress due to unwanted invasion of personal space by a stranger and thus can be considered a defensive response. Distress may be initially expressed as verbal aggression and noncompliance with requests, and, if the staff persist, may lead to physical aggression. Often, normal behavior rapidly follows aggression. Staff need to be trained to "listen" to nonverbal behaviors (e.g. clenching of fists, an angry look) besides verbal indicators of potential physical aggression (e.g. a resident telling the staff, "You'd better stop touching me or I'll

Table 13.5 Bathing: From Frustration to Fun, From Stress to Bonding

Person-Centered Care Practices	Practical Tips	Clinical Pearls
Staff take time to know resident, spend time with resident, develop relationship with resident before engaging in providing personal care, such as bathing	New staff reads one-page biography of resident, spends several minutes chatting with resident while providing soothing hand massage (to facilitate trust and bonding) and have familiar staff accompany first time	Knowing resident in this situation also includes knowing whether he likes tub bath or shower bath, what temperature of water is preferred, and what aroma of soap is favorite
Create pleasant rituals before bath	Staff encourage resident to assist in choice of clothes, putting hand in water to test temperature, and other efforts to prepare resident before bath	Using resident's favorite music (e.g. as background music, sing along favorite songs) is excellent bathing ritual
Therapeutic communication	Staff talk to resident in calm, reassuring, and unhurried manner, apologizing for any discomfort caused	For some residents, talking about their hobbies and interests or having funny moments can lighten tension
Staff education and training using educational DVD *Bathing without a Battle**	Best educational video illustrating PCC care practices; provides several practical tips and strategies to make bathing an event of intimacy and bonding between resident and staff	A must for all nurses and nurse aides Use of innovative bathing equipment and supplies is recommended
Address pain before bathing (both nociceptive and neuropathic pain)	Apply hot packs to sore joints before bath Allow resident to soak in tub with warm water to reduce arthritic pain Consider trial of acetaminophen or low-dose opioid (e.g. 2.5 mg of hydrocodone) or both, one hour before bath for resident who has musculoskeletal pain	Pain in resident who has advanced MNCD may be expressed as aggressive behavior during bathing and personal care Neuropathic pain (e.g. distressing sensation of pins and needles) may become worse with hot/warm water, so lukewarm or slightly cool water may be preferred
Support resident's existing abilities	Staff encourage resident to cleanse herself in areas she is able to and not assume that resident is unable to do so Staff offer choices to resident (e.g. resident can clean painful area first)	Hand-in-hand approach should be used if resident is hesitant and needs a little assistance Staff place warm washcloth in resident's hand and show resident without words what to do with cloth

Table 13.5 (cont.)

Person-Centered Care Practices	Practical Tips	Clinical Pearls
Use creative problem solving	Discuss with family and other team members creative solutions to improve resident's experience of bathing (especially if all efforts have failed or if strategies that worked before are not working anymore due to progression of MNCD)	Switch from standard soap to no-rinse cleanser Use alternative bath (e.g. towel bath, under-the-clothes bath) instead of shower Avoid water dripping on face and over eyes of resident Avoid exposure to cold by covering other parts of body while cleaning one area Wash face and hair at end of bath or at another time Use positive images (e.g. pictures of pets, favorite family or animals) to engage in interaction with resident and reduce distress Try different bathing times (e.g. early morning, late morning, afternoon, evening, late evening) to find ideal time

* Bathing without a Battle: http://bathingwithoutabattle.unc.edu. The website has excellent resources and information on person-centered creative bathing care practices and strategies, innovative bathing equipment, and supplies for purchase.

hit you") and to respond appropriately (e.g. leaving the resident alone and approaching the resident at a later time).

Other psychosocial approaches include having the staff member with the best relationship provide care or be present as a new staff member is taking over, having a staff member of the same sex provide personal or hygiene care, having two staff members provide care (one engaging with the resident using a soothing voice and words or explaining to the resident what is being done and why while the other slowly provides the care), dividing tasks into small, successive steps, being patient and allowing ample time, allowing the resident to perform parts of the task that can still be accomplished, stating instructions one step at a time, and attempting care at a later time.

Models of Understanding the Distress of a Resident Who Has Major Neurocognitive Disorder

Various models have been described to help understand the meaning and causes of biopsychosocial-spiritual distress (BPSD) in a LTC resident who has MNCD. Training caregivers (family and professional) regarding these models may improve the resident's quality of life and improve staff confidence in preventing BPSD.

The Need-Driven Dementia-Compromised Behavior Model views behaviors as stemming from a need or goal of the individual who has MNCD (Algase et al. 1996). The model recognizes that it is difficult to influence background factors (e.g. pathological processes causing MNCD), but proximal factors (e.g. assistance with performing ADLs) are more amenable to modification. The modifications are customized according to individual needs, strengths, and goals. Recreational therapists use this model.

The Progressively Lowered Stress Threshold Model is based on the assumption that the stress threshold is progressively lowered with progression of MNCD and distress is a response to stress (Hall and Buckwalter 1987). The model identifies five stressors: fatigue; change in environment, routine, or caregiver; misleading stimuli or inappropriate stimulus level (over- or understimulation); demands that exceed functional ability; and physical stressors (e.g. pain, constipation).

For example, a resident may be agitated because she is tired and a short nap may be what's needed. Or the resident is stressed and anxious before a dental procedure and may be less resistive during the procedure if she has had a period of relaxation (e.g. soothing music, hand massage with a lotion) before the procedure.

The habilitation approach aims to maximize the functional independence and morale of a resident who has MNCD, stroke, or other disabling condition (Raia 2011). It is a caregiver-controlled environmental therapy that addresses six domains in which positive emotions can be created and maintained: physical environment (providing limited choices of clothing to facilitate dressing); communication (increased use of body language, calm soothing voice, eye contact, use of pictures); functional assistance (prompting to void, to snack); social (resident who can read is encouraged to read aloud to others); perceptual (placing a large stop sign on the door); and behavioral (changing the caregiver's behavior or approach or approaching the resident later for the same task). This approach eliminates attempts at reasoning and replaces the word "no" with distraction and elimination of triggering events.

SPPEICE for Reducing the Distress of a Resident Who Has Major Neurocognitive Disorder

Providing comfort and relieving the resident's distress is an essential responsibility of all HCPs (from frontline staff to the leadership team). Distress is an expression of the resident's unmet needs. (See Box 13.17.) For a resident who has MNCD, personal expression of distress may be through agitation, aggression, expressions of worries, tearfulness, or fear. The perspective

BOX 13.17 The Resident's Biopsychosocial-Environmental Needs

Biological Needs

- Food and water
- Clothing (to protect from cold, heat, sun, insects)
- Comfortable positioning (in chair, in bed, etc.)
- Sexual needs
- Optimal vision and hearing
- Freedom from physical pain
- Treatment of medical conditions and medication-induced BNPS
- Treatment of BNPS associated with MNCD
- Treatment of BNPS due to pre-existing severe and persistent mental illness (e.g. schizophrenia, bipolar disorder)
- Treatment of psychiatric symptoms due to pre-existing other psychiatric disorder (e.g. major depression [single episode or recurrent], obsessive-compulsive disorder, panic disorder, social phobia, generalized anxiety disorder, personality disorder, etc.)

Psychosocial Needs

- To be treated with dignity (to be respected, honored, valued, acknowledged)
- To feel loved
- To be useful
- To engage in meaningful (purposeful) activities
- To be free from boredom
- To have companionship
- Creative expression
- Spiritual expression (includes religious rituals)
- To be appreciated
- To be found attractive
- To be liked
- To be part of community
- To be able to have pets

BOX 13.17 (cont.)

- To be able to interact with children regularly
- To be close to nature
- Cultural needs (language, ethnic food, ethnic clothing, celebration of ethnic festivals)
- Environmental needs

Physical Environment

- Adequate natural light and artificial lighting
- Adequate heating in winter and cooling in summer
- Freedom from excessive noise
- Clean and well-smelling environment
- Esthetics (paintings, sculpture, well-designed architecture that addresses residents' unique cognitive, emotional, and spiritual needs, etc.)
- Ability to walk and wander safely
- Nature and natural surroundings
- Other safety needs (carpeting, etc.)

Caregiving Environment

(includes interpersonal environment involving professional caregivers [staff-resident interaction], family caregivers [family-resident interaction], residents [resident-resident interaction], and volunteers [volunteer-visitor interaction] and need to be protected from negative caregiving environment)

Aspects of a Negative Caregiving Environment

- Caregiver is argumentative with resident or frequently corrects resident's impaired memory
- Caregiver ignores resident's nonverbal communication (e.g. caregiver is "too busy" to realize that resident has decreased social interaction dramatically in last few days)
- Caregiver ignores resident's verbal communication (e.g. staff walk past resident who is calling out, "Help me, help me")
- Caregiver's expectations are beyond resident's capacity (due to cognitive and functional deficits)
- Caregiver does functional activity (e.g. bathing) that resident can do on his or her own (if given time, props, and other help)
- Caregiver provides too much stimulation or too many activities for resident
- Fewer supervisory staff at mealtime
- Lack of consistent care from same caregiver (high staff turnover)
- Two residents arguing with each other
- Resident (who has severe hearing impairment) next door keeps volume of TV too loud
- Volunteer is becoming overly involved and excessively attached to resident who has BNPS
- Abuse of resident by staff, family, another resident, volunteer, or visitor

needs to change to prevention and reduction of distress through PCC practices and SPPEICE, and the perspective of "fixing behaviors" with "interventions" should be abandoned. Words matter, and it is important to replace stigmatizing words with words that reflect compassion and respect. We recommend SPPEICE as the primary approach to honoring LTC residents, improving their well-being, preventing agitation, and helping them live the best life possible (Livingston et al. 2014; Desai and Grossberg 2017).

> If no one turned around when we entered, answered when we spoke, or minded what we did, but if every person we met 'cut us dead,' and acted as if we were non-existing things, a kind of rage and impotent despair would ere long well up in us, from which the cruelest bodily tortures would be a relief; for these would make us feel that, however bad might be our plight, we had not sunk to such a depth as to be unworthy of attention at all.
>
> William James, *The Principles of Psychology*

A common cause of distress is encounters that undermine a resident's self-hood and dignity. Cognitive decline poses a direct threat to a person's dignity and self-hood, especially in our culture that values intellect over capacity to connect and fierce independence over loving interdependence. And yet, many residents who have MNCD rise up to these cultural pressures. The "difficult people" in LTC facilities are those who refuse to be diminished! They demand, threaten, and rage until their needs are met. Their dignity causes trouble in systems of care meant for efficiency. They insist on the prickly assertion of self in places where assertiveness is inconvenient. These are the people who will not let the staff forget what makes them different from others. "You'd better open Martha's drapes the way she likes them or you'll hear about it." Martha's spirit survives in the ways she makes sure her preferences are respected. In the predicament we currently call long-term care, outrage remains one of the best ways for people to preserve themselves. Residents express self-hood in their preferences, in the way they like to arrange things in their room, and the importance they give to having a bed near the window so that they can find peace by looking at the sky through the branches of a tree. Eating when a resident wants (or is used to), sleeping when she wants (or is used to) is to be ensured in order to maintain self-hood, to give the resident some control over life. By sharing our own lives (e.g. telling about our spouse and children, our own quirks), by laughing together, we may even help the resident forget the reality of frailty. We would have a relationship rather than a "clinical encounter." The staff would be engaging in a bonding experience rather than "an intervention to manage agitation." MNCD and disability obscure personhood like a mask. When a physician speaks to the caregiver pushing a wheelchair rather than to its occupant, negation occurs. "How is she feeling today?" The one who has been negated can always shout, "I am fine, Doctor," thereby declaring her continued status as a person, but the harm has already been done. To be overlooked, to be discounted even for a moment, wounds even after apologies have been extracted or a hasty recognition has been won. To have to fight to be seen – that is what causes the damage.

Authentic listening to the resident's wishes and emotional distress in a nonjudgmental manner can be tremendously healing for the resident and can prevent worsening of depression and anxiety. Simple practices such as holding the resident's hand and commitment to presence (being available in person to the resident and family when needed) are central to the role of all professional caregivers as caring and compassionate HCPs (Kleinman 2013).

Helping the resident cope with relationships that are "unhealthy" (e.g. frequently critical and/or insensitive responses by family members) and, when necessary, protecting a resident from an obviously harmful or abusive relationship are essential for the resident's spiritual wellness, as such toxic relationships often cause existential and spiritual angst, which may manifest as agitation.

To help residents experiencing distress and expressing it through agitation, caregivers must try to understand the meaning implied by the behavior as well as investigate the potentially myriad causes (unmet biological, psychosocial, spiritual, environmental, and/or cultural needs). Typically, there are multiple determinants of distress. In this sense, the staff member becomes a detective. Efforts to understand the meaning behind the behavior are critical. If team members are able to decipher the subtle messages in the resident's actions, they may realize that much of the agitated behavior is not meaningless or unpredictable. This is where, once again, knowing the resident well, knowing her rhythms and characteristic ways of expressing distress and commonly experienced triggers (e.g. a nurse familiar with a resident named Dolores [who has been yelling "Help me, help me"] states, "This is not Dolores. Something new is going on") is crucial. We recommend that caregivers learn to replace the words "difficult behavior" with words that indicate some understanding of the meaning. For example, instead of saying that a resident was "resisting personal care" or "acting up again" or "being bad," report that "the resident seemed anxious and did not allow me to clean him properly." Box 13.18 lists some basic "Dos" and "Don'ts" of interacting with an agitated resident.

Boredom and loneliness are pervasive in the lives of LTC residents and often lead to excessive time spent sleeping in daytime, "down time," and time spent not actively engaged in meaningful activity. The first step in bringing back fun and joy for LTC residents is to correct the negative attitude that pervades our society – even among HCPs – that life in a LTC facility is merely a lamentable stage of life and that boredom and loneliness are an inevitable last stage of life. For many residents, SPPEICE may

BOX 13.18 Dos and Don'ts of Interacting with a Resident Who Has Severe Agitation

Do

- take the resident's complaints seriously and validate the resident's feelings
- see agitation as expression of resident's unmet biopsychosocial-spiritual needs that is causing distress to resident and that resident is trying to communicate to caregivers (professional and family)
- try to decipher meaning underneath behavior
- empathize, sympathize, be compassionate and understanding
- allow resident to vent
- show patience
- say "I am sorry that you are feeling this way"

Don't

- argue with resident or try to "make the resident understand"
- ignore the resident's complaints
- take insults personally
- overreact to false claims against you made by resident

provide not only relief from suffering but also avoidance of as-needed psychotropic medication and prevention of complications such as escalation of agitation to physical aggression. These approaches may also improve the milieu for other residents by calming the agitated resident in a loving manner.

Hunger and thirst can often cause distress that is expressed as agitation, and staff who are well attuned to the resident's needs can often abort the "behavioral disturbance" by offering food or beverage of the resident's choice at the first sign of hunger or thirst.

Physically aggressive behavior by a resident who has MNCD can often lead to serious injury to a staff member and/or other resident. Box 13.19 lists some simple strategies staff may use to prevent staff and resident injury and de-escalate the behavior of a resident who is angry and physically aggressive.

BOX 13.19 Safe and Essential Strategies for the Staff to De-Escalate the Behavior of a Resident Who Is Angry and Physically Aggressive

- Allow at least a leg's length (or three to four feet) between you and resident. For some residents, personal space requirements may be different.
- Look for clenched fists, movement away from you, expressions such as "Stay away from me" or "Get out of my face" as indicator that resident's personal space is violated. If so, move farther away.
- Keep your body position slightly to side of resident, because resident may interpret face-to-face position as challenging or threatening.
- Do not cross your arms tightly across your chest. This sends an authoritative message. Position your hands loosely, one in the other, in front slightly above waist, with your elbows at your side. This position will allow you to respond to a strike to chest, face, or groin by blocking with your arms.
- Your stance should be with feet apart, one slightly behind the other, and your knees slightly bent. This posture gives you control over your center of gravity and allows for quick movement.
- If resident lunges toward you or tries to strike, do not grab and hold resident's arm. Instead, block and yield to resident's force of movement as you step out of the way. This directs the momentum away from you as you move away from resident. Ignore verbal insults, name calling, etc., and direct your concentration to the message behind the insult.
- If grabbed, initially resist but then quickly give in to it. This causes resident to momentarily relax grip or throws the resident off balance (mentally) enough for you to escape the grasp.
- Plan what you will do as the level of aggression escalates. Teamwork and decisiveness with which you move is critical.

Summary

The portrait of residents who have MNCD needs to change from "exuberant life, gloomy descent" to one of "exuberant life, dignified and happy descent." There is no reason for residents who have MNCD living in LTC facilities not to experience the fullness of life. A holistic, person-centered approach to caring for persons who have MNCD that values emotional and spiritual well-being as much as physical and cognitive health is key to ensuring that their life is filled with dignity, purpose, meaning, and happiness. Person-centered long-term care communities (PCLTCCs) are communities where residents want to live, where staff would want to work, and where both choose to stay. In PCLTCCs, residents are experts regarding life in their homes. For residents of PCLTCCs, strong positive relationships with staff members are the medium in which happiness is experienced and healing occurs. Every resident who has MNCD should have SPPEICE (strength-based, personalized, psychosocial sensory spiritual and environmental initiatives and creative engagement) as part of a formal care plan. The goal of SPPEICE is to enhance each resident's emotional and spiritual well-being, strengthen resilience, foster psychological and spiritual growth, and prevent and reduce distress due to unmet psychological, social, spiritual, environmental, and/or cultural needs. Caring for the professional caregiver is a key component of any effort to improve the psychosocial-spiritual wellness of LTC residents.

Key Clinical Points

1. A holistic, person-centered approach to caring for persons who have MNCD that values emotional and spiritual well-being as much as physical and cognitive health is key to ensuring that their life is filled with dignity, purpose, meaning, and happiness.
2. We recommend SPPEICE (strength-based, personalized, psychosocial sensory spiritual and environmental initiatives and creative engagement) as part of a formal care plan for all residents who have MNCD in order to honor them, improve their psychosocial and spiritual well-being, prevent distress and agitation, and help them live the best life possible.
3. Person-centered long-term care communities (PCLTCCs) are communities where residents want to live, where staff would want to work, and where both choose to stay.
4. Staff training programs and environmental modifications appear to be the most effective initiatives in promoting the wellness of residents who have MNCD and preventing distress expressed as tearfulness, agitation, and aggressive behavior.
5. Caring for the professional caregiver is a key component of any effort to improve the psychosocial-spiritual wellness of LTC residents.

Resources

Kitwood, T., *Dementia Reconsidered: The Person Comes First.* Philadelphia, PA: Open University Press. 1997. This book is an excellent resource to learn the basics of person-centered approaches for persons with dementia from the father of person-centered care movement.

McFadden S., and McFadden, J.T. *Aging Together: Dementia, Friendships and Flourishing Communities.* 2011. Johns Hopkins Press, Baltimore, MD. This book is the best resource for understanding why it is important for all of us (HCPs, neighbors and other members of a community) to embark upon the journey of becoming friends with our community members who have developed dementia and in that process deeply enrich the life of the person with dementia as well as our own.

American Geriatrics Society Expert Panel on Person-Centered Care. 2015. Person-Centered Care: A Definition and Essential Elements. *Journal of the American Geriatrics Society*, retrieved online on January 4, 2016 at http://onlinelibrary.wiley.com/doi/10.1111/jgs.13866/pdf. Excellent resource to understand person-centered care practices.

University of Buffalo Institute of Person Centered Care: Excellent resource to learn practical programs that reflect Person-Centered Care http://www.buffalo.edu/ipcc.html/contact.html.

Teepa Snow, occupational therapist and a national expert in training staff regarding person-centered care for individuals with MNCD. We strongly recommend inviting Ms. Snow for community and staff education and training programs to improve quality of life of persons with dementia. http://teepasnow.com.

Arts 4 Dementia is an excellent website to inspire caregivers (family and professional) to rejuvenate lives of persons with MNCD through engagement of their creative skills that are retained even as cognitive decline continues. http://www.arts4dementia.org.uk/why-arts-4-dementia.

Dementia Advocacy and Support Network International is an excellent resource for residents with mild MNCD. It is a worldwide organization run by persons with dementia with the goal of improving quality of life of all persons with dementia worldwide. http://dasninternational.org.

Relaxation Response Technique: www.relaxationresponse.org. A useful website providing instructions for eliciting relaxation response that may be printed free of charge. Relaxation response is an excellent intervention to reduce anxiety symptoms that often occur in residents who have mood disorder and may help prevent use of benzodiazepines for the treatment of anxiety symptoms.

Mindfulness Meditation: www.marc.ucla.edu/body.cfm. The website of UCLA Mindfulness Awareness Research Center provides free short audio recordings to engage in guided meditation. Mindfulness meditation is an excellent approach to reduce anxiety and depressive symptoms and to prevent MDD in motivated residents who have relatively good cognitive functioning.

MBSR: Center for Mindfulness in Medicine, Healthcare and Society. This is an excellent resource to learn about MBSR, how one can become a trained MBSR specialist. We recommend each facility have at least one staff who is a trained MBSR specialist who can provide education and training to residents and staff in MBSR. http://www.umassmed.edu/cfm/stress-reduction/.

References

Algase, D., C. Beck, A, Kolanowski, et al. 1996. Need-Driven Dementia-Compromised Behavior: An Alternative View of Disruptive Behavior. *American Journal of Alzheimer Disease.* **11**(6):10–19.

American Geriatrics Society Expert Panel on Person-Centered Care. 2015. Person-Centered Care: A Definition and Essential Elements. *Journal of the American Geriatrics Society.* http://onlinelibrary.wiley.com/doi/10.1111/jgs.13866/pdf (accessed November 22, 2016).

Anderson, K. and G.T. Grossberg. 2014. Brain Games to Slow Cognitive Decline in Alzheimer's Disease. *Journal of the American Medical Directors Association* **15**:536–537.

Bradford Dementia Group. 2005. *DCM 8 User's Manual: The DCM Method,* 8th ed. Bradford, UK: University of Bradford.

Brooker, D.J., E. Argyl, A. J. Sally, and D. Clancy. 2011. The Enriched Opportunities Program for People with Dementia. *Aging and Mental Health.* **15**(8):1008–1017.

Buettner, L. and A. Kolanowski. 2003. Practice Guidelines for Recreation Therapy in the Care of People with Dementia. *Geriatric Nursing* **24**(1): 18–25.

Camp, C. 2010. Origins of Montessori Programming for Dementia. *Nonpharmacological Therapies in Dementia.* **1**(2):163–174.

Chochinov, H. 2007. Dignity and the Essence of Medicine: The A, B, C, and D of Dignity Conserving Care. *British Journal of Medicine* **335**:184–186.

Clare, L. 2010. Awareness in People with Severe Dementia: Review and Integration. *Aging & Mental Health* **14**:20–32.

Dementia Action Alliance. 2016. *Living with Dementia: Changing the Status Quo.* White paper.

Desai, A.K., F. Galliano Desai, S. McFadden, and G.T. Grossberg. 2016. Experiences and Perspectives of Persons with Dementia. In M. Boltz and J.E. Galvin (eds.), *Dementia Care,* pp. 97–112. Switzerland: Springer International Publishing, Switzerland.

Desai, A.K., and G.T. Grossberg. 2017. Psychiatric Aspects of Long-Term Care. In B.J. Saddock, V.A. Saddock, and P. Ruiz (eds.), *Comprehensive Textbook of Psychiatry,* 10th ed., pp. 4221–4232. Virginia: American Psychiatric Press Inc.

Hall, G. and K. Buckwalter. 1987. Progressively Lowered Stress Threshold: A Conceptual Model of Care of Adults with Alzheimer's Disease. *Archives of Psychiatric Nursing* **1**:399–406.

Kleinman, A. 2013. From Illness as Culture to Caring as a Moral Experience. *New England Journal of Medicine* **368**(15):1376–1377.

Livingston, G, L. Kelly, E. Lewis-Homes, et al. 2014. Non-pharmacological Interventions for Agitation in Dementia: Systematic Review of Randomized Controlled Trials. *British Journal of Psychiatry* **205**:436–442.

McFadden S, and J.T. McFadden. 2011. Practicing Friendship in "Thin Places." *Aging Together: Dementia, Friendships and Flourishing Communities,* pp. 163–182. Baltimore, MD: Johns Hopkins Press.

Morley, J. 2016. High-Quality Exercise Programs Are Essential Component of Nursing Home Care. *Journal of the American Medical Directors Association* **17**:373–375.

Nolan, M., J. Brown, S. Davies, J. Nolan, and J. Keady. 2006. The Six Senses Framework: Improving Care for Older People through Relationship Centered Approach. http://shura.shu.ac.uk/280/1/PDF_Senses_Framework_Report.pdf

Raia, P. 2011. Habilitation Therapy in Dementia Care. *Age in Action* **26**(4):1–5.

Reisberg, B. 1988. Functional Assessment Staging (FAST). *Psychopharmacological Bulletin* **24**:653–659.

Chapter 14

Creating a Person-Centered Long-Term Care Community: A Road Map for Long-Term Care Facility Owners and Administrators

Be the light you wish to see in the world.
Mahatma Gandhi

Visionary and determined people are reinventing long-term care (LTC) and LTC facilities. These individuals believe that each of us, no matter how old, sick, frail, disabled, or forgetful, deserves to have a loving home – not a facility, a home where high-quality health care is the norm, not an exception. These individuals have pioneered person-centered long-term care communities (PCLTCCs) to replace LTC facilities. Such PCLTCCs enable their residents' lives to be filled with positive and life-affirming experiences, create a culture that rekindles the human spirit, and mend the frayed social fabric of our current society. Such transformational changes in LTC facilities need to occur as part of a larger change in our culture. Societies based on market-driven economies have deeply embedded value systems that inherently favor economically productive younger people and marginalize nonproductive older and/or disabled people. The wisdom, capacity for love and creativity, and spiritual gifts of older and/or disabled people go unappreciated in our culture.

Many LTC facilities claim to be person centered, but their day-to-day care processes are far from it. Some aspects of their care may be person centered, but they are still a long way from functioning as a genuine PCLTCC on a regular basis. This is not because the staff do not care for the residents' well-being or because the leaders do not want to make the facility truly person centered. Quite the contrary. Staff and leaders in most of these facilities do want to make person-centered care (PCC) for all residents, every day, a reality. The reasons for the lack of significant progress year after year are complex. From more than 20 years of caring for LTC populations in a variety of settings, we have learned that pessimism and neglect can lead to declining standards of care, poor outcomes, and decreasing quality of life for people living in LTC facilities. Complex medical problems, psychosocial issues and family dynamics, unrealistic expectations of residents and families, unrealistic expectations of staff regarding psychotropic medication to "fix" agitation, high workforce turnover, stringent fiscal constraints, a frequently adversarial regulatory process, and heightened legal liability are just some of the barriers that drain energy from the leadership team and prevent them from embarking on a mission to create PCLTCCs. Despite these daunting barriers, some leaders in LTC are determined to make the dream of a PCLTCC a reality. The hope of restoring public confidence in long-term care rests in the hands of such leaders. This chapter provides a road map for these leaders (typically, administrators and owners of LTC facilities) to transform existing LTC facilities into PCLTCCs or to create a PCLTCC from the ground up. Borrowing from the stages of change model, we propose the following five stages in the journey toward creating a PCLTCC: precontemplation, contemplation, preparation, action, and maintenance (Prochaska, DiClemente, and Norcross 1992).

Stage 1: Precontemplation

In stage 1, visionaries (leaders who wish to make PCLTCC a reality) are experiencing deep dissatisfaction with the state of current LTC culture and the quality of life of LTC residents. They recognize the urgent need for radical change but do not yet fully understand what a PCLTCC looks and feels like. Typically, these visionaries are owners and/or administrators of LTC facilities, but they could also be medical directors, directors of nursing, any other member of the facility team (e.g. geriatric psychiatrist, gerontologist, chaplain), or even community leaders. Visionaries respond to their feelings of dissatisfaction and angst by deepening their understanding of what looks and feels like a PCLTCC. Such an understanding propels them to stage 2, contemplation.

There are several remarkable PCLTCCs in the United States (e.g. the VA-directed Community

Living Centers), the Netherlands, United Kingdom, Canada, Australia, New Zealand, Taiwan, Japan, and many other countries led by people with vision and determination and staffed by compassionate, creative, and competent individuals. We encourage owners and administrators of LTC facilities to visit at least one PCLTCC and talk to the staff, owners, and administrators. No amount of description can replace witnessing a PCLTCC.

The primary goal of a PCLTCC is to help each resident live the best life possible. The leaders of a PCLTCC recognize that achieving this goal requires an environment that supports autonomy, diversity, individual choice, and a sense of belonging. Such an environment is filled with opportunities for continuation of normalcy and personal growth. Loving and respectful relationships among residents, families, support systems, and health care personnel are the bedrock of a PCLTCC. The PCLTCC team (from frontline staff to the owners and administrators) commit to responsiveness, spontaneity, and continuous learning. In a PCLTCC, residents and staff celebrate the cycles of life and connect to the local community to continue relationships that nurture the quality of everyday life. In a PCLTCC, residents are considered experts regarding life in their homes. They participate in decisions about the rhythm of their days, the services provided to them, and the issues that are important to them. Their family and other members of their support systems are welcomed.

A PCLTCC is a place where residents want to live, where staff want to work, and where both choose to stay. Residents and staff members of a PCLTCC have more friends than restrictions and rules to follow. The PCLTCC knows that the single most important thing residents and caregivers (both family and professional) value – more than good food, more than good medical care, more than clean facilities – is the warmth of a loving relationship. A PCLTCC sustains high-quality care through relentless adherence to PCC practices.

Stage 2: Contemplation

The second stage on the road to creating a PCLTCC is contemplation. In this stage, visionaries start contemplating why and when to make the formal decision of embarking on this journey. They expand the leadership team to include other key stakeholders (e.g. medical directors, directors of nursing, community leaders, local and nonlocal experts in the PCC movement) to discuss the reasons to take up the challenge of making the dream of PCLTCC a reality. The decision to embark propels them to the next stage, preparation.

Choosing the right reason for embarking on this challenging journey toward a PCLTCC is crucial. Success depends on the reason, as the reason will unite all stakeholders (from frontline staff to physicians to owners), will provide the energy, and will help the team withstand the setbacks that are inevitable on such a complex journey.

The psychological and spiritual challenges of facing decline in health and having to live in a strange place with strangers are daunting for anyone, and especially for older adults and adults who have disability or life-limiting illness (Dementia Action Alliance 2016). Also, loss of independence, fear of becoming a burden, not being involved in decision making, difficulty accessing high-quality health care, and negative attitudes of some caregivers (family and professional), especially when older frail persons feel vulnerable and lack power, all may fracture their sense of dignity. It is a tragedy and a sad reflection on our society that for many LTC residents, the last months and years of life are riddled with a sense of isolation, disenfranchisement, suffering, and loss of dignity. A PCLTCC is primarily driven by compassion for residents whose quality of life now resides in the hands of strangers and for the family members who are heartbroken and worried that their loved one will not receive the loving and respectful care they deserve. The visionaries recognize that the key reason to work to create a PCLTCC is that it is the right thing to do.

Stage 3: Preparation

In stage 3, the leadership team expands further, to include a psychosocial wellness leader (e.g. social worker, recreational therapist) and a spiritual wellness leader (e.g. chaplain). Working together, the expanded leadership team creates a list of essential characteristics of their future PCLTCC. See Box 14.1 for the key essential characteristics of a PCLTCC. This list is long and daunting. Nevertheless, all the characteristics are achievable. The leadership team also creates a list of ethical principles of care for residents in PCLTCCs and shares the list with all stakeholders. (See Box 14.2.) The creation of a PCLTCC requires embracing multiple systematic changes that will promote the quality of life of the residents guided by these ethical principles. The preparation stage also involves tapping into key resources that will accelerate progress toward the goal. (See Table 14.1.)

BOX 14.1 Key Characteristics of a Person-Centered Long-Term Care Community

Characteristics of Leadership Team

- Visionary and driven leadership team (owner, administrator, director of nursing, nursing managers/supervisors, medical director, pharmacist) that adopts the goal of making person-centered care routine rather than rare
- Leadership team exudes optimism, interpersonal warmth, and nonjudgmental approach and sees problems as opportunities to improve
- Leadership team involves at least one clinician with geriatric expertise (e.g. geriatrician, geriatric psychiatrist, nurse practitioner with geriatric training, gerontologist)
- Leadership team includes a psychosocial wellness director (e.g. activities therapist, recreational therapist, social worker)
- Leadership team includes a spiritual wellness director (e.g. chaplain)

Quality of Medical, Psychiatric, Dental, Podiatric, and Vision Care

- High-quality on-site medical, psychiatric, dental, podiatric, and vision care
- Physician, physician assistants, and nurse practitioners are available and involved
- Mental health care is provided on site by a mental health provider with geriatric expertise (e.g. geriatric psychiatrist)
- High level of communication among physician, physician-assistants, nurse practitioners, and staff
- Culture of prevention
- Palliative care is considered at time resident is admitted
- Interdisciplinary team approach

Psychosocial Spiritual Care of Resident

- Every resident has a Psychosocial Spiritual Wellness Care Plan
- Every PCLTCC has an in-house chaplain
- Dignity-conserving care
- Nonjudgmental relationship between staff and residents and between staff and family members
- Routinely addresses the expression of sexual needs and need for intimacy, regardless of sexual orientation
- Cultural sensitivity for residents of all backgrounds

Family of Resident

- Excellent psychosocial support to family of residents
- High participation and involvement of family member(s) in meeting psychosocial needs of resident
- Family members frequently volunteer at PCLTCC, become an integral part of community, befriend other residents, and continue to be involved in PCLTCC even after loved one has passed away

Characteristics of Staff and Staffing

- Staff who love caring for older and/or disabled adults
- Staff well trained and eager to learn more about caring for complex needs of residents
- Leaders provide adequate staffing levels so that frontline staff (nurses, nursing assistants) can provide high-quality care to all residents at all times
- Adequate and ongoing training to improve skills in providing person-centered care and promoting psychosocial and spiritual wellness
- Rigorous training in MNCD and palliative care
- Staff are well paid
- Staff members have permanent assignments (consistent assignments), making it possible for them to form close relationships with residents and families (most important)
- Overarching goal of care is to make each day of the resident's life as pleasant and meaningful as possible
- Culture in which staff members are expected and encouraged to show residents affection

BOX 14.1 (cont.)

- Workload allows staff members to spend time with residents
- Nursing assistants are given much more responsibility and respect than given traditionally
- Excellent communication between staff members and family and between staff members

Design

- Design of the facility is more homelike, clean, and serene
- Ample natural light and appropriate indoor lighting
- Safe wandering areas (indoors and outdoors [e.g. wandering paths in a garden])
- Each resident has a private room

Activity Programming

- High-quality continuous activity programming tailored to strengths, interests, and talents of each resident
- Every resident has a detailed, hour-to-hour, seven-day-per-week, activity plan

Use of Technology

- Electronic medical records
- Computerized physician order entry
- Free access to Wi-Fi/computer

Partnership with key organizations

- Alzheimer's Association (or equivalent organizations in other countries)
- Society for Post-Acute and Long-Term Care Medicine
- Bradford Dementia Group
- Dementia Advocacy and Support Network International

BOX 14.2 Ethical Principles of Health Care for Long-Term Care Residents

- Unconditional respect
- Physical, cognitive, psychosocial, and spiritual well-being
- Participation: irrespective of capacities, resident is enabled to participate as much as possible in own care
- Equal consideration: caring for caregivers (family and professional) is as important as caring for residents
- Nonabandonment: primary care team continues to be intimately involved in all aspects of care of resident from first encounter until death, even if hospice and other clinicians are involved
- Moderation: care should be provided in least-intrusive and least-restrictive yet adequate manner
- Proportionality: care offered at level of organizational capacity that is proportionate to needs and concerns of residents and caregivers

In this stage, the leadership team experiments with small changes in PCC practices to learn from them and begin preparation for large-scale changes. These changes involve the concepts of culture change, continuous quality improvement, and diffusion of innovation. Change is needed at multiple levels: at the institutional level, concerning policy and training; at the unit level, regarding care procedures and follow up; at the individual level (e.g. providing more scrutiny relative to fit and function of hearing aids), and at the societal level (e.g. advocating for better reimbursement to mitigate additional costs of modifying physical environments that support PCC and health care cost issues in this population).

Stage 4: Action

In stage 4, the leadership team begins the actual work of culture change. This is where the rubber meets the road. It is important for the leaders to learn about the current culture before embarking on the culture change journey. This involves taking time first to listen

Table 14.1 Ten Essential Resources to Accelerate the Journey toward a Person-Centered Long-Term Care Community

Resource	Practical Benefits	Therapeutic Pearls
Living Fully with Dementia: Changing the Status Quo. Dementia Action Alliance*	Available for free and should be read by all (from frontline staff to leadership team) to understand fundamentals of person-centered care	Clearly addresses importance of having a holistic approach by addressing biopsychosocial-spiritual distress in people who have MNCD
Words Matter: See Me, Not My Dementia. Dementia Action Alliance**	Available for free and should be read by all (from frontline staff to leadership team) to understand importance of using words that convey respect and understanding and avoiding words that are stigmatizing, disrespectful, and cause distress	Leadership team (especially nurse managers) should take charge of education and training of staff to use words that uplift residents and break habit of using words that compromise resident's dignity and cause distress
Dementia Services Development Center, University of Stirling, UK http://dementia.stir.ac.uk	Excellent resource for flagship courses in PCC and design consultancy	Environmental design to promote wellness of residents who have MNCD is a necessity, not a luxury
Dementia Care Mapping. Bradford Dementia Group***	One of the best tools for developing PCC practices in LTC settings	Recommended for every facility early in its journey of becoming a PCLTCC
Pioneer Network http://pioneernetwork.net	One of the leading authorities in culture change movement in LTC	Website provides a host of resources and information about workshops, conferences, and seminars on culture change
National Consumer Voice for Quality Long-Term Care http://theconsumervoice.org	LTC facilities should encourage use of a host of resources on their website to empower residents and family to become advocates for their own care and for care of their peers	Fact sheets on Culture Change in Nursing Home strongly recommended for sharing with all residents and family as facility embarks on journey of becoming a PCLTCC
Book: *My Mother, Your Mother. Embracing "Slow Medicine"*****	One of the best books to understand what high-quality care means in our fast-paced society	Medical director can be in charge of disseminating to other team members a host of wise and brilliant practical suggestions to provide prudent high-quality care to LTC populations
Book: *Aging Together: Dementia, Friendship and the Aging Community*. Authors: Dr. Susan McFadden (gerontologist) and John McFadden (chaplain). Baltimore: Johns Hopkins University Press, 2011. http://agingtogether.blogspot.com	One of the best books to understand importance of becoming and simple ways to become friends with person who has MNCD	Spiritual wellness leader of PCLTCC takes initiative of sharing with staff, family members, and volunteers pearls of wisdom and simple approaches to befriend vulnerable LTC residents

Table 14.1 (cont.)

Resource	Practical Benefits	Therapeutic Pearls
TimeSlips Creative Storytelling www.timeslips.org/about	One of the best creative engagement programs for LTC populations	Psychosocial wellness leader of PCLTCC (e.g. activities therapist) should become certified in TimeSlips and take leadership role in engaging other staff members to conduct TimeSlips groups regularly (online training available)
Mindfulness-Based Stress Reduction (MBSR)*****	One of the best stress-reduction programs; should be offered to all staff on a regular basis to improve skills to manage stress well	At least one staff member (e.g. activity therapist, social worker) should be trained in MBSR (online training available)

* http://daanow.org/wp-content/uploads/2016/04/Living_Fully_With_Dementia_White-Paper_040316.pdf

** http://daanow.org/wp-content/uploads/2016/03/Words_Matter-See-Me-Not-My-Dementia.pdf

*** www.brad.ac.uk/health/dementia/dementia-care-mapping/

**** Book: *My Mother, Your Mother. Embracing "Slow Medicine." The Compassionate Approach to Caring for Your Aging Loved Ones*, by Dr. Dennis McCullough, a family physician and geriatrician. New York: Harper Collins Publishers, 2008.

***** www.umassmed.edu/cfm/stress-reduction/

to residents, their family, and staff. To determine how to proceed, the leaders need to understand and appreciate what they have heard. Leaders need to explain what they mean, and they need to mean what they say. For example, culture change and PCC need to be defined and explained to all staff in order to achieve engagement of all stakeholders on a journey of transformation. Transformational leaders need to ask questions that will motivate staff members to think critically about their roles and how to solve problems that impede progress toward PCC.

It is important to pace change. It may take three to five years to change the culture to one that is highly person centered. One of the hardest things for the leadership team to do is to give up control. We strongly recommend engaging an outside consultant to work periodically with the leadership team and help them with letting go of control as they continue to empower residents and staff. Once this stage is achieved, then the PCLTCC enters the final stage, maintenance.

Culture Change

Culture change is a philosophy and a process that seeks to transform LTC facilities from restrictive institutions to vibrant and serene communities of older and/or disabled adults and the people who care for them (Foy White-Chu et al. 2009). The first of the three key principles of culture change is that residents and staff will become empowered, self-determining decision-makers. Creating a homelike environment and close relationships are two other key principles of culture change. A table of an organization that embraces culture change is not top down but flatter and likely to depict the resident at the top or in the center of a constellation of services that provide direct and supportive care. Collaborative decision-making and quality improvement projects are also key aspects of culture change. Culture change should include providing an environment that reflects the comforts of home, including accommodations for married couples and significant others regardless of sexual orientation.

More emphasis may be needed on the process of change within organizations. Diffusion of innovation is the process by which change is adopted. The pace of change can be accelerated by paying attention to several dynamics, such as the relative advantage of the innovation, investment in a trial period, the extent to which potential adopters can witness the positive outcomes of other users, communication of opinion leaders, the adaptability of the innovation itself, compatibility with existing technology and systems of care, and the existence of a compatible infrastructure to support the innovation. Effective change requires careful planning and ongoing support. Several models of this approach appear to be effective.

To address the multiple components necessary for system-level change in a person-centered environment,

Quality Partners of Rhode Island developed the *HATCh (Holistic Approach to Transformational Change) model*, which encompasses improvement efforts in care practices, the LTC facility environment, workplace practice, leadership, the regulatory environment, and the community (http://geronet.ucla.edu/sites/default/files/Orientation_Booklet.pdf). The HATCh model has been adopted by the Veterans Administration Community Living Centers all across the United States. We strongly urge all leaders of PCLTCCs to consider adopting the HATCh model.

A *regenerative care model* is based on the view that aging is another stage of life, and a person can still develop. This model is resident centered and seeks to increase residents' autonomy and control. The notion of continued personal growth inherent in this model is supported by a management philosophy that residents should have control over their lives, desire continued learning, and wish to experience a sense of being part of a community. *Learning circles* involve residents expressing opinions, preferences, concerns, and interests in certain activities and events.

A *neighborhood model* of culture change offers smaller units (8–20 residents), consistent staff assignment, separate dining and living room areas, and local (i.e. community) decision-making. Typically, a neighborhood or community "director" (or manager or coordinator), selected or appointed from among the staff, facilitates the discussion and solicits input from each resident. The staff can also attend the meeting.

Continuous Quality Improvement

Continuous quality improvement (CQI) is a philosophy and an attitude for analyzing capabilities and processes and improving them repeatedly to achieve the objective of customer satisfaction. It does not emphasize blame but instead promotes innovation and focuses on a team approach to improve care that incorporates workers at every level of the organization. CQI is one of the primary means of achieving quality improvement in health care delivery in LTC facilities. A culture change should have a strong emphasis on CQI based on established quality indicators. Box 14.3 lists examples of quality indicators. Continued development, innovation, and collaboration are also necessary to fully address the issues that influence residents' psychosocial and spiritual well-being. Implementing CQI may improve job satisfaction and increase the adoption of specific clinical guidelines.

BOX 14.3 Some Quality Indicators that Can Be Tracked to Measure Continuous Quality Improvement

- Reducing occurrence of stage 2 or higher pressure ulcers
- Reducing use of physical restraint
- Reducing risk of falls
- Reducing prescription of inappropriate medication (including inappropriate use of high-risk medication [e.g. opioid, antipsychotic, anticholinergic])
- Improving pain management
- Establishing individual targets for improving quality
- Assessing resident and family satisfaction with quality of care
- Increasing staff retention
- Increasing consistent assignment of frontline staff members, so that residents regularly receive care from same caregiver

Learning and CQI are linked inextricably in the evolution of a safety culture. The leadership team of a PCLTCC develops a culture of safety early in the process of culture change (Simmons et al. 2016). For example, the leadership team aggressively addresses elements of a resident-safety culture by encouraging open communication and nonpunitive responses to error and by building teamwork within units. Such an approach helps LTC facilities avoid catastrophes in an environment in which accidents can be expected because of complexity or other risk factors. The leadership team periodically asks staff members what they have learned as they provide care to residents and what changes are needed to improve current practices. Objective measures to assess successful PCC culture need to be in place, and the data used as learning tools to achieve benchmark goals. Setting reasonable goals and making wise choices to accomplish a critical few things (versus the important many) are some examples of how time can be optimized to achieve objectives. Most successful changes in LTC have involved reducing the frequency of certain poor practices rather than adopting new practices. The primary goal of CQI is to identify and reduce the frequency of poor practices.

System problems, such as overt or covert discouragement of reporting pain and staffing schedules that do not allow for efficient transfer of information from front-line providers to supervisors who can confirm the information and take action, are promptly addressed. One strategy to identify systems problems is asking a sample of residents who have relatively preserved cognitive function what happens if they complain of pain or request pain medicine. The answers can provide insight into the facility's informal and actual, as opposed to written, policy and procedure.

High-Quality Health Care

No resident enters a LTC facility, especially the skilled-nursing component, without having multiple, disabling, and life-limiting physical and mental health conditions and geriatric syndromes (Desai and Grossberg 2017). LTC facilities that have an otherwise strong PCC culture but the quality of health care delivered is poor may not see the benefits of PCC and rehabilitative services (e.g. activity therapy, physical therapy, occupational therapy, speech therapy) on measures of residents' quality of life. Optimal management of these conditions is crucial to achieve the most important goal of PCC: that the resident lives the best life possible. High-quality health care (medical, psychiatric, dental, vision, podiatric), using a holistic approach, is thus an integral component of the action stage. High-quality physical and mental health care in LTC populations rests on close adherence to four basic principles: comprehensive geriatric assessment; rational deprescribing; evidence-based curative, preventive, restorative, and palliative care; and a formal care plan that gives equal value to psychosocial and spiritual well-being and to physical and cognitive well-being (Schubert et al. 2016). The current reality of poor-quality health care for LTC populations is reflected in the high prevalence of inappropriate prescription of medication (point prevalence 50 percent or more), poor management of geriatric syndromes (e.g. urinary incontinence, delirium, MNCD), and palliative and hospice care that comes after too many unnecessary hospitalizations.

Preventive medicine and focus on overall well-being (physical, mental, cognitive, psychosocial, and spiritual) are core concepts of health care services in a PCLTCC. (See Boxes 14.4 and 14.5.) Box 14.4 lists some areas amenable to prevention efforts, and Box 14.5 lists some initiatives geared toward prevention and wellness. Physicians, physician assistants, and nurse practitioners of a PCLTCC may partner with academic centers (local medical schools and universities as well as nonlocal medical schools and universities via telemedicine) to develop evidence-based, state-of-the-art prevention programs. High-quality medical care also involves using and implementing clinical practice guidelines available through the Society for Post-Acute and Long-Term Care Medicine (formerly called the American Medical Directors Association) for geriatric syndromes prevalent in LTC populations. Rehabilitative therapies, dental services, and chiropractic therapies are part of a comprehensive program that is clearly defined in the care plans.

BOX 14.4 Examples of Prevention Programs for a Person-Centered Long-Term Care Community

- Prevention of pain
- Prevention of frailty
- Prevention of delirium
- Prevention of suicide
- Prevention of depression
- Prevention of pressure ulcers
- Prevention of falls
- Prevention of dehydration
- Prevention of undernutrition
- Prevention of constipation
- Prevention of incontinence
- Prevention of dry skin
- Prevention of sarcopenia
- Prevention of pneumonia
- Prevention of dental problems
- Prevention of adverse drug events
- Prevention of medication errors (especially during transition from hospital to LTC facility and vice versa through use of standardized transfer form [www.paltc.org for copy of universal transfer form])
- Prevention of insomnia
- Prevention of unnecessary or inappropriate transfer to emergency department and hospital
- Prevention of prolonged dying process

Due to the complexity of medical and psychiatric conditions in LTC populations, the provision of high-quality health care requires an interdisciplinary team (IDT). IDT means communication, collaboration, cooperation, and coordination among disciplines to address a specific problem, such as persistent pain or persistent distress expressed as agitation. Organizational leaders (especially the medical director) need to set expectations that teamwork will occur. They support its careful

BOX 14.5 Examples of Initiatives for a Person-Centered Long-Term Care Community

- Knowing the resident well
- Medication review (medication safety team/ medication review team [physician, physician assistant, nurse practitioner, consultant pharmacist, nurse] review medications of each resident quarterly)
- Safe patient-handling program
- Introducing mindfulness in routine care
- Program to "extinguish" caregiver burnout
- "Dressing without stressing"
- Bathing: From frustration to fun, from stress to bonding time
- Discussing goals of care

development and ongoing maintenance. Team-building exercises and opportunities for team members to interact in a relaxed and open atmosphere are routinely scheduled. Creative solutions, such as a ten-minute "huddle" during visits, in which key team members (e.g. resident, nurse, nursing assistant, physician, activity therapist, social worker, family member) meet to discuss a problem and further communication and collaboration via telephone and email, may be a practical way to work as an IDT. The resident's nurse can be the team leader and coordinator of the IDT, as she or he is always there and knows the resident better than other team members.

The medical director of a PCLTCC not only provides high-quality care to the residents under care but also inspires and motivates other physicians, physician assistants, and nurse practitioners to provide high-quality care. The primary care team (including medical director, other physicians, physician assistants, and nurse practitioners) of a PCLTCC not only love working with LTC populations but also have experience, training, state-of-the-science knowledge, and relevant skills in providing high-quality care. They strive to keep up with any management guidelines for commonly occurring physical and mental health conditions in LTC populations and routinely involve specialists (e.g. geriatrician, geriatric psychiatrist) in complex cases. Many LTC facilities may need a mental health clinician (e.g. psychiatrist, physician assistant, nurse practitioner) with expertise in LTC (e.g. geriatric psychiatrist) to provide routine care initially and help the facility develop an individualized, strengths-based high-quality psychosocial and spiritual wellness program for each resident and train the staff and the primary care team in early accurate diagnosis and evidence-based treatment of common psychiatric disorders (e.g. MNCD, delirium, major depressive disorder [MDD], persistent distress in the context of MNCD expressed as agitation and aggressive behavior). Once these goals are achieved (usually over one to two years), the need for mental health clinicians should lessen significantly as the primary care team are able to provide high-quality mental health care for common conditions (e.g. MDD, delirium). Further role of mental health clinicians may be limited to the management of behaviors of residents who have severe persistent mental illness (e.g. schizophrenia, bipolar disorder), assessment of decision-making capacity, and consultation for complex cases (e.g. ethical conflict in the context of end-of-life care) and for treatment-resistant psychiatric disorder (e.g. treatment-resistant MDD).

Ensuring the availability and accessibility of the primary care team is another necessary aspect of high-quality care. The medical director of a PCLTCC creates a culture in which all members of the primary care team are expected to be readily available and accessible to residents, their family, and staff. Without readily available and accessible primary care team members, high-quality care cannot be provided, and without high-quality care, other aspects of PCC may not be able to make a significant positive impact on the resident's quality of life. Ready availability and accessibility means that primary care team members are visible and available to residents, families, and staff for questions related to resident care. Primary care team members routinely partner and collaborate with residents and family in coping with health conditions rather than manage the conditions in an authoritarian, "I know what is best" manner. Primary care team members of a PCLTCC are willing to do what is right despite barriers posed by inadequate reimbursement and other system issues and are capable of crossing over to neighboring disciplines (e.g. palliative care, mental health). Providing this high-quality medical care is emotionally and spiritually tremendously gratifying for health care providers (HCPs). We can attest to it.

Fostering Leadership in Staff and Residents

A leader in a PCLTCC exudes kindness, humanity, and respect, the core values of providing care. Leaders lead the charge to create a climate of organizational warmth in which optimism, trust, and generosity can thrive. Leadership work in any field, especially in LTC, is rigorous but immensely rewarding. Leaders are well aware that focusing on one's own health (physical, emotional, and spiritual) is crucial to a professionally and personally balanced life. Leaders serve as role models for staff to focus on self-care. Leaders routinely share with other staff members their methods to prevent burnout (e.g. finding meaning in work, exercise, learning to say no when one is feeling stretched, making time for oneself, having a hobby or a second passion [e.g. playing a musical instrument]). The leaders of PCLTCCs emphasize that every day presents opportunities to communicate, learn, teach, and praise fellow staff members.

The leadership team recognize that they cannot create a PCLTCC by themselves. They need new leaders who can provide much-needed creativity and energy to accelerate the progress toward a PCLTCC. Administrators and directors of nursing of PCLTCCs routinely tap into the nascent leadership pool within their staff community and mentor nurses and nursing assistants who show leadership potential. Networking with experts, in-house leadership seminars, and peer mentoring help sustain leaders at all levels. Leaders of PCLTCC also help motivated residents take leadership roles in various activities and initiatives (e.g. leading the resident council, welcoming new residents, co-running a volunteer program with a staff person).

Improving Enjoyment and Value of Work that Staff Experience

The leadership team of a PCLTCC is aware that they can play a significant role in making staff feel valued and able to enjoy the work. If staff do not feel valued and do not enjoy coming to work because of a stressful work environment, they cannot be expected to engage in PCC practices. Increasing the time that staff members spend with residents is key to improving their job satisfaction. Managers (directors of nursing, unit directors, supervisors) of a PCLTCC always strive for consistent staffing assignments so that staff members take care of the same residents each day and get to know those residents, their schedules, and their preferences. Emphasis on team effort and staff flexibility also helps sustain improvement in job satisfaction. By attending to the welfare and ongoing training of staff who have demonstrated job commitment, managers lessen the tendency of staff to become jaded over time or to seek job opportunities elsewhere. Staff, especially nursing assistants, routinely experience abusive behavior from residents, including but not limited to being yelled at, talked down to, called names, cursed at, being a target of racial slurs, rage reactions, physical aggression, sexually disinhibited behavior (verbal and physical). This is immensely stressful. Supporting staff and validating their distress is an important aspect of PCC. Employee-recognition programs may also improve staff satisfaction. Such programs routinely recognize the hard and creative work of members of an IDT individually and collectively. Sharing success stories regularly with staff and celebrating small successes needs to be done frequently, as it is one of the most important approaches to help staff feel proud of their work and maintain the enthusiasm and determination to stay the course.

Tapping into the Power of Technology

Leaders of PCLTCCs are adept at deploying the potential and power of technology in a wise and efficient manner. Electronic medical records and computerized physician order entry over time may greatly reduce errors and thus enhance the quality of care of residents. Other benefits of health information technology in LTC include timely transfer of data, compliance with regulations, quality improvement, structured clinical documentation, improved medication use process, and clinical data communication (Degenholtz et al. 2016). PCLTCCs make creative use of technology to implement evidence-based practices and maximize the quality of care delivered. The medical director of the PCLTCC is the prime driver in ensuring involvement of the primary care team members in the planning process of implementing electronic medical records and computerized physician order entry. Implementing clinical practice guidelines is another excellent use of technology to achieve and sustain a PCLTCC. Using medication safety teams and implementing technology may substantially reduce medication errors and preventable adverse drug events.

A PCLTCC provides free wireless Internet access to residents and visitors as well as a computer room with free access to computers. This is done to encourage adolescents and young children and grandchildren of residents to spend more time in the PCLTCC, as their presence and involvement in residents' lives is often a crucial determinant of the quality of life. High staff and resident adoption of technology is another key feature of a PCLTCC. Primary care team members of PCLTCCs are eager to work with engineers and software developers to harness the full potential of data science and technology to provide decision-support and self-monitoring tools ideally suited for improving care and care processes in LTC populations.

Partnering with Academic Institutions, Nonprofit Organizations, the Local Government, and the Local Community

PCLTCCs strive to establish thriving and lasting partnerships with academic institutions (especially for teaching future generations of HCPs and for research), nonprofit organizations, experts in LTC, the local government, and the local community. There are many organizations devoted to improving the quality of life of LTC residents. (See Box 14.6.) Each of the organizations listed has a wealth of resources on its website and provides a range of services that can accelerate the journey toward a PCLTCC and help existing PCLTCCs maintain their exemplary work. Partnering with the local government and local community is also key. For example, an older frail adult who has MNCD and lives alone and has no family members may need local government to become the guardian (or appoint a community member to become the guardian) and admit the person to a local LTC facility to better address concerns related to safety and well-being. A local high school can have the students (guided by an English teacher as part of a school learning project) help residents of a local LTC facility write a one-page biography (with family input) as part of a facility-wide initiative for staff to get to know residents well. Local faith-based organizations (e.g. church, synagogue, mosque, temple) can take turns bringing spiritual leaders and congregation members to visit and befriend LTC residents, especially those who do not otherwise receive visitors.

One of the most important organizations to partner is the Bradford Dementia Group. This group continually refines the Dementia Care Mapping method developed by the founder of the PCC movement, the late Tom Kitwood. Dementia Care Mapping is a method of evaluating and improving the care that is given to persons who have MNCD in formal care settings (e.g. LTC facilities). It is a complex tool, and training in this method is available only from Bradford Dementia Group-approved trainers who have undergone rigorous preparation for this role. Dementia Care Mapping is an excellent tool for developing PCC practices in LTC settings (Bradford Dementia Group 2005). The behavior of a resident who has MNCD is mapped (tracked) and the resident's well-being or distress is recorded. Staff behaviors that have the potential to undermine resident self-hood (personhood) (e.g. staff failing to greet a resident properly, staff talking over the resident's head) and staff behaviors that boost a resident's self-hood (e.g. moving to the eye level of the resident, holding the resident's hands) are also recorded. After analysis, the findings are discussed with the team to create an action plan to improve PCC practices and processes.

BOX 14.6 Some Organizations Devoted to Enhancing the Quality of Life of Long-Term Care Residents

- Bradford Dementia Group
- University of Buffalo, New York, Institute of Person-Centered Care
- American Psychiatric Association
- American Association of Geriatric Psychiatry (AAGP)
- Society for Post-Acute and Long-Term Care Medicine (previously called American Medical Directors Association [AMDA])
- American Geriatrics Society (AGS)
- Gerontological Society of America (GSA)
- International Psychogeriatric Association (IPA)
- National Consumer Voice for Quality Long-Term Care (previously called National Citizens Coalition for Nursing Home Reform)
- National Association of Directors of Nursing Administration in Long Term Care
- American Association of Nurse Assessment Coordination
- American College of Health Care Administrators
- Pioneer Network
- Advancing Excellence in America's Nursing Homes Campaign
- American Health Care Association (AHCA)
- Institute for Healthcare Improvement (IHI)

Stage 5: Maintenance

In stage 5, success stories are shared and celebrated, reasons for the journey are revisited, and, with new energy and determination, work is resumed to fortify goals reached and redouble efforts to address issues that were challenging in the action stage. New objective measures to assess successful PCC practices are identified and change in processes is implemented. Many aspects of stage 4 are revisited in this stage.

Preparing PCLTCCs for the Future Residents

LTC is changing more rapidly than ever before primarily because of the aging of the Baby Boomer generation. Some 78 million Baby Boomers will be entering their "senior years" in the next 20 years. This take-charge generation is different from the current generation of seniors. As seniors, Baby Boomers will be more knowledgeable, assertive, computer savvy, and vocal consumers. They will expect more preventive and wellness services, personalized medicine, access to technology, and more sophisticated information from their providers to help them make informed choices about treatment, care, and housing to best match their values and preferences. Baby Boomers will want services based less on aging than on interests, hobbies, and politics. Many of the drivers of well-being of LTC populations will lie upstream from individual approaches to prevention, wellness promotion, and palliation. Baby Boomers will demand that psychosocial and spiritual wellness be deemed a common good and a key outcome in all policies. Baby Boomers will be intimately involved in any and all decisions for creating PCLTCCs.

A PCLTCC will start addressing these needs now because a growing number of current seniors have the take-charge attitude of Baby Boomers. In fact, a future PCLTCC is likely to look completely different from current models, as Baby Boomers will be less inclined to age-segregated lifestyles. Smart home technology may enable many to "age in place" by assisting with emergency assistance, fall prevention/detection, reminder systems, medication administration, and assistance for those who have hearing, visual, and/or cognitive impairment. Smart home technology will make "aging in place" a reality, help in continuous monitoring, and thus improve psychosocial well-being. Future technology in LTC facilities will support "virtual" teamwork, telehealth, disease management, and information sharing through EMR. As families spread out, there will be greater need for long-distance caregiving, which will benefit greatly from robotics and video- and Web-based communication.

Whatever the face of future PCLTCCs, more physicians, physician assistants, and nurse practitioners with geriatric expertise will be needed to work in innovative LTC settings. Future PCLTCCs along with many other health care settings will use health information technology that will be interoperable and implemented across all settings. Sooner or later, our society as a whole will need to grapple with the most difficult issue of meeting the health care needs of older adults: distributive justice (how much of the country's limited resources should be allotted to what aspect of caring for the frail older adult [life-prolonging care versus palliative and preventive care]).

The digital revolution will fundamentally change methods of health care delivery and the way people learn and communicate, and thus inform the precision prevention in LTC populations alongside the goals of precision medicine. Behavioral science, the physical environment, and health informatics will radically alter which medical and psychiatric conditions are addressed with biomedical approaches and which are best managed with psychosocial environmental approaches. The LTC research community will need to work more closely with both the end users (HCPs) and the Baby Boomer generation to ensure that research provides answers that are relevant to both. Ultimately, it is the responsibility of all of us in the academic world (clinicians [as role models of state-of-the-science work practices], teachers [through teaching the next generation], researchers [through relevant research]) to broaden our thinking and work together to lead efforts in making PCLTCCs (in all forms) a reality for all future LTC residents.

Summary

Restoring public confidence in long-term care is long overdue. Vigorous efforts to establish a PCLTCC are a key step in achieving this. The important goals of professional caregivers in PCLTCCs are to maximize residents' independence, ensure dignity, promote choice, create a sense of community, and drive quality and efficiency. These should be incorporated into the mission and vision of the PCLTCC. "Top down" administrative style will have to be replaced by a team approach in which resident (consumer) direction is included as the most important position in all decision-making. The ultimate goal is to make the aging process as dignified, meaningful, and fun as it can be for all. In the future, PCLTCCs will be person centered, driven by technology, and focused on prevention, wellness, and palliation. Even in the best PCLTCCs, there is room for improvement. Creating a genuine PCLTCC is not a destination but a journey. The time to act is *now*.

Key Clinical Points

1. A person-centered long-term care community (PCLTCC) is a place where residents want to live, where staff want to work, and where both choose to stay.
2. The road to creating a PCLTCC goes through five stages: precontemplation, contemplation, preparation, action, and maintenance.
3. A PCLTCC is primarily driven by compassion for residents whose quality of life now resides in the hands of strangers and compassion for the family members who are heartbroken and worried that their loved one will not receive the loving and respectful care she deserves.
4. Loving and respectful relationships among residents, families, support systems, and health care personnel are the bedrock on which to create a PCLTCC.
5. Most successful changes in LTC have involved reducing the frequency of certain poor practices rather than adopting new practices.

Additional Resources

Commission on Long-Term Care. 2013. Report to United States Congress. Excellent resource to understand the demographics and challenging characteristics of LTC populations. http://www.medicareadvocacy.org/wp-content/uploads/2014/01/Commission-on-Long-Term-Care-Final-Report-9–18-13–00042470.pdf.

Guidelines for Care: Person Centered Care for People Living with Dementia Living in Care Homes. Alzheimer Society of Canada. Excellent resource to understand Person-Centered Care practices. http://www.alzheimer.ca/~/media/Files/national/Culture-change/culture_change_framework_e.pdf.

American Geriatrics Society Expert Panel on Person-Centered Care. 2015. Person-Centered Care: A Definition and Essential Elements. *Journal of the American Geriatrics Society*. Excellent resource to understand person-centered care practices. http://onlinelibrary.wiley.com/doi/10.1111/jgs.13866/pdf.

University of Buffalo Institute of Person Centered Care: Excellent resource to learn practical programs that reflect person-centered care. http://www.buffalo.edu/ipcc.html/contact.html.

Models of Dementia Care: Person-Centered, Palliative and Supportive. Alzheimer's Australia. Excellent resource for person-centered palliative and end-of-life care for persons with dementia. https://www.fightdementia.org.au/sites/default/files/NATIONAL/documents/Alzheimers-Australia-Numbered-Publication-35.pdf.

Dementia Friendly Environments. State of Victoria, Australia. Excellent resource to learn in depth about dementia friendly environments (e.g. interior design; bathrooms and privacy; dining areas, kitchen and eating). https://www2.health.vic.gov.au/ageing-and-aged-care/dementia-friendly-environments.

Teepa Snow, occupational therapist and a national expert in training staff regarding person-centered care for individuals with MNCD. We strongly recommend inviting Ms. Snow for staff education and training programs to improve quality of life of persons with MNCD. http://teepasnow.com.

Arts 4 Dementia is an excellent website to inspire caregivers (family and professional) to rejuvenate lives of persons with MNCD through engagement of their creative skills that are retained even as cognitive decline continues. http://www.arts4dementia.org.uk/why-arts-4-dementia.

Dementia Advocacy and Support Network International is an excellent resource for residents with mild MNCD. It is a worldwide organization run by persons with MNCD with the goal of improving quality of life of all persons with MNCD worldwide. http://dasninternational.org.

Relaxation Response Technique: A useful website providing instructions for eliciting relaxation response that may be printed free of charge. Relaxation response is an excellent intervention for staff to reduce work-related stress and prevent burnout. www.relaxationresponse.org.

Mindfulness Meditation: The website of UCLA Mindfulness Awareness Research Center provides free short audio recordings to engage in guided meditation. Mindfulness meditation is an excellent approach for staff to reduce work-related stress, improve emotional and spiritual well-being and prevent burnout. www.marc.ucla.edu/body.cfm.

References

Bradford Dementia Group. 2005. *DCM 8 User's Manual: The DCM Method*, 8th ed. Bradford, UK: University of Bradford.

Degenholtz, H.B., A. Resnick, M. Lin, and S. Handler. 2016. Development of an Applied Framework for Understanding Health Information Technology in Nursing Homes. *Journal of the American Medical Directors Association* **17**:434–440.

Dementia Action Alliance. 2016. *Living with Dementia: Changing the Status Quo. White Paper.*

Desai, A.K., and G.T. Grossberg. 2017. Psychiatric Aspects of Long-Term Care. In B.J. Saddock, V.A. Saddock, and P. Ruiz (eds.), *Comprehensive Textbook of Psychiatry*, 10th ed., pp. 4221–4232. Virginia: American Psychiatric Press Inc.

Foy White-Chu, E., W.J. Graves, S.M. Godfrey, A. Bonner, and P. Slone. 2009. Beyond the Medical-Model: Culture Change Revolution in Long-Term Care. *Journal of the American Medical Directors Association* **10**:370–378.

Prochaska, J.O., C.C. DiClemente, and J.C. Norcross. 1992. In Search of How People Change. *American Psychology* **47**:1102–1104.

Schubert, C.C., L.J. Myers, K. Allen, and S.R. Counsell. 2016. Implementing Geriatric Resources for Assessment and Care of Elders Team Care in a Veterans Affairs Medical Center: Lessons Learned and Effects Observed. *Journal of American Geriatric Society* **64**:1503–1509.

Simmons, S.F., J.F. Schnelle, N.A. Sathe, et al. 2016. Defining Safety in the Nursing Home Setting: Implications for Future Research. *Journal of the American Medical Directors Association* **17**:473–481.

Index